D0116367

Nutrition in Nursing

Linnea Anderson

M.P.H., Associate Professor of Medical Dietetics, School of Allied Medical Professions, The Ohio State University; formerly Associate Professor of Nutrition, School of Nursing and College of Home Economics, Syracuse University

Marjorie V. Dibble

R.D., M.S., Chairman and Associate Professor, Department of Nutrition and Food Science, Nutrition Supervisor, Family Development Research Program, Children's Center, College for Human Development, Syracuse University

Helen S. Mitchell

A.B., Ph.D., Sc.D., Research Consultant, Harvard School of Public Health; Nutrition Consultant, Head Start Program, O.E.O.; Dean Emeritus of the School of Home Economics and formerly Research Professor of Nutrition, University of Massachusetts, Amherst; Exchange Professor Hokkaido University, Sapporo, Japan; Formerly Principal Nutritionist, Office of Defense, Health and Welfare; Professor of Physiology and Nutrition, Battle Creek College

Henderika J. Rynbergen

B.S., M.S., Professor of Science, Emeritus, Cornell University-New York Hospital School of Nursing. Formerly Director of Dietetics, American University Hospital, Beirut, Lebanon; Food Clinic Dietitian, Vanderbilt Clinic, Presbyterian Hospital, New York; Food Clinic Dietitian, Barnes Hospital, St. Louis; and Nutritionist, Community Health Association, Boston

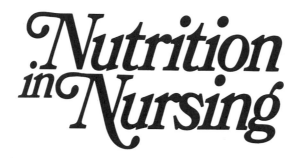

Nutrition in Nursing

Linnea Anderson, M.P.H.

Marjorie V. Dibble, R.D., M.S.

Helen S. Mitchell, A.B., Ph.D., Sc.D.

Henderika J. Rynbergen, B.S., M.S.

J. B. LIPPINCOTT COMPANY

Philadelphia   Toronto

COPYRIGHT © 1972, BY J. B. LIPPINCOTT COMPANY

Distributed in Great Britain by
Blackwell Scientific Publications,
Oxford, London, and Edinburgh

ISBN-0-397-54122-8

Library of Congress Catalog Card Number 74-37296

Printed in the United States of America

Library of Congress Cataloging in Publication Data
Main entry under title:

Nutrition in nursing.

Based on the 15th ed. of Nutrition in health and disease.

Bibliography: p.

1. Diet in disease. 2. Nutrition. 3. Cookery for the sick. I. Anderson, Linnea. II. Nutrition in health and disease.

RM216.N86   613.2′024′613   74-37296

ISBN 0–397–54122–8

3   5   7   6   4   2

Preface

This new nutrition text is designed for students of nursing to help them carry out the nutrition component of nursing care. It is based on the more technical text, Cooper's NUTRITION IN HEALTH AND DISEASE by the same authors, now in its 15th edition (1968), but much of the chemistry and pathology of disease has been deleted. Also the entire section of Modification of Food for Therapeutic Diets has been omitted.

This shorter text should prove particularly useful as core material for any program in nursing education in which the time for the teaching of nutrition and diet therapy has been curtailed.

The authors hope that the text may also prove useful in the teaching of individuals seeking accurate information on nutrition; and to those who must meet the doctor's order for a therapeutic diet, either for themselves or for a member of their family, whether for a cardiac or kidney condition; for those who have diabetes or a problem of weight control, or who have intestinal disease; and for mothers who have a child with a handicap requiring long-term diet modification.

The fundamental principles of nutrition discussed in Part One will guide the student or lay reader who may be confused by the multitude of fad diet books on the market. Part Two is concerned with the application of nutrition in critical periods throughout the life cycle. Part Three deals with diet in disease. Although details of pathology are not included, the essentials for the nutritional care of patients suffering from various diseases are treated in full. Part Four includes a number of reference tables and an extensive bibliography, prepared especially for the teacher. A glossary of less familiar terms is appended.

Wherever necessary the text has been brought up to date to incorporate recent findings. New features are the addition of Chapter 13, dealing with Growth and Development, and Chapter 20, Food Composition as a Basic Tool in Diet Therapy, stressing the use of exchange lists. Discussion of the Frederickson diets for the treatment of hyperlipoproteinemia, Types I to V, has been added to the chapter on Cardiovascular Disease. Chapter 28, Feeding the Handicapped, has been completely rewritten, and offers much new material and many helpful illustrations. Directions for obtaining booklets on food preparation for many of the therapeutic diets, where these are available, have been appended to the appropriate chapters. All references and supplementary readings are up to date and of current significance.

The authors hope that this text may become a valuable tool for all persons associated with any phase of the health field in which nutrition plays a role.

LINNEA ANDERSON, M.P.H.
MARJORIE V. DIBBLE, R.D., M.S.
HELEN S. MITCHELL, A.B., PH.D., SC.D.
HENDERIKA J. RYNBERGEN, B.S., M.S.

Contents

PART ONE

Principles of Nutrition

Nutrition and Food— Their Relation to Health

1

Factors Influencing Food Habits   •   Food Patterns in America
Nutritional Status in the U.S.A.   •   Better Diets Can Improve Nutritional Status
The Role of the Nurse, Dietitian, Nutritionist and Health Aide

Man's hunger drive is basic to his survival. Primitive man learned by experience which foods satisfied his hunger and were not harmful or poisonous. By chance the nutritive value of the foods which primitive man chose supported his nutritive needs, otherwise he and his progeny would not have survived. Today in our complex environment, meeting man's hunger drive cannot be left to chance alone. The modern sciences of food and nutrition teach us the nutritive values of the wide variety of foods we have available and how each nutrient in food, in combination with others, serves specific functions in the growth, development and adaptation of each of us throughout the life span.

The social and behavioral sciences as well as the sciences of food and nutrition play a part in our understanding of what modern man eats. Food has many meanings beside the basic one of the satisfaction of hunger. Home and family traditions, a sense of security and well-being, an expression of love and friendship or of hospitality are all important in establishing the significance of food to an individual. To the person who is ill, familiar and well-liked food has even greater meaning.

FACTORS INFLUENCING FOOD HABITS

The factors that determine individual food habits are varied and complex. The nurse must develop an understanding of them if she is to fulfill her function successfully. Courses in the behavioral and social sciences will increase her knowledge in this area and should be applied to her role in the nutritional care of patients. The following brief discussion indicates some of the influences that help to establish food habits.

Cultural Factors. Culture may be defined as the way of life of a group of people, usually of one nationality or from a particular locality. Food habits are deeply rooted aspects of many cultures. One culture may consider food only as a means of satisfying hunger; another may regard eating as a duty or a virtue, or as gustatory pleasure; still another may feel that food and eating is a means of family or social sharing.

Culture is transmitted from one generation to another by such institutions as the family, school and church. Over periods of time various degrees of change occur within any given culture, some more rapidly than others. The preservation of individual cultures is an important goal of many minority groups today. The revival of interest in the American Indian culture, the "Black is Beautiful" concept, and the activities of Italian-American groups represent attempts to identify and transmit to future generations certain aspects of these cultures. It is important to understand that culturally determined food practices, which vary from group to group, may nevertheless meet the basic biological needs that are similar for all peoples.

Economic Factors. The affluence in America today and the tremendous variety of foods available in our supermarkets make the choosing of the right foods for the family a real challenge. If the homemaker has little or no concept of nutritional value, she bases her choices on cultural and family preferences and on what she can afford. If her food budget is unlimited, so are her choices. In either instance desirable items may be left out, so nutrition guidelines prove helpful.

If the homemaker must shop within a limited budget, she cannot afford to buy "empty calories," as when the children beg for candies and soft drinks. To provide adequate protein, minerals and vitamins as well as calories in her meals, she needs to be aware that some less expensive cuts of meat and lower-cost fish have similar nutritive value to fancy or prepared items; that margarine has essentially the same nutritive value as butter; and dried skim milk may be reconstituted and used in cooking or for drinking in place of whole milk.

A new concept of "consumerism" is rapidly developing in the United States. Consumer groups are active in demanding greater honesty in the marketplace, including more informative labeling, unit pricing and less deceptive packaging. The nurse should take advantage of such consumer education opportunities in her community.

Social Factors. If one recognizes that individuals belong to various social groups, the effect of group behavior cannot be overlooked when considering factors that influence food habits. The organization of society with its many structures and accompanying value systems plays an important part in the acceptance or rejection of food patterns.

The social groups to which one belongs—club, church, union or fraternal organization—often have meals together, and the menus are apt to be typical of the group. For instance, union members such as those who work in heavy industry are used to hearty but simple meals, either at home or in groups. On the other hand, an upper middle class club may be used to exotic foods and delicacies quite unfamiliar to the first group.

If patients accept obesity or overweight as natural—for women as the accompaniment of maturity and for men as a sign of strength—it will be difficult for the nurse or dietitian to persuade them to change their eating habits to accomplish weight loss. By contrast a business executive or professional person, warned of the health hazard of excess weight and too little exercise, will often seek advice and be motivated to follow it. Although socially such people may be exposed to too much or too rich food on occasion, they are able to exert self-control and avoid overeating.

Psychological Factors. Because food has so many meanings besides the satisfaction of hunger, helping a patient to adjust to a new diet regimen is a task requiring patience and skill. To a man, food often means strength to do his work; therefore, it affects his image of himself as the head of the household and its breadwinner. To a woman, food more often means sharing what she has prepared for the satisfaction of her family and her pride in the accomplishment. To a new diabetic the restriction of some carbohydrate foods may indicate that he will lose energy; to an overweight mother the discussion of weight loss may attack the image of herself as a good provider.

When it becomes necessary to make changes in the food patterns for whatever reason, the patient and his family must be helped to understand the problem and must be motivated to follow the prescribed regimen. Here it becomes important for all who are involved in teaching the patient to be aware of the many factors which influence food habits. Because the nurse often has closest contact with the patient, she may best be able to interpret his reactions to dietary change to other medical personnel and herself be able to support and motivate him.

FOOD PATTERNS IN AMERICA

Certain of the factors which influence food habits are important to consider further. The large number of persons of different national backgrounds living together in urban areas have made tamales, frankfurters, pizza, chow mein, sukiyaki and many other dishes of foreign origin as American as apple pie. Thus, it is difficult to define the "typical" American food pattern. As each national group brought its native food habits to this country and adapted them to available foods, they also dispersed them to their neighbors.

Also, because this country stretches across an entire continent, it has a variety of geographic conditions that have resulted in relatively important regional food patterns. Fish, an important source of protein in coastal regions, is less widely used as one moves away from the sea. Soft wheat, indigenous to the South, which makes good "hot breads" but poor yeast breads, has determined regional food preferences that cannot be changed easily.

When large numbers of people of similar national origins or ethnic backgrounds settle in their own communities, they tend to be less influenced by the food habits of indigenous groups or of other cultural groups. Because of the demand for foods they are used to, their own regional stores evolve, such as the German delicatessen, the

Italian fruit and vegetable market, the Chinese restaurant and the Kosher meat market.

It may also be noted that transplanted people usually arrive poor and that it may take several generations before opportunities are available for them to achieve "middle class status." In the meantime, the frugality necessary to stretch the food dollar may develop food habits which are retained even after economic reasons for them have disappeared.

No story of American food practices, however, is complete without mention of the highly developed food technology which makes all foods, in a variety of forms, available in all parts of the country during all seasons of the year. Hence, the choice available to the American public is infinite, even though the individual's selection may normally derive from cultural practices. Also, mention must be made of the effect of mass media advertising on the changing of food habits of the American family. Young children especially are besieged by television commercials that advertise not only a food item but also "prizes" included in the package. Certain display techniques are used in retail stores to intrigue the shopper to buy an item or select a brand that she did not plan to purchase. Such impulse buying can increase the cost of the family's food and may at the same time reduce its nutritive value.

Mention must also be made of the increased use of alcoholic beverages and drugs among certain groups of Americans today. The high cost of such items and the physiological consequences to the people who use them excessively are well known. In cases of true alcoholism and drug addiction the appetite is reduced or perverted and cases of frank malnutrition often result. Such serious problems may be beyond the responsibility of the nurse to cope with, but she needs to be aware of the grave consequences and do whatever she can to help.

NUTRITIONAL STATUS IN THE UNITED STATES

Surveys of large numbers of people are used to determine the nutritional status of the population in any country. In the United States surveys have been made repeatedly, but the full significance of the findings has not always been appreciated.

Between 1968 and 1970 a National Nutrition Survey was conducted in low-income areas in 10 states, widely distributed throughout the nation.

Preliminary reports reveal that "they found every kind of malnutrition that any of us has seen in similar studies in Central America, Africa or Asia."[1] In Texas 50 percent of the Spanish speaking and 30 percent of the black children were significantly below average height for their ages.[2,3] It is indeed alarming to discover that in affluent America the poor suffer from some of the same types of malnutrition as the poor in the underdeveloped countries.

As a result of the increased awareness and concern for the problems of hunger and malnutrition in the United States, President Nixon called for a White House Conference on Food, Nutrition and Health in December of 1969.[4] The recommendations resulting from this conference concerned different facets of the problem, including better surveillance of the nutritional status of Americans, provision of free food stamps for the very poor, realistic family allowances, better health services with emphasis on nutrition for pregnant women, children, adolescents and the elderly, improved nutrition education for all ages from Head Start programs to medical and allied health schools, and more meaningful labeling of nutrition information on packaged foods.

Although much remains to be done, action on certain of these recommendations has been taken. There has been a significant increase in the U.S. Department of Agriculture Food Stamp Program; the cost of stamps has been reduced and the number per family has been increased. The number of children receiving free school lunches has increased notably. In many states, nutrition education has been given more emphasis in the health curriculum in elementary and secondary schools. More nutrition information is being included on labels of common foods, and communications media have joined forces to help explain the nutrition story.

Unfortunately food and nutrition faddists are climbing on the nutrition bandwagon and are promoting much misleading and even wrong informa-

[1] Schaefer, A. E., Johnson, O. C.: Nutrition Today, 4:2, (Spring) 1969.

[2] Ten-State Nutrition Survey in the United States, 1968-70. Preliminary Report to the Congress, April 1971. U.S. Dept. H.E.W., Washington, D.C., 1971.

[3] Congressional Record. Senate, p. S3530. March 23, 1971.

[4] White House Conference on Food, Nutrition and Health. Final Report. U.S. Gov't Printing Office, Washington, D.C., 1970.

tion. Several organizations whose names sound authentic are publishing unreliable books and periodicals. Several paperback books sold in book stores are of this type and have led even some professionally trained people to accept fads and false ideas.

BETTER DIETS CAN IMPROVE NUTRITIONAL STATUS

It may be encouraging to nutrition workers today to recall some accomplishments of the past. The importance attached to proper feeding of industrial workers has come to be appreciated to the extent that provision of adequate foods for employees has become routine where there is progressive union and plant management. The feeding of men in the armed forces is constantly under study to improve both the palatability and the nutritive value of food, resulting in better health and stamina.

Enrichment programs in Newfoundland and in the Philippines are examples of how better diets improved the health of large population groups. In Newfoundland, the enrichment of margarine with vitamins A and D and of white flour with three B vitamins plus iron and calcium resulted in striking improvement in health. Beriberi was virtually eliminated and tuberculosis deaths were reduced by half. Rice enrichment in the Philippines reduced the incidence of beriberi about 90 percent.

Food providing essential nutrients not only can cure deficiencies and allow for optimal growth of children, but also makes the difference between mediocre and buoyant health.

ROLE OF THE NURSE, DIETITIAN, NUTRITIONIST AND HEALTH AIDE IN PROMOTING GOOD NUTRITION ACTIVITIES

The nurse in the hospital may be of great assistance in helping a patient understand and carry out the doctor's diet order, whether normal or therapeutic. She may also consult with the dietitian in planning a menu which the patient will accept. In assisting the patient with his diet she may equally influence his family's food plan, thereby improving the food selection for the whole family.

In the outpatient clinic the nurse, by using an educational approach which the patient understands and accepts, can help in the selection of an adequate and appropriate diet. To change food habits is usually a slow process. Thus, at each clinic visit the nurse has the opportunity to help the patient gradually to make the necessary adjustments.

In the obstetrics unit of the hospital the nurse has a unique opportunity to discuss with the mother her own diet, as well as that of her family, during her prenatal visits to the doctor. After the birth of the baby, new mothers particularly will have many questions on feeding the baby which the nurse can answer (see Chaps. 14 and 15).

The Community Health nurse may be in a position to observe community nutrition problems more closely than any other person. Her function may be largely educational, or it may involve giving some bedside care or directing the home health aide or housekeeper. She has an opportunity to carry practical nutrition into many homes untouched by other services. Her evaluation of family or individual food habits may disclose nutrition problems that might be improved by instruction in food preparation. When such instruction is carried out in the home, suggestions should be made in line with the cooking facilities available.

When money for food is limited, it is particularly important to be able to guide the homemaker in the selection of low-cost foods that will provide adequate nutrition for all members of the household.

The School Nurse has intimate contact with the children, is usually respected by them and sometimes may be more successful than the child's mother in influencing food habits. She may be able to help the mother when a child needs guidance or has eating problems. She often plans or assists with the educational program for the improvement of nutrition either in the classroom or in the lunch room.

Where communities or schools employ "nurse-teachers" with broad responsibilities in school health programs, nurses are often called on to serve on school health committees. They must be prepared to help to coordinate health programs, including nutrition education. They are often the most logical link between the school, the home and the community services.

The dietitian and public health nutritionist, both specialists in human nutrition, are the members of the health team professionally educated to help the nurse provide nutritional care either in the hospital or in the community. The public health nutritionist functions primarily as an educator and resource person, sometimes working with the public health nurses caring for families in their homes and sometimes with school nurses. In any situation the dietitian or nutritionist is ready to assist the nurse, or in complex problems, assume the responsibility for working directly with the individual or his family.

The community or home health aide is the newest member of the health team. Under the supervision of the nurse or nutritionist, the aide (or paraprofessional, as she is called) is trained to provide direct service to the individual patient and his family. She may assist in menu planning, food buying, and preparation of meals and in feeding the patient. As the health worker who often spends the most time with the family, she is in an excellent position to help the patient or his family understand the various aspects of meal management.

Nutritional care and nursing care are closely related not only in function but also in meaning. Both words derive from the same Latin root (nurse = *nutrix*; nutrition = *nutrire*). To be a nurse is to serve in the promotion of health (biologic, psychologic and sociologic equilibrium); to nourish is to provide what is needed for growth, development and health. Thus in one sense *to nurse* is *to nourish*.

STUDY QUESTIONS AND ACTIVITIES

1. How are food habits influenced by economic, psychological, and cultural factors?

2. What groups in the population of the United States are still in need of concern in terms of their nutritional status?

3. List 5 recommendations from the White House Conference on Food, Nutrition and Health. Have any of these recommendations been met?

4. What role does the nurse have in the promotion of good nutrition?

5. What are the current concerns in nutrition in the U.S. today?

6. Class project: Collect clippings on nutrition from newspapers and magazines during the next month. Post on bulletin board.

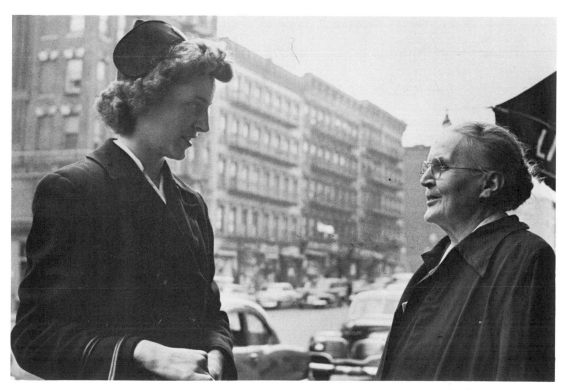

FIG. 1-1. A public health nurse discusses a problem with one of her patients. (Photo from The New York Hospital, New York, N. Y.)

SUPPLEMENTARY READINGS ON NUTRITION AND FOOD—THEIR RELATION TO HEALTH

Ase, K., *et. al.*: Nutrition education for public health nurses. Am. J. Public Health, 56:938, 1966.

Barney, H. S.: The use of nutrition and home economics aides in maternal and infant care and children and youth projects. J. Home Econ., 62:114, 1970.

Beeuwkes, A.: Nutrition education and schools of public health. Am. J. Public Health, 56:926, 1966.

Erlander, D.: Dietetics—a look at the profession. Am. J. Nursing, 70:2402, 1970.

Feeding drug addicts. Hospitals, 45:(Part I) 80, 1971.

Mayer, J.: One year later. J. Am. Dietet. A., 58:300, 1971.

Stiebeling, H. K.: How far have we come? J. Home Econ., 59:341, 1967.

For further references see Bibliography in Part Four.

Carbohydrates

2

Man's Major Source of "Fuel" · Photosynthesis · Simple Sugars · Complex Carbohydrates
Plant Sources of Carbohydrates · Animal Sources of Carbohydrates

MAN'S MAJOR SOURCE OF "FUEL"

Carbohydrates, chiefly in the form of cereal grains and root vegetables, are the major sources of energy for most peoples of the world. They provide from 45 to 50 percent of the calories of the American diet and a far higher percentage for many other peoples. They are the cheapest and the most easily digested form of fuel for human and animal energy. The protein-sparing function of carbohydrates whereby they supply the energy needs and "spare" protein for other purposes is an important consideration if the supply of protein is limited. "Carbohydrate, the fuel of life" applies to more people than does the more common phrase, "Bread, the staff of life."

The proportion of total calories derived from common carbohydrate foods around the world throws light on the respective standards of living in various countries. Most of the peoples of Asia and the middle eastern countries, Africa and Latin America derive over 80 percent of their calories from grains and potatoes or other root vegetables. As economic standards have gone up, especially in the United States and Great Britain, the amount of sugar in the diet has increased while the amount of starch has decreased proportionately (Table 2-1). The grains and other carbohydrate foods used typically in different countries will be mentioned as the food sources are discussed.

Carbohydrates are the chief form in which plants store potential energy. They are compounds of carbon, hydrogen and oxygen and are synthesized from the water of the soil and the carbon dioxide of the air by the green chlorophyll in the leaves which makes use of solar energy. This process is known as photosynthesis. The reaction is so complex that man has yet to understand fully and duplicate the chemical laboratory of the green leaf.

The largest proportion of the sun's energy which is transformed into potential energy by plants appears in some form of carbohydrate. The single sugars (monosaccharides) probably are synthesized first, and then small molecules are combined to form the larger and more complex molecules called polysaccharides (see Fig. 2-1). Small amounts of fats and proteins also are synthesized by plants.

SIMPLE SUGARS

Monosaccharides are the simplest carbohydrate units. Glucose, fructose and galactose, the nutritionally significant single sugars found in foods, require no digestion and are readily absorbed from the intestine directly into the blood stream (see Chap. 9).

Glucose, also called dextrose, is abundant in fruits and vegetables. It is the form of carbohydrate to which all other carbohydrates are converted eventually for transport in the blood and for utilization by the tissues of the body.

Fructose, also called levulose or fruit sugar, is found associated with glucose in many fruits and vegetables, and especially in honey.

Galactose is not found free in nature but is derived by hydrolysis from the disaccharide lactose, found in milk.

Sugar alcohols, sorbitol and mannitol, have a sweetening effect similar to glucose. Sorbitol, which is found in many fruits and vegetables, is very slowly absorbed into the blood stream and can apparently be metabolized without insulin.

TABLE 2-1. CHANGES IN THE PATTERN OF CARBOHYDRATE CONSUMPTION*

| | TOTAL CALORIES FROM CARBOHYDRATE | | CALORIES FROM SUGARS AND SYRUPS | |
	UNITED KINGDOM	UNITED STATES	UNITED KINGDOM	UNITED STATES
1910	56%	48%	13%	11%
1962	57%	47%	18%	16%

* Greaves, J. P., and Hollingsworth, D. F.: Proc. Nutr. Soc., 23:136, 1964.

It has the same caloric value as glucose, the sugar from which it is derived. Mannitol, found in pineapples, olives, asparagus, and carrots, may also be added as a drying agent to other foods. Because it is poorly absorbed, mannitol supplies about one half the caloric value of glucose.

The disaccharides—carbohydrates containing two sugar units—that are commonly encountered in foods are sucrose (cane or beet sugar), maltose (malt sugar) and lactose (milk sugar). Disaccharides are split by specific enzymes in the digestive tract into monosaccharides, or by acid hydrolysis commercially. Each of the three disaccharides has distinct characteristics of interest in human nutrition.

Sucrose—ordinary granulated, powdered or brown sugar—is one of the sweetest forms of sugar and costs the least. On hydrolysis, sucrose yields equal amounts of fructose and glucose, or invert sugar, as this mixture is commonly called.

Maltose, or malt sugar, does not occur free in nature but is manufactured from starch by enzyme or acid hydrolysis. Two molecules of glucose are formed by the hydrolysis of maltose.

Lactose, or milk sugar, is the only one of the common sugars not found in plants. It is formed only in the mammary glands of lactating mothers, animal or human. It is less soluble and more slowly digested than the other two disaccharides. Lactose is only about 1/6 as sweet as sucrose and hence is responsible for the blandness of milk. When it is hydrolyzed, a molecule of glucose and a molecule of galactose are formed.

COMPLEX CARBOHYDRATES

For more stable and efficient storage of potential energy, the plant and animal world packs its fuel in units larger than the sugars—i.e., dextrin, starch, cellulose, and glycogen. All of these are polysaccharides, the molecules of which may contain several hundred times as many glucose units as those of the sugars. Consequently they are much less soluble and more stable but differ markedly among themselves as to digestibility and resistance to spoilage. Because there is so much moisture in all growing plants, one essential characteristic of a storage material is insolubility. To be suitable for human food, however, a carbohydrate must be subject to digestion by the enzymes of the digestive tract. Starches and dextrins fall into this category, but celluloses and hemicelluloses which occur in food are more or less resistant to digestion.

Dextrins occur mostly as intermediate products in the partial hydrolysis of starch by enzymatic

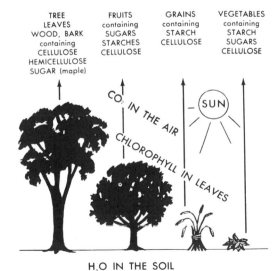

FIG. 2-1. Synthesis of carbohydrates in plants.

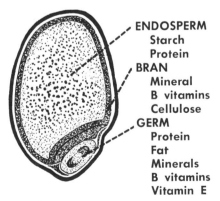

FIG. 2-2. A grain of wheat has three parts. All are used in whole-wheat flour but only the endosperm in white flour. Note what a small part of the grain is germ. (Wellman Food Plannings, Lippincott)

action or in cooking. They are made up of many glucose units joined together with the same linkage as maltose and the straight chains of starch. The individual molecules are smaller than starch and they do not have the thickening property of starch.

Starch, which is composed of 250 to over 1000 glucose units, is the chief form of carbohydrate in the diet. It is found in cereal grains, vegetables and other plants. The starch of the grain is mostly in the endosperm (see Fig. 2-2), encased in a protective covering of cellulose (the bran or the husk). The starch granule in the endosperm consists of tiny particles of starch usually arranged in concentric layers in a pattern of characteristic shape and appearance. The starch granules in turn may be enclosed in cells of larger size. This storage of starch in plants may be compared to warehouse storing of small packages of prepared cereal in cartons, with the cartons in turn packed in larger containers for ease in handling.

Cellulose, found in the framework of plants, is also a polysaccharide of glucose. It is the chief constituent of wood, stalks and leaves of all plants and of the outer coverings of seeds and cereals. Cellulose forms the more or less porous walls of cells in which water, starch, minerals and other substances are stored in the plant much as honey is held in the comb.

No known enzyme secreted in the human intestine can digest cellulose, but bacterial fermentation or disintegration may play a role in dissolving the substances that bind together the cellulose fibers or particles. Thus the cellulose of tender shoots may disappear completely from the intestinal tract.

The indigestibility of cellulose is its major asset, since the undigested fiber furnishes the bulk necessary for efficient and normal peristaltic action (muscular contraction) of the intestines. Research has demonstrated that the normal colon performs better when a reasonable amount (4-7 Gm.) of bulk or residue is present.

Glycogen, or "animal starch," is the form in which the animal stores its carbohydrate. When more glucose than can be immediately metabolized enters the blood stream, the normal individual can combine many glucose molecules (up to 30,000) to form glycogen. By the same token, when glucose is needed, glycogen can be broken down and glucose becomes quickly available (see Chap. 9).

Other polysaccharides, such as the pectic substances, agar, alginates and carrageenens (Irish moss), cannot be digested but are used in various foods because of their colloidal property—i.e., the ability to absorb water and form a gel. Commercial pectin, prepared from cull apple peels and cores or the albedo of lemons and available as liquid or powder, is used primarily for making fruit jellies. Agar is used as a thickening agent in candy manufacturing and in processing meats; the alginates and carrageenens are used in the manufacture of ice cream to give body and smooth consistency; they are also used as stabilizing agents in other food processing.

PLANT SOURCES OF CARBOHYDRATES

Cereal Grains

The ancient Romans called Demeter, the Greek goddess of the grains and harvests, Ceres, and from her name the word cereal is derived. Because of their wide cultivation, their good keeping qualities, bland flavor and the great variety of products that can be manufactured from them, cereals have continued to be the staple of the human diet from prehistoric times to the present. Most of them belong to the botanic family of grasses, with the exception of buckwheat. Each of the cereals has characteristic properties and uses.

Rice has the widest use of any cereal in the world. It is the staple food for Asia, the Near East, some Latin American and African countries and is widely used elsewhere. It provides as much as 70 to 80 percent of the calories for the larger part of the population of these areas.

Rice is usually milled as white rice, the form preferred by most people, although much of the vitamin and mineral content is lost in the milling. When the ancient home milling process, which involves parboiling or steaming before polishing, is used, some of the vitamins are forced into the center of the kernel and thus are conserved. Converted rice, now available in the United States, is commercially processed by a similar method and has a somewhat higher vitamin content than ordinary white rice. Rice enrichment, by the addition of a high vitamin "premix," is being practiced in Japan, the Philippine Islands and parts of the United States. The "premix," which is heavily fortified with certain B vitamins, is applied to the white rice together with a protective coating that is highly resistant to cooking losses.

Unpolished brown rice and "wild rice," both of which contain more of the original minerals and vitamins than does white rice, have limited use because of their different flavor, poor keeping quality and high price. Rice-eating countries do not use rice for bread making but use it in place of bread. Rice flour is used in making a wide variety of delectable snack foods in some of the oriental countries.

Wheat is the next most common cereal used throughout the world and the most widely used in the Americas and Europe. It can be milled for a variety of uses—as breakfast cereals, as flour for bread, cakes, pastries, crackers and for macaroni products. It lends itself to bread making better than other grains because of its high gluten content, which is necessary for yeast breads that demand kneading. Wheat is equally good for baking-powder breads, cakes and cookies. Certain varieties of wheat are preferred for bread flour, others for cake flour, but for both the flour is manufactured by complicated processes designed to produce a pure white flour containing none of the bran or the germ. The final product represents 70 percent or less of the wheat kernel. The outer coatings and the germ, which contain the bulk of the minerals and vitamins, are sold mostly as stock feed. A small amount of pure wheat germ is processed for human consumption. Some bran is also processed for use as high-roughage breakfast cereals.

A small proportion of our wheat crop in the United States is milled as whole-wheat or Graham flour and some as whole-wheat breakfast cereal. Hard winter wheat is milled as semolina for the manufacture of macaroni, spaghetti, vermicelli and noodles. A wide variety of these products are used in Italy and elsewhere in Europe as well as in the Americas and the Orient.

Corn (or *maize*) is used for human food in many countries in a variety of forms: cornmeal, white and yellow; hominy grits; samp, or hulled corn; popcorn; cornflakes or similar ready-to-eat cereals; and as a source of cornstarch, corn syrup and corn oil. All of these products are processed from several varieties of mature field corn. Yellow or white cornmeal is cooked as mush or grits and is used in griddle cakes or in cornmeal breads, corn pone, muffins, johnnycakes and, in Central and South America, for tamales and tortillas. Cornstarch is sold commercially as a thickening agent in cooking. Corn sugar and syrup are made by hydrolyzing the starch in the corn—i.e., breaking it down into dextrins, maltose and glucose. Corn oil is extracted from the corn germ by a carefully controlled commercial process. The special properties of corn oil will be discussed in Chapter 3.

Oats are used chiefly in the form of rolled oats or oatmeal in the United States and western Europe. In recent years some ready-to-eat cereals have been processed from oats. Oat products carry more of the original kernel than do most other processed cereals, and, thus, oats lose fewer nutrients between the field and table.

Rye is similar to wheat in many respects; rye flour may be used with wheat or by itself for bread making. Rye breads such as pumpernickel or Swedish rye are used in northern and central Europe and in Russia more commonly than in the United States.

Barley is used mostly as "pearled" barley, which is the kernel left after the bran and the germ have been removed. Barley flour is made by grinding the "pearls." In the United States pearl barley has limited use in soups. In some other countries such as Korea and Japan barley is raised and used as a low-cost substitute for rice by the poorer people.

Buckwheat is not a true cereal botanically—i.e., it does not belong to the grasses as do the other cereals—but it serves the same purpose for human food. The bran, or the husk, is removed and the rest of the kernel is rolled and bolted to produce buckwheat flour. In the United States its most common use is in buckwheat griddle cakes and waffles; in Japan buckwheat noodles are relished. In Europe buckwheat is used in making heavy breads, gruels, puddings, cakes and beer.

Millet is a staple food for millions of people in India, Russia, China and Africa but is little known in the United States. It can be raised where land is too poor and the climate too dry to grow wheat, rice, corn or most other grains. Millet is used in eastern Europe for making flat bread or porridge. Russian "kasha" (cereal), often made from millet, may also be made from wheat or buckwheat.

Milling of Grains. Natural grains carry not only the store of carbohydrates already mentioned but also protein and certain minerals and vitamins essential for good nutrition. The vitamin-B-complex factors present in the natural whole grains are usually sufficient in amount to help form the enzymes necessary for the metabolism of the carbohydrate of the grain. The balance of nature is upset when we find it desirable to modify natural grains by milling them to produce a whiter, more easily digested flour with better keeping qualities when stored. In so doing some of the minerals and vitamins are lost or discarded in the millings. It is interesting to note that the latter find excellent use as animal feed. Attempts to educate people accustomed to white-flour products to return to the use of whole-grain products have never been successful. Consequently, the expedient of enrichment of bread and flour was initiated in the United States during World War II, with other cereal products of various types added to the list later. Thiamine, riboflavin, niacin and iron are the factors added (see Chap. 10). Bread and flour enrichment is of first importance because bread constitutes one of the main sources of calories in the American diet.

Fruits

Fruits and vegetables constitute a less concentrated source of carbohydrates than do the cereals because of their high water content. In fruits the carbohydrate is mostly in the form of the monosaccharides glucose and fructose. The disaccharide, sucrose, may be found in a few fresh fruits, and most canned fruits contain added sucrose or glucose unless specifically labeled "canned without added sugar." The soluble sugars along with the fruits' acids and traces of volatile oils give fruits their appetite appeal and odor, which is further enhanced by color and texture.

The sugar content of fresh fruits may vary from 6 to 20 percent, those of canteloupe and watermelon being the lowest and that of banana one of the highest. Of course, dried fruits such as prunes, apricots, raisins, dates and figs have a much higher sugar content (near 70 percent) due to their low moisture content. The caloric value of fruits—fresh, canned or frozen—is determined largely by their sugar content.

Although most fruits are considered highly desirable raw, plantains, which are related to the banana except for being larger, are not palatable unless cooked. Because of their high starch content these fruits are an important source of carbohydrates in many tropical countries and when boiled, baked or fried are frequently used in the main course of the meal.

The avocado pear and the olive are different from all other fruits because of their high fat content, which gives them a comparatively high caloric value in spite of their low carbohydrate content.

Most fresh fruits also contain some cellulose or hemicellulose. This type of bulk, along with the fruit acids, seems to serve as a stimulant to intestinal motility for many people.

Vegetables

Under the term *vegetables* are grouped foods representing practically every part of the plant—leaves, stems, seeds, seed pods, flowers, fruits, roots and tubers. They vary as widely in composition as they do in function in the plant and may contain anywhere from 3 to 35 percent of carbohydrate in the forms of starch, sugars, cellulose and hemicellulose.

Obviously, the caloric value of vegetables varies with the percentage of carbohydrate present, but, in general, the high water and cellulose content of leaf, flower and stem vegetables puts them in the low-calorie class. These include all the green leafy vegetables, plus celery, asparagus, cauliflower, broccoli and brussels sprouts. The roots, the tubers and the seeds of plants have a higher starch and sugar content and less water and, therefore, provide more calories per unit of weight. These include all kinds of potatoes, beets, carrots, turnips, parsnips, peas, beans and lentils.

TABLE 2-2. CARBOHYDRATES IN COMMON STARCHY FOODS AND SWEETS

STARCHY FOODS	PERCENT
Barley, pearled	79
Breads, all types	52-58
Cassava, meal and flour	85
Cornmeal and grits	74-78
Crackers	71-74
Macaroni, spaghetti and noodles	73-77
Oatmeal or oat cereals	70
Potatoes, cooked	19
Rice or rice cereals	79
Rye flour	68-78
Wheat flour	69-79
Wheat cereals	72-80

SWEETS	PERCENT
Cakes	56-62
Candies	56-99
Cookies	60-80
Dried fruits	75-88
Honey	80
Jams and jellies	65-71
Syrups	74
Cane or beet sugar	100

The cellulose and hemicellulose found typically in vegetables also varies in amount and digestibility. Some forms of cellulose such as that in certain leafy and stem vegetables and in sweet corn are so resistant even to bacterial digestion and so frequently irritating that they may not be tolerated by some adults or by young children.

Root vegetables often provide much of the carbohydrate in the diets of certain African, Latin American and Asian peoples. Since they are for the most part very poor in protein, their wide use creates certain nutrition problems, particularly in infant feeding where they may take the place of more nutritious foods. Cassava, also called manioc or yucca, has a long root which is 1 to 3 inches thick. It is frequently grated, dried and powdered as a "meal"—tapioca or arrowroot. Taro, which is also grown in tropical and subtropical countries, can be baked or boiled like a potato. The Hawaiians boil the eddoes (as the roots are called), then peel and grind them with water to make *poi,* the sticky pastelike food so popular in the Islands. Other roots and tubers such as sweet potatoes, yams, turnips, and Jerusalem artichokes may also be used as staple foods at certain times by various peoples.

Nuts

Nuts seldom are thought of as a source of carbohydrate because of their high content of fat and protein. However, because of their low moisture content, they contribute from 10 to 27 percent total carbohydrate. They also contain from 1 to 2 percent of fiber. Peanuts, which are really legumes, are usually classed with the nuts because of their composition and common usage.

Because of the high fat content, nuts digest slowly. Chopping or grinding improves digestibility. In the form of nut butter and combined with other foods, there is usually no digestive difficulty. Peanut butter may be used in sandwiches or as an ingredient of a dish.

Other Plant Sources of Carbohydrates

Common table sugar—the refined white granulated or powdered sugar or brown sugar—is processed from either sugar cane or sugar beets.

Sucrose is the chief source of sweetening used in most desserts, ice creams, candies and soft drinks. The average per-capita consumption of sugar in the United States is estimated at approximately 2 pounds per week. This means, of course, that some persons use much more than this, and others consume far less. Sugar is concentrated fuel but furnishes no other nutrients. Because sugar is 99.9 percent carbohydrate and furnishes almost 4 calories to the gram, those who use the average amount or more are getting more than 3,500 empty calories per week. Furthermore, candies and other sweets are known to aggravate dental caries, a major health problem. Sugar consumption in the form of candies, soft drinks and rich desserts is certainly a contributing factor to the great American problem of obesity (Chap. 21).

Molasses is a by-product of sugar refining and carries more of the mineral content of the original plant than do the refined sugars.

Maple syrup and sugar are made by boiling down the sap from sugar maples. This was one of the kinds of sugar used earliest in America—its source known to the Indians and taught by them to the early settlers. Regardless of flavor or color, which are due to traces of other factors, the sugar in all of the above products is the disaccharide sucrose.

Corn syrup, made from field corn by hydrolysis of the starch, is mostly glucose and maltose.

Honey, made by bees from flower nectars, contains a mixture of the two monosaccharides, glucose and fructose. The fructose in honey makes it taste sweeter than corn syrup because fructose has a sweeter taste then either glucose or maltose.

Sorghum syrup is made from the sweet juice of the sorghum stem, and its use is confined largely to the southeastern and south central states. Grain sorghums are also used for food in parts of India, China and Africa.

Other forms of plant life not usually classed as vegetables are the seaweeds used for food in many countries, notably Japan. Certain varieties of seaweed are sources of *agar* and *alginates*.

ANIMAL SOURCES OF CARBOHYDRATES

Most animal foods, such as meats, poultry and fish, contain only traces of carbohydrate in the form of *glycogen* used for muscle contraction. Eggs also contain only traces of carbohydrate. Only liver contains an appreciable amount, and this in the form of glycogen. In all animals the liver serves as a temporary storehouse for quickly available fuel for the body, and it may contain from 2 to 6 percent of glycogen. Another source of glycogen in foods is the seafood, scallops, which are the muscles of shellfish and contain about 3 percent of glycogen.

Fresh milk contains about 5 percent of carbohydrate in the form of *lactose,* a disaccharide.

When consumed in amounts greater than those ordinarily present in milk, some lactose may not be digested. An undigested residue of lactose in the large intestine has a laxative action which may be desirable in certain instances but in excess causes diarrhea. Lactose also seems to increase the absorption or utilization of calcium, and often this finding is cited as the reason for the efficient utilization of calcium from milk. Sometimes lactose is given as an accompaniment of calcium salts prescribed for persons who have an allergy to milk and must obtain their calcium in another form.

STUDY QUESTIONS AND ACTIVITIES

1. Name the monosaccharides and give some food sources of each.

2. What kind of sugar is made from cane or sugar beets? Where else may this same sugar be found in Nature?

3. In what way is the sugar of milk unique?

4. Which carbohydrates are most common in fruits? In root vegetables?

5. What type of food provides the most common source of carbohydrate and calories for the world's people? What are some of the regional or national preferences?

6. What is another name for "animal starch"? Where is it found? Of what significance is it in animal nutrition?

7. Certain polysaccharides are not digested by intestinal enzymes. Which are they? In which foods do we find them? What is their function?

8. Compare the sweetness of the sugars. Why does honey taste sweeter than cane syrup?

9. List the carbohydrate foods you consumed in the past 24 hours. How wide a variety of plant sources is represented?

10. How does your sugar intake compare with that of other carbohydrate sources? If it seems high, how can you replace it with more nutritious but equally desirable foods?

11. Glance at the "ready to eat" cereal shelf in the local supermarket. How many cereal grains are represented? What added ingredients do some of them have? Do you consider this beneficial? What would you judge to be the difference in cost between a serving (1 ounce) of ready-to-eat cereal and a cooked cereal?

SUPPLEMENTARY READING ON CARBOHYDRATES

Harper, A. E.: Carbohydrates. Chap. 8. Food. Yearbook of Agriculture, U.S.D.A., Washington, D.C., 1959.

Hodges, R. E.: Present knowledge of carbohydrates. Nutr. Rev., 24:65, 1966.

For further references see Bibliography in Part Four.

Fats and Other Lipids

3

Fats in the Human Diet   •   Kinds of Fats and Their Characteristics   •   Essential Fatty Acids
Animal Sources   •   Plant Sources   •   Other Lipids

FATS IN THE HUMAN DIET

Fats are a form of stored energy in animals as important as carbohydrates are in plants. Although there are wide differences among individuals and regions, surveys indicate that today Americans as a group consume more than 40 percent of their calories as fat. Visible fats from such sources as butter, margarine, shortening, and salad and cooking oils account for about 40 percent of the fat intake, whereas the fats of meats, eggs, milk, cheese, nuts and cereals, often referred to as invisible fats, contribute about 60 percent of the total fat in the American diet.

Because people differ so widely in their patterns of food preparation and in their eating practices in regard to fat, reliable information as to the actual consumption of this nutrient is difficult to obtain. Some homemakers use considerable amounts of fat for frying and flavoring foods; others may use methods of preparation, especially in the cooking of meats and poultry, which markedly reduce the amount of fat in the cooked food. Habits vary in regard to the eating or discarding of fat on meat, the use of table fats on breads and cream on cereals and the use of salad dressings. People who are accustomed to a large amount of fat in their diet are unhappy when they are deprived of it. The psychological value of visible fat in the diet is far greater than that of the hidden or invisible fat, although physiologically the latter serves an identical purpose.

There is no physiological evidence that the human body needs as much fat as Americans consume, but neither is there proof that such amounts are harmful. Some experts recommend a moderate reduction whereby fat would provide 25 to 30 percent of the total calories in the diet. Even this much fat is not a physiologic necessity for all people, as has been demonstrated by the extremely low-fat diets consumed by large population groups throughout the world. In many countries of the Orient, the Middle East and Africa the average diet provides less than 20 percent of the total calories in the form of fat, as compared with twice that amount in the American diet.

In recent years the American consumer has modified somewhat his selection of fats. For instance, there is an increase in the use of soybean, corn and cottonseed oil, in the consumption of poultry, in the substitution of margarine for butter and the use of non-dairy "creamers" and toppings, instead of cream from milk. These changes have led to differences in the composition of total fat in the diet. Although the amount of saturated fat has not varied in the last thirty years, the percent of polyunsaturated fat has increased.

Fats serve multiple purposes in the diet. In addition to their high fuel value, some act as carriers of essential fatty acids and vitamins. That fat makes a meal more satisfying is due partially to its slow rate of digestion, its satiety value, and to the flavor it gives to other foods.

KINDS OF FATS AND THEIR CHARACTERISTICS

Fats, oils and fat-like substances, because of similar solubilities, are classified as lipids. They are insoluble in water. Like carbohydrates, fats are composed of carbon, hydrogen and oxygen but in proportions that greatly increase their energy value. Fats that are fluid at room temperature are usually called oils, while those that are solid are called fats. Both are primarily mixtures of triglycerides and contain a variety of different fatty acids in varying proportions.

The type of the fatty acids in fats is mainly responsible for differences in flavor, texture, melting points, absorption, essential fatty acid activity and other characteristics.

Fatty acids are also classified as saturated or unsaturated, depending on the amount of hydrogen in their composition. Fatty acids such as oleic are called monounsaturated because they contain 2 less hydrogen atoms than a saturated fatty acid, while linoleic, linolenic and arachidonic acids, which contain 4, 6, and 8 less hydrogens respectively, are called polyunsaturated. The polyunsaturated fatty acids have been shown in certain instances to lower blood cholesterol level, whereas saturated fatty acids may actually tend to raise the serum cholesterol level. Saturated fatty acids have higher melting points and hence tend to be solid in form at room temperature. These fats are found in greater amounts in animal sources.

Oils for the most part contain large amounts of unsaturated fatty acids, have lower melting points and are chiefly of vegetable origin. Coconut oil is a notable exception, however, since it is almost 90 percent saturated, but short and medium chain acids account for its being an oil. Hydrogenation, the addition of hydrogen atoms, increases the degree of saturation and changes a liquid oil to a solid fat.

A clear distinction should be kept in mind between oils which are true fats and the hydrocarbons derived from petroleum, such as lubricating oil or purified mineral oil. The latter contain carbon and hydrogen but no oxygen. Mineral oil is completely indigestible in the animal body and cannot be classified as a food. Formerly, it was used in place of true fats in certain low-calorie diets. This procedure is generally discouraged because mineral oil tends to interfere with the absorption of the fat-soluble vitamins. It is particularly detrimental when used in a food such as salad dressing and when taken with meals. Vegetable gums are now frequently used in low-calorie salad dressings to achieve the desired consistency.

ESSENTIAL FATTY ACIDS (EFA)

An essential fatty acid is one which is necessary for normal nutrition and which cannot be synthesized by the body from other substances. Linoleic acid, the polyunsaturated fatty acid most abundant in nature, is the main essential fatty acid to be considered. Linolenic acid, which was at first classed as one of the essential fatty acids, is not active in relieving the dermatitis of essential fatty acid deficiency; arachidonic acid, which is effective in curing the deficiency, can be synthesized in the body from linoleic acid.

Demonstration of an essential fatty acid deficiency in animals requires the rigid exclusion of fat from the diet. Therefore, it is not surprising that evidence of essential fatty acid deficiencies in adult humans has not been recognized. However, a fatty acid deficiency in infants has been demonstrated, which proves beyond a doubt that essential fatty acids (EFA) are required by humans. The dry and scaly skin of dermatitis was the most frequent finding among the infants receiving formulas low in linoleic acid. Infants also seemed to grow better and required fewer calories for growth when there was an adequate supply of EFA.

Although evaporated milk has proved satisfactory in infant feeding, Wiese *et al.*[1] suggest that the amount of linoleic acid supplied by evaporated milk formulas (1-2 percent of total calories) may be considered minimal, whereas breast milk, which is 4 to 5 times higher in linoleic acid, contains optimal amounts of EFA. Attention was called by these authors to the infrequent incidence of eczema and other skin manifestations in breast-fed infants when compared with those on cow's milk. Analysis of the linoleic acid content of commercial infant formulas and precooked cereals indicates that these also make an important contribution of EFA to the infant diet.[2]

Although the adult human requirement of essential fatty acids is not known, the Food and Nutrition Board of National Research Council recommends that, ". . . the level of linoleic acid in the diet should supply 3 percent of calories."[3]

ANIMAL SOURCES OF FATS
(See Fig. 3-1)

The body fat of each form of animal life is typical of the species but varies with function in the body and the temperature of the environment. The fat of cold-blooded animals—fish, for exam-

---

[1] Wiese, H. F., *et al.*: J. Nutr., 66:345, 1958.
[2] Hughes, G., *et al.*: Clin. Pediat., 2:555, 1963.
[3] National Research Council Publication 1694. Recommended Dietary Allowances. Washington, D.C., 1968.

ple—is a soft fat which remains plastic in the low-temperature environment in which the fish live. The fats of warm-blooded animals have higher melting points but are also plastic at the body temperature of each species. As a rule, the fat of herbivorous animals is harder than the fat of carnivorous animals. When adipose tissue of ani- mals is subjected to heat, the fat liquefies and separates from the connective-tissue cells in which it was stored. Thus pork fat is "tried out" in the manufacture of lard. Sheep have the hardest body fat of any domestic animal; when extracted, it is known as mutton tallow. Poultry fats are inter- mediate between meat and fish fats both in hard-

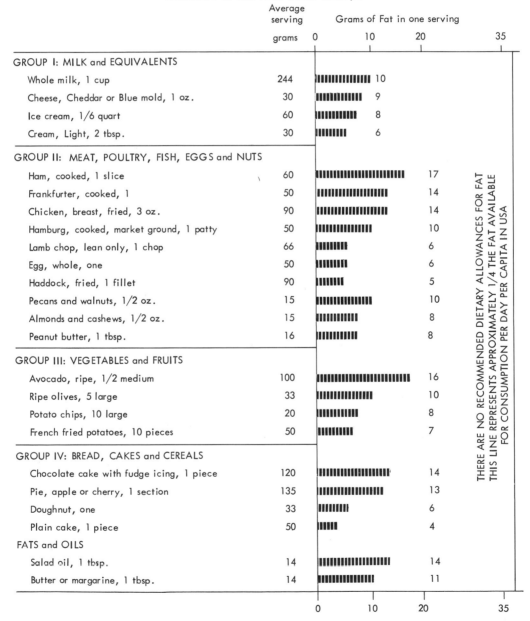

FAT

In Average Servings of Foods
Classified in the Four Food Groups

	Average serving grams	Grams of Fat in one serving
GROUP I: MILK and EQUIVALENTS		
Whole milk, 1 cup	244	10
Cheese, Cheddar or Blue mold, 1 oz.	30	9
Ice cream, 1/6 quart	60	8
Cream, Light, 2 tbsp.	30	6
GROUP II: MEAT, POULTRY, FISH, EGGS and NUTS		
Ham, cooked, 1 slice	60	17
Frankfurter, cooked, 1	50	14
Chicken, breast, fried, 3 oz.	90	14
Hamburg, cooked, market ground, 1 patty	50	10
Lamb chop, lean only, 1 chop	66	6
Egg, whole, one	50	6
Haddock, fried, 1 fillet	90	5
Pecans and walnuts, 1/2 oz.	15	10
Almonds and cashews, 1/2 oz.	15	8
Peanut butter, 1 tbsp.	16	8
GROUP III: VEGETABLES and FRUITS		
Avocado, ripe, 1/2 medium	100	16
Ripe olives, 5 large	33	10
Potato chips, 10 large	20	8
French fried potatoes, 10 pieces	50	7
GROUP IV: BREAD, CAKES and CEREALS		
Chocolate cake with fudge icing, 1 piece	120	14
Pie, apple or cherry, 1 section	135	13
Doughnut, one	33	6
Plain cake, 1 piece	50	4
FATS and OILS		
Salad oil, 1 tbsp.	14	14
Butter or margarine, 1 tbsp.	14	11

THERE ARE NO RECOMMENDED DIETARY ALLOWANCES FOR FAT THIS LINE REPRESENTS APPROXIMATELY 1/4 THE FAT AVAILABLE FOR CONSUMPTION PER DAY PER CAPITA IN USA

FIGURE 3-1

TABLE 3-1. SELECTED FATTY ACIDS IN MARGARINES*

| TYPES OF MARGARINE (first ingredient named on label) | AMOUNT IN 100 GRAMS | | | |
| | TOTAL FAT (Grams) | TOTAL SATURATED FATTY ACIDS (Grams) | UNSATURATED FATTY ACIDS | |
			OLEIC (Grams)	LINOLEIC (Grams)
Hydrogenated or hardened fat	81	18	47	14
Liquid oil	81	19	31	29

* Figures from Composition of Foods: Raw, Processed and Prepared. Agricultural Handbook No. 8. U.S.D.A., Washington, D.C., 1963.

ness and in the content of polyunsaturated fatty acids.

The fat of fish is always fluid at cold temperature and is therefore called an oil. Fish fats contain a higher proportion of polyunsaturated fatty acids than do the meat or poultry fats. However, there is a great difference in the total fat content of fish, which varies from less than 1 percent to more than 12 percent. Thus fish are classified either as low in fat or high in fat. The amount in all fish varies somewhat with the season of the year, with the time of spawning and with changes in feeding conditions. It may be noted that certain fish which have very little fat in the edible portion have a comparatively large amount in the liver. Fish liver oils are extracted and refined for use as rich sources of vitamins A and D.

Milk is an unstable emulsion which breaks (i.e., separates) on standing and allows the cream to rise. Homogenization of milk produces a more stable emulsion with smaller fat globules, and, therefore, the cream does not separate. Butter is the milk fat plus some moisture and milk solids separated by churning; the finished product contains about 85 percent of fat. Butter contains very little polyunsaturated fatty acid. It is valued as a good source of vitamin A.

PLANT SOURCES OF FATS
(See Fig. 3-1)

All fats in the plant kingdom are oils at room temperature. Most vegetables and fruits contain less than 1 percent of fat, with the exception of avocados and olives, as may be seen in Figure 3-1. The nuts and the seeds have a higher fat content. Seed oils are mostly extracted or expressed for use as pure oils for culinary and other purposes. Many of these have a high proportion of linoleic acid.

Margarines and cooking fats are usually made from vegetable oils, cottonseed, soybean and corn oils by the process of hydrogenation. This chemical process involves the introduction of hydrogen into the fat molecule under carefully controlled conditions to produce a fat with exactly the right melting point and other properties for culinary purposes. Fat thus formed is homogenized to form a creamy smooth product, but evidence of its being a mixture is given by the grainy texture of such a fat once it has been melted and allowed to harden again—the high and the low melting point ingredients are no longer evenly mixed.

The public demand for unsaturated fat has prompted margarine manufacturers to reduce the amount of hydrogenation to a minimum in order to retain as much of the unsaturated fatty acid as possible. Margarines are manufactured by either partially hydrogenating the total amount of vegetable oil to the desired consistency or by adding liquid vegetable oil to a more completely hydrogenated solid fat. The latter type contains approximately twice the amount of linoleic acid. The first ingredient named on the label of the margarine package tells the consumer which product he is selecting: "liquid corn oil plus hydrogenated corn oil" means that the margarine has been processed by the second method and hence would have a higher ratio of polyunsaturated to saturated fatty acids (Table 3-1). The fat thus prepared is churned with cultured milk and other ingredients to give the product the flavor of butter. All brands are now fortified with vitamin A to the equivalent of average butter, and some have vitamin D added. Therefore, margarine is nutritionally the equivalent of butter and sometimes is preferred because of the lower cost and the higher content of unsaturated fatty acids.

OTHER LIPIDS

Phospholipids

In addition to fats, the phospholipids play very important roles in metabolism. They are structural compounds in cell membranes, essential components of certain enzyme systems and most probably are involved in the transport of lipids in the body. Their chemical structure is similar to fats. Lecithin, a water-soluble derivative of fats, is the most abundant of the phospholipids in both tissues and foods where, because of its emulsifying properties, it serves as a solubilizer and stabilizer. Other phospholipids, cephalin and sphingomyelin, are also present in most tissues, the latter primarily in brain and lung tissues as a constituent of the myelin sheaths. Foods which contribute phospholipids to the diet include liver, brains, heart and egg yolk. Lecithin may also be added as an emulsifier to margarine, cheese products and other processed foods.

Cholesterol and Other Sterols

Sterols are fat-soluble substances having very complex molecular structures. The two most common sterols are ergosterol, found in plants, and cholesterol, found in animal tissues. Cholesterol, an essential constituent of many cells, especially nerve and glandular tissues, is found in high concentration in the liver, where it is synthesized and stored, and in the blood, where it serves in the transport of fat.

Egg yolks and brains are particularly rich sources of cholesterol in the diet. Other important food sources include butter, cream cheese, heart, kidney, liver, sweetbreads, lobster, shrimp, crab and fish roe. For additional food sources, see Table 2, Part Four.

In normal individuals the body compensates for the level of cholesterol intake in the diet through changes in the synthesis, degradation and excretion of the compound. Cholesterol synthesis may vary from 0.5 Gm. to 2 Gm. per day. Conversion in the liver to bile acids is the chief method of degradation and excretion, but cholesterol as such may also leave the body through the feces by excretion into the bile. Although as much as 50 percent of the cholesterol synthesized each day in the body may be secreted with the bile into the intestines, much of it may also be reabsorbed in the process of fat absorption.

The maintenance of a normal level of blood cholesterol is of great physiologic importance. It is a precursor of vitamin D (see Chap. 7) and closely related to several hormones in the body. It should not, therefore, be considered an abnormal substance in the body but one that has vital functions to perform.

Lipoproteins

Most of the lipids in the body are transported in the blood by combining with proteins. The lipoproteins are classified according to their density as chylomicrons, low-density lipoprotein, or LDL, and high-density lipoproteins, or HDL. The free fatty acids are transported in the plasma bound to the protein albumin.

STUDY QUESTIONS AND ACTIVITIES

1. What can be said about the human requirement for fat in the diet? How does American consumption compare with that of some other countries?

2. What changes have occurred in the consumption and selection of fats by American consumers in the last 50 years? Explain why there may be large differences in the amount of fat consumed by individual families?

3. What is meant by saturated and unsaturated fatty acids? Give illustrations of each.

4. Which of the polyunsaturated fatty acids is most widely distributed in foods? What types of foods contribute the most of this factor?

5. From what sources are margarine and some of the cooking fats manufactured and by what process?

6. Is there evidence that the level of fat in the diet of Americans may be a hazard to health? In what way?

7. Name the essential fatty acids. Why are they called essential? Can any of them be synthesized in the body?

8. Besides its use for energy, what other functions does fat perform in the body?

9. What are the normal functions of cholesterol in the body? How is the excess excreted?

SUPPLEMENTARY READING ON FATS

Coons, C. M.: Fats and Fatty Acids. Chap. 7. Foods. Yearbook of Agriculture. U.S.D.A., Washington, D.C., 1959.

Council on Foods and Nutrition: The regulation of dietary fat. JAMA, 181:411, 1962.

Dietary Fat and Human Health. National Academy of Sciences–National Research Council Publ. No. 1147. Washington, D.C., 1966.

Holman, R. T.: Council on Foods and Nutrition. How essential are fatty acids? JAMA, 178:930, 1961.

For further references see Bibliography in Part Four.

Proteins

4

VITAL IMPORTANCE AND WORLD USE

Every animal, including man, must have an adequate source of protein in order to grow and maintain itself.

Proteins have long been recognized as the fundamental structural element of every cell of the body. In their role as enzymes, proteins control the breakdown of food for energy and the synthesis of new compounds for maintenance and repair of body tissues. When they are supplied in amounts greater than necessary for growth and maintenance, proteins contribute to the energy pool of the body and, similarly, if carbohydrates and fats are not sufficient to meet energy demands, protein will be diverted for this purpose. Thus, protein well deserves its name, which is of Greek derivation, meaning "of first importance." Since proteins are the principal constituents of the active tissues of the body and the body is, in turn, dependent upon food protein for these indispensable substances, the quality and the quantity in the daily diet are of prime importance.

In many parts of the world, the developing countries particularly, food sources of protein, especially proteins of good quality, are extremely scarce. There is some evidence that in countries where the quality and the quantity of protein and other nutrients are inadequate, the stature and well-being of whole groups of people may be affected. When height and weight growth curves of groups of preschool children in Mexico, Lebanon (Arab refugees), Hong Kong, and Thailand were compared with those of United States (Iowa) children, growth retardation was evident in the former groups. Children in Ethiopia, Jordan, and Vietnam were also shorter and weighed less than Iowa children between the ages of one and seventeen years.[1] The increased stature of Japanese youths has paralleled increases in the Japanese diet of both total protein and protein from animal sources[2] (see Chap. 16). Similarly, Japanese who have lived in the U. S. for a generation or more have shown a marked increase in stature—clear evidence that heredity was not the determining factor[3]; and Australians and New Zealanders, perhaps the heaviest meateaters on the globe, have large physiques.

The United States has ample sources of protein available (approximately 100 Gm. per capita per day), and more than two thirds of it comes from meat, fish, poultry, eggs, and dairy products (Fig. 4-1). Although surveys indicate that most of the North American population consumes an adequate amount, there are still people who, for economic or other reasons, may not get enough protein.

COMPOSITION AND SYNTHESIS

Proteins, like fats and carbohydrates, are composed of carbon, hydrogen and oxygen, and, in addition, they must contain nitrogen. Often sulfur and phosphorus and sometimes other elements

---

[1] Pre-school Child Malnutrition–Primary Deterrent to Human Progress. National Academy of Sciences–National Research Council Publ. No. 1282. Washington, D.C., 1966.

[2] Mitchell, H. S.: J. Am. Dietet. A., 40:521, 1962.

[3] Gruelich, W. W.: Science, 127:515, 1958.

TABLE 4-1. CLASSIFICATION OF AMINO ACIDS
WITH RESPECT TO THEIR NEED FOR GROWTH
AND MAINTENANCE OF BODY TISSUE

ESSENTIAL	NONESSENTIAL
Isoleucine	Alanine
Leucine	Asparagine
Lysine	Aspartic acid
Methionine	Cysteine
Phenylalanine	Cystine
Threonine	Glutamic acid
Tryptophan	Glutamine
Valine	Glycine
Arginine*	Hydroxyproline
Histidine†	Proline
	Serine
	Tyrosine

* Arginine can be synthesized by the animal organism, but, since the rate of synthesis may be limited, a dietary supply may be necessary for maximum growth.

† Histidine is required for growth but is not needed for maintenance by the adult human.

such as iron (in hemoglobin) and iodine (in thyroxine) are incorporated into the protein molecule.

Plants can synthesize proteins from the nitrates and the ammonia in soil and decaying vegetable matter. Water and carbon dioxide from the air provide the necessary carbon, hydrogen and oxygen. Animals are dependent on plants for this synthesis because animal cells cannot utilize simpler forms of nitrogen, and animal metabolism of protein, in turn, eventually yields the forms of nitrogen which only plant life and microorganisms can utilize. This sequence of events is called the nitrogen cycle.

Proteins are made up of some 22 or more nitrogen-containing compounds known as amino acids. All the amino acids are organic acids. Protein molecules contain over 100—sometimes several thousand—amino acids. The order in which all these amino acids are arranged is determined by the genetic code found in the nucleus of every cell (see Chap. 9). Protein molecules are so large that they cannot pass through cell membranes. For example, plasma proteins, because they cannot penetrate the capillary membranes, remain in the blood vessels and have an important effect on regulating water balance in the body (see Chap. 6).

Amino Acids: Essential and Nonessential

Amino acids that the body cannot synthesize in adequate amounts are called essential or indispensable because they must be supplied by the diet in proper proportions and amounts to meet the requirements for maintenance and growth of tissue. Nonessential or dispensable amino acids are those the body can synthesize in sufficient amounts to meet its needs if the total amount of nitrogen supplied by protein is adequate (Table 4-1).

Nitrogen balance studies have been used to determine the amounts of essential amino acids required by various groups. An individual is in nitrogen equilibrium or balance when the nitrogen intake from protein is approximately equal to the nitrogen lost in the feces and urine. An adult consuming a diet that contains sufficient amounts of the essential amino acids will be in nitrogen equilibrium providing his energy needs are also met. If an essential amino acid is removed from the diet, negative nitrogen balance results. In this case more nitrogen is being lost than is consumed because tissues requiring the essential amino acid cannot be maintained and hence are broken down

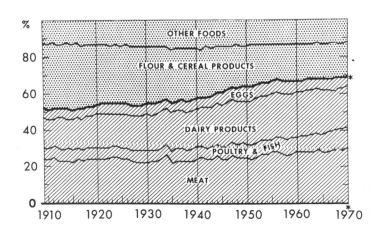

FIG. 4-1. Sources of protein in the diet of the U. S. population from 1910 to 1970. *—Total animal sources. (U.S.D.A. Agricultural Research Service, 1970)

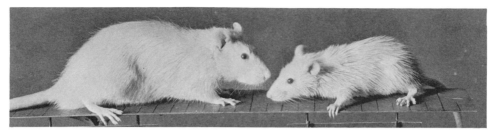

FIG. 4-2. Adequate and inadequate protein (18 percent vs. 4 percent). Rats of the same litter. This deficiency produces stunted growth but no deformities.

and their nitrogen excreted. Nitrogen equilibrium will again be attained when the lacking essential amino acid is supplied in amounts adequate to maintain tissues. Positive nitrogen balance—i.e., nitrogen intake from protein greater than nitrogen loss in urine and feces—occurs only when new tissues are synthesized such as in growth and pregnancy.

According to Rose[4] eight amino acids are essential for maintenance of nitrogen equilibrium in man. In addition, infants probably require histidine as an essential amino acid for growth.

Because of the identification of specific requirements for certain amino acids, it has become necessary to separate consideration of protein needs into two categories. One is the requirement for the essential amino acids, those the body cannot synthesize at a rate to meet its need. The other is the requirement for total protein—or total nitrogen, as it is sometimes called—which must be available to the body for the synthesis of the nonessential amino acids.

QUALITY OF PROTEIN

The effects of proteins on the maintenance or growth of animals are determined by the amounts of each of the eight to ten essential amino acids which are present in the specific protein. Osborne and Mendel in their pioneer work with rats showed that individual proteins differed in their ability to maintain life and support the growth of their animals. Casein (milk protein), when fed at a level of 18 percent of the total calories, both maintained life and supported growth and hence was classified as a complete protein. Gliadin (wheat protein), since it maintained life but did not support growth, was called a partially incomplete protein. Incomplete proteins such as zein (corn protein) were those which could not even maintain life because they were lacking in one or more

of the essential amino acids. Since casein was found to be only half as effective in supporting growth when fed at the 9 percent level as it was at the 18 percent level, it was recognized that quality and quantity were both important in determining the effectiveness of proteins.

Animal proteins, such as meats, poultry, fish, eggs, milk and cheese, provide good quality protein in liberal amounts and are termed complete proteins. The exception to this is gelatin, the protein derived from animal connective tissue which, because of its lack of tryptophan, is classified as an incomplete protein. Proteins from plant sources are usually not of as good quality as those from animal sources because one or more of the essential amino acids are in short supply. They are therefore incomplete or partially incomplete. The best quality plant proteins are found in legumes, such as beans, peas and peanuts, and in nuts. The protein in bread and cereals and in vegetables other than those mentioned and in fruit are all incomplete. These proteins are nevertheless an important part of the food intake, since their amino acids are a part of all tissue protein molecules. If they were not included in the diet, the body would need to synthesize them from the more important essential amino acids.

Fortunately, most of our foods contain a mixture of proteins, one of which often supplements another. More to the point, however, is the fact that we combine several different foods in a meal, the proteins of which tend to supplement one another because of their varying amino acid content. For instance, cereals which are low in the essential amino acid lysine are usually eaten with milk, which provides a generous amount of this factor. Thus, cereal and milk or bread and cheese are good combinations. It is obvious that this type of complementary value among foods makes a varied diet more desirable than a restricted one.

The concept of protein supplementation has also been applied in areas where animal proteins

[4] Rose, W. C.: Nutr. Abstr. and Rev., 27:631, 1957.

TABLE 4-2. PROTEIN IN PATTERN DIETARY FOR 1 DAY*

FOOD GROUP	AMOUNT IN GM.	HOUSEHOLD MEASURE	CALORIES	PROTEIN GM.
Milk or equivalent	488	2 cups	320	17
Egg	50	1 medium	81	7
Meat, fish	120	4 ozs. cooked	376	30
Vegetables:				
Potato, cooked	100	1 medium	65	2
Green or yellow	75	1 serving	21	2
Other	75	1 serving	45	2
Fruits:				
Citrus	100	1 serving	44	1
Other	100	1 serving	85	—
Bread, white enriched	70	3 slices	189	6
Cereal, whole grain or enriched	30	1 oz. dry or		
	130	⅔ cup cooked	89	3
Butter or margarine	14	1 tbsp.	100	—
		Total	1,415	70

* For basis of calculation, see Pattern Dietary in Chapter 10.

are not readily available. Attempts to provide palatable low-cost foods with an adequate amino acid balance from inexpensive indigenous foods has resulted in combinations of various types of vegetable proteins. One such product is "Incaparina" developed by the Institute of Nutrition in Central America and Panama (INCAP). It consists of a mixture of ground maize, sorghum, cottonseed flour, torula yeast and vitamin A.[5] A number of other countries in Asia, the Near East and Africa have developed similar products from local foods to meet the protein needs of young infants. Small amounts of animal protein such as skim milk or fish meal have also been added to mixtures of vegetable proteins to improve their quality. Another example is seen in the enrichment of cereal grains with one or more of the amino acids which are the limiting factors. These mixtures provide a relatively good source of protein, particularly for the growing child, who suffers the most from poor quality and inadequate protein intake.

PROTEIN REQUIREMENTS

Any quantitative estimate of protein requirement must take into account the quality of the proteins involved. The Food and Nutrition Board recommends a daily intake of 0.9 Gm. of protein per kilogram of body weight for the adult. Hence the recommendation for the "reference man and woman" is 65 and 55 Gm. respectively (see Chap. 10). The Board recognized, however, that these were not minimum needs inasmuch as adults can be maintained in nitrogen balance on protein intakes of less than half the recommended dietary allowance when the protein is of high quality. If proteins of low quality are used, the minimum requirement increases proportionately. The recommended allowances for growing children are higher per unit of weight to meet the needs for growth. This is true also for the pregnant woman and the nursing mother, both of whom naturally need an extra supply to provide for the nourishment of two organisms.[6]

It is highly desirable that at least one third of the daily protein intake be derived from animal sources, which is usually the case in the average diet in the United States. It is also strongly recommended that some good quality protein be included in every meal, because the tissues must have all of the essential amino acids present at one time for tissue synthesis. If they are not, they may be metabolized and wasted. This rule applies particularly to breakfast and lunch, for these are the meals most likely to be sketchy, and often contain limited protein. It is also worth noting that, since high quality protein foods are the most expensive class of foods in the diet, there is a tendency among low-income groups to consume less than recommended amounts.

A basic dietary pattern for a day (Chap. 10) is useful in planning menus. This dietary pattern (Table 4-2) of approximately 1,400 calories provides a liberal amount of protein, more than three

[5] Scrimshaw, N. S., and Bressani, R.: Fed. Proc., 20:80, 1961.

[6] Recommended Dietary Allowances. ed. 6. NAS-NRC Publication 1694. Washington, D.C., 1968.

fourths of which is derived from animal sources. Additional foods chosen to supply the extra calories would also provide more protein.

Protein requirement may be modified by certain pathologic conditions. During convalescence from debilitating diseases or surgery, extra protein will hasten recovery and rehabilitation. For this reason the earlier tendency to reduce protein intake in many diseases, with a few exceptions, has been reversed. The nurse should, however, recognize that certain diseases (see Chaps. 24, 25 and 29) may require limiting the total amount of pro-

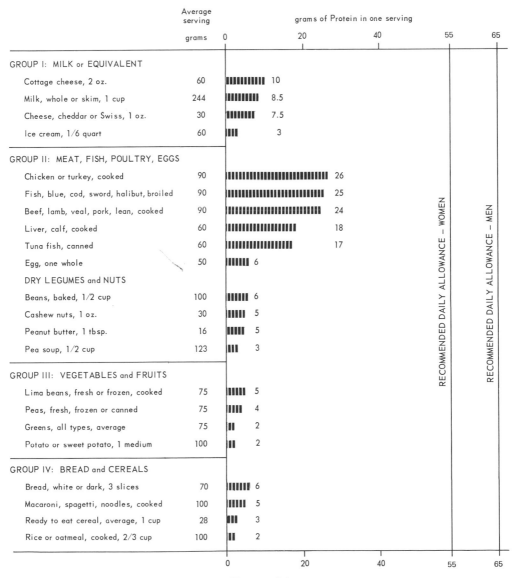

PROTEIN
In Average Servings of Foods
Classified in the Four Food Groups

	Average serving grams	grams of Protein in one serving
GROUP I: MILK or EQUIVALENT		
Cottage cheese, 2 oz.	60	10
Milk, whole or skim, 1 cup	244	8.5
Cheese, cheddar or Swiss, 1 oz.	30	7.5
Ice cream, 1/6 quart	60	3
GROUP II: MEAT, FISH, POULTRY, EGGS		
Chicken or turkey, cooked	90	26
Fish, blue, cod, sword, halibut, broiled	90	25
Beef, lamb, veal, pork, lean, cooked	90	24
Liver, calf, cooked	60	18
Tuna fish, canned	60	17
Egg, one whole	50	6
DRY LEGUMES and NUTS		
Beans, baked, 1/2 cup	100	6
Cashew nuts, 1 oz.	30	5
Peanut butter, 1 tbsp.	16	5
Pea soup, 1/2 cup	123	3
GROUP III: VEGETABLES and FRUITS		
Lima beans, fresh or frozen, cooked	75	5
Peas, fresh, frozen or canned	75	4
Greens, all types, average	75	2
Potato or sweet potato, 1 medium	100	2
GROUP IV: BREAD and CEREALS		
Bread, white or dark, 3 slices	70	6
Macaroni, spagetti, noodles, cooked	100	5
Ready to eat cereal, average, 1 cup	28	3
Rice or oatmeal, cooked, 2/3 cup	100	2

RECOMMENDED DAILY ALLOWANCE – WOMEN (55)
RECOMMENDED DAILY ALLOWANCE – MEN (65)

FIGURE 4-3

tein or the amount of a specific amino acid in a patient's diet.

FOOD SOURCES OF PROTEIN

From the bar chart of average servings (Fig. 4-3), it is evident that the first two food groups supply the most protein per serving and are also the best quality proteins. Dry legumes and nuts are included as meat alternates in Group II because they contain the best quality of plant proteins.

Animal Sources of Protein

Group I. Milk and Milk Products. The foods listed in this group—milk, cheese and ice cream— all derive their protein from milk. Milk is the protein food that Nature provides for the young of the species, and, around the world, milk from many different mammals is used for human food. Milk is almost essential for the infant; it is equally good as a source of protein for older children and adolescents during the growing years. Adults also should get some of their protein from milk and milk products. Nonfat dry milk, better known as dried skim milk, is an excellent source of milk protein and calcium at comparatively low cost.

Cheese is the term applied to any product made from the concentrated curd of milk. Cheese is thought to have been the first manufactured food, the process for which was probably discovered accidentally when milk was stored in a bag made from the stomach of a cow, which contains rennin. The action of rennin on milk causes the curds to form and the whey to separate. Although a certain amount of the milk nutrients remains in the whey, the majority remains in the curd, which provides a large amount of the natural food value in milk in concentrated form. The curd in cottage cheese is formed by the development of or addition of lactic acid bacteria to skimmed milk.

Group II. Meat, poultry and fish are all forms of animal tissue protein synthesized by each species to meet its specific needs for growth and maintenance. Such proteins are remarkably similar in amino acid content to the amino acid requirements of man. Meat, poultry and seafoods vary in protein content from 15 to 30 percent depending on the amount of moisture and fat present.

Variety meats is a term applied to the organs and the glands of animals. They include tongue, liver, kidney, sweetbreads (thymus gland of calf or lamb), beef or calf heart and beef brains. The organ meats tend to be much richer in vitamins and minerals than muscle meats. Popular luncheon meats such as spiced ham, pressed meat loaves, liverwurst and various types of cold sausages such as bologna and frankfurters are sometimes classed as variety meats. They contain from 11 to 17 percent of protein in a convenient form for quick lunches.

Poultry is a general term covering a variety of domestic birds including chicken, turkeys, geese and ducks. After roasting, the protein content of the lean meat of most poultry is about 30 percent; after frying or broiling the proportion of the protein content is slightly less than it is after roasting, because less moisture is lost.

Fish, including shellfish, compare favorably with meats and poultry as good sources of protein and in many countries are the chief source of animal protein. In the United States an effort is being made to stimulate the use of more varieties of both salt and fresh water fish. Shellfish are low in fat and somewhat lower in protein ratio than fish because of their higher water content. In other countries such products as fish sausage, fish flour and meal and other processed fish foods of high protein value are being developed to improve the protein supply.

Eggs are in a class by themselves, a protein food of high nutritive value. They contain 13 percent of protein—less than meats, poultry or fish because of their higher water content. The egg yolk is a more concentrated, much more complex source of protein than the white. It contains lipoprotein, phosphoprotein, nucleoprotein and possibly others, all of which provide nourishment for the embryo chick and are equally valuable as human food.

Plant Sources of Protein

Group III. Vegetables are poor sources of protein; the only ones that provide more than 1 or 2 percent are the legumes—beans and peas. These may run as high as 5 or 6 percent when they are fresh and still higher in the dried form. For this reason, and because they provide one of the better quality of plant proteins, they are listed as meat alternates in the Four Food Group chart. Soybeans, which are the highest in protein content of the legumes, are not used much for human food in the United States, but they are important sources of protein in many countries where animal foods are scarce. Soybean milk, curd, cheese and flour are a few of the soybean products used by Orientals. In India, pulses (legumes) are especially important in a country where animal protein is scarce or the population is largely vegetarian.

Peanuts are really legumes although they are often classed as nuts. Roasted peanuts and peanut butter contain about 26 percent of protein, although roasting reduces the availability or destroys about 10 percent of three of the essential amino acids present.

Nuts in general are good sources of protein of fairly high quality. Because they are expensive, they are seldom eaten in sufficient quantity to make an important contribution to the protein of the diet.

Group IV. Breads and cereals make an important contribution to the protein of the diet, not only because of their liberal consumption but also because many of their uses encourage or increase the consumption of animal proteins such as milk, eggs, meat and fish. The protein of uncooked grains ranges from 7 to 14 percent. The grain proteins are low in one or more essential amino acids. However, plant proteins may supplement each other in such a way that a combination may provide a better balance of amino acids than any one food alone.

Textured Protein Products are a new type of protein food made from one or more of the following sources: cottonseed, peanuts, sesame seed, soybeans, sunflower seed and wheat. These products have similar appearance, taste and texture as the foods they simulate—ground beef, ham, bacon, chicken, fish, cheese.

The textured protein products, also called analogs, are manufactured by making a fiber from one or more of the vegetable sources. Then the fiber can be spun into a form which simulates the texture of meat. Flavor additives are used to make them taste like the products they imitate. They may take the form of fiber, shred, chunk, bit or slice. Some dehydrated forms are also available which may be rehydrated to serve as extenders to mix with ground meat.

The Food and Drug Administration has proposed the establishment of a definition and standard of identity for this new class of foods. Analogs have also been suggested as a food to be considered in nutritional guidelines to be set by the National Research Council. Because they may take the place of meat in the diet, their nutritional value should be comparable. They must supply a specific quantity and quality of protein as well as certain vitamins and minerals.

STABILITY OF PROTEINS IN FOODS

Bacterial Spoilage

Chemically pure proteins are fairly stable, but in the moist state in which they generally are found in foods they decompose readily at room temperature, owing to bacterial action, and may form substances toxic to the body. In this respect, nitrogenous foods are more unstable and will decompose more readily than carbohydrates and fats. Therefore, protein foods such as fresh meat, fish, milk and eggs should be kept in the refrigerator to prevent or delay their decomposition.

Effect of Heat on Protein Foods

Proteins are somewhat modified by heat, both in physical properties and in physiologic availability. In ordinary cooking, proteins such as those in egg, meat and fish are coagulated by heat, but the amino acid content is not changed.

PROTEIN-CALORIE MALNUTRITION

Protein-calorie malnutrition (P-CM) is a term used to describe several different types of deficiency conditions because they are all related to diets low in protein but with varying levels of calories from carbohydrates. P-CM is the most serious and widespread form of deficiency disease in the developing countries today and occurs most frequently in children during the years of rapid growth.

The terms used to describe P-CM are kwashiorkor and marasmus. Kwashiorkor results from a diet very low in protein but generally adequate in calories mainly from carbohydrates, while marasmus results from a diet inadequate in protein and calories. It is impossible to estimate the number of children throughout the world who are affected by these 2 forms of malnutrition. One estimate[7] is that 350 million children—70 percent of the world population under 6—are stunted in their early years by these disorders.

Kwashiorkor

In 1933 Dr. Cicely Williams, a British pediatrician working in West Africa, first described this protein-deficiency disease in children from 1 to 4 years. She called it by its local name, "Kwashiorkor," and found that it was curable by giving the children milk. The name means "the disease the deposed baby gets when the next one

[7] Randal, J.: Current, Jan., 1967.

is born."[8] The picture of a mother from Uganda (Fig. 4-4) is a striking example: the healthy infant in arms and the "deposed" one by her side.

Kwashiorkor is always associated with a low-protein high-carbohydrate diet the small child is given at weaning. In Mexico and Latin America this consists of corn and arrowroot; in Asia, and India, rice; in much of Africa, manioc and cassava; in India, also root vegetables. In these countries there is seldom any food suitable for the weaned child, who needs approximately 2 Gm. of protein per kilogram of body weight per day between the ages of 1 and 2 years.

In developed countries milk is so closely asso-

[8] Went, L. N.: Doc. Med. Geogr. Trop., 7:139, 1955.

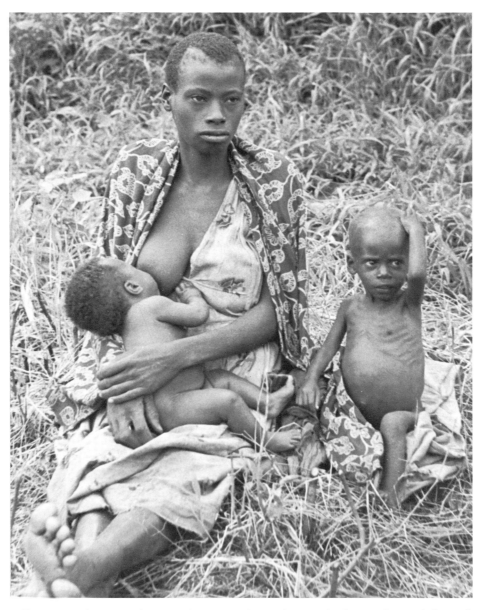

FIG. 4-4. The older child in this picture shows the protein deprivation and the malnutrition that occurred when he was "deposed" or replaced at the mother's breast by the new baby. He is subsisting on starchy foods and a few vegetables. (From Dr. John Bennett, Nutrition Unit, Ministry of Health, Kampala, Uganda)

ciated with the weaning of babies that it is difficult to realize that many of the world's children are weaned directly from human milk to a diet primarily of carbohydrate from grains or roots. Often these foods are unappetizing or are too coarse and bulky for an infant to digest. Either he fails to eat enough or his mother makes a thin gruel from these foods. In either case the infant receives a moderately calorie-deficient and grossly protein-deficient diet.

The signs of kwashiorkor vary from country to country, depending on the nature of the food given at weaning. Invariably growth is retarded and there is some degree of edema, and the muscles are weak and wasted. In addition there may be disorders of pigmentation of the skin and hair. The liver may be enlarged.

Marasmus

In addition to the many children who suffer from Kwashiorkor, there are even more who develop marasmus. The diets of these children are inadequate in calories and protein. It may be described as starvation. Marasmus usually develops in children under 1 year of age when breast-feeding fails or (like kwashiorkor) when the child suffers from some disease, usually diarrhea.

Marasmus differs from kwashiorkor in various ways. According to a WHO account:[9]

The marasmic child is wasted, not swollen. His hair is dull and dry, but not discolored. The skin is thin and wrinkled and has lost its elasticity, but does not break down. The child does not refuse food and does not show the same resentful apathy as in kwashiorkor. The terrible wasting makes the eyes look enormous and staring, and there may be, in some cases, a stiffness of limbs, due to muscle spasm. Why marasmus develops, rather than kwashiorkor, is not understood. . . . The child who has marasmus is much less likely to be depleted of proteins, and dies chiefly because diarrhea and vomiting . . . have brought great losses in body fluids. . . . Only too often marasmic children are brought to the hospital in such a moribund state that nothing can be done to save them.

Synergism Between Malnutrition and Infection

Children who suffer from inadequate protein intake are often exposed to contaminated food and water and unhygienic home conditions. According to Scrimshaw:[10]

Synergism between malnutrition and infection is responsible for much of the excess mortality among infants and preschool children in less developed regions. Two types of relationships can be identified as synergistic. Infections are likely to have more serious consequences among persons with clinical and subclinical malnutrition, and infectious diseases have the capacity to turn borderline nutritional deficiencies into severe malnutrition. Thus malnutrition and infection can be mutually aggravating and can produce more serious consequences for the patient than would be expected from the summation of the independent effects of the two.

P-CM in Older Children and Adults

Older children and adults may also suffer from protein-calorie malnutrition, but fortunately the damage may not be as permanent if food and treatment become available later. In adults emaciation and lethargy are the most common signs of semistarvation and, if protein intake is also inadequate, as is commonly the case, there may be edema and increased susceptibility to infection.

Children deprived of adequate food, especially when the diet is markedly deficient in protein, become emaciated, and growth is definitely retarded. Occasionally they show some edema, but it is less frequent and often less marked than in adults. Even after they have been receiving adequate food long enough to have regained average weight for height, they may still be under height for their age. A relief worker reported surprise on learning that a little fellow who appeared to be about 8-years-old was actually 12, and this happened repeatedly. On the other hand, the facial expression of such children is mature for their age.

In teenagers a protein deficiency in either quantity or quality may result in retarded growth during the adolescent spurt. This situation seems to have occurred in Japan from 1939 to 1948, resulting in shorter stature, especially among teenagers, at the end of the war than before.[11] Yet there were no reports of obvious deficiency disease (see Chap. 16).

TREATMENT OF P-CM

While the emphasis thus far has been on protein and calories, it must be remembered that the quality and quantity of protein as well as all nutri-

[9] Malnutrition and Disease. Geneva, Switzerland, WHO, 1963.

[10] Scrimshaw, N. S.: Recent advances in international nutrition. Presented Oct. 27, 1966. Annual Meeting Am. Dietet. Assoc., Boston.

[11] Mitchell, H. S.: J. Am. Dietet. A., 44:165, 1964.

ents must be considered in the treatment and prevention of P-CM (see Chap. 9). For infants the ideal diet would include a liberal supply of fresh milk or, if necessary, dried skim milk fortified with vitamins A and D, and accompanied by adequate non-protein calories and other nutrients. Unfortunately, milk is not available nor can it be readily distributed in the areas where kwashiorkor and marasmus are prevalent. Therefore, attention is focused on improving the quality of the protein in the diets of infants and children in the first year of life as they progress from human milk to other foods.

In several countries where P-CM is recognized as a public health problem and where milk is not easily available, palatable vegetable protein mixtures have been developed using locally grown and familiar products, for example, the "Incaparina" mentioned previously.

Experience in feeding these vegetable protein mixtures to children suffering from P-CM has demonstrated that recovery, as well as prevention of P-CM, is quite possible if the blend contains a good balance of essential amino acids. Recovery may not be as rapid as is possible when milk or other animal proteins are fed, but these mixtures of locally grown foods have the advantage of being cheap and available to many more people. Through education and an aroused interest in the problem, real progress is now being made toward the eradication of P-CM.

Great credit is due to the technical agencies of the United Nations—FAO, WHO, UNICEF and UNESCO—for their active and practical assistance to the health agencies of the many countries where P-CM is a public health problem. By working cooperatively with local authorities, a better understanding of prevailing food usage and child feeding practices has made it possible to approach a solution without depending on imported foods. The same approach applies to meeting the needs of older children and adults.

STUDY QUESTIONS AND ACTIVITIES

1. Why is good-quality protein important for breakfast and lunch as well as for dinner?

2. For what specific purposes are proteins used in the body?

3. What is meant by "essential amino acids"? Are the same ones essential for maintenance as for growth?

4. Explain three ways that proteins may be supplemented to improve the quality of the diet.

5. What theory is suggested as to why most Australians and New Zealanders are taller than people of similar racial strains living elsewhere?

6. What are the best food sources of complete proteins? Which food groups furnish the most protein? Compare the quality of protein from plant and animal foods.

7. What are the National Research Council recommendations for protein? Which foods must be included in the daily dietary, and how much of each, in order to ensure good nutrition?

8. The high-protein foods listed in Figure 4-3 contain appreciable amounts of other food constituents. Look at the Pattern Dietary in Chapter 10 and see what each supplies.

9. What is the most widespread nutritional deficiency in the developing countries today? In what countries is it most serious?

10. What age group is most susceptible to this deficiency? Why?

11. What are the most likely symptoms of kwashiorkor? What is the meaning of the word kwashiorkor and where did it come from?

SUPPLEMENTARY READING ON PROTEIN AND AMINO ACIDS

Breeling, J. L.: Marketing protein for the world's poor. Today's Health, 47:42, 1969.

Cooley, D. G.: What's so important about proteins? Today's Health, 43:46, 1965.

Leverton, R. M.: Proteins and Amino Acids. Chaps. 5 and 6. Food. Yearbook of Agriculture, U.S.D.A., Washington, D.C., 1959.

McConnell, J. F.: The deposed one. Am. J. Nursing, 61:78, 1961.

Mitchell, H. S.: Protein limitation and human growth. J. Am. Dietet. A., 44:165, 1964.

For further references see Bibliography in Part Four.

Energy Metabolism

5

Energy and Heat · Measurement of Food Calories · Measure of Energy Expended
Basal Metabolism · Factors Influencing Total Energy Requirements

Solar energy is the power that makes life on earth possible. However, of all the sun's energy that reaches the earth only a fraction of 1 percent can be adapted or stored for future use. Even the most efficient man-made devices for harnessing some of the sun's energy are less efficient by far than plants. Here the amazing process known as *photosynthesis* uses the sun's light energy to manufacture carbohydrates from the carbon dioxide of the air and the water from the soil. No animal is capable of accomplishing this synthesis. Thus, the potential or stored energy of the plant world becomes the food of animals who, in turn, spend that energy in the form of heat and work or store the surplus as body fat (see Chap. 2, Fig. 2-1).

Metabolism may be used in a general sense to refer to all types of changes that occur in food nutrients after they have been absorbed from the gastrointestinal tract and to the cellular activity involved in utilizing these nutrients (see Chap. 9). Sometimes the word is used in a more specific sense, as in protein metabolism, to refer to the total picture of what happens to protein in the body. These changes, which result ultimately in the combustion of foodstuffs with the release of heat or energy, constitute what is called energy metabolism.

ENERGY AND HEAT

Energy is expended whenever work is performed by the body in the completion of any function, small or large. It matters not whether the action is voluntary, such as walking, sitting and the various acts involved in the performance of one's daily work, or involuntary, such as in respiration, digestion, the circulation of the blood, and the maintenance of muscular tone.

The body must be supplied with food as a source of energy to maintain its temperature and perform its work. There is a direct relation between the amount of work performed, the heat produced by the body and the total food intake. One cannot perform more work than is provided for by the food intake unless one uses the reserve supply stored as adipose tissue. This latter is dramatically illustrated by the loss of body fat in starvation.

Heat in Relation to Metabolism. Heat is the result of combustion of fuels outside the body and also of the oxidation of foods in our bodies. Because heat is a by-product of all energy spent as work, heat can serve as a measure of energy metabolism. As it is necessary in scientific work to have measures of length (centimeter, inch) and measures of weight (gram, ounce), so is it necessary to have a measure of heat. A Calorie (kilo calorie) is the amount of heat required to raise the temperature of one kilogram of water one degree Centigrade. In our more common measures, it is approximately the amount of heat required to raise the temperature of 4 pounds of water one degree Fahrenheit. This is a large calorie and is 1,000 times the small calorie, the unit used by physicists.

MEASUREMENT OF FOOD CALORIES

A bomb calorimeter is a device for measuring calories, the stored fuel in foods. The apparatus shown in Figure 5-1 is carefully designed for measuring all the heat produced by the complete oxidation of an accurately measured amount of any food. The apparatus is insulated thoroughly against loss of heat, and the amount of heat produced is measured by the change in temperature of a measured amount of water.

Physiologic Calorie Values. The calorie value of nutrients determined by the bomb calorimeter must be modified to take account of losses in digestion and excretion. From a large number of determinations Atwater derived the well-known physiologic fuel values:

	CALORIES PER GRAM
Protein	4
Fat	9
Carbohydrate	4

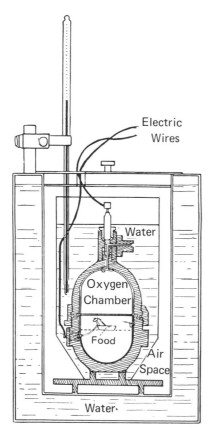

FIG. 5-1. Diagram of the parts of a bomb calorimeter. The water in the inner chamber changes in temperature when the food is burned. The water in the outer chamber acts with the intervening air space as insulation.

These values were approximate only, but they served reasonably well when applied to foods in the average American diet. For practical purposes, it is possible to estimate the caloric value of most foods by applying the physiologic fuel values to the percentage composition for protein, fat and carbohydrate. Some modification of these procedures for calculating calories has been made as a result of more recent research findings, and these are the basis for the calorie values published in Agriculture Handbook No. 8.[1]

Table 1, in Part Four, Composition of Foods, is based on Handbook No. 8 and Bulletin 72.[2]

MEASURE OF ENERGY EXPENDED

The actual energy expended by the body throughout a given period may be determined by placing a human subject in a special calorimeter. The heat given off by the subject is absorbed by the water in the coils surrounding the well insulated chamber, where, by an accurate mechanism, the total heat may be measured. This procedure is known as direct calorimetry. As there

---

[1] Watt, B. K., and Merrill, A. L.: Composition of Foods: Raw, Processed, Prepared. Agriculture Handbook No. 8. U.S.D.A., 1963.

[2] Nutritive Value of Foods. Home and Garden Bull. No. 72. U.S.D.A., Washington, D.C., 1964.

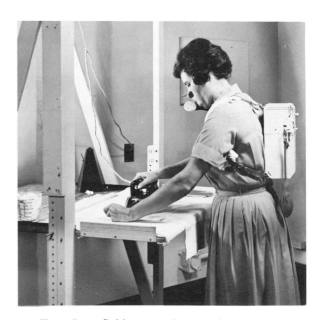

FIG. 5-2. Subject wearing respirometer to measure calorie expenditure while standing to iron at a work-surface level of 36 inches from the floor. (U.S.D.A. Office of Information)

are in existence only a few calorimeters large enough for making direct observations on human beings, and because they are exceedingly expensive, this method is used only for scientific research.

By another method, known as indirect calorimetry, the rate of metabolism is calculated from the oxygen intake or from the oxygen intake and carbon dioxide content of the expired air, as measured by a respiration apparatus. By determining either the oxygen consumed or the carbon dioxide exhaled in a given number of minutes, the caloric expenditure can be calculated. This principle may be applied to persons engaged in various types of activities or when lying at rest. If the subject is moving about, he has to carry his respirator with him (Fig. 5-2). Under basal conditions, or when work is performed in a stationary position, a tank-type apparatus is used.

BASAL METABOLISM

The energy expended under basal conditions includes the work of

1. Maintenance of muscle tone and body temperature
2. Circulation
3. Respiration
4. Other glandular and cellular activity.

In order that there may be some basis of comparison for tests, the rate of metabolism must be studied under standard basal conditions. Therefore, it is specified that the subject be lying down, awake and at complete rest, and that the test be taken at least 12 hours after the last meal and several hours after any vigorous exercise.

In the morning before breakfast is the most convenient time to comply with these conditions. The rate of metabolism as determined under these "standard" conditions is known as the basal metabolic rate (BMR). Marked variations in the basal rate of metabolism are an indication of disease.

Formerly, the basal metabolism test was used extensively as a means of diagnosis, particularly in cases of hyperthyroidism, hypothyrodism, and other endocrine disturbances which may alter the metabolic rate. Because the thyroid hormone, thyroxine, has the greatest effect on the metabolic rate, measurement of protein-bound iodine (PBI) —the combination of iodine-thyroxine with certain proteins in the blood—is a more accurate diagnostic test. It requires only a small sample of the patient's blood and is easier for both the patient and the physician. The normal range for PBI is from 4 to 8 micrograms per 100 ml. of plasma.

Factors Determining Basal Metabolic Rate (BMR)

There are normal variations in basal metabolism, the causes of which lie within the body itself: the size, the shape and the composition of the body, the age of the individual and the activity of certain internal glands. It is generally accepted that a variation of from 10 to 15 percent either way from the accepted metabolism rate (all variables considered) is within normal limits. Complete tables of average metabolic rates for men and women of different age, height and weight are used for comparison with the measured rate. The basal metabolism of an average man and woman would be about 1,650 and 1,350 calories, respectively.

The surface area of the body is used as a measure of size in these studies. The skin of the body is a radiating surface from which heat is given off continually. Therefore, the greater the skin area, the greater will be the amount of heat lost by the body and, in turn, the greater the necessary heat production by the individual. It has been found that a tall, slender person has a greater surface area than a shorter, stout person of the same weight; that is, surface area is proportional to height multiplied by weight.

The higher the proportion of active muscular tissue the higher the metabolic rate will be, because fatty tissue has a much lower rate. Thus, the athlete will tend to have a higher rate than a sedentary man of the same age and size.

Age and growth are responsible for normal variations in basal metabolism. The relative rate is highest during the first and the second years of life and decreases after that, although it is still relatively high through the ages of puberty, in both girls and boys. During adult life there is a steady decrease in rate, with a marked drop in old age, due undoubtedly to decrease in muscle mass.

Sex probably has little effect on metabolism, although women in general have a lower metabolism than men. This may be accounted for by habitually less activity or by a difference in body composition, women usually having more fat and less muscular development than men.

The state of nutrition may effect the BMR. In order to conserve energy during severe starvation or prolonged undernutrition, the body adapts by decreasing its metabolic rate, possibly by as much as 50 percent.

Diseases such as infections or fevers raise the BMR in proportion to the elevation of the body temperature, approximately 7 percent for each degree Fahrenheit rise in temperature.

The secretions of certain endocrine glands such as the thyroid, the adrenals and the pituitary affect metabolism. The secretion of the thyroid gland has the most marked effect. Hyperthyroidism is that condition in which the metabolism is accelerated by increased production of thyroxine, while hypothyroidism is characterized by a decrease resulting in subnormal metabolism. Adrenalin, a secretion of the adrenals, causes a temporary increase in the BMR. Those pituitary hormones which stimulate thyroid and adrenal secretions also affect the metabolic rate.

FACTORS INFLUENCING TOTAL ENERGY REQUIREMENTS

For all voluntary activities the energy needed is in direct relation to the intensity of the exercise. For instance, a moderate amount of energy is needed for walking, whereas for the heavy labor of digging a ditch or for the active exercise of tennis a much greater number of calories is needed.

Muscular work is the greatest factor influencing energy requirements. Mental work, strange as it may seem, does not affect the total metabolism sufficiently to be detected easily. Investigators, working with very delicate apparatus, found that nerve tissue, when active, does expend some energy, but that the amount is minute compared with the total energy output of the body. In exceptional cases, physical work may be the means of increasing the metabolism by as much as 4,000 calories per day. In every case the food intake should equal in caloric value the heat units expended by the body (except, of course, in overweight individuals who find it necessary to reduce). A man doing sedentary work may require only 2,500 calories per day, while a man doing exceedingly hard manual labor may require as much as 5,000 calories. The calorie allowances given for different age and sex categories in the Recommended Daily Dietary Allowances apply to individuals engaged in moderate physical activity (see Chap. 10). For men, the range is from 2,800 down to 2,400; for women, from 2,000 to 1,700 calories, the lower figures being for the older age groups.

Table 5-1 gives the average energy expenditure per pound or per kilo per hour for several everyday activities. Obviously, not all types of activity

TABLE 5-1. ENERGY EXPENDITURE FOR EVERYDAY ACTIVITIES*

	CAL./ KG./HR.	CAL./ LB./HR.
Sleeping	.9	.4
Bicycling, mod. speed	3.8	1.7
Cello playing	2.5	1.1
Dancing, foxtrot	5.2	2.4
Dancing, waltz	4.4	2.0
Dishwashing	2.2	1.0
Dressing and undressing	1.9	.9
Driving an automobile	2.1	1.0
Eating a meal	1.5	.7
Horseback riding, trot	5.8	2.6
Ironing	2.2	1.0
Laundering, light	2.5	1.1
Lying still and awake	1.2	.5
Painting furniture	2.8	1.3
Playing Ping-pong	5.9	2.7
Piano playing, moderate	2.6	1.2
Reading aloud	1.5	.7
Running	8.8	4.0
Sewing by hand	1.5	.7
Sewing, elec. mach.	1.5	.7
Sitting quietly, watching TV	1.4	.6
Skating	4.9	2.2
Standing, relaxed	1.7	.8
Sweeping, vacuum cleaner	4.1	1.9
Swimming (2 mi./hr.)	9.8	4.5
Tailoring	2.1	1.0
Typing rapidly	2.2	1.0
Walking, 3 mph	3.3	1.5
Walking, 4 mph	4.9	2.2
Writing	1.5	.7

* Adapted from Taylor, MacLeod & Rose: Foundations of Nutrition. ed. 5. New York, Macmillan, 1956. (Calculated by adding to original figures 1 cal./Kg./hr. for BMR plus 10 percent for influence of food.)

have been measured but, in using this table to estimate energy expenditure, the data requiring similar exertion may be used for an activity for which no figure is given.

Individual variation in the amount of energy spent in performing a given task or activity may be considerable. One person may sit so relaxed that he spends no more energy than another may spend lying down. One person makes more motions in doing a job than another. Thus, in calculating the energy expenditure for a day from such a table one can expect only an approximate figure because of the many variables and the difficulty of estimating the exact length of time spent in each activity.

A quick estimate of the energy needs of a moderately active person may be made as follows:

Basal needs = 1 cal./Kg./hr.

Weight in Kg. × 24 = BMR for 1 day

BMR plus 50 percent = total energy needs for light activity.

The increase above the basal is proportional to the degree of activity, as indicated in Table 5-2 for the rough estimation of energy needs.

Habitual muscular exercise not only increases the total energy metabolism but affects the basal rate, because energy is required to maintain muscle tone. On the other hand, sleep lowers metabolism because the muscles are relaxed. A prolonged period of absolute rest in bed means loss of muscle tone and lowered metabolism.

A person who habitually consumes more calories than he expends for work plus body heat tends to store the extra food as body fat (adipose tissue). This is easy to do, especially when one's activities are less than they were previously. Frequently, eating habits are not adjusted to fit reduced activities. Therefore, it is not surprising that people tend to gain weight with age; it is more surprising that they do not gain more weight. A fuller discussion of weight control and the treatment of obesity is given in Chapter 21.

Age and body weight affect total energy requirement as well as the BMR. Of course, activity is the biggest variable, but, in general, activity decreases with age as does the metabolic activity of the tissues.

The ingestion of food increases the metabolic rate. It was demonstrated that a fasting man had a metabolism averaging 9 percent lower than that on the days when food was consumed. However, metabolism goes on during fasting, showing that the body must continue metabolizing even though the tissues are called on to make up the deficit. This explains the loss of weight and wasting in severe illness and starvation.

With prolonged fasting and subsequent loss of weight, the body tends to adjust itself by lowering the metabolic rate. This is comparable with setting back a thermostat so that the organism runs at a lower rate. This adjustment is true of adults, but children who are undernourished may have a higher rate, which makes undernutrition in children even more serious than in adults. So far there is no satisfactory explanation of this difference.

Specific Dynamic Action of Protein. Not all kinds of food are oxidized with an equal effect on metabolism. Protein stimulates metabolism, so that a greater amount of heat is produced in its metabolism than in that of similar quantities of fats and carbohydrates. This effect is commonly known as the specific dynamic action of protein. Carbohydrates and fats have a much less marked effect, but the slight stimulation that results from the intake of food of any type accounts for the fact that metabolism tests usually are taken before breakfast when no food has been eaten for at least 12 hours. For a person on an average diet the specific dynamic action of food may account for a rise of about 10 percent above the basal.

Climate, season, housing and clothing affect metabolism, chiefly through their bearing upon the regulation of body temperature. The heat produced in the body by metabolic processes must be conserved or given off in such a way as to maintain the body temperature at a remarkably constant figure. If no heat were lost from the body during average daily activity, the temperature would rise about 2° F. an hour. In winter we purposely curtail our heat loss from the body by wearing heavier clothing and living in heated houses; in summer we wear thinner clothing to expedite greater losses. However, nature has provided for a carefully controlled loss of heat that may vary as climate and environment dictate. A thinly clothed person on a cold winter day may shiver. This process is a series of rapid muscular contractions set up involuntarily in the body to increase heat production in order to make up for the rapid heat loss. Evaporation of perspiration from the skin is a mechanism employed by the body to reduce temperature. Insensible perspiration is evaporating continuously with a slight loss of heat, but sensible perspiration means greater heat loss and affords a welcome cooling effect when the body is overheated in warm weather or after strenuous exercise.

Caloric Needs. Although essential nutrients should be considered in the selection of an adequate diet, it must be remembered that the caloric value is fundamentally one of the most important points. "No supplements of [amino acids], vita-

TABLE 5-2. APPROXIMATE INCREASE ABOVE BASAL NEEDS FOR LISTED ACTIVITIES

	PERCENT ABOVE BASAL
Bed rest (hospital patient)	10
Sedentary activity, knitting	30
Light activity, tailor or nurse	50
Moderate activity, carpenter, painter	75
Severe activity, lumberman, stone mason...	100

mins or mineral elements can alter the laws of the conservation of energy. Calories are still needed . . . to furnish energy for muscular work"[3] and maintain body functions.

When emergencies arise in war or famine, it is total calories which must be provided first to keep people alive and satisfied. The quality and the nature of the calories can be adjusted later to meet specific needs.

For a discussion on the effects of calorie deficiency see Chapter 4, Protein-Calorie Malnutrition.

STUDY QUESTIONS

1. Explain the use of the word *metabolism* in the expressions "energy metabolism" and "protein metabolism."

2. What is the unit of measure for energy and how is food energy measured? Define it specifically.

3. What are the so-called physiologic fuel values? How can they be used to estimate food values?

4. What is measured in a basal metabolism test? Under what conditions must the test be performed? Name the factors that affect the basal metabolic needs of any given individual.

5. What is the largest single factor affecting the total energy requirements? List other factors that play a part in the total calories needed.

6. When there are acute food shortages, which should relief agencies supplying a minimum of food to relieve starvation consider first—calories, protein or vitamins?

SUPPLEMENTARY READING ON CALORIE REQUIREMENTS AND ENERGY METABOLISM

Konishi, F.: Food energy equivalents of various activities. J. Am. Dietet. A., 46:186, 1965.
Review: Food intake and energy expenditure. Nutr. Rev., 14:48, 1956.
————: Variability in Basal Metabolic Rate. Nutr. Rev., 25:12, 1967.
————: Variability in caloric intakes. Nutr. Rev., 24:39, 1966.

For further references see Bibliography in Part Four.

---

[3] DuBois, E. F., and Chambers, W. H.: JAMA, 119: 1183, 1942.

Water and Mineral Metabolism

6

Water in Relation to Body Function · Water Intake and Output
Electrolytes and Non-electrolytes · Acid-Base Balance · Vital Minerals and Their Distribution
Mineral Content of Foods · Calcium and Phosphorus · Magnesium · Iron
Sodium and other Mineral Elements · Trace Elements or Micronutrients

FLUIDS AND ELECTROLYTES

Water in Relation to Body Function

Water is more essential to life than is food, for a person may live weeks without food but only days without water. It is an essential component of blood, lymph, the secretions of the body (extracellular fluid) and of every cell in the body (intracellular). About half the adult weight is water, 60 percent for men, 54 percent for women. The internal environment of the body is bathed in fluids that are held in compartments of the body divided by semipermeable membranes. The extracellular compartment (the space outside the cell membrane) accounts for ⅓ of the body water and includes the fluid in plasma and in interstitial spaces; intracellular fluid contains ⅔ of the body water.

Fluid is necessary for the functioning of every organ in the body. It is the universal medium in which the various chemical changes of the body take place. As a carrier it aids in digestion, absorption, circulation and excretion; it is essential in the regulation of body temperature; it plays an important part in mechanical functions, such as the lubrication of joints and the movement of the viscera in the abdominal cavity. Waste products from the tissues are transferred to the blood in watery solutions; they are carried by the blood, which is about 80 percent water; and they are excreted via the kidneys in the urine, which is about 97 percent water (Fig. 6-1).

The same water is reused many times and for different purposes. Approximately 8 liters of digestive juices are produced and secreted by the glands in 24 hours (see Chap. 9). The water that carries the enzymes into the digestive tract is used during absorption to carry the digested nutrients into the blood and lymph. Over 4 liters of water are always circulating in the blood stream. Water is the carrier of nutrients throughout the body. It is estimated that some 50 liters of water cross cell membranes in a day. In the kidney large volumes of water carry the dissolved waste material through the capsule of the uriniferous tubules, but, in passing through the tubules, most of the water, with some of its useful dissolved material, is reabsorbed. The urine which is excreted is the concentrated aqueous solution of the waste products.

Water Intake and Output

Water normally is lost from the body by four routes: from the skin, as sensible and insensible perspiration; from the lungs, as water vapor in the expired air; from the kidneys, as urine; and from the intestines, in the feces. A minimum of 800 ml. of water is lost daily through the skin and lungs, and this amount may increase in hot, dry environments. The kidney eliminates approximately 1,000 to 1,500 ml. of water in the urine; fecal losses approximate 200 ml. daily but increase greatly when diarrhea occurs. Large water losses also result from excessive perspiration due to

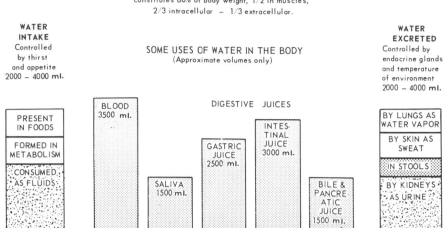

THE STORY OF WATER IN THE BODY

Water functions in every tissue of the body. It
constitutes 60% of body weight, 1/2 in muscles,
2/3 intracellular — 1/3 extracellular.

| WATER INTAKE Controlled by thirst and appetite 2000 – 4000 ml. | SOME USES OF WATER IN THE BODY (Approximate volumes only) | WATER EXCRETED Controlled by endocrine glands and temperature of environment 2000 – 4000 ml. |

PRESENT IN FOODS
FORMED IN METABOLISM
CONSUMED AS FLUIDS

BLOOD 3500 ml.

DIGESTIVE JUICES

SALIVA 1500 ml.
GASTRIC JUICE 2500 ml.
INTESTINAL JUICE 3000 ml.
BILE & PANCREATIC JUICE 1500 ml.

BY LUNGS AS WATER VAPOR
BY SKIN AS SWEAT
IN STOOLS
BY KIDNEYS AS URINE

FIGURE 6-1

fever, or from vomiting, burns or hemorrhage (see Fig. 6-2).

Fluids are replaced by the ingestion of liquids and foods containing water. Although some water (14 ml. per 100 calories) is formed within the body as an end product of food metabolism, from

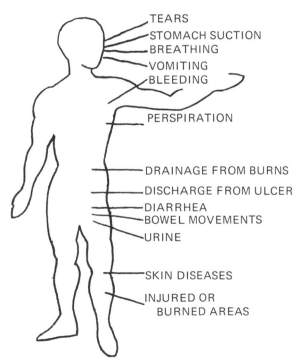

TEARS
STOMACH SUCTION
BREATHING
VOMITING
BLEEDING
PERSPIRATION
DRAINAGE FROM BURNS
DISCHARGE FROM ULCER
DIARRHEA
BOWEL MOVEMENTS
URINE
SKIN DISEASES
INJURED OR BURNED AREAS

FIG. 6-2. Ways in which water and electrolytes may be lost. (Snively, W. D.: Sea Within. Philadelphia, J. B. Lippincott, 1960)

4 to 6 cups (1-1½ liters) of water or other liquids should be consumed daily in order to ensure a sufficient amount of water for body functions. Many foods contain a high percentage of water (Fig. 6-3) and may provide as much as 1 liter a day. Once ingested, water is absorbed rapidly from the digestive tract into the blood and lymph, although enough water is retained with food residues in the colon to produce a soft stool.

Homeostasis—Water Balance. Water balance is carefully regulated within the body and normally a balance between intake and output is maintained, provided that there is free access to water. Thus the weight of a man varies by approximately only ⅓ pound in a 24-hour period.

When water losses are increased owing to excessive sweating or diarrhea, for example, the kidneys conserve water by making less urine.

Excessive loss of water results in sensations of extreme thirst. Thirst is a sensation of dryness at the root of the tongue and the back part of the throat and is Nature's signal that liquid intake must be increased. Monitoring the patient's fluid intake and output may be an important aspect of patient care.

Dehydration. Dehydration may be fatal, a fact that further emphasizes the importance of water in the body. The German physiologist Rubner stated that we can lose all our reserve glycogen, all reserve fat and about one half of the body protein without great danger, but that a loss of 10 percent of the body water is serious and from 20 to 22 percent loss is fatal.

The term **dehydration** implies more than change in water balance—there are always accompanying changes in electrolyte balance. When the water supply is restricted or when losses are excessive, the rate of water loss exceeds the rate of electrolyte loss. The extracellular fluid becomes concentrated, and osmotic pressure draws water from the cells into the extracellular fluid to compensate. This condition is called intracellular dehydration and is accompanied by extreme thirst and nausea.

Electrolytes and Non-electrolytes

Chemical compounds that dissociate in water, breaking up into separate particles called ions, are known as electrolytes, and the process is referred to as ionization. Salts, acids and bases are electrolytes; compounds such as glucose, urea and protein are called non-electrolytes because they are molecules that do not ionize.

Electrolyte Composition of the Body Fluids. Sodium and chloride are the major ions in plasma and interstitial fluid. The major ions in intracellular fluid are potassium and phosphate. Other ions are present in varying amounts in the different body fluids. Functions of these minerals will be discussed later in this chapter.

Osmotic Pressure. As previously stated, the fluid compartments of the body are separated by semipermeable membranes. These permit free exchange of water molecules but partially or completely prevent passage of dissolved particles such as glucose or electrolytes. If there is a solution containing a relatively large number of dissolved particles on one side of a semipermeable membrane and a solution containing a relatively small number of dissolved particles on the other, the force of osmosis is brought into play. Osmotic pressure causes water to pass across the semipermeable membrane from the less concentrated to the more concentrated solution, until the concentration of dissolved particles on both sides is equal.

Hence, exchanges of water between the various fluid compartments of the body occur as a result of osmotic pressure, which, in turn, is due chiefly to the concentration of electrolytes. Osmotic pressure in the cellular fluid is regulated mainly by the concentration of potassium and in the extracellular fluid by the concentration of sodium. If there is a loss or gain in either of these electrolytes in one compartment, the osmotic pressure is disturbed, and an increased amount of water will then be found in the compartment of greater osmotic pressure.

Plasma protein also plays an important role in maintaining osmotic equilibrium in the extracellular compartments. By remaining in the plasma it tends to prevent the leakage of water into the interstitial spaces, where an excess of extracellular fluid is known as edema.

Excess water losses may also result in excess loss of electrolytes. These are not always replaced through water intake, in which case serious problems may result.

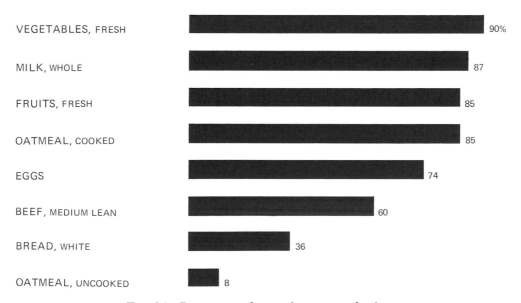

Fig. 6-3. Percentage of water in common foods.

Acid-Base Balance

Electrolytes play an important part in maintaining the acid-base balance in the blood and throughout the tissues. The maintenance of this balance is a function of normal metabolism. The reaction of the blood is slightly alkaline (pH 7.3-7.45), varying only within narrow limits, regardless of the amount of acid products formed in metabolism. This equilibrium is maintained by a series of buffers in the blood and the tissue fluids which have a tendency to resist changes in their pH.

Acid products formed in metabolism are disposed of through either the lungs or the kidneys. The respiratory mechanism reacts quickly but the renal system adapts itself over longer periods of time. The respiratory system controls the removal from the blood of CO_2 and can either increase or decrease its loss by regulating the depth and rate of respiration. The kidneys excrete acids and, at the same time, return bicarbonate to the blood.

When the supply of buffers becomes depleted due to starvation or inability to metabolize food properly, a condition known as acidosis may result. Actually, the blood does not become acid, but the term *acidosis* is used to indicate the lowered alkaline reserve which results when the basic elements are used up faster than they are replenished. This may happen in severe diabetes, when the organic acids from faulty fat metabolism accumulate.

Alkalosis is the opposite of acidosis. This may occur when severe vomiting over a period of time causes a great loss of hydrochloric acid. The body quickly adjusts when the acute condition is relieved.

Acid-Base Reaction of Foods. Conclusive evidence is not as yet available in regard to the practical importance of the acid-base balance of foods in relation to health. Experience and scientific evidence indicate a wide range of adaptability on the part of the human body and do not support the "scare" propaganda with which certain food faddists promote the sale of "alkalizing" compounds to prevent acidosis.

The usual mixed diet contains a good balance of acid and basic factors. The mineral elements are sometimes referred to as "ash" because they do not "burn" up. When foods are metabolized in the body, the mineral elements are released to function in maintaining the acid-base balance; the organic acids are mostly oxidized to carbon dioxide and water. Foods are said to be acid or basic according to whether the acid or the basic

elements in the ash predominate. Most fruits contain organic acids combined with basic inorganic elements. When such compounds are oxidized in the body, they leave an alkaline ash. Some other foods, such as cereals and meats, not at all acid in taste, yield end products that are strongly acid. Thus, by potential acidity or alkalinity of foods is meant the reaction that they will ultimately yield after being oxidized in the body.

MINERALS

Vital Minerals and Their Distribution

Although mineral elements constitute but a small proportion (4 percent) of the body tissue, they are essential both as structural components and in many vital processes. Some form hard tissues such as bones and teeth; some are in the fluids and soft tissues. For some functions it is the balance of mineral ions that is important—for example, in bone formation, the amount and the ratio of calcium and phosphorus; for normal muscular activity, the ratio between potassium and calcium in the extracellular fluid. Electrolytes, of which sodium and potassium ions are the most important, are the major factors in the osmotic control of water metabolism as discussed earlier in this chapter. Other minerals may act as catalysts, in enzyme systems, or as integral parts of organic compounds in the body, such as iron in hemoglobin, iodine in thyroxine, cobalt in vitamin B_{12}, zinc in insulin and sulfur in thiamine and biotin.

Plant life and animals, as well as bacteria and other one-celled organisms, all require proper concentrations of certain minerals to make life possible. In fact, changes in concentration of minerals, small in themselves, can be fatal to various forms of life. Thus, common salt, which in dilute solution is necessary for most forms of animal life, becomes a preservative when foods are salted or kept in brine because the concentration kills bacteria. In the human body also, the maintenance of a normal concentration of minerals in body fluids is essential.

The principal minerals which the body requires are calcium, phosphorus, potassium, chlorine, sodium, sulfur, magnesium, iron and iodine. These elements are present in the body in amounts as given in Table 6-1. Several minerals are used by animals in trace quantities and are sometimes called micronutrients; these are copper, manganese, cobalt, zinc, fluorine, molybdenum, selenium and chromium. Aluminum, arsenic, boron, cadmium and silicon also are present as trace elements in animal tissue, but their function is uncertain.

Mineral Content of Foods

In unrefined foods, minerals are present in various forms mixed or combined with proteins, fats and carbohydrates. Processed or refined foods, such as fats, oils, sugar and cornstarch, contain almost no minerals. The total mineral content of a food is determined by burning the organic or combustible part of a known amount of a food and weighing the resulting ash. The ash then is analyzed for individual mineral elements. Most foods have been analyzed for 10 or more mineral elements, but in dietary practice the figures most commonly used are those for calcium, phosphorus and iron and, for therapeutic purposes, sodium, potassium and magnesium (Tables 1 and 4, Part Four).

Minerals such as iodine, copper and other trace elements which are essential for life may be found abundantly in drinking water in certain areas or in foods grown in the soil of those areas, whereas in other parts of the country they are deficient in both soil and water. Still other mineral elements, such as sodium, potassium, chlorine and sulfur—all necessary in human nutrition—are so universally present in foods that we recognize no need to worry about deficiencies.

Calcium and Phosphorus

FUNCTIONS OF CALCIUM AND PHOSPHORUS

Structures of Bones and Teeth. The adult human body contains approximately 2 percent of calcium and 1 percent of phosphorus. Ninety-nine percent of the calcium and 75 percent of the phosphorus in our bodies are found as constituents of bone and teeth, giving to them strength and rigidity.

Bone is constantly being synthesized and broken down. In children, bone synthesis—the formation of new bone—is greater than the destruction or resorption of bone; on the other hand, the skeletal changes frequently observed in old age occur when bone resorption dominates and there is a decrease in the absolute amount of bone (osteoporosis). In the normal adult the two processes—mineralization (incorporation of calcium in bone) and demineralization (resorption of calcium)—are equally balanced.

Hormones control these processes. The parathyroid hormone controls the resorption of cal-

TABLE 6-1. MINERAL COMPOSITION OF AN ADULT HUMAN BODY

ELEMENT	PERCENT OF TOTAL ASH	GM./70 KG. MAN
Calcium (Ca)	39	1,160
Phosphorus (P)	22	670
Potassium (K)	5	150
Sulfur (S)	4	112
Chlorine (Cl)	3	85
Sodium (Na)	2	63
Magnesium (Mg)	0.7	21
Iron (Fe)	.15	4.5
Iodine (I)	.0007	.02

cium from bone, and recently a thyroid hormone—thyrocalcitonin—that prohibits release of calcium from bone has been identified.

Bone, like other tissue, is in a state of dynamic equilibrium with the constituents of the plasma and other tissue. Calcium and phosphorus, when the food supply is abundant, can be stored in the trabeculae at the ends of the bones. From this storehouse these minerals are readily available to meet the needs of other tissues of the body when the dietary intake of calcium or phosphorus is inadequate. However, if calcium has not been stored in the trabeculae, calcium will be withdrawn from bone structure itself. Prolonged removal of calcium from bone naturally results in bones more easily bent or broken. When calcium phosphate is removed from bone, the remaining tissue is as flexible as cartilage; in fact, it is essentially the same as cartilage. Osteomalacia is the term used to describe this condition in adults. Cartilage precedes bone in the development of the fetus, and normally the calcium phosphate is deposited in it as growth and strain demand. When nature's plan is thwarted by an inadequate supply of these minerals in food, or by an inability to utilize them, growth may be retarded, or, as more often happens, growth in size continues, but the new bone is abnormal in structure and poorly calcified. This may result in the bowed legs, enlarged ankles and wrists, prolapsed thorax and other bone deformities characteristic of rickets. Osteomalacia and rickets are discussed with Vitamin D in Chapter 7.

Tooth structures, particularly the dentine and enamel, are metabolically more stable than the bones. There is little turnover of calcium from the teeth.

Functions in Serum and Soft Tissues. When compared with the amounts in bones and teeth the concentrations of calcium and phosphorus in the blood are small, but their presence in normal amounts is essential for body function. Although they are often associated because they function together in the skeletal structures, elsewhere in the body their functions are quite distinct. A normal calcium level in the blood is necessary for blood clot formation. Calcium has a vital role in maintaining muscle tone and irritability; it is required for normal nerve transmission; it is an activator of several enzymes; and it influences the permeability of cell membranes. The neuromuscular hyper-

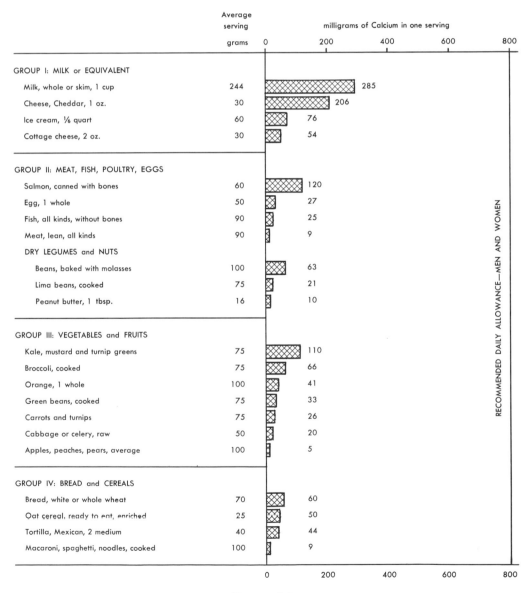

CALCIUM

In Average Servings of Foods
Classified in the Four Food Groups

	Average serving grams	milligrams of Calcium in one serving
GROUP I: MILK or EQUIVALENT		
Milk, whole or skim, 1 cup	244	285
Cheese, Cheddar, 1 oz.	30	206
Ice cream, ⅙ quart	60	76
Cottage cheese, 2 oz.	30	54
GROUP II: MEAT, FISH, POULTRY, EGGS		
Salmon, canned with bones	60	120
Egg, 1 whole	50	27
Fish, all kinds, without bones	90	25
Meat, lean, all kinds	90	9
DRY LEGUMES and NUTS		
Beans, baked with molasses	100	63
Lima beans, cooked	75	21
Peanut butter, 1 tbsp.	16	10
GROUP III: VEGETABLES and FRUITS		
Kale, mustard and turnip greens	75	110
Broccoli, cooked	75	66
Orange, 1 whole	100	41
Green beans, cooked	75	33
Carrots and turnips	75	26
Cabbage or celery, raw	50	20
Apples, peaches, pears, average	100	5
GROUP IV: BREAD and CEREALS		
Bread, white or whole wheat	70	60
Oat cereal, ready to eat, enriched	25	50
Tortilla, Mexican, 2 medium	40	44
Macaroni, spaghetti, noodles, cooked	100	9

RECOMMENDED DAILY ALLOWANCE—MEN AND WOMEN

Figure 6-4

TABLE 6-2. CALCIUM, PHOSPHORUS, MAGNESIUM AND IRON IN PATTERN DIETARY FOR 1 DAY*

FOOD GROUP	AMOUNT IN GM.	HOUSEHOLD MEASURE	CALORIES	CALCIUM MG.	PHOSPHORUS MG.	MAGNESIUM MG.	IRON MG.
Milk or equivalent	488	2 cups	320	576	452	63	.2
Egg	50	1 medium	81	27	102	5	1.2
Meat, fish, poultry	120	4 ozs. cooked	376	13	212	104	3.3
Vegetables:							
Potato, cooked	100	1 medium	65	6	48	22	.5
Green, leafy, and yellow	75	1 serving	21	44	28	29	.9
Other	75	1 serving	45	16	41	18	.9
Fruits:							
Citrus	100	1 serving	44	18	16	12	.3
Other	100	1 serving	85	10	21	16	.8
Bread, white, enriched ...	70	3 slices	189	59	68	15	1.7
Cereal, whole grain or							
enriched	30	1 oz. dry or					
	130	⅔ c. cooked	89	12	95	34	.9
Butter or margarine	14	1 tbsp.	100	3	2	2	..
			1,415	784	1,085	320	10.7

* For basis of calculation, see Pattern Dietary in Chapter 10.

irritability characteristic of tetany occurs when the blood calcium level falls below normal.

Phosphorus is a necessary constituent of every cell in the body. It is part of the nucleic acids DNA (deoxyribonucleic acid) and RNA (ribonucleic acid) which determine the genetic code (see Chap. 9). Phosphorus is part of the ATP (adenosine triphosphate)-ADP (adenosine diphosphate) energy-transporting systems in the cells (see Chap. 9) and is also a component of the phospholipids which are involved in the emulsification and transport of fats and fatty acids. Phosphates also assist in maintaining the acid-base balance of the blood.

FOOD SOURCES OF CALCIUM AND PHOSPHORUS

It is apparent in Figure 6-4 that milk and milk products are the most important sources of calcium in readily available form. A few of the green, leafy vegetables used commonly in the Southern states are good sources of calcium, but others such as spinach, chard, beet greens and rhubarb contain sufficient oxalic acid to form insoluble calcium oxalate, thus rendering the calcium unavailable. In most sections of the country greens are not used regularly enough or in sufficient quantity to be relied upon to replace milk, but they are important when milk is scarce or unobtainable. Meats and poultry are poor sources of calcium. Cereal products contribute little, except where breads are enriched with calcium or are made with a high percentage of milk solids.

The pattern dietary of 1,400 calories provides almost the recommended allowance of 800 mg. (0.8 Gm.), which will be supplemented by the calcium of the foods added to make up the needed calories (see Table 6-2 and Chap. 10).

Phosphorus, as seen in the pattern dietary, is more widely distributed than calcium and less likely to be deficient in the average diet. Poultry, fish, meats, eggs, cereals, nuts and legumes, as well as milk and milk products, are all good sources. In the cooking of vegetables, there may be slight losses of calcium and phosphorus, especially if the cooking water is discarded.

FACTORS AFFECTING ABSORPTION AND RETENTION

All of the calcium and phosphorus in foods is not available to the body. Approximately 20 to 40 percent of the calcium and 70 percent of the phosphorus consumed by an individual is absorbed from the intestinal tract into the blood stream to become available. The amounts absorbed, however, may be greatly increased during periods of rapid growth when mineral needs are high. Individuals on limited intakes of calcium also are more efficient in their utilization than those on more liberal intakes.

Various factors, in addition to need, influence the efficiency of calcium and phosphorus absorption. Adequate amounts of vitamin D, an acid pH in the upper part of the intestinal tract, and a normal motility of the gastrointestinal tract enhance the absorption of these minerals. On the other hand, large amounts of fats, phytates (phosphorus compounds found in cereals) or oxalates which can form insoluble compounds with calcium may interfere with intestinal absorption.

In cases of parathyroid disturbances variations in calcium absorption and retention are even greater than under normal conditions. Hypercalcemia (high serum calcium) may occur in hyperparathyroidism, and hypocalcemia (serum calcium below normal) may result after operative removal of the parathyroid glands.

DIETARY REQUIREMENTS

The 1968 Recommended Dietary Allowances for calcium and phosphorus are 0.8 Gm. (800 mg.) each per day for adults. The same allowance is recommended for women, despite their smaller average size, as for men, to ensure ample stores in preparation for maternity. These recommendations are both increased to 1.2 Gm. during pregnancy and 1.3 Gm. for lactation.

Special attention should be given to the calcium intake of older people, especially women, because of their tendency commonly to decrease their intake when there may be even an increased need. For this group, a population at high risk for development of osteoporosis, the RDA of 800 mg. may allow little margin of safety (see Chap. 17).

The calcium and phosphorus requirements for growth have been investigated in children of different ages by observing the level of intake at which maximum retention of calcium and phosphorus is attained. Growth of bone requires the storage of new calcium and phosphorus as well as replacement. For infants up to 2 months a calcium-phosphorus ratio of 2:1 is recommended instead of the 1:1 ratio for adults. This is in keeping with the calcium-phosphorus ratio in human milk. The phosphorus recommendation is gradually increased until at 1 year it is the same as that for calcium. The growth requirement varies with age, being highest in relation to weight in the infant, lower and fairly constant after the first year and until puberty, when there is a rise again during the period of rapid growth. The recommended allowances of calcium and phosphorus for children take into account the different ages and sex needs.

A careful selection of foodstuffs rich in calcium and phosphorus is necessary to meet the needs of the body. For infants, the intake requirements may well be stated in terms of the amount of milk, because this is the chief food source. For pre-

school and early schoolage children, the intake should be from 1 to 1½ pints of milk a day. For older children and adolescents, the requirements for calcium and phosphorus are most easily met by including a quart of milk a day or its equivalent in milk products. In adult life, 1 pint of milk plus calcium and phosphorus from other sources provides the daily requirement.

The calcium and the phosphorus content of milk is not only high but in good proportion, and these factors are more readily available from milk than from most other foods. During all periods of growth vitamin D, or sunshine, is essential for the most efficient absorption and utilization of these two minerals. Compare this with the story of vitamin D in Chapter 7.

Magnesium

FUNCTIONS OF MAGNESIUM

Magnesium in the body is divided between the bone and other tissue; about 70 percent is combined with the calcium and the phosphorus in the structure of the bone, while the rest is unevenly distributed in the soft tissues and fluids. The highest concentrations occur in the muscles and the red blood corpuscles.

Magnesium is an activator for the enzyme systems involving carbohydrate, fat and protein in energy producing reactions. It also functions in the metabolism of other minerals such as calcium, phosphorus, sodium and potassium. Proper levels of magnesium are necessary for normal neuromuscular contractions. The synthesis of protein and fat requires magnesium.

Magnesium salts taken by mouth are both diuretic and laxative. The cathartic action is due to the slow absorption of magnesium from the intestines and the consequent drawing of water into the gut.

DIETARY REQUIREMENTS AND FOOD SOURCES OF MAGNESIUM

For the first time in the 1968 revision of the Recommended Dietary Allowances, recommended allowances were made for magnesium. The allowances were set at 350 mg. per day for the adult man and 300 mg. per day for the woman. During pregnancy and lactation the recommended allowance is 450 mg. per day. Allowances based on the magnesium content of human milk and cow's milk were also established for infants and children.

Magnesium is widely distributed in foods: it is a part of the chlorophyll in green vegetables and is also found in cocoa, nuts, cereal grains, meat, milk and seafood. Table 4, Part Four, gives the magnesium content of various foods.

The recommended dietary allowance of the adult woman for magnesium (300 mg.) is met by the pattern dietary of 1,400 calories. The additional foods necessary to meet caloric requirements will further supplement the magnesium for the adult man (see Table 6-2 and Chap. 10).

Seelig,[1] in reviewing the published data on magnesium, has suggested that diets in western countries, which contain less magnesium (less than 5 mg. per Kg. per day) than do oriental diets (more than 6 mg. per Kg. per day), may be marginal in their magnesium content. There is also evidence that bone magnesium is not readily available for replacement in soft tissues when dietary magnesium is severely reduced. These two factors have contributed, no doubt, to the magnesium deficiencies that have been observed in patients with certain clinical conditions where magnesium intake or absorption have been decreased or magnesium excretion has been increased. These include the following conditions: chronic alcoholism, diabetes, malabsorption syndrome, renal disease, disorders of the parathyroid gland and postsurgical stress. The symptoms of magnesium deficiency are similar to the tetany seen when blood levels of calcium are reduced. There is hyperneuromuscular activity which, if untreated, results in convulsive seizures.

The relationships between high levels of magnesium intake and the decreased incidence of calcium deposits in soft tissues and the reduced susceptibility to cardiovascular disease await further research on the functions of magnesium in metabolism.

Iron

There is less than 5 Gm. of iron in the body of a normal healthy adult, but its importance to our well-being is strikingly out of proportion to the quantitative figure. Sixty to 70 percent of the iron in the body is found in hemoglobin; iron stores in the liver, spleen, and bone marrow account for the next largest concentration of iron (30-35 percent). Small but essential amounts of iron are found in muscle myoglobin; in transport form (bound to protein-transferrin) in the blood serum; and in every cell as a constituent of certain enzymes and chromatin (colored) materials.

[1] Seelig, M. S.: Am. J. Clin. Nutr., 14:342, 1964.

FUNCTIONS OF IRON

Hemoglobin Synthesis. Iron is a necessary constituent of hemoglobin, the coloring matter of the red blood cells, and as such is vital to the processes of nutrition. Hemoglobin is a compound composed of the protein, globin, and the iron-containing pigment, heme. The heme is responsible for the characteristic color and oxygen-carrying capacity of blood. Hemoglobin combines with oxygen in the lung capillaries to form oxyhemoglobin, which travels in the blood stream to the tissues where the oxygen is released to take part in oxidative processes. Part of the carbon dioxide formed is carried back by the same hemoglobin, which drops its load in the lungs and starts out with a new supply of oxygen. Hemoglobin values below 12 to 14 Gm. per 100 ml. of blood are considered low.

The iron of our bodies is used very efficiently and normally is not used up or destroyed but is conserved and utilized again and again. Small amounts of unabsorbed iron may be lost in the stools, a very small quantity is excreted in the urine, and traces may be lost through the skin in perspiration. Loss of blood due to hemorrhage, menstruation, or blood donations is responsible for the major losses of iron from the body.

Hemoglobin synthesis depends on the presence of traces of copper. Adequate protein must also be available for synthesis of the complex compound hemoglobin. Other dietary essentials, especially certain vitamins, seem to aid in this process.

Myoglobin. Myoglobin, found only in the muscle tissue, is related to blood hemoglobin in both structure and function. It is an oxygen-carrier capable of supplying oxygen to the muscles and removing carbon dioxide.

Cellular Iron. As part of the various enzymes that catalyze oxidation-reduction processes in the cell, iron has an important role in tissue respiration.

IRON TRANSPORT AND STORAGE

All of the iron in the plasma is transport iron. It is absorbed from the intestinal mucosa into the blood stream, where it is bound to a protein compound which transports iron to the bone marrow for hemoglobin synthesis, to the liver or spleen for storage or to other tissues for their use.

Iron is stored in the liver, spleen, intestinal mucosa, and in all reticulo-endothelial cells (connective tissue cells which ingest solid particles). The stores of iron, as well as the iron released from the disintegration of the red blood cells, are available to the body for hemoglobin synthesis. Hence, the iron actually used daily by an individual far exceeds that supplied by the dietary intake for the same period.

FOOD SOURCES OF IRON

The best food sources of iron are found in the meat, fish, poultry and egg group. The green, leafy vegetables, potatoes, dried fruits and enriched bread and cereal products are the best plant sources. Milk and milk products are conspicuously low in iron (Fig. 6-5). Foods such as molasses and raisins, popularly featured as good sources of iron, are rich on a percentage basis, but small servings of these foods used infrequently do not constitute as important a source of food

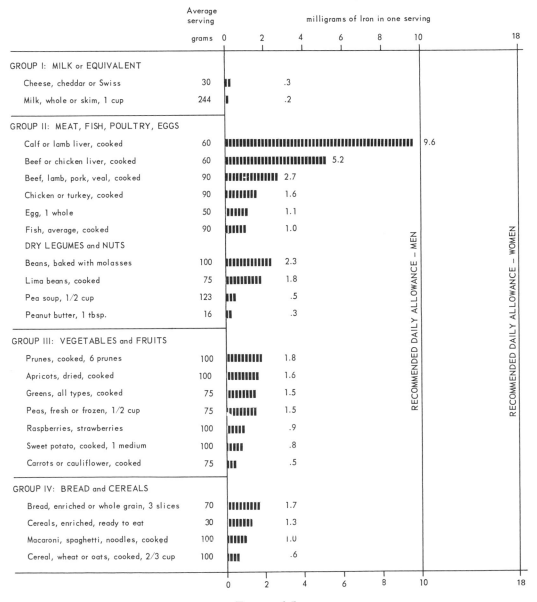

IRON

In Average Servings of Foods
Classified in the Four Food Groups

	Average serving grams	milligrams of Iron in one serving
GROUP I: MILK or EQUIVALENT		
Cheese, cheddar or Swiss	30	.3
Milk, whole or skim, 1 cup	244	.2
GROUP II: MEAT, FISH, POULTRY, EGGS		
Calf or lamb liver, cooked	60	9.6
Beef or chicken liver, cooked	60	5.2
Beef, lamb, pork, veal, cooked	90	2.7
Chicken or turkey, cooked	90	1.6
Egg, 1 whole	50	1.1
Fish, average, cooked	90	1.0
DRY LEGUMES and NUTS		
Beans, baked with molasses	100	2.3
Lima beans, cooked	75	1.8
Pea soup, 1/2 cup	123	.5
Peanut butter, 1 tbsp.	16	.3
GROUP III: VEGETABLES and FRUITS		
Prunes, cooked, 6 prunes	100	1.8
Apricots, dried, cooked	100	1.6
Greens, all types, cooked	75	1.5
Peas, fresh or frozen, 1/2 cup	75	1.5
Raspberries, strawberries	100	.9
Sweet potato, cooked, 1 medium	100	.8
Carrots or cauliflower, cooked	75	.5
GROUP IV: BREAD and CEREALS		
Bread, enriched or whole grain, 3 slices	70	1.7
Cereals, enriched, ready to eat	30	1.3
Macaroni, spaghetti, noodles, cooked	100	1.0
Cereal, wheat or oats, cooked, 2/3 cup	100	.6

RECOMMENDED DAILY ALLOWANCE – MEN
RECOMMENDED DAILY ALLOWANCE – WOMEN

FIGURE 6-5

iron as some staple foods, such as whole-grain or enriched breads and cereals. The iron content of all common foods is given in Table 1, Part Four. Note that foods poor in iron have a noticeable lack of pigment, which is significant, because iron salts are all colored and usually lend color to a food rich in this element. Compare, for instance, egg yolk with egg white, molasses with white sugar, whole with milled grains, and spinach with celery. With a few exceptions, such as the potato and enriched white bread, it may be helpful to remember that white foods are not good builders of red blood.

The basic dietary of 1,400 calories provides 10.7 mg. of iron which meets the RDA for the adult male. Additional foods to supply extra calories increase only slightly the amount of iron consumed by the menstruating woman for whom the recommended allowance is 18 mg. per day. Therefore, because usual food patterns will not supply this need, supplementation of iron is suggested until the iron content of the diet is increased by additional fortification of foods (see Table 6-2 and Chap. 10).

FACTORS AFFECTING IRON ABSORPTION

As was the case with calcium and phosphorus, not all the iron present in foods is absorbed into the body. In fact, in the normal adult with adequate iron stores usually less than 10 percent of the iron in food is absorbed; infants and young children absorb greater amounts of the iron from their food.

The form of the iron in food also affects its availability; ferrous (Fe^{++}) salts are absorbed more efficiently. Hence, because most food iron is in the form of ferric (Fe^{+++}) salts, they must be reduced for efficient absorption. Ascorbic acid and other reducing agents have been shown to enhance iron absorption. Iron from liver, muscle meats and enriched bread was absorbed better than that from eggs or various vegetables.

Large amounts of fiber, or substances that form insoluble complexes with iron such as phytates and certain sulfur-containing compounds, reduce absorption. As might be expected, diarrhea also results in poor absorption.

DIETARY REQUIREMENTS FOR IRON

Adults. The recommended allowance for women is 18 mg. of iron per day and for men 10 mg. per day. After menopause in women, when menstruation has ceased, the sex difference in the iron requirement no longer exists.

Children. During the period of rapid growth, when an increase in red cells and hemoglobin is taking place, provision for new material as well as replacement requires a more liberal supply of iron. The anemias of infancy and childhood are evidence of the shortage that frequently occurs, although nature seems to have made provision for the period of nursing. Milk is essentially low in iron, but a reserve of this mineral provided by the high hemoglobin level of the infant at birth is economically conserved for repeated utilization. The potential shortage of iron that may occur by the sixth or the seventh month may be forestalled by the use of iron-fortified commercial formula, fortified infant cereals, egg yolks, vegetable and meat purées, and other suitable sources of iron.

Adolescents. Few data are available for the requirements of this age group. The allowance of 18 mg. recommended was estimated on the assumption that needs are at least as much as for the adult female. Menstruation in adolescent girls means loss of hemoglobin and, consequently, an increased demand for all blood-building elements. Chlorosis or adolescent anemia in girls may be due to a low reserve of iron, or of other factors necessary for blood building, when menstruation begins. Boys are growing rapidly at this age and also need iron for hemoglobin building; but even before menstruation starts girls seem to need more iron than boys of the same age.

ANEMIAS

Anemia may be defined as a condition in which there is a decrease in the quantity of hemoglobin, of the number of red cells, of the volume of packed cells (hematocrit) or a combination of these. From the strictly nutritional aspects, anemias may be classified as follows:

1. Hypochromic anemias (too little hemoglobin)
   Due to hemorrhage, acute or chronic
   Due to inadequate intake of iron
2. Hyperchromic macrocytic anemias, due to deficiency of substances essential to red cell formation, and the release of these cells from the bone marrow. (See Folic Acid Deficiency and Pernicious Anemias in Chap. 8.)

Anemia Due to Loss of Blood

Severe Hemorrhage. In severe hemorrhage the immediate treatment is restoration of blood volume by transfusion. The blood must be further restored by an increase in the production of red blood cells and hemoglobin. In an otherwise normal individual, recovery is spontaneous, but the red cells are replenished more rapidly than is the hemoglobin. The latter will be restored gradually, but the speed of its restoration seems to depend largely on the diet of the individual. The necessary food materials must be supplied in the diet in order that each of these red cells may contain the normal amount of hemoglobin (see under Iron Deficiency Anemia).

Chronic Hemorrhage. Chronic blood loss may accompany such conditions as gastric ulcer, colitis or long untreated hemorrhoids. The important aspect of treatment is to determine the cause of the blood loss and to control it. The dietary care is the same as that described under Iron Deficiency Anemia.

Iron Deficiency Anemia

Iron deficiency anemia is characterized by a low hemoglobin, giving less color than normal to the red blood cell (hypochromic). Red cells are in sufficient number, but are smaller than normal (microcytic) due to inadequate hemoglobin to fill the cell. It is most often due to a diet inadequate in iron, although poor absorption of iron from the intestinal tract may be a factor.

An inadequate iron intake may result owing to insufficient money to buy food; to consumption of food low in iron such as often occurs in children 6 months to 2 years of age, teen-age girls at the time of the menarche and pregnant women; to severe reducing fads, especially if undertaken without the supervision of a physician; and to poor food intake and anorexia accompanying illness.

Food iron is absorbed at any level of the intestinal tract from the stomach on, but is greatest in the duodenum. In malabsorption syndromes, such as are described in Chapter 25, there may be poor absorption of iron as of other nutrients. In disease accompanied by low gastric acidity there may also be insufficient iron absorption, since an acid medium is essential to keep iron in solution. Medications of hydrochloric acid as well as iron may be necessary to maintain a normal level of hemoglobin, although the dietary intake of iron should also be investigated.

Iron deficiency anemia in infants is discussed in Chapters 15 and 29; in pregnancy in Chapter 14

Dietary Treatment of Iron Deficiency Anemias

An increased supply of iron and protein is the important factor to stress in a diet which must be adequate also in all other dietary essentials.

Whipple[2] and his coworkers found liver, high in both iron and protein, to be at the top of the list of foods that promote blood regeneration. Other investigators have shown experimentally that diets high in iron but inadequate in protein will not promote hemoglobin regeneration (see Figures 4-3 and 6-5 for food sources of protein and iron).

Medications. When it is necessary to restore the hemoglobin level promptly, iron medication as well as a diet high in protein and iron are indicated. Fortunately, most patients respond well to such a regimen. Simple ferrous sulfate is as effective as more elaborate preparations. Since iron tablets sometimes cause irritation when taken on an empty stomach, they should be taken after meals.

Sodium and Other Mineral Elements

Sodium is the most abundant cation in the extracellular fluid of the body. It acts with other electrolytes in the regulation of the osmotic pressure and the acid-base equilibrium. Sodium is a major factor in maintaining a proper water balance within the body and also functions in preserving the normal irritability of muscles.

The sodium intake of Americans has been estimated to be between 3 and 7 Gm. per day (equivalent to 7.5-18 Gm. of table salt per day), which is more than adequate for usual body needs. This amount may need to be reduced in certain diseases where water or electrolyte balance is disturbed. The sodium content of various foods is given in Table 4, Part Four, but it must be remembered that drinking water may also be an important consideration in determining sodium intake.[3,4]

Most of the salt consumed is excreted by the kidneys, with variable amounts lost through the skin and stools. In the normal individual, sodium is almost completely absorbed from the gastrointestinal tract but substantial losses may occur with vomiting and diarrhea. The skin losses may increase greatly when there is profuse perspiration from strenuous physical exertion in a hot environment. Under such circumstances salt depletion may be accompanied by heat exhaustion. Salt tablets taken with a liberal amount of water may be advised under these conditions.

---

2 Whipple, G. H., and Robscheit-Robbins, F. S.: Am. J. Physiol., 72:408, 1925.

3 White, J. M., *et al.*: J. Am. Dietet. A., 50:32, 1967.

4 Cooper, G. R., and Heap, B.: J. Am. Dietet. A., 50:37, 1967.

Potassium is found principally in the intracellular fluid, where it plays an important role in cell metabolism, enzyme reactions and the synthesis of muscle protein from amino acids in the blood. Potassium ions maintain osmotic equilibrium with the sodium ions in the extracellular fluid. However, a small amount of potassium in the extracellular fluid is necessary for normal muscular activity.

Potassium requirements have not been established, but an intake of 0.8 to 1.3 Gm. per day is estimated as approximately the minimum need. Potassium is widely distributed in our foods, the average intake varying from 0.8 to 1.5 Gm. of potassium per 1,000 calories. Although potassium deficiency is most unlikely in the healthy individual, medications such as certain diuretics and adrenal cortical hormones may cause potassium depletion if efforts are not made to replace potassium in the diet. As with sodium, potassium losses may also be increased with vomiting and diarrhea. Meats, cereals, fruits, fruit juices and vegetables are good sources of potassium. Values for the potassium content of foods are given in Table 4, Part Four.

Chloride is the anion most commonly combined with sodium in the extracellular fluid and, to some extent, it is also found with potassium in the cells. The chlorides are among the electrolytes that help to maintain the osmotic pressure and acid-base equilibrium in the body. During digestion some of the chloride of the blood is used for the formation of hydrochloric acid in the gastric glands and is secreted into the stomach where it functions temporarily with the gastric enzymes and is then reabsorbed into the blood stream along with other nutrients. The approximate intake of 3 to 9 Gm. daily from foods and from added table salt easily meets the requirement. The only time when the body may be depleted of chloride is after the loss of gastric contents due to vomiting. Excess chloride is readily excreted by the kidneys and the skin, mostly as sodium chloride.

Sulfur is part of the protein in every cell of the body and occurs in most food proteins. Thus, the sulfur intake is usually sufficient if the protein is adequate. Sulfur occurs in a number of physiologically important organic compounds; in amino acids; in insulin, glutathione, heparin, thiamine and biotin. Keratin (the protein of hair, fur, nails and hoofs) is rich in sulfur.

Trace Elements or Micronutrients

Many inorganic elements occur in animal tissues in extremely small quantities and are known as micronutrients or trace elements. However, this does not mean that they are unimportant, for it is now known that some of them are absolutely essential, usually in some enzyme system, although the functions of others are not well understood.

ESSENTIAL MICRONUTRIENTS

Iodine was one of the first micronutrients to be recognized as vital in nutrition, and it is still one of the most important.

Function of Iodine and Thyroid Activity. Before surveys were made of the iodine content of soil, it had been noted that the disease of common goiter was unevenly distributed over the United States and that it seemed to be most prevalent in the very regions where there was the least iodine. This early suspicion was confirmed, and we now recognize that common goiter is primarily an iodine-deficiency disease.

As an essential constituent of the thyroid gland in man, sufficient iodine must be supplied if that gland is to synthesize enough of the hormones to function normally.

Dietary iodine is absorbed from the gastrointestinal tract into the blood; about 30 percent is removed by the thyroid gland for the synthesis of thyroid hormone and the rest is excreted by the kidneys. The amount of iodide present in the body of an adult is estimated to be about 25 mg., most of it concentrated in the thyroid. When the amount of thyroid hormone in the serum is decreased, the pituitary gland releases a thyroid-stimulating hormone (TSH) which causes the thyroid gland to produce more cells and increase in size in an attempt to manufacture more hormone. This results in enlargement of the thyroid gland, or simple goiter.

Natural Food Sources of Iodine. The fact that goiter is not evenly distributed throughout the world or even in the United States indicates that some areas must provide natural protection through food or drinking water. People who live near the coasts and consume generous amounts of seafood probably get an adequate amount of iodine from these sources.

Because growing plants pick up iodine when it is present in the soil, plant foods vary widely in iodine content according to the soil in which they are grown. Thus, plant foods grown near sea coasts and in our southern states contain more iodine than those grown in the Great Lakes area or other regions where the surface soil is low in iodine. For this reason it is impossible to list the iodine content of foods in tables of food composition or to estimate the amount in the pattern dietary. Since our urban markets today abound in foods grown in many different regions there is less likely to be a severe iodine deficiency even in so-called goitrous regions. It is a very different situation where rural people confine their diet chiefly to home-grown products in mountainous regions where the soil is notably low in iodine. It should also be noted that many commercially prepared foods do not use iodized salt; hence, the extensive use of these products may contribute to the problem of goiter.

Dietary Requirements for Iodine. A recommended dietary allowance was set for iodine in the 1968 revision of the Recommended Dietary Allowances. It is 0.14 mg. (140 mcg.) per day for adult males and 0.1 mg. (100 mcg.) per day for adult females. An increase to 0.125 mg. (125 mcg.) per day for pregnancy and to 0.15 mg. (150 mcg.) per day during lactation is recommended. The need for iodine during growth is great and hence the recommendations for children are higher.

Goiter Prophylaxis. In an experiment, iodine was administered to school children in Akron, Ohio, with remarkably successful results. By a similar project, in three cantons in Switzerland the incidence of goiter was diminished during 3 years from 87 to 13 percent. These demonstrations suffice to show that the body requirements for iodine, although they are exceedingly small, must be met in order to prevent goiter. Many sections of the country, notably the east coast and the southern states, as well as California on the west coast, need pay little attention to this factor because iodine is indigenous. However, in the goitrous regions this was a problem requiring attention, and Michigan led the way in its solution by promoting education in goiter therapy as a public-health measure.

Administration of iodine as a prophylactic measure against goiter had to be planned as a public-health activity so that it would reach all people in an area in safe but significant amounts. Common salt is used by nearly everyone in somewhat comparable amounts. Therefore, a small percentage of an iodine compound was added to table salt to be marketed in goitrous regions, and an educational campaign was conducted to inform people why they should buy and use iodized salt.

This plan was adopted by Michigan in 1924, and all salt manufacturers in the state put on the market a table salt containing 0.02 percent of sodium iodide. Eleven years later the results of this plan adopted by the Michigan Department of Health far exceeded the hopes of those who instigated it. The incidence of endemic goiter or enlarged thyroid had been reduced almost to nil. The decrease in the sale of iodized salt that has occurred since publicity on the subject has fallen off is paralleled by a slight increase in the number of goiters in school children. The discontinuance of iodized salt in one county in Michigan was followed by a marked rise in the incidence of goiter within 3 years.

In states where the use of iodized salt was not encouraged, the incidence of thyroid enlargement has remained fairly constant over the same period of years.

Since 1941, iodized salt has been continuously available in groceries in parts of the country where it is needed and at no increased cost to the consumer. However, education is still necessary if all people are to understand why it is desirable to choose iodized salt when shopping.

Goitrogens are substances that tend to produce goiters, and it has been demonstrated experimentally that such a substance is present in vegetables such as cabbage, brussels sprouts, cauliflower, rutabagas and peanuts. Goitrogenic action is prevented by cooking, and an adequate supply of iodine inhibits or prevents it.

Copper is essential for the utilization of iron in the synthesis of hemoglobin and as a constituent of many enzymes that function in tissue metabolism. Copper may function in the formation of bone and the maintenance of the myelin sheath in the nervous system. It is absorbed from the gastrointestinal tract and transported to the various tissues loosely bound to plasma proteins. Copper compounds are found in the liver, kidney, heart, brain and blood.

The average American diet contains about 2.5 to 5.0 mg. of copper, and it has been estimated that the human requirement may be 2.0 mg. or less per day for adults. A copper deficiency has not been noted in humans. Food sources of copper include liver, kidney, shellfish, nuts, cereals, cocoa and chocolate.

Manganese plays essential roles in both plant and animal nutrition. The human body contains about 10 to 20 mg., but little is known of its distribution. Manganese is absorbed rapidly and is also exchanged rapidly between the blood and tissue cells. It seems to function in blood formation and is found in high concentration in the mitochondria of the cells. Manganese is an important element in many enzyme systems. It is a normal part of the enzyme which is necessary for the formation of urea, and it functions as an activator of certain other enzymes as well. The manganese requirement of man is not known, but the average diet probably supplies enough. Blueberries and wheat bran are the richest known sources; nuts come next. The manganese content of plants is dependent on soil content.

Cobalt is a component of vitamin B_{12}, a nutritional factor necessary for the formation of red blood cells. There is ample cobalt present in the average diet.

Zinc occurs in animal and plant tissue in slightly smaller amounts than iron. Insulin is known to contain zinc, as does the enzyme which plays an important role in the maintenance of equilibrium between carbon dioxide and carbonic acid. Recent studies in Egypt and Iran have indicated that zinc deficiency does occur in humans.[5,6] Although there are differences among the authorities in interpreting these findings, dwarfism, hypogonadism, and iron-deficiency anemia were symptoms found in these populations where zinc intake was presumed inadequate. Zinc insufficiency may also result from chronic alcoholism where zinc excretion is greatly increased even when zinc levels in the serum are low.[7]

Studies at the University of Rochester have shown a relationship between zinc and wound healing.[8] When daily doses of zinc were given to a group of patients undergoing surgery, their wounds healed considerably faster than another group not receiving zinc supplements.

The average diet contains approximately 10 to 15 mg. of zinc, and excretion figures indicate that this amount is adequate.

Fluorine has long been recognized as a normal constituent of bones and teeth, the dental enamel being especially rich in this element. The fluorine content of surface soils and water supplies varies widely; this, naturally, influences the fluorine content of food grown in the region and, in turn, the level of human consumption.

Excess fluorine is now recognized as the cause of mottled enamel in the permanent teeth of children in certain areas of the world. This condition is endemic in limited areas—i.e., in the Texas Panhandle and adjacent areas—and is commonly known as dental fluorosis. The mottling occurs when fluorine is present in the drinking water in concentrations of 1.5 ppm. (parts per million) or more. In these same areas the low incidence of dental caries attracted comment. Subsequently, the relation of traces of fluorine in local water supplies to the low incidence of dental caries has been studied extensively. The question of finding a level of fluorine in drinking water low enough to eliminate mottled enamel but high enough to reduce the incidence of dental caries had to be answered. It is now estimated that 1 ppm. is about the critical level, and if this amount is added to the water in a community, a reduction of 50 to 60 percent in dental caries in children may be anticipated. Large-scale experiments now in progress in several communities point the way to effective use of fluorine prophylaxis. Mass control of dental caries in children is indeed a possibility in the future.

While fluorine, says Hodge,[9] cannot "be listed literally as an element essential to life . . . it is now established beyond reasonable doubt that optimal quantities of fluorides are desirable and beneficial in improving tooth health."

There is also some evidence that fluoride is effective in the prevention and treatment of osteoporosis. Increased retention of calcium accompanied by a reduction in bone demineralization was observed in patients receiving fluoride salts.[10]

Molybdenum is an essential micronutrient associated with or functioning as a constituent of oxidative enzymes. The few foods known to contain as much as 0.6 ppm. of molybdenum are legumes, cereals, organ meats and yeast. Molybdenum may be active metabolically in deriving energy from fats.

Selenium also has joined the ranks of essential micronutrients within the last decade. It is closely associated with vitamin E in some of its metabolic action.

Chromium is the latest micronutrient that has been recognized as essential in animal nutrition and is associated with carbohydrate metabolism—the ability of the body to use glucose.

When low chromium diets were fed to rats, they developed, first, diabetes and then vascular lesions similar to atherosclerosis. Evidence that chromium levels are higher in human infants than in adults and that the concentration in human tis-

[5] Prasad, A. S., *et al.*: Am. J. Clin. Nutr., 12:437, 1963.
[6] Reinhold, J. G., *et al.*: Am. J. Clin. Nutr., 18:294, 1966.
[7] Sullivan, J. F., and Lankford, H. G.: Am. J. Clin. Nutr., 17:57, 1965.
[8] Strain, W. H., *et al.*: Surg. Forum, 11:291, 1960.

[9] Hodge, H. C.: JAMA, 177:313, 1961.
[10] Bernstein, D. S., *et al.*: J. Clin. Invest., 42:916, 1963.

sues varies greatly in different parts of the world (depending both on dietary habits and the amount of chromium in water supplies) raises many questions, which are currently under investigation, as to the role of chromium depletion in the incidence of chronic diseases such as diabetes and atherosclerosis in man.

Chromium appears to function by increasing the effectiveness of insulin, thereby facilitating the transport of glucose into the cell. (See Chapter 22 for a discussion of the role of insulin and diabetes.)

TOXICITY AND TOLERANCE OF HIGHER LEVELS OF MICRONUTRIENTS

It is intriguing and worthy of note, says King, that eight of these trace elements "fit the pattern of discovery as an essential nutrient after several decades of biologic study that had been undertaken originally because in high concentrations [the element] had been dangerous" to some form of animal life. These findings of recent years "show how urgent the need is for the public as well as scientists to understand the concept that all nutrients are safe or useful to the body within a limited quantitative range."[11]

TRACE ELEMENTS OF DOUBTFUL SIGNIFICANCE

No one has yet been able to demonstrate that aluminum, arsenic, boron, cadmium and silicon are essential to animal life. However, all are found in traces, both in animal and in plant tissues.

Contrary to an earlier popular misconception, traces of aluminum from cooking utensils or in baking powders are harmless.

Arsenic is found in seafoods and in the human body. It accumulates in hair and in nails, but its biologic function is not understood. It has been used therapeutically since the Middle Ages. Overdoses cause gastrointestinal disturbances, but there is no danger of an excess from natural foods.

STUDY QUESTIONS AND ACTIVITIES

1. If water in the body is not sufficient for metabolic needs, what makes a person aware of this particular need?

2. What happens in growth if calcium and phosphorus are inadequate in the dietary? Why are these two minerals usually discussed together?

3. Milk is the single best source of calcium in the diet. See if you can write a diet which meets the calcium requirement for the adult, allowing cheese but omitting milk. Repeat, omitting both cheese and milk.

4. What situation results when the iron intake of the diet is low? Name four good food sources of iron other than liver.

5. Give the reasons underlying the supposition that adult men may need very little iron in their intake. Why will adult women continue to need larger amounts?

6. How does iodine function in the body? Where in the United States is iodine lacking in surface soil and water? What is being done to overcome such shortages?

7. Compare the calcium and iron supplied by the 1,400-calorie Pattern Dietary (Table 6-2) with the recommended allowances for these minerals.

8. Which minerals are most important in maintaining the electrolyte balance in the body? How is this accomplished?

9. Which of the micronutrients are known to be essential for animal life. Discuss the function of four of these nutrients.

10. For what tissues is fluoride important? How is this nutrient supplied to the body?

11. Are the blood and the tissues basic or acid in their reactions? How would you answer someone who said that she could not eat tomatoes "because they made her blood acid"? How does the body maintain its acid-base balance?

12. What nutrients are involved in the synthesis of hemoglobin?

13. How do water and electrolytes function together in blood and tissue metabolism?

SUPPLEMENTARY READING ON WATER AND MINERAL METABOLISM

Baker, E. M., *et al.*: Water requirements of men as related to salt intake. Am. J. Clin. Nutr., 12:394, 1963.

Brown, E. B.: The absorption of iron. Am. J. Clin. Nutr., 12:205, 1963.

Cartwright, G. E., and Wintrobe, N. M.: Copper metabolism in normal subjects. Am. J. Clin. Nutr., 14:224, 1964.

Council on Foods and Nutrition: Symposium on human calcium requirements. JAMA, 185:588, 1963.

Finch, C. M.: Iron metabolism. Nutrition Today, 4:2, (summer) 1969.

Knutson, J. W.: Fluoridation. Am. J. Nursing, 60:196, 1960.

Krehl, W. A.: The potassium depletion syndrome. Nutrition Today, 1:20, 1966.

---

[11] King, C. G.: J. Am. Dietet. A., 38:223, 1961.

Water and Mineral Metabolism 53

Lowenstein, F. W.: Iodized salt in the prevention of endemic goiter: a world-wide survey of present programs. Am. J. Public Health, 57:1815, 1967.

Luecke, R. V.: Significance of zinc in nutrition. Borden Rev. Nutr. Res., 26:45, 1965.

Magnesium in Human Nutrition. National Dairy Council Digest, 42:2, (Mar.–Apr.) 1971.

Peden, J. C., Jr.: Present knowledge of iron and copper. Nutr. Rev., 25:321, 1967.

Swanson, P. P.: Calcium in Nutrition. Pamphlet. Chicago, National Dairy Council, 1965.

For further references see Bibliography in Part Four.

SUMMARY OF MINERAL ELEMENTS IN NUTRITION

(The information summarized here is given in more detail in the text.)

ELEMENT	RICH SOURCES	DIETARY ALLOWANCE FOR ADULTS	FUNCTION IN THE BODY	ELIMINATION
Calcium	Milk, cheese some green vegetables	0.8 Gm. daily	Bone and tooth formation; coagulation of blood. Regulates muscle contractibility including heartbeat; activates enzymes	Feces chiefly; some in urine and sweat
Phosphorus	Milk, poultry, fish meats, cheese, nuts, cereals, legumes	0.8 Gm. daily	Forms high-energy phosphate compounds for muscular and tissue cell activity, constituent of DNA, RNA, phospholipids and buffer system	Urine and feces
Magnesium	Nuts, cereals, legumes, green vegetables	Women, 300 mg.; men, 350 mg.	Constituent of bone; in soft tissue related to carbohydrate, protein and lipid metabolism, regulates muscles and nerves	Feces chiefly; some in urine
Iron	Liver, meat, legumes, whole or enriched grains, potatoes, egg yolk, green vegetables, dried fruits	Women, 18 mg.; men, 10 mg.	Constituent of hemoglobin, myoglobin and tissue cells	Feces (mostly unabsorbed iron), small amounts in sweat
Sodium	Common salt, animal products	Estimated—about 0.5 Gm.	In extracellular fluid, regulates electrolyte and water balance, muscle irritability	Urine chiefly, and sweat
Potassium	Meats, cereals, vegetables, legumes, fruits	Estimated — 0.8-1.3 Gm.	In intracellular fluid, regulates electrolyte and water balance and cell metabolism	Urine chiefly, and sweat
Chlorine	Common salt, animal products	Estimated—about 0.5 Gm.	Forms acid in gastric juice; helps to regulate electrolyte and water balance	Urine chiefly, and sweat
Sulfur	Protein foods	Adequate if protein is adequate	Constituent of all body tissues —hair and nails especially and of specific organic compounds	Urine and feces
Iodine	Seafoods, water and plant life in nongoitrous regions; sodium iodide in iodized salt	Women, 0.10 mg.; men, 0.14 mg.	Necessary for formation of thyroxine, a hormone of the thyroid gland	Urine
Copper	Liver, nuts, legumes	Estimated—about 2.0 mg.	Aids in utilization of iron in hemoglobin synthesis; constituent of many enzymes	Feces chiefly
Micronutrients	Leafy foods, cereals, fruits, legumes, meats, seafoods	Minute traces	Enzyme, hormone or vitamin constituents; act as catalysts	Urine and feces

Fat-Soluble Vitamins

7

**All Vitamins: Definitions · Vitamin Content of Foods · The Fat-Soluble Group: Vitamin A
Vitamin D · Vitamin E · Vitamin K**

GENERAL DISCUSSION
OF ALL VITAMINS

The term *vitamine,* meaning a vital amine, was proposed by Funk in 1911 to designate a new food constituent necessary for life which he thought he had identified chemically. Other terminology was proposed as new factors were discovered, but the word *vitamin,* with the final "e" dropped to avoid any chemical significance, met with popular favor.

At first the individual vitamins were named by letter or according to their curative or preventive properties, but present opinion favors names descriptive of the substance. However, the lettered nomenclature may still be used to some extent, especially in popular discussions of the subject.

When a supposedly single vitamin proved to be more than one chemically and physiologically unrelated compound, the term *complex* was incorporated as additional identification, as in the B complex.

Sometimes it is convenient to group the vitamins according to solubility. Vitamins A, D, E, and K are fat-soluble. Two water-soluble groups are recognized—those having vitamin C activity and the large group known as the vitamin B complex.

Definitions. *Vitamins* are potent organic compounds that occur in small concentrations in foods; they perform specific and vital functions in the cells and the tissues of the body. They cannot be synthesized by the organism, and their absence or improper absorption results in specific defi-ciency diseases. They differ from each other in physiologic function, in chemical structure, and in distribution in food.

Vitamins may be classified according to their function as biological catalysts in the many and varied enzyme systems of the body or as constituents of body compounds such as the visual pigments.

There are also terms that apply to vitamins in general. A *provitamin,* or *precursor,* is a compound structurally related to a vitamin which the body can convert to a vitamin active compound. The word *avitaminosis* means literally without vitamins, although it is generally used with a letter following (e.g., avitaminosis A) to indicate a specific deficiency of that factor. The word *deficiency* may be used to indicate varying degrees of shortage: mild, moderate, severe or complete. Early symptoms of vitamin deficiencies so vague that they are rarely noted except by a medical nutritionist are called *marginal.* The possibility of an excess intake of certain vitamins has been postulated, and in some instances a large excess has proved to be harmful; such a condition is termed *hypervitaminosis.*

Vitamin Content of Foods. Determination of the specific vitamin activity of natural foods becomes an increasingly difficult task as the number and the complexity of the vitamins increase. Table 1, Part Four, gives figures for some of the vitamins in foods. Vitamin losses in the cooking and the storage of food will be mentioned more specifically under each vitamin, but, in general, certain principles of vitamin conservation are worth noting. Fat-soluble vitamins (A, D, E, K) are not easily lost by ordinary cooking methods and they do not dissolve out in the cooking water. Water-soluble vitamins (B complex and C) are dissolved easily in cooking water and a portion of the vitamins actually may be destroyed by heating; therefore, cooking food only until tender in as little water as feasible is, in general, the best procedure. Vitamin losses due to storage of vegetables tend to parallel the degree of wilting; such losses are progressive in the long storage of fresh fruits and vegetables.

THE FAT-SOLUBLE GROUP

The four fat-soluble vitamins, A, D, E, and K, have nothing in common as to chemical structure except that they are all soluble in fat and fat solvents. Absorption from the intestinal tract follows the same path as the fats; thus, any condition that interferes with fat absorption may result in poor absorption of these vitamins. They can all be stored in the body to some extent, mostly in the liver, and as a consequence of storage manifestation of deficiencies is likely to be slower than for most of the water-soluble group. Fat-soluble vitamins have distinct functions but all are involved in some phase of protein metabolism. In several instances, vitamin activity is not confined to a single substance and several related substances produce a similar effect on the body.

Vitamin A

Nomenclature. A group of structurally related compounds are recognized as having vitamin A activity. Those found in animal products are colorless or only slightly pigmented and the most common of these *preformed vitamins* is vitamin A alcohol, or *retinol*.

A number of forms of *provitamin A* are found in the yellow carotenoid plant pigments. *Betacarotene* has the highest biological activity of the carotenes.

Some animal products such as cream and butter may contain both preformed vitamin A and carotene, because some of the provitamin may remain unchanged.

Vitamin A values in most food composition tables are given as International Units. International Units can be converted to micrograms as follows:

1 I.U. (or U.S.P. unit) of vitamin A
= 0.3 mcg. retinol
= 0.6 mcg. beta-carotene

Constituents of Visual Pigments. The best-defined function of vitamin A is its role in the visual process. Vitamin A combines with the protein opsin to form rhodopsin, or visual purple, in the rods of the retina of the eye which are responsible for vision in dim light (scotopic vision). When light strikes the eye, the rhodopsin is bleached to yield the original protein opsin and vitamin A. Although most of the vitamin A can be combined again with opsin, some is lost and must be replaced. Adaptation to dim light depends on the completion of the cycle. When bright light has caused excessive bleaching of the visual purple, the eyes' ability to regenerate it appears to be directly related to the amount of vitamin A available. The "dark adaptation" test which measures the eyes' ability to recover visual acuity in dim light has been used as a means of determining vitamin A status. Insufficient vitamin A for the synthesis of rhodopsin results in night blindness, or *nyctalopia*.

The cones of the retina which are responsible for vision in bright light (photopic vision) also contain a light-sensitive vitamin A–protein complex, iodopsin.

Maintenance of Epithelial Tissue. Vitamin A functions in maintaining normal epithelial membranes and the mucus-secreting activity of these cells. When vitamin A is deficient, the membranes lining the nose, the throat and other air passages, the gastrointestinal and the genito-urinary tracts show changes in the epithelial cells known as keratinization. Rough, dry and scaly skin, especially on the arms and thighs, may also occur with vitamin A deficiency. The biochemical explanation of these symptoms is that newly formed cells undergoing differentiation at a time when vitamin A is limited do not become mucus-producing; instead, they synthesize fibrous keratinizing protein.

Whenever these tissue changes occur, the natural mechanism for protection against bacterial invasion is impaired and the tissue may easily become infected. Clinical observations show that normal mucous membranes lining nose, throat, sinuses and ear passages are the best defense against infections and that adequate vitamin A is an important factor in maintaining the normal functions of these membranes.

Damage to the epithelial layer of the eye is one of the most important clinical signs of vitamin A deficiency in humans, particularly children. There is a drying and thickening of the conjunctiva; the tear ducts fail to secrete; keratinization results, with the epithelial cells of the cornea becoming opaque and sloughing off. Infection and permanent blindness may follow if vitamin A is not administered.

Growth and Development. Failure to grow occurs in vitamin A deficiency, as it does in many other nutrient deficiencies, before any other symptoms appear. Therefore, growth retardation indicates a problem which may be nutritional but, by itself, it does not indicate a specific cause.

Bones also depend on vitamin A for normal development. Control of bone deposition and resorption is not coordinated in a growing animal on a vitamin-A–deficient diet and structural defects in epiphyseal bone formation result. Tooth formation may be impaired.

ABSORPTION, TRANSPORT AND STORAGE OF VITAMIN A AND CAROTENE

Vitamin A. Dietary vitamin A is hydrolyzed in the gastrointestinal tract and is absorbed across the mucosal cell membrane into the cell. Vitamin A then travels by way of the lymphatic system and blood stream to the liver, where it is stored.

Liver stores of vitamin A are hydrolyzed and transported to the tissues of the body wherever a metabolic requirement exists. The liver stores can maintain the blood at relatively constant vitamin A levels even when the diet is deficient. Hence, vitamin A deficiencies may not develop for long periods of time, depending on the reserve stores in the liver and the ability of the body to mobilize these reserves of vitamin A.

It is estimated that the liver may contain as much as 95 percent of the vitamin A of the entire body, with small amounts in adipose tissue, lungs and kidneys. Infants and young animals probably have low reserves of vitamin A at birth, but if they are well fed, they store it rapidly. The liver gradually acquires, over a period of years, an increasing reserve of vitamin A which normally reaches its peak in adult life. The advantage of this reserve is chiefly to take care of temporary shortages or increased requirements. Obviously, an intake above minimum requirement must be maintained most of the time if such a reserve is to be built up.

Carotene. In the presence of fat and bile acids carotene is absorbed into the intestinal wall, where some is converted to vitamin A. The carotene that is not converted is absorbed into the lymph and carried to the blood stream. Some carotene is stored in adipose tissue. Approximately one third of the carotene in food is available to the body. Moreover, the amount of available carotene which is then converted to vitamin A varies considerably, but, in general, only about half is converted to vitamin A.

Inadequate protein intakes decrease the absorption, transport and metabolism of both vitamin A and (to an even greater extent) carotene.

DIETARY REQUIREMENTS FOR VITAMIN A

The National Research Council's recommended allowance of 5,000 I.U. daily for the average adult is approximately double the minimum requirement. The requirement assumes that the American diet provides at least ⅓ of the vitamin A as preformed vitamin A and ⅔ or less from carotene.

To permit adequate stores of vitamin A and to meet the needs of growth, liberal allowances of vitamin A are recommended for infants and children, ranging from 1,500 I.U. in infancy to 5,000 I.U. during adolescence. In addition to the 5,000 I.U. for women, an extra 1,000 I.U. is recommended during pregnancy and an extra 3,000 I.U. during lactation. (For complete table of vitamin A allowances for all ages and sex categories see Chap. 10.)

Hypervitaminosis A. An overdose of vitamin A may cause serious injury to health. It is most likely to happen when children are given too much of a high potency supplement. The symptoms of hypervitaminosis A are loss of appetite, abnormal skin pigmentation, loss of hair, dry skin (with itching), pain in long bones and increased fragility of bones in general. Such symptoms have been observed in children who were given 50,000 to 75,000 I.U. of vitamin A daily for some time.

In three cases of adolescent girls reported by Morrice and Havener,[1] massive doses of 90,000 and 200,000 I.U. of vitamin A caused symptoms of brain tumor, pseudotumor cerebri, along with most of the syndrome described above.

Food Sources. The richest natural sources of vitamin A are the fish-liver oils, which usually are classed as food supplements rather than as foods. They vary according to species and season when caught, but commercial brands are well standardized for our convenience.

---

[1] Morrice, G., Jr., and Havener, W. H.: JAMA, 173: 1802, 1960.

All animal livers are good sources of vitamin A, but they are not as rich as fish liver. All milk products that include milk fat, such as whole milk, butter, cream or full cream cheese, are rich in vitamin A. Margarine and some skimmed milk are fortified with vitamin A.

Carotene is abundant in carrots, from which it derives its name, but it is also present in even higher concentration in certain green, leafy vegetables and grasses in which the color of the chlorophyll masks the yellow of the carotene. In certain species such as corn there is more carotene —hence, more vitamin-A activity—in yellow varieties than in white. In certain African countries red palm oil is used extensively and contributes greatly to the carotene intake.

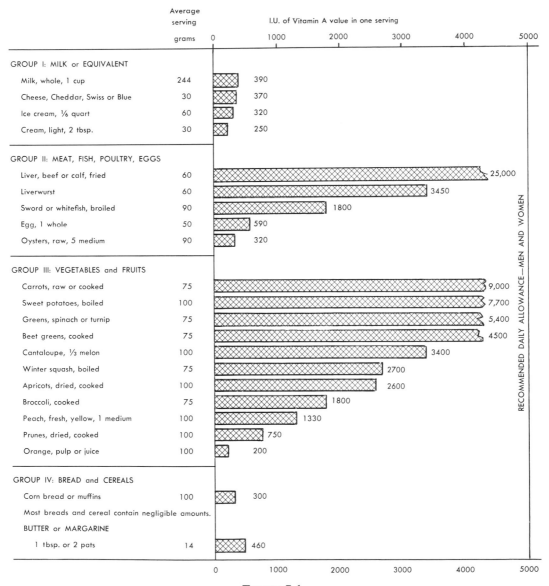

FIGURE 7-1

Animal foods that contain mostly preformed vitamin A seem to be more efficient sources of this factor for humans than are the precursors found in plants. However, the ample supply of carotenes in plant foods may well contribute a large share of the vitamin A requirement. (See Table 8-1 and Chap. 10 for sources of vitamin A in the pattern dietary.) Cooking, puréeing or mashing of vegetables rupture the cell membranes and thereby make the carotene more available. Figure 7-1 shows the relative vitamin A values of some common foods in 4 food groups.

Vitamin D

Nomenclature. About 10 compounds with vitamin-D activity have been identified; the two most important are vitamin D_2, or *ergocalciferol,* and vitamin D_3, *cholecalciferol.* These active vitamins are formed by the irradiation of two provitamins: ergosterol, found in lower forms of plants (such as yeast and fungi) and a form of cholesterol found in the skin and other animal tissues. They appear to be equally effective in man.

Measurement of Vitamin D. The International Unit (I.U.) of vitamin D is the activity of 0.025 mcg. of pure crystalline vitamin D_3. One U.S.P. unit equals one I.U.

Functions. Recent research has helped explain the role of vitamin D in bone metabolism. Vitamin D activates the production of a protein in the intestinal wall which carries the calcium from the small intestine into the blood, thereby increasing the availability of calcium for bone deposition. In vitamin D deficiency, not only is calcium absorption from the small intestine decreased, but the mobilization of calcium from the bone is depressed, resulting in hypocalcemia (see Chap. 6). In addition there is an increase in the urinary losses of phosphorus and amino acids.

The role of vitamin D in the prevention of rickets and other deficiency diseases will be discussed later in this chapter.

Absorption, Transport and Storage. Vitamin D is absorbed in the presence of bile primarily from the jejunum and is transported to the liver where some vitamin D is converted to the active form. It is further activated in the kidneys and then carried by the bloodstream to the intestinal wall and to the bone. Reserves of vitamin D are stored as such in the liver and kidneys.

Human Requirements. Because vitamin D may be supplied either by ingesting it in foods or supplements or by exposure to certain wavelengths of sunlight, its requirement has been difficult to determine.

There is good evidence that vitamin D is needed throughout the growth period. The recommended daily allowance of 400 I.U. permits maximum calcium retention during childhood and adolescence, and similar recommendations (400 I.U.) are made for both formula-fed and breast-fed infants. The premature infant who is growing rapidly and is usually not exposed to sunlight for a considerable length of time is more prone to develop rickets than the full-term infant and hence should be assured an adequate amount of vitamin D.

The adult requirement is not known but it is assumed to be so small that the average individual will receive sufficient vitamin D in the diet and by exposure to sunlight. During pregnancy and lactation, however, 400 I.U. daily are recommended, and small amounts of vitamin D may also be desirable for others who get little exposure to sunlight.

Hypervitaminosis D. Vitamin D has been demonstrated to have specific toxicity when administered in overdosage. Usually toxicity is not manifest except after huge doses. Estimations are that 20 percent of adults receiving a daily dose of 100,000 I.U. of vitamin D for several weeks or months would develop hypercalcemia. A comparable amount for infants based on weight would be 10,000 to 30,000 I.U. per day. Cases of vitamin D toxicity occur "because of unjustified and indiscriminate medical use of the vitamin, lack of appreciation of its toxicity and the self-administration of highly concentrated preparations."[2]

The maximum safe level of vitamin D for infants has yet to be precisely established, although intakes of 1,600 I.U.—four times the recommended dietary allowance—have not interfered with the rate of growth in either length or weight of infants.[3] However, evidence that certain infants may be more sensitive to the toxic effects of vitamin D and may develop hypercalcemia on intakes of 2,000 I.U. has caused considerable concern regarding the infant's total intake of this vitamin.[4] It is particularly important that the mother recognize the need for vitamin D but even more important that she be aware of the harmful effects of

---

[2] Fomon, S. J., *et al.*: J. Nutr., 88:345, 1966.
[3] Review: Nutr. Rev., 19:158, 1961.
[4] Report: Pediatrics, 31:512, 1963.

overdosage. This means, of course, that the physician and the mother should be aware of the sources of vitamin D in the diet as well as in supplements.

In adults, hypercalcemia has been accompanied by symptoms such as anorexia, nausea, weight loss, polyuria, constipation and azotemia. Similar symptoms are seen in infants, and, in certain rare severe forms, mental retardation also occurs.

SOURCES OF VITAMIN D

Sunshine. The low incidence of rickets in tropical climates suggested that sunshine might play a role in its prevention. Even after it had been demonstrated conclusively that the ultraviolet light from sunshine aided in the healing of rickets, it was difficult to understand the connection between this effect of light and that of vitamin D from sources such as cod-liver oil. Eventually, the puzzle was solved when it was discovered that vitamin-D activity could be produced by irradiation. In the skin a form of cholesterol is activated to vitamin D_3 when exposed to sunlight; by absorption into the circulation vitamin D protects the body against rickets. The amount of ultraviolet light in sunlight varies with the season and the locality, as does the total amount of sunlight. These rays are also filtered out by fog, smoke and ordinary window glass. Thus, it is obvious that an adequate natural source of ultraviolet light is impossible in northern climates during the winter months. Therefore, some other source of vitamin D is needed.

Similarly, the pigments in the skin which protect against overproduction of vitamin D in the dark-skinned peoples living in the tropics also reduces the effectiveness of the smaller amount of irradiation in temperate climates.

Foods and Supplements. The natural distribution of vitamin D in common foods is limited to small, often insignificant, amounts in cream, butter, eggs and liver. Thus, we have come to depend upon fortified foods, fish-liver oil or concentrates for preventive and therapeutic use.

It was necessary to decide on one food, commonly used by children, to be fortified with a standard amount of vitamin D. Thus, the Council on Foods and Nutrition of the American Medical Association made the following decision:

"Of all the common foods available, milk is the most suitable as a carrier of added vitamin D. Vitamin D is concerned with the utilization of calcium and phosphorus, of which milk is an excellent source."[5]

Vitamin D milk on the market is produced by adding a vitamin D concentrate to homogenized milk; the present standard of 400 I.U. per quart means that a quart of milk provides a day's requirement of vitamin D. All brands of evaporated milk also have vitamin D added, and strong recommendations to fortify nonfat milk solids with vitamins A and D have also been made by the American Medical Association.[6] Promiscuous fortification of a variety of other foods with vitamin D does not seem to be either necessary or desirable.

In the numerous fish-liver oils investigated there is a wide range of potency. This seems to vary with the season of the catch and the oil content of the livers. The highest potency oil often is yielded from fish that give the lowest amount of oil. Concentrates are made from the natural fish-liver oils or by irradiating pure ergosterol and cholesterol. Such preparations are labeled with the exact units per dose or per capsule and are prescribed accordingly. A protective dose to meet the daily requirement is considerably less than what may be prescribed as a curative dose.

In a recent study of the consumption of vitamin D by children (birth to 18 years) the average daily intake for all age groups was above 400 I.U. Fortified milk supplied the largest amount of vitamin D, the percentage increasing with age. Vitamin preparations were more important in the infant and preschool groups than with the older children. Fortified foods contributed to intakes of vitamin D over the recommended dietary allowance, particularly in the school age group (Fig. 7-2).[7]

Stability. Vitamin D in foods and in food concentrates is remarkably stable to heating, aging and storage. Vitamin D milk that is warmed for the baby is still a reliable source of this factor.

Vitamin D Deficiency—Rickets

"The disappearance of rickets" is the title of an article[8] reviewing the history and prevention of vitamin D–deficient rickets as a triumph of medi-

[5] Council on Foods and Nutrition A.M.A., Decision. JAMA, 159:1018, 1955.

[6] Council on Foods and Nutrition A.M.A., Statement. JAMA, 197:1107, 1966.

[7] Dale, A. E., and Lowenberg, M. E.: J. Pediat., 70: 954, 1967.

[8] Harrison, H. E.: Am. J. Public Health, 56:734, 1966.

cine and nutrition. As late as 1940 rickets was still a common disease of early childhood in northern climates.

One cannot be complacent, however, about the overall decrease in rickets, for within the last decade a survey by the Committee on Nutrition of the American Academy of Pediatrics[9] reported 843 cases of rickets in 5 years among hospital pediatric admissions. It would seem that the general use of antirachitic supplements in infant feed-

---

[9] Report: Pediatrics, 29:646, 1962.

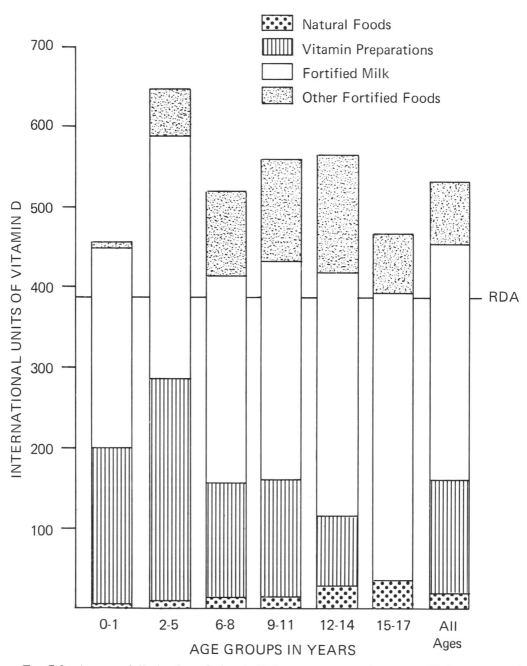

FIG. 7-2. Average daily intakes of vitamin D by age groups and sources. (Dale, A. E., and Lowenberg, M. E.: J. Pediat., 70:954, 1967)

ing would have precluded the possibility of this deficiency still being a public health problem. Of course, the widespread use of vitamin D supplements in infant feeding has reduced the incidence in northern climates. It is rare in our southern states and in tropical countries in general, where children spend more time out of doors and expose more of their skin to the sun. However, children of darkskinned races living in northern climates are even more susceptible to rickets than those of the white race.

Symptoms and Pathology. Rickets is a disease of infancy and early childhood in which the bones do not calcify properly as they grow. They become pliable, malformed and distorted, the result being such evident deformities as pigeon chest, enlarged wrists and ankles, and bowed legs or knock knees which result when the leg bones are not strong enough to support the child learning to walk. The enlargement or beading of the ribs, frequently called "the rachitic rosary," may be less evident in a plump infant than in an emaciated one, but it is characteristic. Profuse sweating and restlessness are early symptoms of rickets in infants. Growth may not be retarded at first, since nature seems to allow the bones to increase in length to keep up with growth in soft tissues if other nutrients are adequate. Prolonged and severe cases usually show stunted growth.

OSTEOMALACIA

Incidence and Pathology. Prolonged deficiency of dietary calcium and vitamin D or sunlight may result in osteomalacia, sometimes called adult rickets. This condition is characterized by poor calcification of the bones with increasing softness, so that they become flexible, and leading to deformities of limbs, spine, thorax or pelvis. These bone changes may be accompanied by rheumatic pains and exhaustion.

Osteomalacia is rare in western countries but still occurs in the Middle East and the Orient, especially among women following several pregnancies and when they nurse their infants for extended periods of time. The high incidence of osteomalacia among women in certain parts of India where the rite of purdah is still practiced and among Bedouin Arab women who wear long black garments and live in dark tents testifies indirectly to the protective action of sunshine on exposed skin. In many of these same areas the diet consists largely of cereals and root vegetables low in calcium.

Osteomalacia is often confused with osteoporosis, which may occur in older people in any country, even the most prosperous. The etiology of osteoporosis is not well understood but is more likely due to a metabolic or endocrine disturbance than to a deficiency.

Vitamin E

Nomenclature. Eight naturally occurring compounds have vitamin-E activity. Alpha-tocopherol is the most active form—1 mg. d-α tocopherol = 1.49 I.U. vitamin E. It deteriorates on exposure to light and decomposes upon irradiation with ultraviolet light. Contact with lead and iron hastens destruction. Tocopherols, because they are readily oxidized themselves, have antioxidant properties and prevent deterioration of certain foods by oxidation. This same characteristic probably exerts a protective action upon vitamin A.

Functions and Physiologic Significance of Vitamin E in Humans. Vitamin E appears to function as an antioxidant in the body, protecting the unsaturated fatty acids from oxidation. Possibly as a result of this function, vitamin E helps maintain the structural integrity of cell membranes. Other antioxidants, including the mineral selenium, may replace or spare vitamin E in certain of its functions.[10]

Red blood cells from subjects on low vitamin E and high polyunsaturated fatty acid (PUFA) dietary intakes have less resistance to hemolysis in the presence of hydrogen peroxide than those from individuals on higher vitamin E and lower PUFA intakes. This test is one of the measurements used to determine the vitamin E status of individuals. Although vitamin E deficiencies in man are rare, considerable interest has been shown because of the relationship of vitamin E to PUFA and the present trend toward increasing the latter in the diets of certain individuals.

Macrocytic anemia in infants with kwashiorkor was greatly improved by administering vitamin E.[11] Premature babies tend to have very low levels of vitamin E, owing to limited transfer through the placenta. When such infants were fed formulas high in PUFA, Hussan and his associates reported the occurrence of a skin condition which also responded to vitamin E therapy.[12]

Human Requirement. The Food and Nutrition Board's 1968 revision of the Recommended Dietary

---

[10] Roels, O. A.: Nutr. Rev., 25:33, 1967.
[11] Majaj, A. S.: Am. J. Clin. Nutr., 18:362, 1966.
[12] Hussan, H., *et al.*: Am. J. Clin. Nutr., 19:147, 1966.

TABLE 7-1. FOOD SOURCES OF VITAMIN E*

Food	MILLIGRAMS PER 100 GM.
Fats and Oils	
Corn oil	
Unhydrogenated	100
Hydrogenated	105
Cottonseed oil	
Unhydrogenated	91
Hydrogenated	80
Soybean oil	
Unhydrogenated	101
Hydrogenated	73
Coconut oil	8
Mayonnaise	50
Margarine (made with corn oil)	47
Butter	1
Fruits and Vegetables	
Tomatoes, fresh	0.85
Green peas, frozen	0.65
Banana	0.42
Carrots	0.21
Orange juice, fresh	0.20
Potatoes, baked	0.085
Cereal Grains	
Yellow cornmeal	3.4
Whole-wheat bread	2.2
Cornflakes	0.43
White bread	0.23
Meat, Fish, Poultry, and Eggs	
Beef liver, broiled	1.62
Egg	1.43
Fillet of haddock, broiled	1.20
Ground beef	0.63
Pork chops, pan-fried	0.60
Chicken breast	0.58

* From Bunnel, R. H., *et al.*: Am. J. Clin. Nutr., 17:1, 1965.

Allowances included recommendations for vitamin E. The RDA for the reference man is 30 I.U. per day and for the reference female 25 I.U. per day. Allowances for pregnancy and lactation are 30 I.U. per day. The recommendation for infants, 5 I.U. per day, is in keeping with the vitamin E content of human milk (2-5 I.U. per liter).

Food Sources. Wheat germ and wheat germ oil afford the richest sources of this factor, but it is so widely distributed in common foods that it is actually difficult to obtain a food mixture for experimental purposes that is deficient in vitamin E.

Herting[13] reported that, in individual vegetable oils and fats, the tocopherol levels varied according to source of the plant, time of harvest, stability after harvest, refining procedure and commercial hydrogenation procedures. Table 7-1 lists some common food sources of vitamin E. Satisfactory food tables for the analysis of vitamin E are not available; hence, this nutrient is not included in the pattern dietary, Table 8-1 and Chapter 10.

Vitamin K

Nomenclature. Vitamin K is a yellowish crystalline substance. At least two forms (K_1, phylloquinone, and K_2, farnoquinone) occur naturally and a number of simpler substances with antihemorrhagic properties have been synthesized. Menadione, from which vitamin K_2 is synthesized, is the most potent and is also available in water-soluble analogues. The K vitamins are heat resistant but are destroyed by alkalis, strong acids and certain oxidizing agents. In the concentrated form vitamin K seems to be sensitive to light.

Function. Vitamin K is essential in blood coagulation for the maintenance of normal prothrombin time through its effect on prothrombin and other clotting factors. Prothrombin levels regulate the rate of blood coagulation; when they are low, the coagulation is depressed. Coumarin drugs, vitamin K antagonists, are used in anticoagulation therapy.

Human Requirement. For most people the vitamin K in the average diet plus that available from bacterial synthesis in the intestines is adequate, and no quantitative estimate of human requirement has been attempted.

Because a food deficiency of vitamin K is rare, the deficiency state is more likely caused by failure to absorb or utilize the vitamin. The absorption of vitamin K seems to be dependent on the presence of bile and the normal digestion and absorption of fats. The use of mineral oil in reducing diets or as a laxative interferes seriously with the absorption of vitamin K as well as with the other fat-soluble vitamins. The prophylactic use of vitamin K in the prevention of hemorrhage in the newborn is practiced in some hospitals. A vitamin K preparation may be administered orally to the mother before delivery and a single dose of 1 mg. parenterally to the infant immediately after birth. If mothers have received anticoagulant

[13] Herting, D. C., and Drury, E.-J. E.: J. Nutr., 81:335, 1963.

therapy, their infants should be given 2 to 4 mg. of vitamin K immediately after birth.

Hypervitaminosis K. Vitamin K can be toxic if given in large doses over a prolonged period of time. Symptoms of vitamin K toxicity reported by Smith and Custer[14] are hypoprothrombinemia, petechial hemorrhages and renal tubule degeneration, and, in premature infants, hemolytic anemia.

In 1963 the Food and Drug Administration recommended the removal of menadione from all food supplements. Vitamin K is still permitted in carefully regulated amounts.

---

[14] Smith, A. M., Jr., and Custer, R. P.: JAMA, 173:502, 1960.

Food Sources. Vitamin K is fairly widely distributed in foods. It appears abundantly in cauliflower, cabbage, spinach, pork liver and soybeans and, to a lesser extent, in wheat and oats. It can be synthesized in the lower gastrointestinal tract by the bacterial flora. However, because vitamin K is absorbed mainly from the upper section of the tract, only limited amounts are probably absorbed. Medication such as antibiotics which reduce intestinal flora decrease the synthesis of vitamin K.

Storage. Vitamin K is not stored easily in the body, but, according to clinical reports, whatever is stored is found in the liver.

TABLE 7-2. FAT-SOLUBLE VITAMINS

	A	D	E	K
Active Chemical Forms	Retinol Retinal Retinoic acid Carotenes	Cholecalciferol Ergocalciferol	Tocopherols α, β, γ, etc.	Phylloquinone, menaquinone, menadione, watersoluble synthetic forms
Important Food Sources	Liver Egg yolk Butter, cream Margarine Green and yellow vegetables Apricots Cantaloupe	Irradiated foods Small amounts in: Butter Egg yolk Liver Salmon Sardines Tuna fish	Wheat germ Leafy vegetables Vegetable oils Egg yolk Legumes Peanuts Margarine	Cabbage Cauliflower Spinach Other leafy vegetables Pork liver Soybean oil and other vegetable oils
Stability to Cooking, Drying, Light, etc.	Gradual destruction by exposure to air, heat and drying, more rapid at high temperatures	Stable to heating, aging and storage Destroyed by excess ultraviolet irradiation	Stable to methods of food processing Destroyed by rancidity and ultraviolet irradiation	Stable to heat, light and exposure to air Destroyed by strong acids, alkalis and oxidizing agents
Function	Maintains function of epithelial cells, skin, bone, mucous membranes, visual pigments	Calcium and phosphorus absorption and utilization in bone growth	Antioxidant in tissues, related to action of selenium	Necessary in formation of prothrombin, essential for clotting of blood
Deficiency: Signs and Symptoms	Night blindness Glare blindness Rough, dry skin Dry mucous membranes Xerophthalmia	Rickets Soft bones Bowed legs Poor teeth Skeletal deformities	Increased hemolysis of red blood cells Macrocytic anemia and dermatitis in infants	Slow clotting time of blood Some hemorrhagic disease of newborn Lack of prothrombin
Recommended Dietary Allowances	5000 I.U., when 1/3 from animal sources	Children and adolescents, 400 I.U.	Adult male, 30 I.U. Adult female, 25 I.U.	Unknown

STUDY QUESTIONS AND ACTIVITIES

1. How was the word *vitamin* derived? Can you define a vitamin as distinct from any other food nutrient?

2. Describe the function of each of the fat-soluble vitamins and good food sources of each, if there are any.

3. Does the depth of yellow color in butter or egg yolks indicate the vitamin A potency? Why, or why not?

4. Since the supply of vitamin D is small in natural foods, what commercial process is used to produce vitamin D foods? Which foods are commonly fortified with vitamin D?

5. How does vitamin E function in animal nutrition? Is it essential for humans?

6. When is a deficiency of vitamin K most likely to occur and what prophylactic measures are sometimes recommended?

7. Are any of the fat-soluble vitamins toxic if used in too large quantities? For which one is special caution necessary when concentrates are administered to infants?

SUPPLEMENTARY READING ON FAT-SOLUBLE VITAMINS

Council on Foods and Nutrition: Fortification of non-fat milk solids with vitamins A and D. JAMA, 197: 1107, 1966.

Dale, A. E., and Lowenberg, M. E.: Consumption of vitamin D in fortified and natural foods and in vitamin preparations. J. Pediat., 70:952, 1967.

DeLuca, H. F.: Vitamin D: a new look at an old vitamin. Nutr. Rev., 29:179, 1971.

Olson, R. E.: The mode of action of vitamin K. Nutr. Rev., 28:171, 1970.

Recent developments in vitamin D. Dairy Council Digest, 41:1, 1970.

Roels, O. A.: Present knowledge of vitamin A. Nutr. Rev., 24:131, 1966.

————: Present knowledge of vitamin E. Nutr. Rev., 25:33, 1967.

————: Vitamin A physiology. JAMA, 214:1097, 1970.

Wefring, K. W.: Hemorrhage in the newborn and vitamin K prophylaxis. J. Pediat., 63:663, 1963.

For further references see Bibliography in Part Four.

Water-Soluble Vitamins

Ascorbic Acid · **The Vitamin B Complex** · **Thiamine** · **Riboflavin** · **Niacin**
Vitamin B$_6$ · **Pantothenic Acid** · **Vitamin B$_{12}$** · **Folacin**
Biotin · **Vitamin Antagonists**

ASCORBIC ACID

Introduction. The chemical name for vitamin C is ascorbic acid, because it is a specific cure for scurvy—a common deficiency disease for many centuries. Man, the primates and guinea pigs do not possess the ability to synthesize vitamin C when it is missing from their diets and must rely totally on the vitamin C ingested with their food.

Functions. Vitamin C has a variety of roles in the life processes, but to date the specific biochemical functions of ascorbic acid are not well understood. One of the most significant is its role in the formation of *collagen,* the protein substance that cements the cells together. Failure to synthesize collagen results in delayed healing of wounds. There is an actual increase in the amount of ascorbic acid present at the site of the wound during healing.

Because of failure of the osteoblasts to function properly in scurvy, bone disorganization results. Tooth dentin may also be adversely affected by vitamin C deficiency, although structural defects in the teeth rarely occur in man. Shortages of this vitamin also result in weakened capillary walls, which in turn leads to hemorrhages of varying degree.

Ascorbic acid functions in the metabolism of certain amino acids. It is also necessary in the conversion of the inactive form of the vitamin, folic acid, to the active form, folinic acid. Ascorbic acid enhances the absorption of iron by reducing the ferric to the more readily absorbed ferrous form.

Clinical experience with a number of infections accompanied by fever shows a decreased blood level of ascorbic acid, indicating either increased need for this vitamin or increased destruction of it at this time. It appears, however, that a suboptimal intake of vitamin C is not a predisposing cause of any of these diseases. It has also been observed that the normally high concentration of ascorbic acid in the adrenal cortex is depleted whenever the gland is stimulated by hormones or certain toxins.

Administration of large doses of ascorbic acid appears to protect an individual exposed to very low environmental temperatures. However, the recent controversy involving the use of large doses of ascorbic acid to prevent and cure the common cold has not been resolved. Although there is not complete agreement regarding the relationship of ascorbic acid and stress, Baker in a review stated that he believed "there is definitely an increased requirement for ascorbic acid in all forms of stress; however, we do not, at this time, have sufficient knowledge to state an absolute or quantitative level of increased requirement."[1]

Absorption, Storage and Excretion. Absorption of ascorbic acid takes place in the upper part of the small intestines. It is circulated in the blood stream to the tissues of the body. The amount of ascorbic acid in different tissues varies; adrenal and pituitary tissue, brain, pancreas, kidney, liver and spleen have relatively high concentrations; blood cells contain more than blood serum. When tissues have attained their maximum concentration of vitamin C, they have reached the state known as *saturation,* and excess ascorbic acid is

---

[1] Baker, E.: Am. J. Clin. Nutr., 20:583, 1967.

65

excreted in the urine. It is generally believed that a habitual intake of vitamin C of between 80 and 100 mg. daily will keep a person in a state approaching saturation, which condition is probably more conducive to optimum health than one in which there is no reserve.

Human Requirement. Elaborate studies have been made to determine human requirements for ascorbic acid at different ages, under different conditions of environment, under physical exertion, in fevers and in infections. The amount necessary to prevent frank symptoms of scurvy

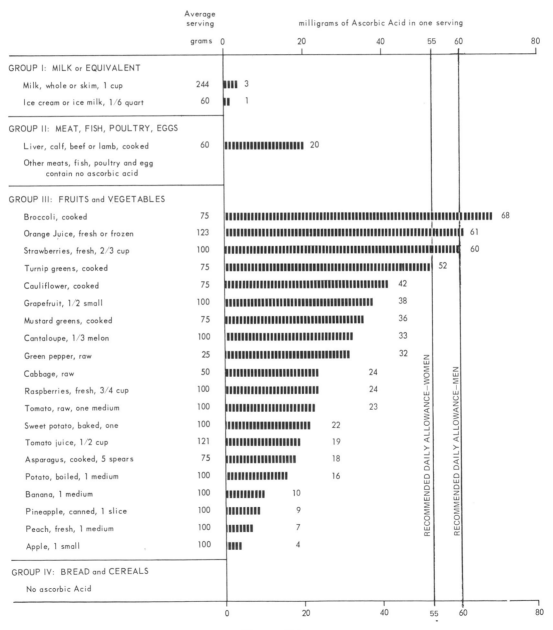

ASCORBIC ACID

In Average Servings of Foods
Classified in the Four Food Groups

Average serving — grams

milligrams of Ascorbic Acid in one serving

Food	grams	mg
GROUP I: MILK or EQUIVALENT		
Milk, whole or skim, 1 cup	244	3
Ice cream or ice milk, 1/6 quart	60	1
GROUP II: MEAT, FISH, POULTRY, EGGS		
Liver, calf, beef or lamb, cooked	60	20
Other meats, fish, poultry and egg contain no ascorbic acid		
GROUP III: FRUITS and VEGETABLES		
Broccoli, cooked	75	68
Orange Juice, fresh or frozen	123	61
Strawberries, fresh, 2/3 cup	100	60
Turnip greens, cooked	75	52
Cauliflower, cooked	75	42
Grapefruit, 1/2 small	100	38
Mustard greens, cooked	75	36
Cantaloupe, 1/3 melon	100	33
Green pepper, raw	25	32
Cabbage, raw	50	24
Raspberries, fresh, 3/4 cup	100	24
Tomato, raw, one medium	100	23
Sweet potato, baked, one	100	22
Tomato juice, 1/2 cup	121	19
Asparagus, cooked, 5 spears	75	18
Potato, boiled, 1 medium	100	16
Banana, 1 medium	100	10
Pineapple, canned, 1 slice	100	9
Peach, fresh, 1 medium	100	7
Apple, 1 small	100	4
GROUP IV: BREAD and CEREALS		
No ascorbic Acid		

RECOMMENDED DAILY ALLOWANCE—WOMEN (55)

RECOMMENDED DAILY ALLOWANCE—MEN (60)

FIGURE 8-1

in humans is far less than that recommended for an optimum state of health. Saturation tests after graded levels of intake and observations on blood ascorbic acid have been the chief techniques used for studying human requirements.

The National Research Council recommends 60 mg. daily for men and 55 mg. daily for women. The allowance for pregnancy and lactation is 60 mg. per day. The recommended allowances for infants are related to the amount of ascorbic acid and protein in human milk. Growing children need relatively more than adults (see Table 10-1, Chap. 10). During and following fevers and infections the demand for ascorbic acid seems to be increased, either because of rapid destruction or because of an increased need. A regular and adequate intake of ascorbic acid is emphasized because of the limited storage and constant need.

Opinions differ more widely as to what constitutes an adequate or optimal intake of ascorbic acid than for any other nutrient.

Food Sources. It is obvious from Fig. 8-1, that the commonly used fruits and vegetables of Group 3 are the richest sources of ascorbic acid, with citrus fruits, strawberries, cantaloupe and a number of raw, leafy vegetables topping the list. Canned or frozen citrus juice may be the cheapest source of vitamin C when fresh citrus fruit is scarce or expensive, and may even be cheaper than tomato juice, because it takes 3 times as much tomato as citrus juice to supply the same amounts of vitamin C.

Many factors affect the ascorbic acid content of fruits and vegetables; variety, maturity, length of storage, part of the plant, seasonal and geographical factors all have their influence. Exposure to sunlight also tends to increase the plant's ascorbic acid content. Food value tables give average representative amounts, whereas any individual food may vary considerably from this value.[2]

In some countries indigenous fruits high in vitamin C are overlooked, even though they are readily available. For example, in Puerto Rico the acerola (*azarole,* or West Indian cherry) has the highest ascorbic acid content of any known food.[3] Depending upon diet, mother's milk may contain more ascorbic acid than average cow's milk and considerably more than is found in pasteurized milk, thus affecting the amount and the timing of additional sources needed in an infant's diet.

[2] Merrill, A. L.: J. Am. Dietet. A., 44:264, 1964.

[3] del Campello, A., and Asenjo, C. F.: J. Agriculture, 61:161, 1957.

Stability in Foods. Of all the vitamins, ascorbic acid is the least stable to heat, oxidation, drying and storage.

Alkalinity, even in a slight degree, is distinctly destructive to this vitamin; therefore, soda should never be added to food in cooking. Acid fruits and vegetables lose much less ascorbic acid on heating than nonacid foods. Vitamin C is extremely soluble in water and dissolves out of some vegetables during the first few minutes in the process of cooking.

To reduce as much as possible the loss of ascorbic acid in cooking vegetables, the use of the least possible amount of cooking water, short cooking time (water should be boiling when vegetable is added) and little chopping or cutting is recommended. Studies have shown that baked, boiled or steamed potatoes retain a large proportion of their vitamin C if cooked whole. Fresh fruits and more especially vegetables lose vitamin C activity rapidly when stored at room temperature and somewhat less rapidly at refrigerator temperatures. Expert advice is not to shell peas, cut beans, or peel vegetables until ready to cook. Quick freezing of fruits and vegetables destroys little if any of this factor. To retain a maximum of the ascorbic acid, frozen fruits should be used promptly after thawing, and frozen vegetables should be plunged directly into boiling water for immediate cooking.

Ascorbic Acid Deficiency and Scurvy

History and Incidence. Scurvy is probably the oldest recognized deficiency disease. Although its specific relationship to ascorbic acid was not recognized until the 20th century, its prevention by the use of fresh foods was practiced much earlier. Prevalent in Europe during the 19th century and earlier, for centuries scurvy was attributed to a limited food supply. On the long voyages which followed the discovery of America, sailors were often obliged to subsist for long periods on salt fish and meats, hardtack or other breadstuffs, entirely deprived of any fresh food. The outbreaks of scurvy on such voyages were frequently so severe that there was scarcely enough of the crew left to man the vessel. Subsequently, limes or lemons were included in the supplies, because they had been found to be antiscorbutic; i.e., scurvy preventive.

Other outbreaks of the disease have been associated with famine or war areas, when the food supply was limited. Its occurrence in earlier years was reported during polar expeditions or other circumstances in which supplies of fresh food were unavailable. Expert dietetic advice was sought in planning the food supplies for the more recent polar expeditions in order to avoid the possibility of a vitamin C shortage, because scurvy is greatly dreaded by explorers.

Eskimos seldom have scurvy on their native diets but are susceptible to it when they adopt the "white man's diet." On their native diets they may include organ meats and mosses that supply some ascorbic acid. It is also reported that some groups eat meat raw or undercooked, thus retaining the slight amount of ascorbic acid that may be present.

The only cases of scurvy in adults reported in this country are in men living alone and preparing inadequate meals or in psychoneurotic individuals on bizarre diets.

Frank scurvy is so rare in the U. S. today that medical students seldom have a chance to observe the disease. Yet the history of this disease and its prevention is worthy of note.

Symptoms and Pathology. The principal symptoms of scurvy are restlessness, loss of appetite, general soreness to touch, sore mouth and gums with bleeding and loosening of the teeth, petechial skin hemorrhages, and swelling of the legs with special tenderness about the knee joints. Anemia may occur as a result of the loss of blood.

Marginal symptoms of this disease are sallow skin, muddy complexion, lack of energy, and fleeting pains in limbs and joints, so often noted in adolescence. Irritability, retarded growth and tooth defects may also accompany this dietary deficiency.

Mild manifestations of ascorbic acid deficiency in adults may easily be overlooked or ignored. Tendency to bruise easily, slow healing of minor wounds and pin-point hemorrhages may be indications of tissue depletion of this factor.

VITAMIN B COMPLEX

Subdivision into Separate Factors. Numerous workers began to observe a complexity of symptoms due to deficiencies among peoples with different dietary patterns. These reports were confusing until the discrepancies in experimental findings and the diversity of physiologic properties ascribed to this so-called vitamin B led to the recognition of several factors instead of one. From then on the group was known as the vitamin B complex, and each fraction received separate designation—letter, descriptive name or chemical term—as research progressed to disclose the chemical nature of each.

At present some 12 fractions of the vitamin B complex are generally recognized, and others are postulated. Those discussed in this chapter are thiamine, riboflavin, niacin, vitamin B_6, vitamin B_{12}, folacin, pantothenic acid and biotin, with brief comments about several others.

Distribution and Properties. Certain properties, the solubility in water and the distribution in many common foods, are similar for all members of the B complex. The very fact that several of the fractions occurred together in the same food gave rise to the early idea that there was only one substance. New factors when identified are classified as belonging to the B complex if they are water-soluble and are abundant in liver and yeast; dry yeast is the richest natural source of the B complex.

Thiamine

Functions. Thiamine functions as a coenzyme in at least 24 enzyme systems. In carbohydrate metabolism (see Fig. 9-3) thiamine is necessary for the formation of acetyl coenzyme A from pyruvate and for the removal of CO_2 in the Krebs' Cycle. In thiamine deficiency pyruvic acid tends to accumulate in the body.

The enzyme transketolase also requires thiamine as a coenzyme. Present in red blood cells, liver, kidney and other tissue, transketolase is necessary for the synthesis in the body of the five-carbon sugars, such as ribose, found in DNA, RNA and other nucleotides.

There is no well-defined relationship at the present time between the biochemical abnormalities and the clinical manifestations which result from thiamine deficiency. Loss of appetite, constipation, irritability and fatigue are all symptoms that have been associated with low thiamine intakes. Changes in the central nervous system affecting peripheral nerves, eye-hand coordination and mental ability are found among chronic alcoholics who have inadequate intakes of thiamine. The various forms and symptoms of beriberi are discussed later in this chapter.

Absorption, Storage, Excretion and Synthesis. Thiamine is absorbed from the small intestine and undergoes phosphorylation in the intestinal mucosa. Thiamine cannot be stored to any extent in the animal body, although certain tissues—heart, brain, liver, and kidney—tend to have higher concentrations than others. These amounts decrease quickly when thiamine is not supplied, so an adequate daily intake is important. When excess thiamine is ingested, it is excreted in the urine.

Although some thiamine may be synthesized by bacterial action in the large intestine of humans, very little is believed to be absorbed there.

Human Requirement. Because thiamine functions primarily in terms of carbohydrate metabolism, the recommended allowances suggested by the National Research Council's Food and Nutrition Board are based on calorie levels. The recommended daily allowance was set at 0.5 mg. per 1,000 calories for males (1.4 mg. daily) and females (1.0 mg. daily). Increased amounts are suggested by the Food and Nutrition Board for

THIAMINE

In Average Servings of Foods
Classified in the Four Food Groups

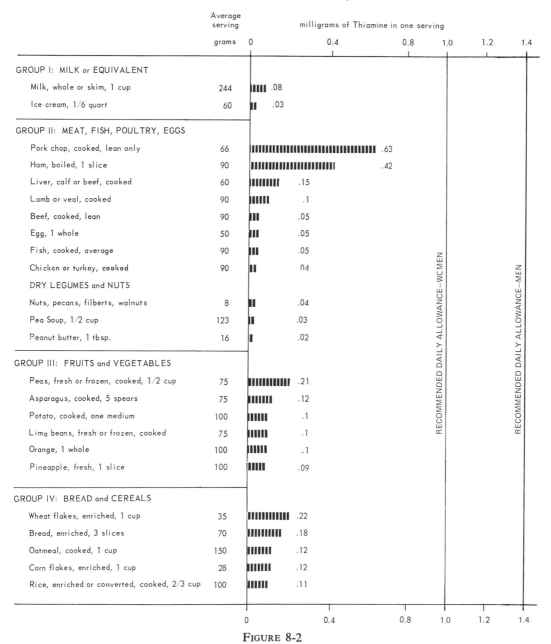

FIGURE 8-2

pregnancy and for lactation, 0.1 mg. per day and 0.5 mg. per day respectively, in addition to the allowance recommended for the nonpregnant woman. Recommendations for infants and children are the same as adults, 0.5 mg. of thiamine per 1,000 calories (see Chap. 10).

Food Sources. Thiamine is widely distributed in a large variety of animal and vegetable tissues, but there are few foods in which it occurs in abundance. This is strikingly emphasized in Figure 8-2, which shows the thiamine content of average servings of some common foods. Obviously, several servings of even the better sources of thiamine are needed to meet the recommended allowance. Therefore, enrichment of bread and cereals was instigated to make it easier for the average person to meet his requirement economically. Because bread constitutes about 1/5 of the calories in the average American diet and because only a very small fraction of the bread consumed in this country is made from whole wheat, the enrichment of white flour and bread with thiamine, riboflavin, niacin and iron was a logical step. On the basis of the average per capita consumption of flour and bread in the United States, as much as 35 percent of the daily thiamine requirement is now supplied by these foods. (For more details about enriched flour and bread see Chap. 10.)

Dry yeast and wheat germ are the richest natural sources of thiamine, but they are eaten only in relatively small amounts. Except for pork, which is outstanding, muscle meats contain less than the organs, such as liver, heart and kidney. Fruits in general are poor sources of this vitamin.

Stability in Foods. The losses of thiamine in cooking are dependent upon several factors, such as type of food, method of preparation, temperature, length of cooking and the acidity or alkalinity of the cooking medium. In the dry state thiamine is stable and is not easily destroyed by heat or oxidation. In water solution it is less stable, more so in a neutral or alkaline medium than in an acid one. Research indicates that on the whole fresh vegetables retain thiamine well during cooking. From a trace to 15 percent is dissolved in the cooking water, and up to 22 percent may be destroyed by cooking. If the cooking water is discarded, thiamine losses may be from 20 to 35 percent.

In acid foods this vitamin is quite stable, but its activity is destroyed rapidly by sulfite, a fact which may explain the loss of thiamine in dried fruits, such as apricots and peaches, treated with sulfur.

Thiamine is well-retained in cereals, since they generally are cooked slowly and at a moderate temperature and the cooking water is used. Baked products lose about 15 percent of their original thiamine. Generally, the losses in cooking meat are greater than in other foods, ranging from 25 to 50 percent of the raw value.

Thiamine Deficiency

BERIBERI

The frank deficiency disease known as beriberi is of special significance among the rice-eating peoples of the Orient, where it still occurs, although less frequently than formerly. The story is well-told by Dr. R. R. Williams in his book entitled *Toward the Conquest of Beriberi.*[4]

Symptoms and Pathology. Beriberi in adults and older children is of three main types: the chronic dry, atrophic type generally found only in older adults, often associated with prolonged consumption of alcohol; the fulminating acute type which is more serious and dramatic but rarely found; and the mild subacute form which is most common. This third type

> . . . has characteristic nervous manifestations, including alterations in tendon reflexes. Paresthesia is common. . . . Sensations of fullness and tightening of the muscles and muscle cramps are common at night. Cardiovascular signs and symptoms range from breathlessness on exertion and palpitation to tachycardia, cardiac dilation and some degree of congestive heart failure. Coexisting deficiencies of ascorbic acid, riboflavin, niacin and vitamin A are common.[5]

The enrichment of rice in the Philippines and some other oriental countries has resulted in marked reduction in the incidence of beriberi.

NUTRITIONAL DISORDERS OF THE CENTRAL NERVOUS SYSTEM

Several acute disorders of the central nervous system have been associated with alcoholism. Similar disturbances may also occur in the absence of alcoholism when there is a prolonged deficiency of food intake, as in gastric carcinoma

---

[4] Williams, R. R.: Toward the Conquest of Beriberi. Cambridge, Harvard University Press, 1961.

[5] Scrimshaw, N. S.: New Eng. J. Med., 272:137, 1965.

or when anorexia is a complication of other conditions such as pregnancy.

Polyneuropathy is defined as a disease which involves many nerves and affects the peripheral nerves. The symptoms are remarkably similar to those of classical beriberi and are usually relieved by thiamine or vitamin-B–complex therapy. Under some circumstances a deficiency of pyridoxine or pantothenic acid may give rise to similar symptoms. The chief ones are weakness, numbness, partial paralysis and pain in the legs. The legs are affected earlier than the arms. Motor, reflex and sensory reactions are lost in most cases. Recovery is a slow process involving weeks or months, and a year may pass before a patient is able to walk unaided.

Wernicke's disease is closely associated with Korsakoff's psychosis, and the combination is often referred to as the Wernicke-Korsakoff syndrome. The specific nutritional factor mostly concerned is thiamine. This syndrome may occur apart from alcoholism but is most frequently encountered in chronic alcoholics. The chief symptoms are ophthalmoplegia (paralysis of the eye muscles), nystagmus (involuntary rapid movement of the eyeballs) and ataxia (failure of muscular coordination). The ophthalmoplegia is relieved promptly after a few adequate meals; the other symptoms respond more slowly to thiamine therapy, indicating, perhaps, some structural damage to the nerve tissue. Wernicke's disease is a medical emergency and massive doses of thiamine (as much as 250 mg. per day) may be prescribed. Mental symptoms such as apathy, drowsiness, inattentiveness, inability to concentrate or sustain a conversation seem to clear up upon thiamine administration.

The Korsakoff syndrome is characterized by memory defect and confabulation (a form of mental confusion consisting of giving answers and reciting experiences without regard to truth). These symptoms may not respond to thiamine therapy as do the other mental symptoms mentioned in the preceding paragraph. There is evidence that the damage to the nervous system in the Korsakoff syndrome may be structural rather than biochemical and that thiamine deficiency of long standing may be responsible.

Riboflavin

Introduction. The second member of the B complex—riboflavin—was recognized in the 1920's when it became evident that some growth-promoting properties of vitamin B were retained after heat had destroyed the antiberiberi properties.

Functions. Riboflavin functions as a part of a group of enzymes called flavoproteins which are involved in the metabolism of carbohydrates, fats and proteins. These enzymes transfer hydrogen from the niacin-containing enzymes to the iron-cytochrome system, after which the hydrogen is combined with oxygen to form water. Thus riboflavin is essential for the release of energy within the cell (see Chap. 9).

Because riboflavin takes part in a number of chemical reactions within the body, it is essential for normal tissue maintenance. Deficiency of riboflavin causes damage to a variety of different types of tissues.

Riboflavin also plays an important role in relation to the eye. Ocular symptoms appear consistently on a low riboflavin diet and may precede all other manifestations. Eye-strain and fatigue, itching and burning, sensitivity to light and frontal headaches are the most frequent complaints. In man, riboflavin deficiency is apt to occur along with a deficiency of other members of the B complex.

Absorption, Storage and Excretion. Riboflavin is absorbed through the walls of the small intestines where it is phosphorylated before entering the blood stream. It is carried to the tissues of the body and incorporated into cellular enzymes. There is no great storage capacity in the body for this vitamin. It has been suggested that under stress the body can conserve its store of riboflavin much better than it can conserve thiamine. The excess riboflavin is excreted in the urine.

Human Requirements. The Food and Nutrition Board of the National Research Council has set the recommended dietary allowance for riboflavin at 1.7 mg. for the reference 22- to 35-year-old male and 1.5 mg. for the average 22- to 35-year-old female. Allowances of 1.8 mg. and 2.0 mg. per day are suggested for pregnancy and lactation respectively. The recommended dietary allowance for infants and children is 0.6 mg. per 1,000 calories. The actual recommendation for each age and sex group is given in Chapter 10.

Food Sources. Riboflavin is widely distributed in animal and in vegetable foods, but only in small amounts in most of them. Organ meats, milk and green leafy vegetables are the outstanding food sources. This is strikingly emphasized in

Figure 8-3, which shows the riboflavin content of average servings of some common foods and the contribution they make toward the day's requirement.

The average person is not apt to get an optimum amount of riboflavin unless he consumes a generous amount of milk. The addition of ribo-flavin in the enrichment of flour and bread has helped to raise the average intake.

Stability in Foods. Riboflavin is stable to ordinary cooking processes but unstable in alkaline solutions. It is stable in milk—an important source—if the milk is distributed in cartons or dark bottles or otherwise protected from light.

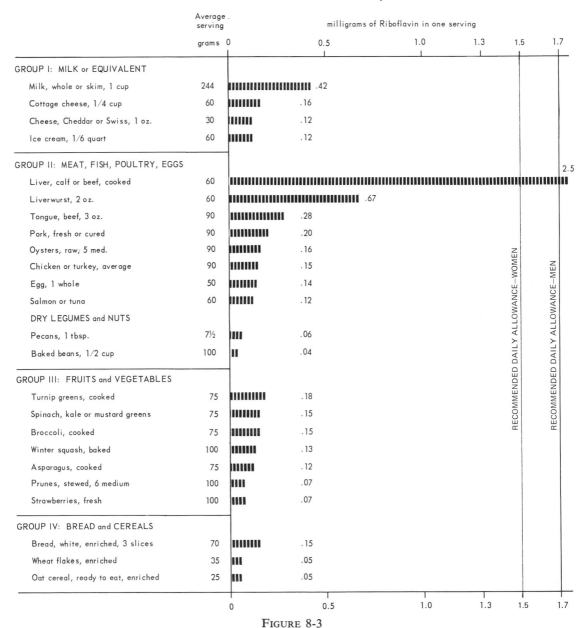

FIGURE 8-3

TABLE 8-1. VITAMINS IN PATTERN DIETARY FOR 1 DAY*

FOOD GROUP	AMOUNT IN GM.	HOUSEHOLD MEASURE	CALO- RIES	VITA- MIN A I.U.	THIA- MINE MG.	RIBO- FLAVIN MG.	NIACIN MG.	ASCORBIC ACID MG.
Milk or equivalent ...	488	2 c.	320	700	.16	.84	.3	5
Egg	50	1 medium	81	590	.06	.15	..	..
Meat, fish, fowl	120	4 ozs. cooked	376	280	.14	.23	6.1	..
Vegetables:								
Potato	100	1 medium	65	..	.09	.03	1.2	16
Green or yellow ...	75	1 serving	21	4,700	.05	.10	.5	25
Other	75	1 serving	45	300	.08	.06	.6	12
Fruits:								
Citrus	100	1 serving	44	140	.06	.02	.3	43
Other	100	1 serving	85	365	.03	.04	.5	4
Bread, white enriched..	70	3 slices	189	..	.17	.15	1.7	..
Cereal, whole grain or enriched	30	1 oz. dry or						
	130	⅔ c. cooked	89	..	.08	.03	.7	..
Butter or margarine ...	14	1 tbsp.	100	460	..	..	..	..
		Totals	1,415	7,535	.92	1.65	11.9	105

* For basis of calculation, see Pattern Dietary in Chapter 10.

One half or more of the riboflavin in milk may be lost in two hours if exposed to light.

Riboflavin Deficiency

Incidence. No well-defined deficiency syndrome or disease with a long history, such as scurvy or beriberi, is associated with a lack of riboflavin. However, dietary and clinical evidence of ribo- flavin deficiency or borderline intake have been reported from Taiwan, Korea, the Philippines, East Pakistan and Turkey[6] within the last 15 years. Riboflavin deficiency was the deficiency most commonly reported from these countries, which are predominantly rice-eating. Aribofla- vinosis as it exists today is seldom fatal, but it is a serious handicap. It must be remembered that a person with a riboflavin deficiency is likely to have associated deficiencies of thiamine and niacin.

Symptoms and Pathology. Before any true clinical symptoms appear, a mild riboflavin defi- ciency may be responsible for a type of light sensitivity and dimness of vision, followed later by itching, burning and eyestrain. Later clinical manifestations are a shiny red mucosa of the lips with cracking at the corners of the mouth, known as cheilosis, a beefy red tongue and roughened skin around the mouth and the nose, often accom- panied by sebaceous exudate.

---

[6] Williams, R. R.: J. Am. Dietet. A., 36:31, 1960.

Niacin

Functions. Niacin, like thiamine and riboflavin, also functions as a coenzyme in energy metabo- lism. It is essential in the release of energy from carbohydrates, fats, and protein. Niacin-contain- ing enzymes transfer hydrogen from the oxidizable material (i.e., carbohydrate) to the riboflavin- containing enzymes (see Functions of Riboflavin). They are also involved in the synthesis of pro- teins and fats. Hence a variety of tissues, includ- ing the skin, gastrointestinal tract and nervous system, are affected by niacin deficiency.

Relationship of Tryptophan to Niacin. Re- search studies have indicated that approximately 60 mg. of the amino acid tryptophan are equiva- lent to 1 mg. of niacin. Animal and vegetable protein contain about 1.4 percent and 1 percent of tryptophan respectively. Total niacin equiva- lents equal the preformed niacin plus the niacin equivalents available from protein.

Recommended Dietary Allowances. The Food and Nutrition Board has established the recom- mended dietary allowance for niacin equivalents at 6.6 mg. per 1,000 calories for all age groups. The 1968 NRC-RDA for the reference male is 18 mg. of niacin equivalents daily and for the reference female 13 mg. daily. An increase of 3 mg. and 7 mg. respectively above the allowance for the nonpregnant woman is recommended dur- ing pregnancy and lactation. Infants and children follow the same recommendations as adults.

Storage and Excretion. Little is known regarding the extent of storage of niacin in the body, but probably it is stored in the liver. Excess is eliminated in the urine.

Food Sources. In general, meat, poultry and fish are better sources of niacin than plant products, as emphasized in Figure 8-4, showing average servings. The use of meat drippings is recommended, because niacin is easily dissolved out of foods in cooking. Whole grain and enriched products make an appreciable contribution. Fruits and vegetables other than mushrooms and legumes

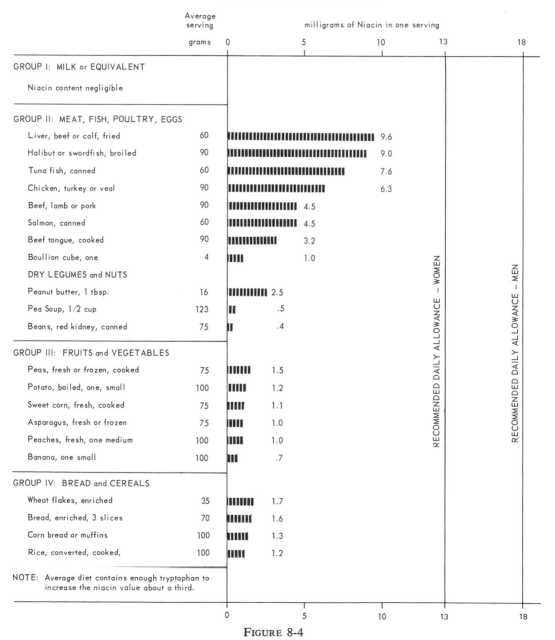

NIACIN

In Average Servings of Foods

Classified in the Four Food Groups

	Average serving grams	milligrams of Niacin in one serving
GROUP I: MILK or EQUIVALENT		
Niacin content negligible		
GROUP II: MEAT, FISH, POULTRY, EGGS		
Liver, beef or calf, fried	60	9.6
Halibut or swordfish, broiled	90	9.0
Tuna fish, canned	60	7.6
Chicken, turkey or veal	90	6.3
Beef, lamb or pork	90	4.5
Salmon, canned	60	4.5
Beef tongue, cooked	90	3.2
Boullion cube, one	4	1.0
DRY LEGUMES and NUTS		
Peanut butter, 1 tbsp.	16	2.5
Pea Soup, 1/2 cup	123	.5
Beans, red kidney, canned	75	.4
GROUP III: FRUITS and VEGETABLES		
Peas, fresh or frozen, cooked	75	1.5
Potato, boiled, one, small	100	1.2
Sweet corn, fresh, cooked	75	1.1
Asparagus, fresh or frozen	75	1.0
Peaches, fresh, one medium	100	1.0
Banana, one small	100	.7
GROUP IV: BREAD and CEREALS		
Wheat flakes, enriched	35	1.7
Bread, enriched, 3 slices	70	1.6
Corn bread or muffins	100	1.3
Rice, converted, cooked,	100	1.2

RECOMMENDED DAILY ALLOWANCE – WOMEN (13)

RECOMMENDED DAILY ALLOWANCE – MEN (18)

NOTE: Average diet contains enough tryptophan to increase the niacin value about a third.

FIGURE 8-4

are insignificant sources of niacin. Milk and eggs are poor sources of preformed niacin but good sources of its precursor tryptophan. Niacin is more stable to heat and alkali than many other B complex vitamins.

Food values as given in Fig. 8-4 and in most food tables (Table I, Part Four) are not in *niacin equivalents* because such values are almost impossible to determine. Thus, when the listed niacin content of foods in a diet fails to meet the niacin equivalent recommendations, one may calculate the approximate amount available from tryptophan. In the average diet in the United States, with adequate amounts of protein, the niacin value may be increased by ⅓ or more.

Niacin and Tryptophan Deficiency—Pellagra

Incidence. "Pellagra is still found seasonally in Egypt, Yugoslavia and some parts of Africa, where corn supplies more than 60 percent of the daily calories. Because of the niacin supplied by beans and coffee it is not seen in Mexico and Central America, even among populations deriving up to 80 percent of the calories from corn."[7]

Isolated cases of pellagra may occur in any area in a person confined to a restricted diet low in protein and niacin. This can happen in older people with self-imposed restrictions or in a person with allergies to a number of protein foods. Alcoholic pellagra is essentially identical with endemic pellagra. It is caused by the substitution of alcohol for food.

Symptoms and Pathology. On exposure to sun, persons whose diets supply inadequate tryptophan and are deficient in niacin acquire a scaly, pigmented dermatitis over the exposed areas. Depending on the type of clothing and exposed skin, the areas most affected are face, neck, back of hands, elbows, knees and ankles. The classic "three D's" *dermatitis, diarrhea* and *dementia* may still describe the symptoms although dementia is rare. Anemias are frequent, probably owing to associated deficiencies.

Vitamins in Pattern Dietary for One Day

The contribution made by the Pattern Dietary (see also Chap. 10) to the 5 vitamins for which we have specific recommendations is given in Table 8-1. Because the pattern dietary provides only 1,400 calories, the foods chosen to supplement these will also provide additional vitamins

to bring the totals up to the recommended allowances.

Vitamin B₆ Group

Introduction. Vitamin B₆ is a complex of 3 closely related chemical compounds—*pyridoxine, pyridoxal* and *pyridoxamine*—all of which are active physiologically.

The need for and the function of vitamin B₆ in humans has been demonstrated conclusively in both adults and infants. The accidental destruction of this factor in a canned-milk formula resulted in the occurrence of nervous irritability and convulsive seizures in young infants.[8] Rapid recovery followed injection of the vitamin, proving conclusively that the symptoms noted were a result of a deficiency.

Functions. The mechanism of the action of pyridoxine and its several analogues is associated closely with the synthesis and metabolism of amino acids. About half of the vitamin B₆ found in the body is in muscle. The coenzyme form of vitamin B₆ is necessary for transamination, the process by which the amino group (NH_2) from one amino acid is transferred to another to produce a different amino acid needed for protein synthesis.

Vitamin B₆-containing enzymes are also involved in removal of CO_2 and H_2S groups from amino acids. The conversion of tryptophan to niacin requires vitamin B₆. Folic acid metabolism is also dependent on pyridoxine-containing enzymes.

Coursin recently discussed several different aspects of vitamin B₆ deficiency in man. He points out that in extreme cases of vitamin B₆ deficiency there have been clearcut symptoms of anemia, oxalate stone formation or central nervous system abnormalities. In addition, consideration must be given to what appear to be suboptimal intakes by some people and increased needs of pregnant females and those taking certain birth control pills.[9]

A vitamin B₆ Dependency Syndrome of genetic origin has been identified in which the patient requires large amounts of the vitamin to prevent convulsive seizures and mental retardation. Similar deficiencies of other B₆-dependent enzymes have also been identified where only massive doses of the vitamin facilitated enzyme activity.[10]

---

[7] Scrimshaw, N. S.: New Eng. J. Med., 272:137, 1965.

[8] Coursin, D. B.: JAMA, 154:406, 1954.
[9] Coursin, D. B.: Am. J. Clin. Nutr., 20:558, 1967.
[10] Review: Nutr. Rev., 25:72, 1967.

Human Requirements. The National Research Council's Recommended Dietary Allowances for vitamin B_6 was set at 2.0 mg. per day for adults. This would provide a margin of safety and permit an intake of 100 Gm. or more of protein. The allowance for pregnancy and lactation is 2.5 mg. per day. In infancy the requirement is related to the amount of protein in the milk. The ratio of vitamin B_6 to protein may be critically low in both human milk and cow's milk. Hence, the early introduction of solid foods containing vitamin B_6 is beneficial for the infant not receiving commercial formula supplemented with this vitamin. A complete list of the recommended dietary allowances for each age and sex group is given in Chapter 10.

Food Sources. Of the animal foods, liver and kidney are the richest, although pork, veal, lamb, beef and fish are also good sources. Milk and eggs are only fair sources. Of the plant foods, legumes, nuts, potatoes, oatmeal, wheat germ and bananas are the richest, with cabbages, carrots and other vegetables providing fair amounts.

Pantothenic Acid

Functions. Pantothenic acid is a part of coenzyme A which plays a basic role in metabolism —in the release of energy from carbohydrates, fats and proteins, and also in the synthesis of amino acids, fatty acids, sterols, and steroid hormones. It is also essential for the formation of porphyrin, the pigment portion of the hemoglobin molecule, and for the production of antibodies.

Human Requirement. A definite dietary requirement for pantothenic acid has not been established. In a survey by Chung, *et al.*[11] it was found that pantothenic acid activity of high-cost diets averaged 16.3 mg. per day and for the poorest diets 6.0 mg. per day. These workers estimate that the average American diet provides from 10 to 20 mg. per day, which is liberal in terms of the estimated need of 10 mg. per day.

Food Sources. The word pantothenic, meaning widespread, indicates that the distribution of this vitamin is extensive. Figures on the pantothenic acid content of foods are limited in number. Yeast, liver, kidney, heart, salmon and eggs are the best sources. Other good sources are broccoli, mushrooms, pork, beef tongue, peanuts, wheat, rye and soybean flour. About one half of

the pantothenic acid is lost in the milling of grains, which constitute an important, if not a rich, source of this factor in the average diet. Fruits are relatively poor sources of this vitamin.

Vitamin B_{12}

Introduction. Ever since the discovery that liver was effective in the treatment of pernicious anemia research workers have been hunting for the active principle, or "extrinsic" factor, in liver. At first it seemed that folic acid was the answer, but it proved to be ineffective in relieving many of the symptoms of the disease. In 1948 a more active substance, B_{12}, isolated from liver, was found to be effective in microgram quantities in the therapy of pernicious anemia as well as in other types of macrocytic anemias. Thus, vitamin B_{12} is probably identical with Castle's "extrinsic" factor. Its oral effectiveness is enhanced by the "intrinsic" factor found in normal gastric juice, as was true of the active factor in liver extracts. The "intrinsic" factor is essential for the absorption of the vitamin B_{12}.

Properties. Two of the active forms of this vitamin are cyanocobalamin (Vitamin B_{12}) and hydroxocobalamin (vitamin B_{12a}). Vitamin B_{12} coenzymes are called cobamides. Cobalt, long known as a trace element essential for some animals, never before had been found in a natural organic compound.

Functions. Vitamin B_{12} functions as a coenzyme in various chemical reactions in the cell. It is particularly important in the bone marrow where the red blood cells are formed, in nervous tissue and in the gastrointestinal tract. The synthesis of nucleic acids and, hence, of DNA, depend on B_{12}-containing enzymes. Cobamides are also involved in folic acid metabolism and fatty acid metabolism.

Absorption, Transport and Storage. Because vitamin B_{12} is the largest and, probably, the most complicated molecule of any of the water-soluble nutrients, it is not surprising that its deficiency is caused more frequently by problems of absorption than by dietary inadequacy. Of equal interest is the fact that its absorption requires the presence in the gastric secretions of an even larger molecule, a mucoprotein called Castle's "intrinsic factor" (IF). The B_{12}-IF complex forms in the stomach, passes through the upper part of the small intestine to the ileum, where the IF attaches itself to the epithelial cells specific to this area of the gut and thereby facilitates the transfer of vitamin B_{12} into the ileal epithelium. Calcium is also

---

[11] Chung, A. S. M., *et al.*: Am. J. Clin. Nutr., 9:573, 1961.

necessary for this transfer. Three hours are required for the transport of B_{12}, whereas only seconds are required for most water-soluble compounds. Because the IF is not found in lymph or plasma, it must remain in the intestinal tract.[12]

When cobalamin is released into the bloodstream, it is attached to another protein and carried to the various tissues. Protein-bound vitamin B_{12} not immediately needed is stored in the liver, which is capable of storing relatively large amounts of this nutrient. As the quantity of the vitamin increases in the diet, the percentage absorbed decreases.

Although in some instances very large therapeutic doses of B_{12} given by mouth to pernicious anemia patients have caused some of the nutrient to be absorbed, in the absence of IF, vitamin B_{12} usually must be administered parenterally.

Human Requirement. The Food and Nutrition Board recommends 5 mcg. vitamin B_{12} per day for adults. Allowances during pregnancy and lactation are 8 mcg. and 6 mcg. respectively. (See Chap. 10 for a complete list of recommendations for each age and sex category.)

In pernicious anemia patients who have been treated to replenish their stores 1.5 mcg. daily given parenterally will meet the body needs; continuous treatment at predetermined intervals is indicated.

Food sources of vitamin B_{12} have not been widely investigated, but on present evidence liver and kidney are the best sources and it is also found in milk, muscle meats and fish.

In surveys of typical diets the remarkable difference in the vitamin B_{12} content between the adequate and the poor diets emphasizes the importance of the contribution made by meats and other animal products to the B_{12} intake.

Folacin (Folic Acid)

Introduction. Folic acid is transformed within the living organism to a biologically active form called folinic acid.

Functions. There are five known enzyme forms of folacin, and their major role is in the transfer of 1-carbon units to various compounds in the synthesis of DNA, RNA, and in amino acid metabolism.

Folic acid deficiency in man results in megaloblastic anemia, glossitis, and gastrointestinal disturbances. Because of the interdependence of vitamins B_{12}, B_6, ascorbic acid and folic acid the anemia found in these deficiency diseases may be similar and may respond to treatment with one or several of these nutrients. It should be pointed out, however, that even though the anemia in pernicious anemia may be relieved by folic acid, only vitamin B_{12} cures the neurologic symptoms.

Absorption, Excretion and Storage. Folic acid is readily absorbed by the gastrointestinal tract and carried by the blood to the tissues of the body. It is stored primarily in the liver, and excess is excreted in the urine.

The questions of both dietary folic acid deficiency and secondary folic acid deficiency have been raised. In the case of the latter numerous possible causes have been cited: failure to absorb dietary folate; increased urinary excretion of folic acid; increased folate destruction; interference in the synthesis or activation of enzymes necessary for its utilization; and production of anti-folates.[13]

Human Requirements. For the first time, in the 1968 revision, Recommended Dietary Allowances for folacin were established. The adult recommendation is 0.4 mg. per day. Because of the increased needs of the fetus, the allowance for pregnancy was set at 0.8 mg. per day; 0.5 mg. per day is the RDA for lactation. The infant allowance is 0.05 mg. per day for the first 6 months, at which time it is increased to 0.1 mg. per day until 2 years. The recommendation for folic acid from 2 to 6 years is 0.2 mg. per day; from 6 to 8 years it is 0.3 mg. per day. The adult recommendation (0.4 mg. per day) starts at 8 years and is continued throughout life for both sexes.

Chung et al.[14] found that high-cost and low-cost diets averaged 0.193 and 0.157 mg. of total folic acid activity respectively. A total folic acid content of 0.15 mg., which should supply at least 0.05 mg. of active folic acid, is considered adequate. However, the actual amount of folacin in foods which is available for absorption is not well-established. Therefore, the NRC-RDA has included a large margin of safety for this nutrient.

Because more than 0.1 mg. of folic acid per day may prevent anemia but not cure the neurologic symptoms of pernicious anemia, vitamin preparations which contain more than 0.1 mg. of folic acid cannot be sold without prescription.

Food Sources. The presence of this group of factors in green leaves was the basis for the name

---

[12] Wilson, T. H.: Nutr. Rev., 23:33, 1965.

[13] Review: Nutr. Rev., 24:289, 1966.

[14] Chung, et al.: op. cit. (ref. 11).

TABLE 8-2. WATER-SOLUBLE VITAMINS

VITAMIN	C ASCORBIC ACID	FRACTIONS OF THE VITAMIN B COMPLEX		
		THIAMINE	RIBOFLAVIN	NIACIN
Important food sources	Citrus fruits Strawberries Cantaloupe Tomatoes Sweet peppers Cabbage Potatoes Kale, parsley Turnip greens	Pork Liver Organ meats Whole grains Enriched cereal products Nuts Legumes Potatoes	Liver, milk Meat, eggs Enriched cereal products Green, leafy vegetables	Liver, poultry Meat, fish Whole grains Enriched cereal products Legumes Mushrooms
Stability to cooking, drying, light, etc.	Unstable to heat and oxidation, except in acids. Destroyed by drying and aging	Unstable to heat and oxidation	Stable to heat in cooking, to acids and oxidation Unstable to light	Stable to heat, light and oxidation, acid and alkali
Function: Essential in	Formation of intercelluar substance, cellular oxidation and reduction	Carbohydrate metabolism, coenzyme form cocarboxylase	Carbohydrate, fat and protein metabolism, coenzyme forms FMN and FAD	Carbohydrate, fat and protein metabolism, coenzyme forms NAD and NADP
Deficiency manifest as	Scurvy Sore mouth Sore and bleeding gums Weak-walled capillaries	Beriberi Poor appetite Fatigue Constipation	Eye sensitivity Cheilosis (man)	Pellagra Dermatitis Nervous depression Diarrhea
Recommended Dietary Allowance	Men, 60 mg. Women, 55 mg.	Men and women 0.5 mg./1000 calories	Men, 1.7 mg. Women, 1.5 mg.	Niacin equivalent men and women 6.6 mg./1000 calories

TABLE 8-2. WATER-SOLUBLE VITAMINS (*Continued*)

FRACTIONS OF THE VITAMIN B COMPLEX

VITAMIN	PANTOTHENIC ACID	VITAMIN B_6	VITAMIN B_{12}	BIOTIN	FOLACIN
Important food sources	Liver Organ meats Eggs, peanuts Legumes Mushrooms Salmon, whole grains	Pork Organ meats Legumes, seeds Grains Potatoes Bananas	Liver and other organ meats, milk, eggs	Liver Organ meats Peanuts Mushrooms	Green leafy vegetables Liver and organ meats Milk Eggs
Stability to cooking, drying, light, etc.	Unstable to acid, alkali, heat and certain salts	Stable to heat, light and oxidation	Stable during normal cooking		Unstable to heat and oxidation
Function: Essential in	Carbohydrate, fat and protein metabolism, coenzyme form coenzyme A	Metabolism of amino acid—coenzyme form PALP	Growth, blood formation, choline synthesis, amino acid metabolism	Fatty acid synthesis, carboxylation reactions	Blood formation Synthesis DNA, RNA, choline Amino acid metabolism
Deficiency manifest as		Convulsions Anemia Renal calculi	Macrocytic anemias, sprue and pernicious anemia	Lassitude Anorexia Depression Anemia	Megaloblastic anemia Glossitis Diarrhea
Recommended Dietary Allowance	No RDA figure Probably 10 mg./day	Men and women 2 mg.	Men and women 5 mcg.	No RDA figure Probably 150-300 mcg./day	Men and women 0.4 mg.

folacin (*folium,* meaning *leaf*). In addition to their presence in green leaves, these factors are found in liver, meats and fish, nuts, legumes and whole grains.

Many of the folates in food are easily destroyed by storing, cooking and other processing. Because of the destruction of folic acid activity in dried milk, it has been suggested that ascorbic acid be added as a preservative to the milk before processing.[15]

Biotin

Functions. Biotin plays an essential role as a coenzyme in adding and removing CO_2 in carbohydrate metabolism. It also functions in fatty acid synthesis and amino acid metabolism.

There is also some evidence that biotin is necessary for the utilization of vitamin B_{12}.

Biotin deficiency results in lassitude, anorexia, depression, malaise, muscle pain, nausea, anemia, hypercholesterolemia and changes in the electrocardiograph.

Human Requirements. Most American diets contain 150 to 300 mcg. of biotin per day which is entirely adequate for good health.

Food Sources. Few foods have been analyzed for this factor. It is abundant in liver and other organs, in mushrooms and peanuts. Lesser amounts occur in milk, eggs and certain vegetables and fruits.

Other B-Complex Factors

Para-aminobenzoic acid (PABA) is a moiety of pteroylmonoglutamic acid (PGA), one of the forms of folic acid, and is no longer considered a vitamin.

Inositol was first considered to be a vitamin in 1940, but there is no evidence today that humans cannot synthesize all that is needed by the body.

Choline and Betaine. The classification of these two nitrogenous compounds as vitamins is questioned by some. They are structural components of body cells rather than catalysts. Choline occurs in foods as well as in the body in relatively large amounts and has never been associated with a deficiency disease in man. The body can make choline from methionine, an amino acid, with the aid of vitamin B_{12} and folacin. The action of choline, betaine or methionine in the prevention of "fatty livers" is known as lipotropic (fat moving). Choline is distributed widely in plant and animal tissues, and a deficiency is not likely in the average diet. Betaine is formed by the oxidation of choline.

ANTIVITAMINS OR VITAMIN ANTAGONISTS

Research in the chemical structure of vitamins has led logically to more understanding about their characteristic reactions. Some are destroyed by oxidation or light or are inactivated by reaction with other compounds. Any substance which prevents the absorption or metabolic functioning of a vitamin in the body is called an antivitamin or a vitamin antagonist; avidin is an antagonist to biotin.

One type of antagonist is a compound so similar in chemical structure that it starts to react like the true vitamin but cannot finish the reaction, thus blocking the space where the real vitamin could function. An interesting example of this type of reaction is a folic acid antagonist which has been used clinically in the treatment of malignant growths. The theory is that rapidly dividing cells may need more folic acid than normal cells, and therefore an antagonist might inhibit growth of the abnormal cells. Unfortunately, the folic acid antagonist inhibits growth in normal as well as abnormal cells.

Antibiotics and, possibly, some of the sulfa drugs used in the treatment of infections may be vitamin antagonists. Normally, bacteria in the intestinal tract have the ability to synthesize certain vitamins. When a sulfa drug or an antibiotic is given orally, it may make some of the intestinal bacteria incapable of vitamin synthesis, thus inhibiting growth. Conversely, in other animals antibiotics seem to stimulate growth by changing the balance of the intestinal microorganisms.

STUDY QUESTIONS AND ACTIVITIES

1. List properties and food sources of ascorbic acid.

2. How many fractions of the vitamin B complex are recognized today? Which ones are listed in the Recommended Dietary Allowances?

3. Which vitamins of the B complex group function in the release of energy from carbohydrates, fats and proteins?

4. What single food is the best source of riboflavin in the diet?

5. Is it easy to obtain sufficient quantity of thiamine in the diet? Which two common foods are good sources? Will these supply adequate amounts? (See Pattern Dietary in Chap. 10.)

---

[15] Ghitis, J.: Am. J. Clin. Nutr., 18:452, 1966.

6. What is meant by the term "niacin equivalent"?

7. Which vitamins are likely to be reduced in foods under following treatment:
   (A) Bottled milk exposed to sunlight
   (B) Cabbage kept overnight after shredding
   (C) Vegetables to which soda has been added in cooking
   (D) Potatoes peeled and allowed to soak 2 to 3 hours before cooking?

8. Which group of vitamins are preventive and curative of macrocytic anemias? Which one is called the "extrinsic factor" and is the one most potent in pernicious anemia?

9. What is meant by an antivitamin, and how is the vitamin activity destroyed or prevented?

SUPPLEMENTARY READING ON WATER-SOLUBLE VITAMINS

Baker, E. M.: Vitamin B_6 requirement for adult men. Am. J. Clin. Nutr., 15:59, 1964.

Bridges, W. F.: Present knowledge of biotin. Nutr. Rev., 25:65, 1967.

Food and Nutrition Board: Recommended Dietary Allowances. National Academy of Sciences–National Research Council Publ. 1694. Washington, D.C., 1968.

Horwitt, M. K.: Nutritional Requirements of man, with special reference to riboflavin. Am. J. Clin. Nutr., 18:458, 1966.

King, C. G.: Present knowledge of ascorbic acid (vitamin C). Nutr. Rev., 26:33, 1968.

Review: Present knowledge of folacin. Nutr. Rev., 24:289, 1966.

Revlin, R. S.: Riboflavin metabolism. New Eng. J. Med., 13:636, 1970.

Schwartz, F. W.: Ascorbic acid in wound healing—a review. J. Am. Dietet. A., 56:497, 1970.

Sherlock, P., and Rothschild, E. O.: Scurvy produced by a zen macrobiotic diet. JAMA, 199:794, 1967.

Wilson, T. H.: Intrinsic factor and B_{12} absorption—a problem in cell physiology. Nutr. Rev., 23:33, 1965.

For further references see Bibliography in Part Four.

Digestion, Absorption and Metabolism

9

Digestive-Absorptive Processes • Metabolism • Catabolism
Anabolism • Disposal of End Products

DIGESTIVE-ABSORPTIVE PROCESSES

Because the organs and the processes of digestion and absorption may have already been studied in anatomy, physiology and chemistry courses, this section will focus primarily on the nutrients which form the substrates, the specific enzymes involved in the hydrolysis reactions and the products that are formed by the digestive process. The mechanisms of absorption will also be discussed. One should remember, however, that foods are eaten in a variety of forms and combinations; cooking and other processing methods may, therefore, begin the breakdown of complex compounds such as starch and collagen (protein) before foods are ingested.

Digestion

The two major and interrelated processes of digestion—i.e., the mechanical and the chemical—proceed simultaneously. In the first category are the muscular contractions of the walls of the gastrointestinal tract which move the food in solution (chyme), making contact possible between the food and the digestive enzymes. The second —chemical digestion—is the process of hydrolysis by which carbohydrates, fats and proteins are divided into simpler units which can be absorbed through the walls of the small intestine. Table 9-1 reviews briefly the chemical digestion of carbohydrates, fats and proteins. Each enzyme involved in the process is specific for the substrate —e.g., pepsin (gastric protease) acts only on proteins and is capable of breaking them down only as far as polypeptides.

In addition to the enzymes listed in Table 9-1 there are other chemical substances which affect digestion. The stomach secretes hydrochloric acid (HCl) which (1) activates the gastric protease pepsinogen to pepsin, (2) creates the proper acidity for the digestion of protein, (3) acts as a bacteriocidal agent, and (4) increases the solubility of certain minerals such as iron and calcium. Gastric secretions also contain *mucin* which protects the lining of the stomach from the HCl both by neutralizing the strongly acid contents and by forming a protective covering on the gastric epithelium.

Bile, excreted by the liver into the duodenum, emulsifies the fat, breaking it down into smaller globules to provide a larger surface area so that it can be acted upon more readily by the lipase. Bile, which is slightly alkaline, also neutralizes the acidity of the chyme. Hormones, which also affect the digestive process, are produced in the mucosa of the gastrointestinal tract.

Absorption

SITES OF ABSORPTION

Absorption consists primarily of the transfer of nutrients from the lumen of the small intestine through the intestinal epithelium into the *lamina propria,* where the nutrients enter the blood and lymph vessels. Although limited amounts of water, alcohol, simple salts and glucose are absorbed through the gastric mucosa, the small intestine is by far the more important organ for absorption.

TABLE 9-1. DIGESTION OF CARBOHYDRATES, FATS AND PROTEINS

SOURCE OF ENZYME	ENZYME	+	SUBSTRATE	→	PRODUCTS
Mouth Salivary glands	Salivary amylase ptyalin		Starch	→	Dextrins and maltose
Stomach Gastric mucosa	Gastric protease pepsin rennin		Proteins Casein	→ →	Polypeptides Paracasein (insoluble)
	Gastric lipase		Emulsified fat	→	Fatty acids and glycerol
Small Intestine Pancreas	Pancreatic proteases trypsin chymotrypsin carboxypeptidases		Proteins and Polypeptides	→	Smaller polypetides and amino acids
	Pancreatic lipase steapsin		Fats	→	Mono and diglycerides fatty acids and glycerol
	Pancreatic amylase amylopsin		Starch	→	Maltose
Intestinal mucosa Brush border	Intestinal peptidases aminopeptidase dipeptidase		Polypeptides Dipeptides	→	Smaller polypeptides and amino acids
	Intestinal disaccharidases sucrase maltase lactase		Sucrose Maltose Lactose	→ → →	Glucose and fructose Glucose (2 molecules) Glucose and galactose

Specifically, the most active absorptive area in the small intestine is the lower part of the duodenum and the first part of the jejunum[1] (see Table 9-2).

Structure of Intestinal Wall. The inner lining, or mucosa, of the small intestine is gathered up into folds and covered by a mass of fingerlike projections (villi) which increase its surface area tremendously (Fig. 9-1). With the development of the electron microscope and biopsy methods, the villi can now be studied in much greater detail. The epithelial cells which cover them have a so-called brush border consisting of thousands of tiny rodlets, or *microvilli,* which further increase the surface area available for absorption. A triple-layered membrane, made up of two layers of protein with a layer of fat in between, defines the outside edge of the microvilli. The single layer of epithelial cells lining the lumen rests on a con-

[1] Davenport, H. W.: Physiology of the Digestive Tract. Chicago, Year Book Publishers, 1971.

TABLE 9-2. SITES OF ABSORPTION OF NUTRIENTS FROM GASTROINTESTINAL TRACT

NUTRIENT	SITE IN SMALL INTESTINE
Glucose	Lower duodenum Upper jejunum
Amino Acids	Lower duodenum Jejunum
Fats	Lower duodenum Upper jejunum
Iron	Duodenum
Calcium	Duodenum
Sucrose	Lower jejunum Ileum
Lactose	Jejunum Upper ileum
Maltose	Jejunum Upper ileum
Vitamin D	(?) Ileum
Vitamin B_{12}	Ileum

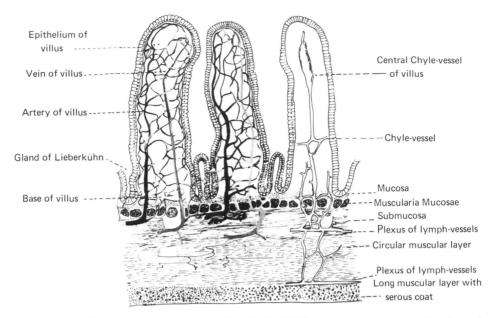

Epithelium of villus

Vein of villus

Artery of villus

Gland of Lieberkühn

Base of villus

Central Chyle-vessel of villus

Chyle-vessel

Mucosa
Muscularia Mucosae
Submucosa
Plexus of lymph-vessels
Circular muscular layer

Plexus of lymph-vessels
Long muscular layer with serous coat

Fig. 9-1. Diagrammatic drawing (after F. P. Mall) showing the great extension of absorbing surface of the intestinal lining due to projecting villi.

nective tissue structure (lamina propria) which contains blood and lymph vessels (see schematic drawing, Figure 9-2).

For normal absorption to occur the substrate—for instance, glucose—must enter the intestinal epithelial cell and make its way across the cell where it sometimes undergoes a chemical change. Then the substrate, glucose in this case, not only must leave on the opposite side of the cell but must pass through two additional layers of tissue before it is finally within a blood vessel. If the substrate were a fat-soluble nutrient such as a long-chain monoglyceride, the process would be similar, except that it would enter a lacteal or lymph vessel rather than a blood capillary. Figure 9-2 schematically represents nutrients in the process of absorption.

MECHANISMS OF ABSORPTION

Several current theories explain the various mechanisms used to accomplish the process of intestinal absorption.[2] Because the lipoprotein membrane of the microvilli makes the cell relatively impervious to water and water-soluble substances, there is a need to explain how large amounts of water constantly enter and leave the cell.

Pores. It is postulated that this bulk-flow of water is permitted by the presence of so-called pores, or channels, throughout the epithelium. These pores are just large enough to allow water,

---

[2] Ingelfinger, F. J.: Nutrition Today, 2:2, (March) 1967.

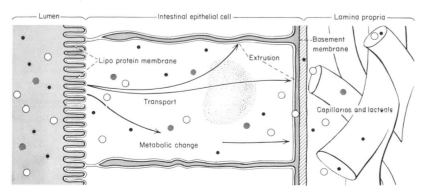

Lumen — Intestinal epithelial cell — Lamina propria

Basement membrane

Lipo protein membrane

Extrusion

Transport

Capillaries and lacteals

Metabolic change

Fig. 9-2. Diagrammatic drawing, showing the process of absorption of nutrients from the lumen through the intestinal epithelial cell into the blood and lymph vessels of the lamina propria. (Ingelfinger, F. J.: Gastrointestinal Absorption. Nutrition Today, 2:3, 1967)

certain electrolytes and very small water-soluble molecules to enter the cell.

Carriers. Larger molecules are thought to enter the cell by the action of carriers. These carriers, located in the lipoprotein membrane, can attach themselves to a water-soluble compound and temporarily render it fat-soluble and, thereby, ferry it across the lipid layer of the membrane. Some carriers may be involved with two types of compounds such as glucose and galactose. These sugars then compete for the available carriers. The number of carriers are also probably limited, and hence carrier transport will slow down or cease as vehicles become unavailable. This passive carrier-mediated diffusion continues only until there is a balance between the solutes in the cell and those in the lumen.

Pumps. In order to achieve continued absorption when there is a greater concentration in the cell or in the blood than in the lumen, a nutrient must be actively transported or pumped across the membrane barrier. These "pumps" require energy to operate, but they do permit a very large and rapid transfer into the body of such nutrients as glucose, galactose, many amino acids, sodium and probably calcium, iron and vitamin B_{12}.

Pinocytosis, which is an amoeba-like action of the epithclial cell membrane whereby a food particle or molecule is encompassed and thus brought into the cell, accounts for the absorption of large molecules such as those of a protein or a fat.

The roles which these mechanisms play in the absorption of monosaccharides, glycerides, fatty acids and amino acids will be briefly discussed.

CARBOHYDRATES

In the process of absorption, carbohydrates (disaccharides) are hydrolyzed to monosaccharides by the disaccharidases in the brush border of the epithelial cell. The very large quantities of the three monosaccharides, glucose, galactose and fructose, which the body is able to absorb calls for an explanation over and above the fact that they are water-soluble. Because they are larger molecules than would be able to pass through the so-called pores, a carrier mechanism has been suggested for all three. In addition, glucose and galactose may also be pumped across the intestinal barrier. Because the latter mechanism is active transport, which does not depend on the concentration of the sugar in the blood being less than in the intestines but actually permits the sugar to go from a lower to a higher concentration, it requires energy. This energy in turn is

supplied by the metabolism of the glucose within the cell. The transfer of sodium and hence of fluid also depends on the metabolism of glucose.

Glucose, galactose and fructose are transported from the capillaries to larger blood vessels and finally to the portal vein, which carries them to the liver where galactose and fructose are converted to glucose. From the liver glucose is transported to the tissues as needed or converted into glycogen for storage.

FATS

Bile salts and phospholipids aid in the absorption of fatty acids into the lacteals. They are transported by the lymph vessels to the thoracic duct, which empties into the left subclavian vein. Here the triglycerides enter the blood stream slowly and are carried to the liver and adipose tissue for metabolism and storage. Very hard fats, those with completely saturated long-chain fatty acids, are absorbed less readily than softer fats. Other fat-soluble substances such as cholesterol and vitamins A, D, E, and K are absorbed with the triglycerides.[3]

Short-chain and medium-chain fatty acids (see Chap. 3) are absorbed directly into the blood capillaries in the villi and carried by the portal vein to the liver. Here they may be metabolized or carried to the tissues for metabolism. Fats which have been specially processed to produce only the medium-chain fatty acids can be used for patients when normal fat absorption is impaired.

PROTEINS

Proteins are absorbed chiefly as amino acids by much the same route as monosaccharides are transported, primarily by specific carriers and by the so-called pump mechanisms. Some protein may also be absorbed as peptides or even as polypeptides. The latter may account for certain allergic reactions to specific food proteins. Although most amino acids enter the capillaries and are carried to the liver by the portal vein, some may remain in the epithelial cell to be used in the synthesis of intestinal enzymes and new cells.

OTHER NUTRIENTS

Simultaneously with the absorption of amino acids, monosaccharides, fatty acids, and monoglycerides, the vitamins, minerals, and fluids are also being absorbed through the intestinal mucosa.

---

[3] Mead, J. F.: Nutr. Rev., 24:33, 1966.

About 8 liters of fluid from the body pass back and forth across the membrane of the gut each day to keep the nutrients in solution. This fluid is being continuously reabsorbed. If diarrhea occurs, this fluid is lost to the body, resulting in dehydration and poor absorption.

METABOLISM

When the nutrients in the blood stream pass through the cellular membranes of the body, they enter into the metabolic processes of the cell. Metabolism can be defined as the process by which the cells convert the nutrients from food into useful energy and at the same time create new molecules for tissue synthesis and other vital compounds. The conversion of nutrients into useful energy is called catabolism and the synthesis of new molecules is called anabolism. Because anabolic processes depend on energy from catabolic processes, both proceed simultaneously.

Catabolism

In this metabolic pathway energy is released from the molecules of food—glucose, fatty acids, glycerol and amino acids—through a complex sequence of stepwise chemical enzymatic reactions which take place in the cell. The energy released in the cell as a result of oxidation is conserved as chemical energy by the compound adenosine triphosphate (ATP). Chemical energy is carried by ATP from the energy-yielding oxidation of food molecules to those processes or reactions of the cell which require it.

The entrance of glucose into the cell is facilitated by insulin. In the cell, glucose is activated and broken down in a series of reactions to pyruvate. This process is known as glycolysis. As previously mentioned, cellular enzymes, some of which contain vitamins, are required to catalyze these reactions.

In the presence of oxygen, pyruvate can be converted to the two-carbon compound acetyl CoA, which is a key substance in the metabolism not only of glucose but also, as will be shown, of fatty acids and certain amino acids. Thiamine is required as part of the coenzyme in this reaction. Also involved in the conversion of pyruvate to acetyl CoA is an enzyme containing the vitamin pantothenic acid (coenzyme A). Acetyl CoA combines with other substances to form citrate and enters the oxidative cycle (Citric Acid, or Krebs Cycle) where the greatest amount of the potential energy from the food is released. In this cycle carbon dioxide and water are produced when energy is released. Figure 9-3 illustrates schematically this pathway of glucose metabolism. The intermediary steps in this cycle require, as in glycolysis, vitamin-containing enzymes—in this case, riboflavin and niacin (see Chap. 8).

The potential energy in fat is also released in a similar catabolic pathway. The glycerol of fat is converted to pyruvate and follows the glucose pathway (Fig. 9-3). Through a series of complex stepwise reactions also involving coenzyme A, fatty acids are broken down into acetate or acetyl CoA. In the presence of normal glucose metabolism, the acetate formed from fatty acids enters the oxidative cycle and follows the same pathway as the acetate from glucose. The two-carbon compound acetate is also a key substance in the synthesis of ketone bodies (see Chap. 22) and cholesterol (see Chaps. 3 and 23).

About 50 percent of the protein of the diet can enter the metabolic pathways which yield energy. After the removal of nitrogen (deamination) certain of the amino acids enter directly into the oxidative cycle, while others contribute to the cycle through pyruvate or acetate (Fig. 9-3). Thus, like carbohydrate and fat, the potential energy in amino acids can be released in the oxidative cycle.

Anabolism

In the anabolic pathways of the cell the amino acids are utilized in the synthesis of proteins. This applies not only to the synthesis of new cells but also to the maintenance of already formed cells in tissues and organs. There is a continuous turnover of the amino acids in the cell, with amino acids available from dietary protein to replace similar amino acids being discarded. Not only single amino acids are replaced in anabolic activities; cells also are constantly being renewed. The red blood cell, for instance, is estimated to have a "life" of approximately 120 days. The maintenance of this state of dynamic equilibrium, which is essential for health, is the reason why protein must be included in the diet with each meal. When new tissue is being synthesized, the demand for protein is even greater—for example, the recommendation of protein per kilogram for an infant is 2 to 3 times greater than that for the adult. It is important to recognize that protein synthesis also requires energy, vitamin-containing enzymes, particularly vitamin B_6, and minerals.

Protein Synthesis—DNA-RNA Genetic Con-

trol. The ability to produce the many different kinds of proteins needed by the body is determined by the pattern for protein synthesis which is carried in the DNA (deoxyribonucleic acid) of the cell's nucleus. Because this pattern is genetically determined, the various diseases which result from enzyme deficiencies are often referred to as "inborn errors of metabolism" (see Chap. 29). Because the cells of the body are constantly manufacturing a wide variety of proteins, each of which must have available all the amino acids it requires for synthesis, the need of the body for a regular supply of the essential amino acids becomes obvious.

Other Anabolic Processes. Glycogen may be synthesized from glucose (glycogenesis) in liver or muscle cells to be available when needed. This is a limited but essential supply of energy when compared with the potential in adipose tissue. Glucose at the pyruvate level with the addition of

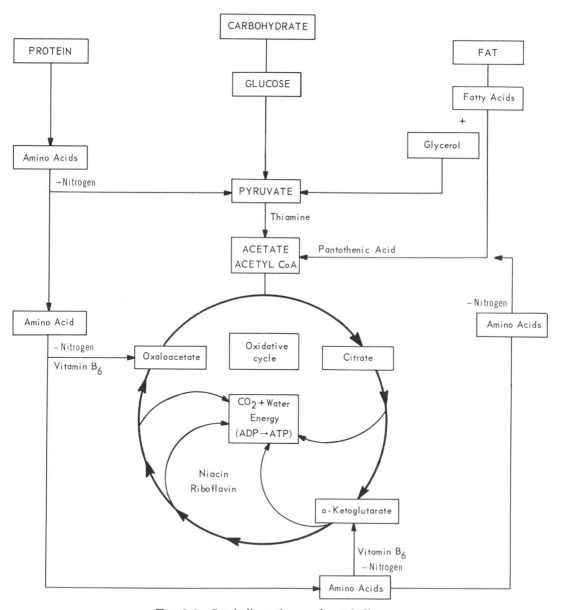

FIG. 9-3. Catabolic pathway of metabolism.

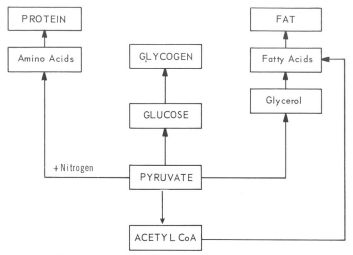

FIG. 9-4. Anabolic pathway of metabolism.

nitrogen may be utilized to synthesize a non-essential amino acid (Fig. 9-4).

Various lipid compounds are also synthesized by the cells of the body. The fatty acids are synthesized by combining acetate molecules in the numbers which are needed to make up a specific fatty acid. Biotin, a B vitamin, is required for this synthesis. Adipose tissue contains fatty acids synthesized by this method as well as fatty acids obtained directly from food sources. This tissue is the major way in which the body stores reserve energy. Phospholipids also contain fatty acids made available through the same pathways. The glycerol required by both these substances may be synthesized from pyruvate.

The Body's Use of Energy

In the constant round of catabolism and anabolism within the cell, chemical energy is used to perform work. Much chemical energy is converted to mechanical energy for the work performed by the musculature of the body. When a nerve impulse is transmitted, chemical energy is transformed into electrical energy. Chemical energy as such is used for the synthesis of new compounds. All chemical energy produced in the body is eventually converted to heat energy. The heat energy is used to maintain body temperature, and when more heat than necessary is produced for this purpose, the body rids itself of such by way of the skin, the lungs and the excreta.

DISPOSAL OF END PRODUCTS OF METABOLISM

As the blood transports nutrients to support cellular metabolism, it also participates at the same time in the disposal of the end products of metabolism. The carbon dioxide formed in the

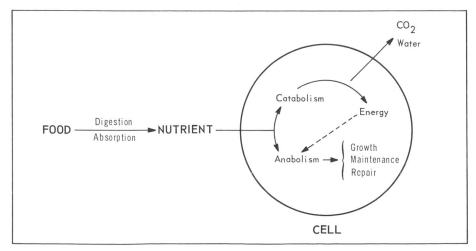

FIG. 9-5. How the cell utilizes nutrients from food.

oxidative cycle is transported to the lungs where it is lost to the body in the expired air. The nitrogen, from amino acids which have undergone deamination, is synthesized into urea in the liver and is excreted by the kidney in urine, together with the water formed in cellular metabolism. Water and some other nutrients may also be lost to the body through the skin and lungs.

SUMMARY OF DIGESTION, ABSORPTION AND METABOLISM

Figure 9-5 summarizes the sequence of processes food undergoes to support the cellular processes we know as growth, maintenance and repair, as well as to supply the chemical energy required for these processes. The ingestion of food followed by the digestive-absorptive processes are basic to the support of the body's metabolic processes.

STUDY QUESTIONS AND ACTIVITIES

1. How does the structure of the mucosal cell in the gastrointestinal tract aid in absorption?

2. Describe the suggested mechanisms for absorption in the gastrointestinal tract.

3. How are short-chain fatty acids absorbed? Long-chain fatty acids?

4. Where in the gastrointestinal tract does most of the absorption take place? Exceptions?

5. What is the meaning of the word catabolism? Of anabolism?

6. What is the relationship between enzymes and vitamins?

7. What happens to ingested carbohydrate, fat, or protein if it is more than the body can use for energy at that time?

8. What are the sources of fat in adipose tissue?

9. What is meant by an "inborn error of metabolism"?

10. Which vitamins are essential for the catabolic metabolism of carbohydrate? Of fatty acid synthesis? Of protein synthesis?

SUPPLEMENTARY READINGS ON DIGESTION, ABSORPTION AND METABOLISM

Chaffee, E. E., and Greisheimer, E. M.: Basic Physiology and Anatomy. ed. 2. Chaps. 16, 17. Philadelphia, J. B. Lippincott, 1969.

Danielsson, H.: Influence of bile acids on digestion and absorption of lipids. Am. J. Clin. Nutr., 12:214, 1963.

Ingelfinger, F. J.: Gastric function. Nutrition Today, 6:2, (Sept.-Oct.) 1971.

————: Gastrointestinal absorption. Nutrition Today, 2:2, (March) 1967.

Jukes, T. H.: Present status of the amino acid code. J. Am. Dietet. A., 45:517, 1964.

Mead, J. F.: Present knowledge of fat. Nutr. Rev., 24:33, 1966.

Review: Carbohydrate digestion and absorption. Nutr. Rev., 21:279, 1963.

————: Factors affecting amino acid absorption. Nutr. Rev., 24:332, 1966.

————: Metabolic interrelationships of dietary carbohydrate and fat. Nutr. Rev., 22:216, 1964.

————: The role of carbohydrates in the diet. Nutr. Rev., 22:102, 1964.

For further references see Bibliography in Part Four.

Meeting Nutritional Norms

10

Interpretation and Use of Recommended Dietary Allowances
Foods Fortified or Enriched to Help Meet Nutritional Norms • A Daily Food Guide
Pattern Dietary • Meal Management • Food Fads

In the discussion (in preceding chapters) of the various nutrients needed for health, references have frequently been made to the Recommended Dietary Allowances. These represent the establishment of a nutritional norm for planning and assessing dietary intake.

INTERPRETATION AND USE OF RECOMMENDED DIETARY ALLOWANCES

When the Food and Nutrition Board was appointed by the National Research Council in 1940, it undertook as one of its most important projects the establishment of a set of figures for human needs in terms of specific nutrients. As a result of long and careful consideration, Recommended Dietary Allowances (RDA) were first published in 1943. Since then, they have been revised many times as new research data have become available. The objectives are stated as follows in the latest revision:[1]

The allowances are intended to serve as goals for planning food supplies and as guides for the interpretation of food consumption records of groups of people. The actual nutritional status of groups of healthy people or individuals must be judged on the basis of physical, biochemical and clinical observations combined with observations of food or nutrient intakes. If the RDA are used as reference standards for interpreting records of food consumption, it should not be assumed that malnutrition will occur

whenever the recommendations are not completely met. . . .

The RDA are those that, in the opinion of the Food and Nutrition Board, will maintain good nutrition in practically all healthy persons in the United States.

Excepting calories, the allowances are designed to afford a margin sufficiently above average physiological requirements to cover variations among practically all individuals in the general population. The allowances provide a buffer against increased needs during common stresses and permit full realization of growth and productive potential, but they are not necessarily adequate to meet the additional requirements of persons depleted by disease, traumatic stresses, or prior dietary inadequacies. However, the allowances are generous with respect to temporary emergency feeding of large groups under conditions of limited food supply and physical disaster.

The margin above normal physiological requirements varies for each nutrient because of differences in body storage capacity, in individual requirements, and in the possible hazard of excessive intake of certain nutrients.

With the exception of iron, patterns of food consumption and food supplies in the United States permit ready adaptation to and compliance with the RDA. The primary objective of the RDA is to permit and encourage the development of food practices by the population of the United States that will allow for greatest dividends in health and in disease prevention.

The RDA (see Table 10-1), as adopted by the U. S. Food and Nutrition Board, are expressed in nutrients rather than in specific foods because these particular goals can be attained from a

---

[1] Food and Nutrition Board: Recommended Dietary Allowances. National Academy of Sciences–National Research Council Publ. No. 1694. Washington, D.C., 1968.

Table 10-1 FOOD AND NUTRITION BOARD, NATIONAL ACADEMY OF SCIENCES—NATIONAL RESEARCH COUNCIL
RECOMMENDED DAILY DIETARY ALLOWANCES,[a] Revised 1968

Designed for the maintenance of good nutrition of practically all healthy people in the U.S.A.

	Age[b] (years) From Up to	Weight (kg)	Weight (lbs)	Height cm	Height (in.)	kcal	Protein (gm)	Fat-Soluble Vitamins Vitamin A Activity (IU)	Vitamin D (IU)	Vitamin E Activity (IU)	Water-Soluble Vitamins Ascorbic Acid (mg)	Folacin[c] (mg)	Niacin (mg equiv)[d]	Riboflavin (mg)	Thiamin (mg)	Vitamin B₆ (mg)	Vitamin B₁₂ (μg)	Minerals Calcium (g)	Phosphorus (g)	Iodine (μg)	Iron (mg)	Magnesium (mg)
Infants	0–1/6	4	9	55	22	kg × 120	kg × 2.2[e]	1,500	400	5	35	0.05	5	0.4	0.2	0.2	1.0	0.4	0.2	25	6	40
	1/6–1/2	7	15	63	25	kg × 110	kg × 2.0[e]	1,500	400	5	35	0.05	7	0.5	0.4	0.3	1.5	0.5	0.4	40	10	60
	1/2–1	9	20	72	28	kg × 100	kg × 1.8[e]	1,500	400	5	35	0.1	8	0.6	0.5	0.4	2.0	0.6	0.5	45	15	70
Children	1–2	12	26	81	32	1,100	25	2,000	400	10	40	0.1	8	0.6	0.6	0.5	2.0	0.7	0.7	55	15	100
	2–3	14	31	91	36	1,250	25	2,000	400	10	40	0.2	8	0.7	0.6	0.6	2.5	0.8	0.8	60	15	150
	3–4	16	35	100	39	1,400	30	2,500	400	10	40	0.2	9	0.8	0.7	0.7	3	0.8	0.8	70	10	200
	4–6	19	42	110	43	1,600	30	2,500	400	10	40	0.2	11	0.9	0.8	0.9	4	0.8	0.8	80	10	200
	6–8	23	51	121	48	2,000	35	3,500	400	15	40	0.2	13	1.1	1.0	1.0	4	0.9	0.9	100	10	250
	8–10	28	62	131	52	2,200	40	3,500	400	15	40	0.3	15	1.2	1.1	1.2	5	1.0	1.0	110	10	250
Males	10–12	35	77	140	55	2,500	45	4,500	400	20	40	0.4	17	1.3	1.3	1.4	5	1.2	1.2	125	10	300
	12–14	43	95	151	59	2,700	50	5,000	400	20	45	0.4	18	1.4	1.4	1.6	5	1.4	1.4	135	18	350
	14–18	59	130	170	67	3,000	60	5,000	400	25	55	0.4	20	1.5	1.5	1.8	5	1.4	1.4	150	18	400
	18–22	67	147	175	69	2,800	60	5,000	400	30	60	0.4	18	1.6	1.4	2.0	5	0.8	0.8	140	10	400
	22–35	70	154	175	69	2,800	65	5,000	—	30	60	0.4	18	1.7	1.4	2.0	5	0.8	0.8	140	10	350
	35–55	70	154	173	68	2,600	65	5,000	—	30	60	0.4	17	1.7	1.3	2.0	5	0.8	0.8	125	10	350
	55–75+	70	154	171	67	2,400	65	5,000	—	30	60	0.4	14	1.7	1.2	2.0	6	0.8	0.8	110	10	350
Females	10–12	35	77	142	56	2,250	50	4,500	400	20	40	0.4	15	1.3	1.1	1.4	5	1.2	1.2	110	18	300
	12–14	44	97	154	61	2,300	50	5,000	400	20	45	0.4	15	1.4	1.2	1.6	5	1.3	1.3	115	18	350
	14–16	52	114	157	62	2,400	55	5,000	400	25	50	0.4	16	1.4	1.2	1.8	5	1.3	1.3	120	18	350
	16–18	54	119	160	63	2,300	55	5,000	400	25	50	0.4	15	1.5	1.2	2.0	5	1.3	1.3	115	18	350
	18–22	58	128	163	64	2,000	55	5,000	400	25	55	0.4	13	1.5	1.0	2.0	5	0.8	0.8	100	18	350
	22–35	58	128	163	64	2,000	55	5,000	—	25	55	0.4	13	1.5	1.0	2.0	5	0.8	0.8	100	18	300
	35–55	58	128	160	63	1,850	55	5,000	—	25	55	0.4	13	1.5	1.0	2.0	5	0.8	0.8	90	18	300
	55–75+	58	128	157	62	1,700	55	5,000	—	25	55	0.4	13	1.5	1.0	2.0	6	0.8	0.8	80	10	300
Pregnancy						+200	65	6,000	400	30	60	0.8	15	1.8	+0.1	2.5	8	+0.4	+0.4	125	18	450
Lactation						+1,000	75	8,000	400	30	60	0.5	20	2.0	+0.5	2.5	6	+0.5	+0.5	150	18	450

[a] The allowance levels are intended to cover individual variations among most normal persons as they live in the United States under usual environmental stresses. The recommended allowances can be attained with a variety of common foods, providing other nutrients for which human requirements have been less well defined. See text for more detailed discussion of allowances and of nutrients not tabulated.

[b] Entries on lines for age range 22–35 years represent the reference man and woman at age 22. All other entries represent allowances for the midpoint of the specified age range.

[c] The folacin allowances refer to dietary sources as determined by Lactobacillus casei assay. Pure forms of folacin may be effective in doses less than ¼ of the RDA.

[d] Niacin equivalents include dietary sources of the vitamin itself plus 1 mg equivalent for each 60 mg of dietary tryptophan.

[e] Assumes protein equivalent to human milk. For proteins not 100 percent utilized factors should be increased proportionately.

variety of different food patterns. One should remember also that the allowances are goals for groups of people; failure to achieve these nutrient intake levels should not be interpreted as malnutrition unless additional nutritional status information (physical, biochemical or clinical assessments) is available and is also indicative of deficiencies.

A Canadian committee, working independently and with a different philosophy of interpretation, arrived at somewhat lower figures for certain nutrients than the U. S. Food and Nutrition Board. The Canadian standard represents a minimum for each nutrient, in other words, a probable physiologic requirement below which maintenance of health could not be assumed.

Calorie Allowance

The body requires calories for resting metabolism, physical activity, synthesis of tissues in growth and maintenance, and maintaining body temperature. Although calorie allowances should be sufficient to maintain body weight or rate of growth at levels best for health and well-being, energy needs vary greatly with the size and activity of the person. Thus, it was necessary to adopt the device of using a "reference" man (age 22, weight 70 Kg. or 154 lb.) and a "reference" woman (age 22, weight 58 Kg. or 128 lb.). They are presumed to live in an environment with a mean temperature of 20° C. (70° F.) and are considered to perform "light" physical activity. Their caloric allowances are somewhat lower than previous estimates in order to conform to modern American living patterns.

Adjustments must be made when individuals or population groups differ from the physical size or activity pattern defined above. Planning caloric needs for varying activities is not simple. Dictates of appetite in relation to maintenance of body weight help. For extreme degrees of activity such as heavy physical work, the allowance may be increased as much as 1,500 calories; for sedentary activities it may be reduced by 500 to 700 calories. For example, a large teen-age boy, active in athletics, may require 3,600 calories, whereas his grandmother, aged 70, cannot use more than 1,200 calories (one third as many) without gaining weight.

The allowances for children are listed separately for the sexes after age 10, when differences in growth rates between boys and girls occur. Allowances are based on needs for the middle years in each age group and for the normal activity and weights as given in the table.

Allowances for Other Nutrients

The specific nutrients included in the 1968 RDA and the quantities of each for the several categories of persons were based upon the best consensus of authorities at the time the table was published. Other nutrients not listed in the tabulation are apt to be present in adequate amounts in the usual diet, or they are trace elements or vitamins for which there are insufficient data to serve as a basis for recommendations at this time (see Chaps. 6, 7 and 8). Some adjustments may need to be made for unusual situations, but, in general, less adjustment is necessary for specific nutrients than for calories. The margins provided take care of ordinary variations.

In the evaluation of diets to see if they meet the recommended allowances, food consumption figures should be for food as it is actually consumed, allowing for losses in storage, cooking and serving. The allowances do provide for incomplete availability or absorption of nutrients such as iron and carotene.

Emergency conditions necessitate some modification in the interpretation of recommendations. The liberal margins of safety, desirable in normal times, may become untenable when whole nations are starving. It then becomes desirable to raise the food allowance of as many people as possible to maintenance levels. Rationing at such times should give special attention to the most vulnerable groups, such as children and pregnant women.

FOODS FORTIFIED OR ENRICHED TO HELP MEET NUTRITIONAL NORMS

About 50 years ago nutritionists began to investigate how certain nutritional limitations in our food supplies could be corrected. The first large scale experiment was the addition of iodine to salt to prevent goiter. This program was so successful that iodized salt is available in most markets today (see Chap. 6).

In the 1930's the fortification of homogenized milk with vitamin D was started in an attempt to prevent rickets in infants. Today most of the homogenized milk in our markets is fortified with 400 I.U. of vitamin D per quart. Much of the dry, skimmed milk is also fortified with vitamins A and D (see Chap. 7).

In the 1940's the increased use of margarines prompted the addition of vitamin A to make the content equivalent to average butter. Today all margarines in our markets are fortified with 15,000 I.U. of vitamin A per pound. Some margarines also have 2,000 I.U. of vitamin D per pound added.

During World War II the enrichment of bread and flour with iron, thiamine, riboflavin and niacin was initiated when it was realized that repeated attempts to persuade people to use whole grains were unsuccessful. The modification of natural grains by milling had produced a more acceptable flour—whiter, with better keeping qualities and more easily digested—but reduced the vitamin and mineral content. Now the practice of enrichment of milled grains and breads has expanded to include not only wheat, but also corn and rice and ready-to-eat breakfast cereals. Some macaroni, spaghetti and noodle products are also enriched. Dry infant cereals have relatively large

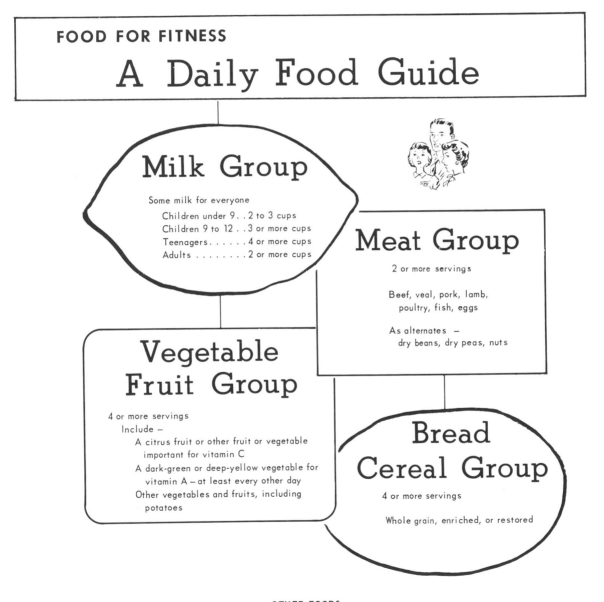

FOOD FOR FITNESS

A Daily Food Guide

Milk Group

Some milk for everyone
> Children under 9 . . 2 to 3 cups
> Children 9 to 12 . . 3 or more cups
> Teenagers . . . . . . 4 or more cups
> Adults . . . . 2 or more cups

Meat Group

2 or more servings

Beef, veal, pork, lamb,
> poultry, fish, eggs

As alternates —
> dry beans, dry peas, nuts

Vegetable Fruit Group

4 or more servings
> Include —
>> A citrus fruit or other fruit or vegetable
>> important for vitamin C
>> A dark-green or deep-yellow vegetable for
>> vitamin A — at least every other day
> Other vegetables and fruits, including
>> potatoes

Bread Cereal Group

4 or more servings

Whole grain, enriched, or restored

OTHER FOODS

To round out meals and meet energy needs, most everyone will use some foods not specified in the Four Food Groups. Such foods include breads, cereals, flours; sugars, butter, margarine, other fats. These often are ingredients in a recipe or added to other foods during preparation or at table. Try to include some vegetable oils among the fats used.

FIG. 10-1. (Modified from Leaflet 424, Institute of Home Economics, U.S.D.A., Washington, D.C.)

amounts of iron as well as certain B-complex vitamins added to them. The feasibility of increased iron enrichment in flour and cereal products is presently under study, and current levels may be doubled or tripled in the near future. Enrichment of white flour and bread is now mandatory in 30 states and in Puerto Rico, and enrichment of cornmeal is common in 12 states. Actually most of the bread and all-purpose flour sold in the United States today is enriched, although this is not mandatory in all states. However, many of the prepared foods, such as packaged mixes, frozen baked products, refrigerated doughs and crackers are made from nonenriched flour (see Chap. 20).

Although the indiscriminate fortification of foods has been discouraged, a number of other food products have had vitamins and minerals added to them in varying amounts. Careful consideration must be given to any new proposal for fortification; for example, too enthusiastic fortification with vitamin D might be harmful for young children consuming excess amounts of this nutrient.

A DAILY FOOD GUIDE

The recommended allowances for nutrients for most people can be obtained from a well chosen variety of ordinary foods, including those in our markets which are commonly fortified or enriched with vitamins and minerals. The Daily Food Guide[2] (Fig. 10-1), prepared by nutritionists in the U.S.D.A., presents one way to select food. With this aid almost anyone can get the nutrients needed from everyday foods.

Most foods contain more than one nutrient, but no single food contains all the nutrients in the amount we need. The Daily Food Guide suggests the kinds that together supply nutrients in the amounts needed. In using the Guide one selects the main part of his diet from the four broad food groups. To this one adds other foods as desired to make meals appealing and satisfying. The additional foods should add enough calories to meet energy needs, which will vary widely for different members of the family.

PATTERN DIETARY

The accompanying pattern dietary (Table 10-2) planned according to the Daily Food Guide provides only about 1,400 calories—less than needed by an active person—but meets or approaches the

² Consumer and Food Economics Research Div. Agr. Res. Service. Washington, D.C., (rev.), 1964.

recommended allowances for all nutrients for an adult male. Supplementary foods, such as extra milk for children, will help meet the calcium level recommended for them. In general, the foods added to meet caloric needs of individuals will provide additional nutrients as well as contribute to taste and satisfaction of meals.

The iron provided in the pattern dietary is low for women when compared with the 18 mg. recommended. This amount of iron is impossible to obtain unless a special effort is made to include iron-rich foods. It is suggested that perhaps women might use dried fruits for snacks instead of candy if calories permit, and try to include some type of liver in the diet at least once a week. Iron supplements may still be needed. The level of B-vitamins, which appears to be slightly low for men and boys, will be raised to RDA when calories are increased to meet their needs.

In Part Three, the hospital diets discussed are also based upon this pattern dietary but modified as required to meet specific needs.

MEAL MANAGEMENT

If mealtimes are to fulfill the many purposes associated with such occasions in our culture, the homemaker, particularly the inexperienced young woman, may need assistance from the nurse in meal management. The following steps briefly outline the factors which may be helpful. As skill in this area is developed, some of the steps may be combined.

1. **Menu planning.** Using a guide such as the Daily Food Guide (Fig. 10-1), the homemaker may plan a week's menus which take into consideration the family's preferences as well as the time, energy and money available. Because it is possible to obtain the recommended dietary allowance of nutrients in many different diet patterns, anyone attempting to evaluate or teach nutrition should be conscious of this fact and avoid the use of stereotyped diet yardsticks for judging individual diets. It is possible for some people to get enough calcium from the daily use of cheese, canned fish with bones, legumes and leafy vegetables, even though the more usual pattern would be from the use of whole or skim milk. Thus, although nutrition guides such as the Four Food Groups are valuable, their limitations when applied to an individual must be recognized (see Chap. 20).

2. **Shopping lists.** Until some experience has been gained in knowing the types and amounts of food required for the various menu items, the

TABLE 10-2. EVALUATION OF A PATTERN DIETARY FOR ITS NUTRITIVE CONTENT[1]

Food Group	Amt. in Gm.	Household Measure	Calories	Protein Gm.	Fat Gm.	Carbohydrate Gm.	Minerals				Vitamins				
							Calcium Mg.	Phosphorus Mg.	Magnesium Mg.	Iron Mg.	A I.U.	Thiamine Mg.	Riboflavin Mg.	Niacin Mg.	Ascorbic Acid Mg.
Milk or equivalent[2]	488	2 c. (1 pint)	320	17	17	24	576	452	63	.2	700	.16	.84	.3	5
Egg	50	1 medium	81	7	6	..	27	102	5	1.2	590	.06	.15	Tr.	..
Meat, fish or fowl[3]	120	4 ozs., cooked	376	30	31	..	13	212	104	3.3	280	.14	.23	6.1	..
Vegetables:															
Potato, cooked	100	1 medium	65	2	..	15	6	48	22	.5	..	.09	.03	1.2	16
Deep green or yellow, cooked[4]	75	½ c.	21	2	..	6	44	28	29	.9	4,700	.05	.10	.5	25
Other, raw or cooked[5]	75	½ c.	45	2	..	10	16	41	18	.9	300	.08	.06	.6	12
Fruits:															
Citrus[6]	100	1 serving	44	1	..	10	18	16	12	.3	140	.06	.02	.3	43
Other[7]	100	1 serving	85	..	..	22	10	21	16	.8	365	.03	.04	.5	4
Bread, white, enriched	70	3 slices	189	6	2	35	59	68	15	1.7	..	.17	.15	1.7	..
Cereal, whole grain or enriched[8]	130 30	⅔ c. cooked or 1 oz. dry	89	3	1	18	12	95	34	.9	..	.08	.03	.7	..
Butter or margarine	14	1 tablespoon	100	..	11	..	3	2	2	..	460	..	..	..	..
Totals			1,415	70	68	140	784	1,085	320	10.7	7,535	.92	1.65	11.9[9]	105
Compare with recommended allowances[10]														Niacin Equiv.	
Reference man (70 Kg., 22 yrs. old)			2,800	65	..	..	800	800	350	10.0	5,000	1.40	1.70	18	60
Reference woman (58 Kg., 22 yrs. old)			2,000	55	..	..	800	800	300	18.0	5,000	1.00	1.50	13	55

[1] Calculations from Composition of Foods. Handbook No. 8. U. S. Department of Agriculture, Rev. 1963.
[2] Milk equivalents means evaporated milk and dried milk in amounts equivalent to fluid milk in nutritive content; cheese, if water-soluble minerals and vitamins have not been lost in whey; and food items made with milk.
[3] Evaluation based on the use of 700 Gm. of beef (chuck, cooked), 200 Gm. of pork (medium fat, roasted), 200 Gm. of chicken (roaster, cooked, roasted) and 100 Gm. of fish (halibut, cooked, broiled) per 10-day period.
[4] Evaluation based on figures for cooked broccoli, carrots, spinach and squash (all varieties).
[5] Evaluation based on figures for raw tomatoes and lettuce, and cooked peas, beets, lima beans, and fresh corn.
[6] Evaluation based on figures for whole orange and grapefruit, and orange and grapefruit juices.
[7] Evaluation based on figures for banana, apple, unsweetened cooked prunes and sweetened canned peaches.
[8] Evaluation based on figures for shredded wheat biscuit and oatmeal.
[9] The average diet in the United States, which contains a generous amount of protein, provides enough tryptophan to increase the niacin value by about a third.
[10] From the National Research Council Recommended Dietary Allowances, revised 1968.

homemaker may save time, money and heartache by making a shopping list based on her week's menu plan. Most local markets usually advertise in the Wednesday or Thursday newspaper and these are most helpful in indicating the foods available and their prices. Shopping lists are good deterrents to impulse buying in the supermarket, especially if the husband and children accompany the shopper.

3. **Food purchasing.** Most communities offer the homemaker a variety of different markets, and the wise shopper soon learns where to buy certain items. The newspaper advertisements also inform her where to find the specials on various items.

Modifications in the family menus may be made when necessary to reduce costs. Intelligent adjustments can ensure that meals are still nutritionally adequate and acceptable to the family.

Milk and Dairy Products. Either evaporated milk or dried skim milk (fortified with vitamins A and D) is cheaper than fresh milk and is entirely satisfactory for cooking. Both products also have use as a beverage. Inexpensive cheese is as good a source of protein as more expensive types.

Meats, Poultry, Fish and Eggs. Less expensive cuts of meat may be used when it is necessary to cut food costs. A rough estimate of the cost of the edible portion of some of the apparently cheapest cuts may disclose that the cheapest is not always the cut which has the lowest price tag per pound. Variety meats, such as pork or lamb liver, pork heart and beef tongue, are often good buys. Fish may be cheaper than meat. Poultry today is less expensive per pound than good-quality meats. When meats are high, main dishes of beans or peas and peanut butter for sandwiches may be used. Grade B eggs are as nutritious as Grade A and usually are cheaper. Eggs of graded size show considerable variation in price—sometimes small eggs are the best buy, sometimes large ones.

Fruits and vegetables in season and when plentiful are usually cheaper than canned or frozen. However, home-frozen foods are good economy if home produced. As a rule, carrots and cabbage are inexpensive and can be used raw or cooked. Fresh greens in season and wild greens in some areas may be used in place of more expensive green vegetables. Canned fruits and vegetables can replace fresh products when these are expensive or out of season. Canned tomatoes are cheaper and often higher in vitamin C than raw tomatoes out of season. During some seasons either canned or frozen orange juice is cheaper than fresh and has about the same nutritive value. Canned tomatoes, tomato juice, grapefruit juice and low-cost fresh fruits may be used in place of orange juice. The nutritive value of cheaper standard grades of canned fruits and vegetables is essentially the same as that of the more expensive fancy grades, and they are equally wholesome.

Bread, Cakes and Cereals. In general, foods prepared at home are less expensive than foods purchased ready to eat. Sweet rolls, buns, and coffee cakes are expensive types of bread. Breakfast cereals cooked at home are cheaper than the ready-to-eat varieties. Large packages are economical for big families but not for small ones, as the contents may become stale and have to be discarded. Day-old bakery products may represent savings to large families who consume many loaves of bread each week.

4. **Food storage.** Special attention should be paid to the storage of perishable items. Many food dollars are wasted on foods that must be discarded before they can be consumed. This is particularly true of frozen foods when there is not adequate freezer space to store them in the home. The manner in which foods are stored or prepared may alter nutritive values. Table I in Part Four gives the average values for nutrients in most foods. Averages, however, do not tell, for example, that half of the ascorbic acid in potatoes is lost after several months' storage and that an additional amount is lost in cooking and reheating.

5. **Food preparation.** A good, reliable cookbook is a must for the new homemaker. Careful attention should be given to recipe amounts and instructions until the cook has developed sufficient skill to make her own adjustments. Food values for prepared dishes are based on standard recipes, but people do not always use standard recipes. Obviously, a fish chowder made with salt pork and heavy cream will have a higher calorie and fat value per serving than a chowder made with diluted evaporated or dried skim milk. Water-soluble vitamins and minerals may be lost in cooking water.

6. **Meal service.** The temperature and appearance of food as it is placed before the family can be the determining factors as to whether or not a certain dish will be consumed. The homemaker who wishes to please her family will take special pleasure in presenting attractive offerings. Children and ill people especially react to the appearance of the plate.

FOOD FADS

In this scientific age quackery still flourishes in the field of nutrition as well as in the area of drugs and medical devices. Quacks thrive by misinterpreting scientific authorities in order to sell their ideas and their products. It is estimated that some 10 million Americans spend $1 billion a year on worthless and sometimes dangerous drugs, treatments, dietary fads and other quackery. This section focusses attention on those nutrition fads that are most widespread.

Vitamin Concentrates and Food Supplements. The promotion of vitamin and mineral supplements and special diet foods is misleading millions of people who have little need for such products. This type of deceptive advertising, which until recently appealed mainly to the "golden-agers," is now deceiving people of all ages, even teen-agers. Many people are attempting self-medication for imaginery or real illnesses with a multitude of irrational products. They are apt to spend much more for such products than they would for beneficial nutrients provided in an adequate diet.

"Natural" Foods. So-called "natural" foods have become especially popular of late years. Natural food enthusiasts use raw in place of refined sugar or sea salt in place of table salt and do not realize that the trace minerals which may be present in the impurities of such natural products are widely available in most foods. The use of olive oil in place of other fats or stone ground wheat instead of whole wheat may be taste preferences but have little nutritional significance.

Certain vegetable juices have been credited with virtues they do not possess, such as celery juice for rheumatism and garlic juice for high blood pressure. Juices, extracted from vegetables or fruits, have essentially similar nutritive value as the original product except for the cellulose. There is no evidence that certain vegetables or their juices have special curative properties other than as sources of nutrients.

Although it must be admitted that the number and variety of processed foods now available is often confusing, the prejudice expressed against processed foods is quite unwarranted. In general, processing is for the purpose of improving keeping quality, flavor, texture, nutritive value or convenience in preparation. Seldom does such processing significantly reduce nutritive value. Moreover, all additives must be approved by the Food and Drug Administration which has strict requirements.

"Organic" Foods. The craze for "organic" foods has reached such a point that even wayside markets are advertising food grown "organically." This means that crops are grown without chemical fertilizers or pesticides. People seldom realize that all organic material—compost, manure—used in growing foods "organically" must be broken down to inorganic elements before plants can absorb the nutrients from the soil. Scientific tests have shown that such foods show no significant difference in nutritive value from those grown with commercial fertilizers.

Pesticides aid in the production of good quality foods and of increased yields, thus making larger quantities of products ever more widely available to our growing population. The use of pesticides to prevent destruction of crops by infestations of fungi, microorganisms or insects is carefully controlled so that no dangerous residues will remain when the food reaches the market.

Meat is considered organically grown when produced from animals raised without antibiotics or hormones and dressed without the use of chemicals. People should be aware that our regular market meats are inspected regularly; also, the constant vigilance of law-enforcing agencies regulates the use of all additives and medical agents to be sure that they are harmless and within safe limits.

The whole cult of "natural" and "organic" foods has puzzled scientific nutritionists for years, because all the evidence points to the fact that fertilizers and pesticides increase yield and that plant genetics determine the color, flavor and nutritive value of the crop.

According to an article that appeared in the New York Times, the FDA takes the following position concerning "organic" foods:

Organic or natural foods are not considered to be significantly different from other foods, in terms of their nutritional qualities. The FDA feels that if you want them and can afford them, they're there is the marketplace for you to buy. But they must be labeled in a manner that's neither false or misleading, and no attempt can be made in promoting these foods to suggest that they offer special health benefits. There's just no evidence to show that people living on organic or natural foods will be protected from chronic disease problems, or that they can expect better health. Nevertheless, the interested and alert consumer can get food and nutritious food either from the so-called organic food store or the modern supermarket. The choice is and should remain open to the individual. But the main point is that we cannot hope to feed today's population with yesterday's production methods. We must use the technical advances that science and chemistry have given us if we hope to produce and preserve enough food to meet today's requirements.

Macrobiotic Diet. Among college students today the macrobiotic diet is by far the most important diet craze. It is an outgrowth of an interpretation of Zen Buddhism introduced into the United States and Europe from Japan by Ohsawa. According to the macrobiotic system there are 10 diet plans (Diet No. -3 to Diet No. 7) which may be followed to establish a healthy and happy life. In progressing from Diet No. -3 to Diet No. 7, one gradually gives up in the following order: desserts, salads and fruits, animal foods, soups, and finally vegetables, at the same time increasing the amount of cereal grains to be consumed. There is no scientific basis for the restrictions or recommendations of the macrobiotic system. Part of the plan for all the diets is the consumption of as little beverage as possible. Only "organically" produced fresh vegetables, fruits or animal products are used. Foods are classified into Yang (the male principle) or Yin (the female principle), and a 5:1 balance between these is considered to be important. Because sweets and many fruits are Yin foods, the amount of these in the macrobiotic diet is small.

Most of the diet plans are low in ascorbic acid. Diet No. 7 (in which whole grain cereal, usually brown rice, is the only food consumed) is grossly inadequate in many of the essential minerals and vitamins as well as in good quality protein. Fortunately not too many students follow No. 7 diet plan for very long. Another danger in the macrobiotic concept is that, since the various diet plans promise to cure the body of disease and purge it of all poisons, adequate medical care may be postponed when it is needed.

Because it is possible to have an adequate intake of nutrients on certain of the macrobiotic diet plans, emphasis should be placed on the role of essential nutrients in maintaining health and well-being and in counseling the followers of this system to select their macrobiotic foods in keeping with this principle of good nutrition.

Fact and Fancy. There is no magic in any specific food item. It makes little difference whether one obtains his nutrients from fluid milk or milk powder, from milk products such as cheese, yoghurt or ice cream, or whether he gets them from meat, fish or fowl, wheat germ, whole grains or blackstrap molasses. The essential point is to get an adequate supply of each nutrient from food that tastes good.

Complicating and encouraging the food fads today are the growing number of false nutrition ideas, or folklore, built up by pseudo-scientific books, pamphlets and periodicals on diets of various sorts. Some tell us that calories don't count or that arthritis can be cured by oils to lubricate your joints; others tempt the unwary with a drinking-man's diet or with martinis and whipped cream. In some unreliable books there is enough of the true mixed with the false regarding food values and human needs to make it difficult for the average person to judge what is valid.

Many dietary fads may be relatively harmless but senseless. Too often they detract from the pleasure of eating, an important element in good nutrition. Variety is in itself a safeguard, and, when variety is severely limited, as it is by some fads and self-imposed restrictions, certain nutritive factors are apt to be low or absent. When fads lead to delay in seeking necessary medical advice, they can be dangerous indeed. In any event food fads may increase food costs unduly and result in the omission of foods really needed. The consequences are the same whether one is led to food faddism by the enthusiasms of the uninformed neighbor or of the profit-seekers.

Hence, attention is again called to the Recommended Dietary Allowances as the nutritional norms against which any dietary pattern may be measured. If a given food plan compares favorably with the RDA, the basic nutrients for health and well-being will be supplied, and one need not be concerned with the specific dietary pattern of the individual.

STUDY QUESTIONS AND ACTIVITIES

1. The Food and Nutrition Board of the National Research Council has recommended dietary allowances for certain specific nutrients. Which ones are listed in this table?

2. For which factor do the allowances vary directly with the caloric requirements?

3. The recommended allowances for children are estimated for age groups. How is the average value for each age group computed, and what values would you use for a 13-year-old boy large for his age?

4. Which nutrients are most difficult to obtain in sufficient quantities in low-cost meals in your locality at the season of year when you are studying this chapter?

5. List the food you ate yesterday and check to see whether all four food groups were adequately represented.

6. Visit a local bookstore or your local library and look at the available books on nutrition and diet. Do any of them seem to be reliable or unreliable? Can you state why?

7. What food fads have you heard discussed or seen practiced? How would you help a layman to distinguish between fact and fad or between true and false ideas about food?

8. From what sources could you get reliable information about a new food product advertised for a specific diet purpose?

9. Can the average person obtain sufficient vitamins and minerals from food or should supplements be taken regularly?

SUPPLEMENTARY READING ON MEETING NUTRITIONAL NORMS

Council on Food and Nutrition—American Medical Association: Zen macrobiotic diets. JAMA, 218: 397, 1971.

Food and Nutrition Board: Recommended Dietary Allowances. National Academy of Sciences–National Research Council Publ. No. 1694. Washington, D.C., 1968.

Food for the young family. Home and Garden Bulletin No. 85. U.S.D.A., Washington, D.C., (April) 1971.

Jalso, S. B., Burns, M. M., and Rivers, J. M.: Nutrition beliefs and practices. J. Am. Dietet. A., 47:263, 1965.

Kaplan, J.: A therapy of chaos. Today's Health, 41: 38, 1963.

Mitchell, H. S.: Don't be fooled by fads. Food, The Yearbook of Agriculture, pp. 660-668. U.S.D.A., Washington, D.C., 1959.

Monge, B., and Throssell, D.: Good nutrition on a low income. Am. J. Nursing, 60:2190, 1960.

Moore, M. L.: When families must eat more for less. Nurs. Outlook, 14:66, 1966.

Sailor, N. M.: Nutrition knowledge applied to everyday living. Nurs. Outlook, 9:756, 1961.

Stare, F. J.: Good nutrition from food, not pills. Am. J. Nursing, 65:86, 1965.

For further references see Bibliography in Part Four.

Regional, Cultural and Religious Food Patterns

11

Regional Food Patterns in the United States • Cultural Food Patterns
Religious Food Patterns

Characteristic food habits of every regional or national group should be respected, because there are good nutritional practices in each of them and nutritional needs may be met by many different patterns of eating. Emphasis should be placed on the desirable features of the established food pattern and on methods of preparation that preserve maximum food values. Although the choice of foods and the methods of preparation may differ from those to which we are accustomed, it often happens that the foods used fall into the Four Food Groups and provide nutrients that meet recommended allowances.

Unfamiliar foods and methods of preparation need to be studied and possible values recognized before changes are suggested. A family may be encouraged to continue its own methods of preparation and seasoning when these are not incompatible with health and then gradually be helped to institute necessary changes to correct poor practices, if these exist.

Therapeutic diets should be interpreted for the patient or the homemaker in terms of the regional or the national food pattern. A woman of foreign birth or one from a different part of the country may have little contact outside her home and little opportunity to learn how to use foods that are new to her. The marked improvements in homes where the mother has had the opportunity to learn to adjust to local foods and customs show that instruction as well as understanding is an important phase of nutrition work.

In this chapter special attention is given to regional, cultural and religious food patterns which are distinctive. A knowledge of these food preferences and attention to them may help to build the bridge of understanding between the health worker, the nurse or the nutritionist and the family that she is trying to assist.

REGIONAL FOOD PATTERNS IN THE UNITED STATES

Anyone who has traveled in different parts of the United States and has eaten meals typical of various regions is aware of differences in menus, food preparation and local terms for foods or special dishes. Part of the joy of travel is in eating the traditional foods of each locality. However, national advertising in magazines and on TV has tended to popularize certain foods so that diets are not as regional as they once were.

People who are ill are much more likely to want familiar foods cooked in a traditional manner with familiar seasoning. Therefore, the dietitian and the nurse should recognize some of these regional differences which exist in our own country so that they can make some adjustments of the diet on the basis of the essential nutrients in terms of familiar foods.

In the South, hot breads are served at nearly every meal, and baker's yeast breads are not popular. Corn and rice are popular sources of carbohydrates. There is a preference for vegetables that have been cooked a long time and often with fat pork. Undoubtedly some vitamins are destroyed by this process, but the common use of pot liquor conserves the nutrients which are in solution. The wide variety of greens used compensates in a measure for the low consumption of milk and cheese as sources of calcium and vitamins. The scarcity of fresh milk and refrigeration in some localities has encouraged the use of evaporated and dry milk. Buttermilk is liked and is used when available. Because many black Americans, now living elsewhere, came from the South, their food customs reflect some of the practices of this region, as discussed later in the chapter.

In the Southwest, the Mexican influence is shown in the use of beans and highly seasoned dishes. Again, milk production is limited, and, while the drinking of fresh milk was not part of the original pattern of eating, it is being introduced gradually. Mexican foods such as tortillas, tamales, enchiladas and a wide variety of beans are popular in American homes of the Southwest as well as in Mexican families. More details of Mexican foods are given later in this chapter.

In the Far West, the infiltration of oriental cultures has influenced food habits. The use of a wide variety of garden produce and locally grown citrus fruits, the short-time cooking of vegetables typical of oriental cooking, and the serving of generous salads as the first course are features to be commended.

In the north central states, there is a mixed cultural background with a strong northern European and Scandinavian heritage in many localities. Homes still maintain characteristic native dishes, perhaps modified by regional choice of ingredients. Many of these states produce and use large quantities of dairy products, especially cheeses of several varieties closely resembling European types. The so-called typical American diet is really an adaptation of much of the northern European food pattern. This is only natural since climatic conditions and crops are similar. Locally grown fruits and vegetables are used in season and preserved for winter use. This is a good custom and should be encouraged.

On the east coast and in New England, many traditional dishes have come down from the Pilgrim settlers. The use of corn meal in Indian pudding and johnnycake was acquired from the Indians by their new neighbors. Baked beans, codfish cakes, clam or fish chowder and turkey for festive occasions are all old New England traditions, some of which have been adopted nationally. A smaller variety of green, leafy vegetables is used in New England than in many other areas, but yellow vegetables, such as squash, turnips and carrots, are popular.

In isolated communities in any part of the country, unusual food habits may be encountered. Malnutrition may result from a limited variety of foods grown locally, especially if the economic status prohibits extensive use of foods from other producing areas. Sporadic outbreaks of actual deficiency diseases have been reported occasionally. National attention has been called to such problems in Appalachia, on Indian Reservations and among the Eskimos in Alaska. State and Federal agencies are recognizing their responsibilities for these conditions quite as much as for the control of communicable disease.

In metropolitan areas a great variety of food patterns may be found. In large cities, there may be whole sections in which the inhabitants follow as closely as possible the food customs of the country of their origin. This influence is retained to some extent by the second generation. People who come to the city from regions of the United States where definite types of foods are preferred continue to attempt to follow the diet to which they have been accustomed. Usually they can be persuaded to supplement their meals with the foods that are more generally available in the city than they were in the part of the country where their food habits were established.

CULTURAL FOOD PATTERNS

The Black Experience

The food habits of the black American reflects the region of the country from which he comes. Southern blacks have the same distinctive food habits that are typical of the geographic locale in which they reside. The northern black may evidence little identification with the regional patterns of the South, or on the other hand, he may have adapted many of these in his present environment. This fact was made exceptionally clear to one of the authors when planning menus with a group of paraprofessionals in a preschool center in the North. In developing a feeding program which would be supportive of the cultural backgrounds of black children, many of the "Soul Food" items planned and prepared by black staff were new and strange to many northern blacks and whites alike, although completely familiar to blacks and whites with considerable experience in the South.

With many exceptions, the following represents what, in general, might be considered the black experience with food customs. Breakfast patterns are similar to the breakfasts of many other groups except for the very frequent use of grits in some form. If eggs and bacon or other form of pork are available, they are served with the grits. Hot breads, biscuits, muffins and cornbread take the place of yeast bread at most meals.

The family usually has one main meal at a time

determined by the activities of the family members. Greens—mustard, turnip, collard and kale—cooked in a pot liquor with some form of pork are popular. Although fresh greens are used in the South, a wide variety of frozen greens are available in northern markets. Sweet potatoes, squash, lima beans, snap beans, fresh corn and cabbage are also popular vegetables. Sweet potatoes and squash are often used in pies as the New Englander uses pumpkin. Fruits, such as oranges, watermelon and peaches are enjoyed when available.

Grits, rice or potatoes provide the chief source of carbohydrate, while black-eyed peas and other dried beans may be used and contribute both carbohydrate and protein. Fried fish of all kinds, particularly that caught by members of the family in streams and lakes, are considered most acceptable. Poultry, cured and fresh pork, and some wild game, such as rabbit, woodchuck and pheasant, are served when available. Frying, barbecuing and stewing are the most popular methods of preparation even when an oven is available. Milk, milk products and cheese are not used extensively; however, buttermilk, evaporated milk and ice cream are the preferred forms. Sweets—particularly molasses, other syrups, cakes, pastries and candy—are consumed in large quantity. Sweetened flavored drinks often take the place of fruit juice and milk as a beverage.

"Soul Food," a descriptive term for many of these dishes, connotes special feelings and emotions. It is the spirit of the provider or cook to create an atmosphere of love and well-being for those she is feeding. There is also the implication that from limited food resources, much happiness and enjoyment can be achieved by giving special care to the preparation of food.

Because of the large amounts of fat and carbohydrate consumed, adequate or more than adequate calories are, as a rule, provided. However, because relatively small amounts of meat, milk and fish may be available, the protein content of the diet of the poor family is often limited. Minerals, iron and calcium, have also been found inadequate in many Southern black dietaries, as have vitamins A and C.[1]

Dietary Habits of Mexicans and Other Latin Americans

The Mexicans use freely many varieties of beans, especially the pinto, as well as rice, pota-

---
[1] Mayer, J.: Nutr. Rev., 23:161, 1965.

toes, peas and some vegetables. Chili, a variety of pepper, is also popular. The chili plant is sacred to the Mexican, who is supposed to be blessed in health if he uses it plentifully. The tomato always is prominent in Mexican cookery. Mexicans use little meat and practically always cook it with vegetables. They have a strong aversion to meat that is not perfectly fresh and slaughtered in the approved Mexican style. Chili con carne is a favorite meat dish. It consists of beef seasoned with garlic and chili peppers and cooked several hours. Tamales also are popular. They are made of corn meal and ground pork, highly seasoned; they are rolled in corn husks and steamed. Tortillas, made with ground whole corn which has been soaked in lime water and baked on a griddle, serve as a bread. Enchiladas, another favorite, are made by filling tortillas with cheese, onion and shredded lettuce. Tacos, a similar dish, is prepared by adding meat and a sauce to the tortilla. Thus some calcium is provided in tortillas and in beans in a diet which includes very little milk or cheese. The use of milk for the children should be encouraged when and if a change to the American type of bread is made.

The influx of Cuban refugees into our southern states creates a need to recognize and adjust nutrition advice and special diets to Cuban preferences when counseling these people. Their food pattern is similar to that of other West Indian groups where the Spanish influence predominates.

It is notable, however, that many of the more prosperous eastern South American peoples have a meat and milk consumption as high or higher than the United States. Spanish and Portuguese influences are evident in the liberal use of peppers and spices.

On the west coast of South America the situation is quite different. A few cities are prosperous, but agriculture is handicapped by desert, mountains and jungles. The native Indian populations of the Andes in Ecuador, Peru and Chile are short of food and especially of some adequate sources of protein.

Puerto Rican Dietary Habits

The dietary pattern in Puerto Rico is similar to that in other Caribbean Islands and to some of the Latin American countries. From the extensive work of Dr. Lydia Roberts in Puerto Rico information is available on a typical moderate-cost food supply for an adult for one day (Table 11-1). The nutrient value comes close to meeting the U.S. recommended allowances.

When Puerto Ricans migrate to the United States, as they have in great numbers, they may modify this pattern considerably according to what is available and what they can afford.

Rice, beans and viandas (starchy root vegetables and plantains) are the staple foods, used daily. Salt codfish is used more often than fresh fish and is served with viandas, oil and vinegar. Chicken, pork and beef are favorite meats and used when there is money to purchase them. Tomatoes, peppers, onions, garlic, salt pork and seasonings (sofrito) cooked with different varieties of dried peas and beans is a common dish. Bananas, oranges and pineapple are popular and relatively inexpensive in Puerto Rico. Even more important are some of the native fruits which are not familiar in the north, such as the mango, papaya and the West Indian cherry, or acerola, which is now recognized as the richest known natural source of ascorbic acid.

Milk is not popular as a beverage except perhaps when income permits, as café con leche, a combination of coffee and hot milk. Sweetened cocoa and chocolate made with milk is also consumed occasionally.

Puerto Ricans living in the northern United States may have to adjust to different fruits in season and to canned fruits. They may well be encouraged to use more milk and cheese, and cheaper cuts of meat to supplement the protein at meals when rice and beans are served. Acceptance of canned tomatoes in place of more expensive fresh ones out of season, margarine in place of butter and cheaper cuts of meat would provide better nutrition for less cost.

Puerto Ricans in New York City and other urban areas are often among the lower economic groups because many of them are unskilled laborers. Their poor and crowded housing may provide inadequate cooking and refrigeration facilities. Thus they may be unable to provide their families with as good food as they had at home. Malnutrition, rickets and tuberculosis are not uncommon among Puerto Rican children living under such conditions. The nurse or the social worker can offer suggestions as to how they can improve their nutrition within their budgets.

Italian Dietary Habits

Italian-Americans, few of whom today were born in Italy, have adopted many food customs of the United States. Likewise, the popularity of Italian spaghetti and pizza in this country testifies to the influence that Italian food customs have

TABLE 11-1. MODERATE-COST FOOD FOR A DAY FOR A PUERTO RICAN ADULT

FOOD	AMOUNT OF EDIBLE PORTION	WEIGHT GM.
Rice	3 cups cooked	668
Plantain or root veg.	1 serving	200
Bean, broad, kidney or other type	1 cup	256
Onion	1 medium	110
Egg Plant	1 small	100
Green Pepper	2 small	100
Tomato	1 medium	100
Mango	1 medium	200
Banana	2 medium	300
Salt Codfish	1 oz. dry	30
Goat's Milk	1 cup	244
Lard	½ cup	50
Olive Oil	2 Tbsp.	28

The value of this diet is approximately:

Calories	2,506	Vitamin A	33,500 I.U.
Protein	69 Gm.	Thiamin	1.0 mg.
Fat	77 Gm.	Riboflavin	1.0 mg.
Calcium	0.6 Gm.	Niacin	13.3 mg.
Iron	12.5 mg.	Vitamin C	195 mg.

Adapted from information provided by Dr. Lydia Roberts, University of Puerto Rico, and Miss Ethel Robinson, formerly a teacher in rural Puerto Rico.

had on Americans. Italians here continue to use pastas in a great variety of shapes and with many different sauces and cheeses. Similarly, bread is still an essential part of an Italian meal, although crusty white bread is now more popular than the dark breads that were a former standby.

Southern Italians may use more fish and highly seasoned foods, while northern Italians use more root vegetables and more meat. The liberal use of eggs, cheese, tomatoes, green vegetables and fruits by all Italians is to be commended. They may well be encouraged to use more milk and meat, both of which they like. In general, the northern Italians have better food habits than those from the south.

Italians have a strong sense of individuality. We may think of spaghetti as a typically Italian food, but not all Italians like spaghetti. They dislike foods that are not prepared to their particular tastes. They are particularly sensitive to the lack of close family ties in a hospital and therefore dread hospitalization more than one may suspect. Most Italians eat a very light breakfast: black coffee for adults and milk for children, with perhaps bread without butter. Some like the main meal at noon, others at night, but bread and cheese with coffee or wine are an acceptable light meal.[2]

Western European and Scandinavian Dietary Habits

Most of the western European peoples, including the Scandinavians, have food patterns not unlike those of northeastern and central North America where immigrants from these areas have settled during the past two centuries. Many American food customs of today have been derived from these countries. The lists of meats, vegetables, fruits and grain products used by them would be a mere recital of those in our markets. To be sure, they make more frequent use of dark breads, potatoes, fish and cheese than native Americans do. For western Europeans the differences in culinary methods, seasonings and attitudes toward food are never serious hurdles in adjusting to American food patterns.

Central European Dietary Habits

In many of the central European countries grains and potatoes provide 60 to 70 percent of the total calories for the rural and the lower income groups. They use rye and buckwheat as well as wheat for their breads. Pork and pork products including highly seasoned sausages are popular. Cabbage may be used raw, cooked or as sauerkraut, and other vegetables—onions, turnips, peppers, carrots, beans, squash and greens—are often cooked with a little meat. Eggs, fresh milk, sour cream and yoghurt (called by a different name in each country), cottage cheese and other cheeses are widely used. Central Europeans bring with them many good food habits which are to be encouraged.

Dietary Habits of the Middle East— Lebanese, Armenian, Turkish, Greek and Syrian

The inhabitants of the Middle East are outdoor people. Most of them are farmers: they raise their own sheep, goats, cattle, chickens, ducks and geese; they produce their own grains and grow fruits and vegetables in abundance, wherever water is plentiful. Grains, rice or wheat, furnish the major source of calories. The whole wheat is parboiled and cracked for use as a staple starchy food at the main meal. Eggs, butter and cheese also are produced on the farm. Lamb is the favorite meat. The food is not highly spiced but is rich in fat.

The fat is cooked with the food and this serves in place of butter. Matzoon, leban or yoghurt, a sour-milk preparation, is used almost universally by these people; sweet milk is seldom used. Black coffee, heavily sweetened, in which the pulverized bean is retained—often called Turkish coffee—is the preferred beverage in many countries of the Middle East.

Chinese Dietary Habits

The Chinese diet is varied, consisting of eggs, meat, fish, cereals and a large variety of vegetables. Many plants and weeds, such as radish leaves and shepherd's purse, are used, as well as various sprouts (bean, bamboo, etc.). None of these vegetables is ever overcooked, and no cooking water is discarded; thus, nutrients are well retained. The soybean is abundant, and some 30 or more products are manufactured from it. The protein content is high and of good quality for a vegetable protein.

Rice is used freely and takes the place of American bread, particularly in southern China. In northern China, wheat, corn and millet seed are used in abundance. The millet seed (ground or whole) is made into cakes or a thin mush, the latter being the form in which it is given to children. Noodles are widely used. Grains and, in some areas, sweet potatoes constitute the chief source of calories in the Chinese diet; grain and potato together provide from 70 to 90 percent of the total calories.

The quantity of meat eaten is small, and usually it is served with vegetables. All ingredients are cut into small pieces in conformity with an ancient law laid down by Confucius, the philosopher, specifying that food should not be eaten unless it had first been chopped or cut into small pieces. Pork is the chief meat of the poorer classes. Lamb and goat meat and other animal foods are used when available, but beef is uncommon.

In certain parts of China, a child rarely tastes cow's milk, but water-buffalo milk is used to some extent. Soybean milk and cheese are more common. When transplanted to this country, the Chinese readily accepts the use of dairy products for children and adults.

The Chinese use practically every part of the animal as food (with the exception of the hair and the bones); even the brain, the spinal cord and the various internal organs, as well as the skin and the blood, are utilized. Coagulated blood is sold on the market in pieces similar to liver, and since this

---

[2] Abstr. J. Am. Dietet. A., 40:342, 1962.

is one of the inexpensive foods, it is used freely. Fish and shellfish are also in common use. They are sold alive, for the Chinese have a strong aversion to dead fish and consider them unfit for food.

Eggs, including hen, duck and pigeon eggs, are used in abundance, when they can be afforded. The Chinese prepare what are known as fermented eggs, much relished by them, as well as other types of "preserved" eggs, which are eaten much as we in this country eat sweets.

Soy sauce, highly flavored and salted, is a frequent accompaniment with meals. It may present problems to the Chinese patient who must omit salt from his diet. This is true also of the Japanese diet.

Japanese Dietary Habits

During the past 20 years there have been spectacular changes in Japanese food habits, influenced by Western culture. Typical diets formerly included rice, bean paste soup, raw or cooked fish and pickles. Now the trend is to bread as well as rice, milk, cheese, meat, eggs, vegetables and fruits. Instant foods and frozen items are avail-

able. Seafoods are served raw, smoked, fried and, recently, as fish sausage. Japanese make a whole meal of wheat or buckwheat noodles cooked in broth and garnished with a few bits of vegetables and fish sausage and served with salty pickles. Although they are traditional tea drinkers, many of them now prefer coffee, and they like to drink milk when it is available. Many kinds of crisp salty snack foods made from rice or wheat flour, seaweed and other delicacies are popular. A Japanese or Chinese meal is complete without dessert, but at New Years' and other holidays the Japanese relish their "decoration cakes." Even the simplest one-dish meal is attractively served, and an elaborate party meal, served in 10 or 12 separate and colorful dishes of different shapes, is truly a work of art.

RELIGIOUS FOOD PATTERNS

Jewish Dietary Habits and Laws

In the United States today Jewish family food habits differ according to whether they belong to Orthodox, Conservative or Reform groups. Their

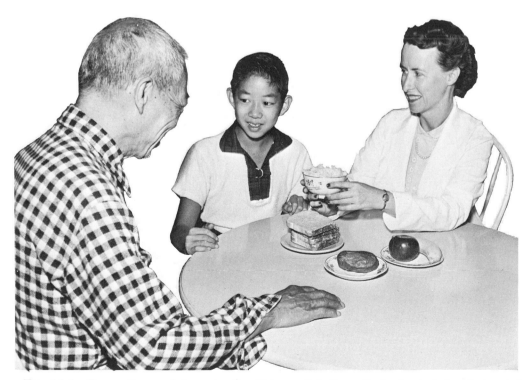

Fig. 11-1. Boy acting as interpreter for Chinese diabetic patient who is being instructed regarding the carbohydrate equivalent of his favorite bowl of rice. (Frances Stern Food Clinic of the Boston Dispensary)

food habits may also be influenced by the country from which they or their forefathers came, as well as by Biblical and rabbinical regulations, known as the Jewish dietary laws.

According to Kaufman[3]:

> Variations in observance are due largely to differences in interpretation and importance placed on dietary laws by the three schools of thought among American Jews today. Orthodox Jews still place great value on traditional and ceremonial practices of their religion, and observe the dietary laws under all conditions. Reform Jews place much less emphasis on rules which they consider to be purely ceremonial and tend to minimize the significance of the dietary laws. Conservative Jews stand between these two groups and, while nominally adhering to dietary laws, sometimes draw the distinction between the observance of the rules in the home and outside.
>
> Regulations include selection, preparation and service of the foods involved. The Bible gives no reason for these rules, but observant Jews feel that the rules known as Kashruth and hallowed since the time of Moses, are a positive means of self-purification and of service to their God. Although many hygienic and ethical bases have been alleged for these rules, the spiritual factors of sanctification and self-discipline are the primary motivations for those who adhere to them.

Miss Kaufman also gives some definitions of Jewish terms and special foods.

A brief outline of some of the specific rules to which the Orthodox Jews conform follows:

Foods Allowed or Prohibited. MEATS AND POULTRY. Quadrupeds with the cloven hoof who chew a cud are allowed. These include cows, sheep, goats and deer. Pork in all forms including lard and bacon is prohibited. The poultry allowed includes chicken, turkey, goose, pheasant and duck. All meats and poultry must be freshly slaughtered according to prescribed ritual and soaked in salted water to remove all trace of blood. This process is known as koshering (meaning clean), and many Jewish markets sell koshered meat and poultry. Prescribed methods of preparing meats and other foods are given in most Jewish cookbooks.

FISH. The fish prescribed in the Bible are those with fins and scales. Thus all shellfish and eels are excluded.

Food Combinations Allowed or Prohibited. The command "Thou shalt not seethe a kid in its mother's milk," repeated several times in Exodus and Deuteronomy, is the basis for never combining meat and milk in the same meal, or even cooking them in the same utensils. Eggs, fruits, vegetables, cereals and all other foods may be used without restrictions.

A striking characteristic of the Jewish diet is the richness of the food, including pastries and cakes, foods rich in fats, and preserves and conserves, as well as stewed and canned fruits. Butter, being a product of milk, must not be served with meat. Most vegetables, therefore, are cooked with the meat. Cooked vegetables are more often served in soup than otherwise. Borscht, a soup made with "sour salt" (tartaric acid) and vegetables to which sour cream is added, is a favorite dish but is not served with the meat meal. Cereals, especially barley and millet, are frequently served as a vegetable with meat or in soup.

Noodles and other egg-and-flour mixtures are used extensively. Rye and whole wheat breads are well-liked, as well as crusty rolls.

Dried fruits, as well as fresh, are used by those who can afford them.

Fish is served frequently, especially cod, haddock, carp, salmon and whitefish, as well as the smoked and the salted fishes—herring, salmon and sturgeon. Gefüllte fish is a delicacy prepared in almost all Jewish homes. Chicken is considered almost an essential for the Sabbath evening meal.

Because milk in any form cannot be served with meat at the same meal, the diet of children in Jewish families that rigidly observe the dietary laws may lack the proper amount of milk. The use of more green vegetables and canned vegetables and fresh and canned fruits for the whole family and more milk for the children should be stressed. The continued use of rye bread, legumes, coarse cereals, dried fruits and a variety of fish which are characteristic of the Jewish diet is advantageous.

Dietary laws for the Jewish Sabbath and religious holidays are often observed by even the less orthodox groups and therefore merit comment.

Sabbath: No food may be cooked on the Sabbath. This means that all cooking for both days is done on Friday. This need has led to the development of foods such as Sabbath Kugel or Sholend, Petshai, and many others.

Passover: During Passover week no leavened bread or its product, or anything which may have touched leavened bread, may be used. A complete new set of dishes is used during the week. Cutlery, silver, or metal pots may be used during this holi-

³ Kaufman, M.: Am. J. Clin. Nutr., 5:676, 1957.

day if properly koshered or sterilized. In actual practice this means that in every orthodox Jewish household there are four sets of dishes—the usual set for meat and the set for milk food, in addition to duplicate Passover sets.

Fast days: Yom Kippur (the Day of Atonement); no food or drink may be taken for 24 hours. Fast of Esther: this precedes the Feast of Purim and is now observed only by the very pious. The Feast of Purim is universally observed.

Roman Catholic

The Pope liberalized the dietary restrictions and fast days; thus customs vary in different localities. It is well to conform to local custom with regard to foods allowed on fast days and days of abstinence.

Greek Orthodox

The Orthodox laws have not changed in recent years but are interpreted somewhat more liberally. The use of meat, fish, poultry, eggs and dairy products is still restricted on Fridays and certain Wednesdays and during the first and last weeks of the Greek Orthodox Lent.

Seventh Day Adventists

Adventists in general are lacto-vegetarians; thus, they allow the use of eggs, milk and cheese as good sources of animal protein but, they use no meat, fish or poultry. They also use nuts and legumes as sources of protein.

Latter-Day Saints

The Mormons make no food restrictions but prohibit the use of alcohol, tobacco, tea and coffee.

STUDY QUESTIONS AND ACTIVITIES

1. Why is it essential that a public health nurse or a nutritionist be able to adjust her advice on nutrition to various regional and cultural food patterns?

2. After noting the regional dietary habits in the United States, which ones in the South and in the Southwest would you recommend and encourage, and what changes would you recommend?

3. How has the transplanting of various cultures influenced the food habits of those in various regions of the United States?

4. Why is the Jewish diet one of the most difficult problems for the health worker? What are some of the dietary laws which must be respected?

5. How does the use of grains, potatoes and animal protein vary among the different regions of Europe and Asia?

6. How can you help others to gain respect for the food habits and the favorite dishes of cultural groups other than their own?

SUPPLEMENTARY READING ON REGIONAL, CULTURAL AND RELIGIOUS FOOD PATTERNS

Anderson, L., and Browe, J. H.: Nutrition and Family Health Service. Chap. 2. Philadelphia, W. B. Saunders, 1960.

Cantoni, M.: Adapting therapeutic diets to the eating patterns of Italian Americans. Am. J. Clin. Nutr., 6:548, 1958.

Fathauer, G. H.: Food habits—an anthropologist's view. J. Am. Dietet. A., 37:335, 1960.

Hacker, D. B., and Miller, E. D.: Food patterns of the Southwest. Am. J. Clin. Nutr., 7:224, 1959.

Kaufman, M.: Adapting therapeutic diets to Jewish food customs. Am. J. Clin. Nutr., 5:676, 1957.

Macgregor, F. C.: Uncooperative patients: some cultural interpretations. Am. J. Nursing, 67:88, 1967.

Mayer, J.: The nutritional status of American Negroes. Nutr. Rev., 23:161, 1965.

Phillips, M. G., and Dunn, M. M.: Toward better understanding of other people: Their folkways and foods. Nurs. Outlook, 9:498, 1961.

Torres, R. M.: Dietary patterns of the Puerto Rican people. Am. J. Clin. Nutr., 7:349, 1959.

Valassi, K. V.: Food habits of Greek-Americans. Am. J. Clin. Nutr., 11:240, 1962.

For Further References see Bibliography in Part Four.

Ecology of Food

12

Safeguarding the Food Supply • **Food-borne Diseases and Toxins**

INTRODUCTION

The production and processing of food in the United States today is a highly developed scientific business. The 296 billion pounds of food produced each year to feed the 206 million people in this country is accomplished almost entirely by scientific farming methods using chemical fertilizers and pesticides. It would be impossible to achieve these production levels using so-called "organic farming" methods alone (the growing of food without the use of chemical aids). In the first place, the gigantic quantities of manures and composts which would be required for our vast farm system do not exist; hence, the crop yield would be drastically reduced. Without the insecticides and herbicides, the amount of crop loss from insect and fungi infestation would increase and food shortages such as exist in the underdeveloped countries would occur.

Selective breeding of plants, another aspect of scientific farming, has developed strains of cereals, fruits and vegetables appropriate for varying climatic and soil conditions. Other specific characteristics, such as increased resistance to certain diseases, increased amino acid content and decreased perishability also result from selective breeding. The nutritive value of individual foods is determined chiefly by their genetic character and not by the soil or type of fertilizer used.

Animals too, have been bred for certain desired characteristics, namely the lean, meat-type hog and steer, and the tenderer, meatier chicken and turkey. Antibiotics and some hormones have been employed in scientific feeding techniques and in the control of animal diseases which have markedly increased the animal food production; in the United States the per capita consumption of beef

has increased by approximately 70 percent and of chicken by 100 percent in the last 20 years.

Most of the food consumed in American homes today has undergone some form of commercial processsing—canning, freezing, drying, or irradiation. The TV dinner is perhaps the ultimate in commercial processing, but even the fresh fruits purchased in the supermarket may have had a heat and/or chill treatment before shipping to preserve their quality. In the processing of foods to produce specific properties there may be significant changes in the characteristics and composition of the original food such as happens in the milling of the whole wheat kernel to make white flour with good bread-making properties. Food additives may also be used as preservatives, antioxidants, stabilizers, emulsifiers, coloring and flavoring agents.

All of these factors involved in the production and processing of food provide the American consumer with an almost limitless choice of food items throughout the year, but they also make laws and regulations essential in order to protect the safety of this food supply.

SAFEGUARDING THE FOOD SUPPLY

The food industry is the nation's largest industry and depends upon the work of thousands of scientists and experts to predict needs and regulate food production and processing in the United States. People in general do not have the means or the skills to examine how meats are handled, to check fruits and vegetables for residues of pesticides or processed foods for harmful preservatives or accidental contaminants or packaged goods for insect infestation. Through Congress, however, laws have been passed making certain federal agencies

HOW FOODS GET TO THE CONSUMER—THE PRINCIPAL SUPPLY ROUTES

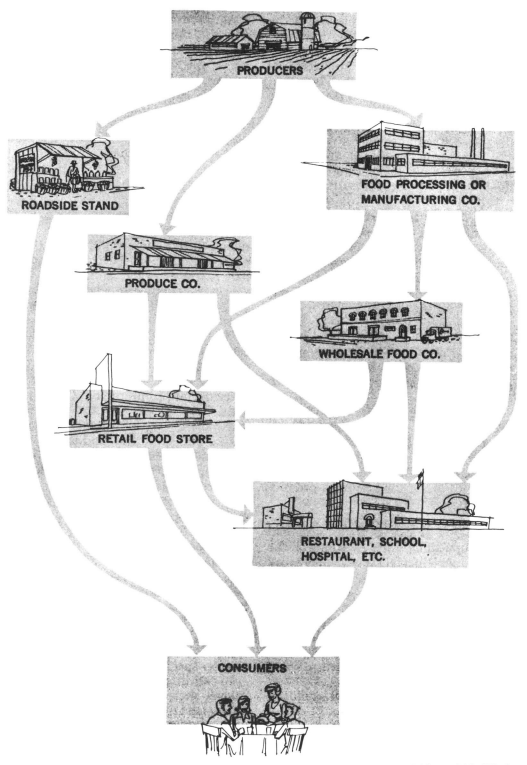

FIG. 12-1. (From Protecting Our Food, Yearbook of Agriculture, 1966. p. 239, Washington, D.C., U.S.D.A.)

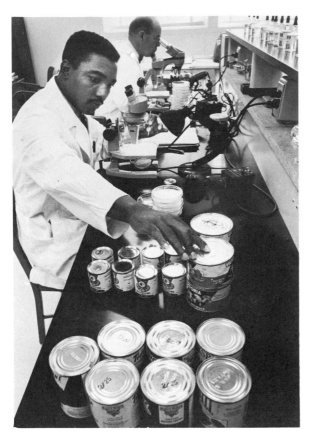

FIG. 12-2. FDA's enforcement effort for foods is mainly concerned with food plant sanitation and the wholesomeness of ingredients and finished products. The Federal Food, Drug, and Cosmetic Act (1938) makes it illegal to ship in interstate commerce a food that comes from unsanitary premises. To enforce this section of the Act, FDA inspects food processors to insure that the factories are sanitary. FDA is responsible for establishing safety standards for additives in foods. (FDA Publ. No. 1. U.S. Dept. HEW, Washington, D.C.)

responsible for protecting the safety of our food supplies. Such agencies as the Food and Drug Administration, the Federal Trade Commission and the Department of Agriculture have extensive programs for safeguarding our foods.

U.S. Department of Health, Education and Welfare—Food and Drug Administration

Federal Food, Drug and Cosmetic Act. Under the Food, Drug and Cosmetic Act, the Food and Drug Administration (FDA) of the Department of Health, Education and Welfare has jurisdiction over the safety of foods shipped interstate or man-ufactured in a territory of the United States or the District of Columbia. Federal regulations also control imported and exported foods. Foods manufactured and sold within a state's boundaries are not subject to Federal regulation but are controlled by the food regulations of the state in which they are produced.

ADULTERATION OF FOODS. A food is considered to be adulterated if it is filthy, putrid or decomposed, if noncertified colors are used, if the container is made of a substance injurious to health (e.g., lead), if there is dilution or substitution, or if there is omission of a valuable ingredient. Food is also considered to be adulterated if it contains meat from a diseased animal or one that died by means other than slaughter.

STANDARDS. Standards of identity, quality and fill have been established under federal regulations. A **standard of identity** defines what a food product is. It determines what ingredients must be included, the minimum and maximum amounts of each and additional ingredients that are optional. Standards of identity have been set for such products as milk and cream; cheese and cheese products; eggs and egg products; margarine; mayonnaise, French dressing and salad dressing; frozen desserts; flours; macaroni and noodle products; jellies and preserves; canned fruit and fruit juices; vegetables and vegetable products. Only the optional ingredients used in these products must appear on the label. Hence, the nurse needs to know that even though salt may not appear in the list of ingredients on the label of the catsup bottle, it is included in the standard of identity; therefore, catsup is a food to be avoided on a sodium-restricted diet.

Standards of quality have been established chiefly for canned fruits, vegetables and meats. Foods that do not meet the minimum standards for quality must be labeled substandard. These foods are not usually sold on the retail market.

Standards of fill are specifications for the amount of food that must be in a container. They were established to prevent the use of deceptive containers and to provide guidelines for foods such as cereals and crackers that tend to "shake down" after being packaged.

PESTICIDE CONTROL. An amendment to the Food, Drug and Cosmetic Act of 1938 was passed in 1954 to establish safe limits of pesticide chemical residues on fresh fruits and vegetables. The chemical pesticide sprays range in toxicity to man from virtually harmless to extremely toxic and dangerous poisons. To control their use the FDA has published a list of more than 2,000 tolerance levels for pesticide chemicals and has established a zero tolerance for certain pesticides such as cyanides, mercury-containing compounds and selenium-containing compounds, which are extremely dangerous.

To protect the consumer, foods which are shipped in violation of FDA regulations are subject to seizure. The manufacturers may be fined and/or imprisoned, depending on the circumstances.

FOOD ADDITIVES. The Food Additives Amendment of 1958 and the Color Additive Amendment of 1960 govern the use of intentional and incidental food additives. These amendments are designed to protect the public from the presence in foods of any substance not demonstrated to be safe under the recommended conditions of use as judged by competent experts.

Food additives are prohibited specifically by the Food, Drug and Cosmetic Act where they are used to mask faulty processing and handling technics, to deceive the consumer and to aid processing at the expense of a substantial reduction of the nutrition value of the product, and where good manufacturing practices do not require the use of an additive to produce a food item economically.

Intentional food additives include preservatives, antioxidants, stabilizers, emulsifiers, coloring and flavoring agents. Well over 1,000 such additives are being used in food processing today, and these are continually being investigated by the Food and Drug Administration.

The GRAS list, published by the FDA, is a list of substances used in food which are *Generally Recognized As Safe*. Other approved food additives not on the GRAS list are known as regulated food additives. All GRAS list items are currently under review to determine their usage rates in the American food supply and their relative safety in terms of amounts consumed. The FDA has recently proposed removing saccharin from the GRAS list and issuing a food additive regulation for it.

The manufacturer has the burden of proof for the usefulness and safety of a proposed additive. Usually, judgment of safety is based on the result of experiments on three or more types of animals to determine acute toxicity and chronic toxicity at levels far above those intended for use in foods. The maximum level of consumption of an additive in a day's food must be determined or estimated. The minimum level which will produce deviations from normal in animals is studied carefully to determine what effects in humans may be expected, and an adequate margin of safety must

be established to reduce to a minimum any hazard to the health of people of varying ages and physiologic states. Any additive shown to be a carcinogen (produce malignant tumors) in any experimental animal is automatically not approved. The removal of cyclamates from the approved list of additives was based on this regulation.

Although safety of food additives is a problem of extreme importance, it is practically impossible to demonstrate absolute proof of safety of an additive for all people in a population which may include a few very sensitive individuals and others in poor physiologic condition, as well as those suffering from a disease of one sort or another.

The incidental additives, usually undesirable, which may appear in food products include:

1. Pesticides (used for plant and animal pest control)
2. Fertilizers (utilized by plants)
3. Feed adjuvants and drugs (antibiotics, hormones, tranquilizers and enzymes)
4. Chemicals used in packaging materials (may migrate into the food)

These regulations are monitored by FDA officials and the public is protected when foods are found which do not conform to them.

Pollution. The hazards of environmental pollution to our food supply have become a national concern. The rapid increase in the contamination of air, water, and soil as a result of increased population and technological advances requires diligent monitoring by those persons responsible for safeguarding the nation's health.

Of special concern is the possible presence of *radioactive materials* in food. For example, the milk supply requires constant radiation surveillance because of the possible presence of strontium-90 or iodine-131, two potentially harmful substances, especially for infants and children. Although most of the Sr-90 is excreted from the body, small amounts may be deposited in bones. Larger amounts of I-131 are absorbed and have a carcinogenic effect on the thyroid gland. Currently the amounts of radioactive fallout in our food supply are well below danger levels.

Very recently, the FDA alerted the public to the excessive amounts of *mercury* in certain types of fish. Swordfish, in particular, has been identified as containing potentially harmful levels and is no longer available on the market. Although the presence of mercury has been detected in tuna fish, these amounts were not as alarming and tuna fish may still be purchased. In fact, most of the fresh tuna fish is now examined before it is canned and only that fish which is below guideline levels is canned for the consumer market.

The pollution of inland lakes and streams and coastal waters from industrial wastes and sewage has not only reduced the available supply of fish from these sources but also has increased the health hazard from the consumption of that supply which remains.

Fair Packaging and Labeling Act. The Fair Packaging and Labeling Act of 1966, known as the "truth in packaging" laws, provides for more informative and more prominent labeling of packaged foods. The regulations concerning labeling include the following requirements: (1) the common name of the food with appropriate descriptions such as whole, sliced, diced or chopped, must appear in bold type on the principal display panel; (2) the name and address of the manufacturer, packer, and distributor must be conspicuous on the package; (3) the net contents of the package must be stated in terms of standard measure and the number and size of servings (no misleading statements such as "giant quart" or "jumbo pound" may be used); (4) the common names of ingredients must be listed in legible type in decreasing order of their prominence in the food.

Nutritional labeling of precooked and processed foods is currently under study by the FDA. It is evaluating various labeling alternatives to determine the most meaningful way of presenting to the consumer the nutrient content of foods. This will be an important first step in a comprehensive nutrition education program for consumers.[1]

Nutritional Guidelines for Classes of Food. At the present time the FDA is in the process of deciding the various classes of food for which nutritional guidelines will be determined. Two of these classes have tentatively been established— complete dinners and formulated main meals— and the guidelines for the complete dinners have recently been published. They include minimum levels for protein, vitamin A, thiamine, riboflavin, niacin and iron. A minimum of 340 calories per precooked meal has also been established for the dinners. Similar guidelines for the formulated main meals should soon be available. The complete dinners include the various frozen, heat-and-serve dinners made from traditional foods, whereas the formulated main meals will be made of the food analogs previously discussed in Chapter 4.

Although the nutritional labeling of these foods will be voluntary, the regulation requires that the declared amount of nutrients on the label must be in the actual item or the product will be declared misbranded.[2] These guidelines should be of considerable help to the nurse in evaluating the nutritional adequacy of an individual's food intake.

U.S. Public Health Service

Standards have been established for the chemical quality of drinking water by the U.S. Public Health Service.[3] The toxic or other physiologic effects from ingestion of excessive quantities of given substances are outlined and limits for their permissible concentration in drinking water are indicated. The chemicals listed include: alkyl benzene sulfonate (detergent), arsenic, barium, cadmium, carbon-chloroform extract, chloride, chromium, copper, cyanide, fluoride, iron, manganese, lead, nitrate, phenols, selenium, silver, sulfate, zinc and total dissolved solids.[4]

Traces of these chemicals and others can get into food in dangerous amounts through ignorance or accident in the home: antimony, cadmium, mercury, insecticides, detergents, kerosene, lye, washing soda and silver polish, to name the more obvious. The swallowing of poisons is a common cause of death among children in the United States. It is imperative that poisonous chemicals be plainly marked and kept as far as possible from food supplies.

Federal Trade Commission

False advertising of foods, drugs and cosmetics through media such as television and radio is under the jurisdiction not of the FDA but of the Federal Trade Commission.

U.S. Department of Agriculture

Federal Meat Inspection Act. Through the Bureau of Animal Industry (BAI), the Secretary of Agriculture administers regulations concerning the meat industry. Formerly, laws provided for the inspection of all cattle, sheep, swine and goats slaughtered for transportation or sale as articles of interstate or foreign commerce. A new law, passed in late 1967, provides for similar inspection and regulation of all meats sold for human consumption anywhere in the United States. The

---

[1] Cooke, J. A.: J. Am. Dietet. A., 59:99, 1971.

[2] Breeling, J. L.: J. Am. Dietet. A., 59:102, 1971.

[3] U.S. Public Health Service: J. Am. Water Works A-53:935, 1961.

[4] Wright, C. V.: Public Health Rep., 77:628, 1962.

carcasses and parts of all such animals found to be sound, healthful, wholesome and fit for human food are stamped "Inspected and Passed." Animals found to be unfit for human food are separated and stamped "Inspected and Condemned." Carcasses which have been condemned for food purposes must be destroyed under the supervision of a Federal inspector.

The Secretary of Agriculture also enforces the regulations concerning imported and exported meat and meat products, as well as the regulation concerning the labeling of horsemeat. Horsemeat may be used for human food, but strict labeling is required to prevent its use as a substitute for beef.

A law passed in 1957 provides for compulsory inspection of poultry and poultry products and is similar in nature to the Meat Inspection Act.

USDA Grade Standards and Inspection Service for Processed Foods. The Fruit and Vegetable Division of the Agricultural Marketing Service, United States Department of Agriculture, develops grade standards for processed foods and supplies an inspection service for processed fruits, vegetables and related foods.

The Federal grading of foods aids in informing processors, sellers, brokers, distributors and buyers concerning the class, the quality and the condition of the product. The grades serve as a basis for arriving at a value of the product for purposes of securing a loan, payment of damages or sale of the product.

State Regulations

It is the responsibility of the states to regulate food production and processing of certain products which do not leave the state. The state also controls such things as pasteurization of milk, inspection of cattle and goats for brucellosis and tuberculosis, and regulations concerning sale of margarine. Many state food regulations are similar to the Federal regulations, but others may prohibit some things which are allowed by Federal law. Food processors must satisfy the regulations of the state in which they operate and the states in which the food is sold, as well as the Federal regulations.

Local municipal sanitary codes may also regulate food production and processing to the extent that they may be more restrictive than state or federal but not less so.

FOOD-BORNE DISEASES AND TOXINS

Foods may be contaminated by a variety of pathogenic organisms. These contaminants may be various worms, molds, bacteria, viruses, and other organisms or the toxins produced by them. The appearance, taste and smell of the food so infected may show no change and thus give no warning to the consumer.

These infections may be present in the food at its source, such as animals infected with tuberculosis, brucellosis, salmonellosis, tularemia, tapeworms or trichinae, and may be carried to the consumer if the food is undercooked.

Food may also be infected by food handlers who are convalescent from infectious diseases. They may be in apparent good health but still carry infectious organisms. The organisms may be distributed on food by hands soiled with urine or feces or by spray of oral and nasal secretions by coughing and sneezing over the food being prepared. Contamination may also come from the butcher block or from the handling of an infected animal before working with the food in question.

Dust falling on uncovered foods and the feces and the bodies of insects may also convey pathogenic organisms to a food supply. Covering of cooked foods and refrigeration can do much to cut down on the number of pathogenic organisms in foods. It is wise to put cooked foods promptly into an efficient refrigerator rather than to allow them to cool thoroughly before refrigerating. Often the period required for cooling in a warm kitchen is sufficient for bacteria to grow rapidly.

Bacterial Contamination of Food and Water

Salmonella infection is a term used to cover a large group of infections caused by several species of the Salmonella organism and common to man and several animals and birds. Salmonellosis is an infection of the intestinal tract, and symptoms begin to appear from 12 to 48 hours after contaminated food has been eaten. Symptoms typically are headache, vomiting, diarrhea, fever and cramps. An attack may last a few hours or several days. Infants and debilitated older people may be most seriously affected and death may result. Antibiotics do little to relieve an attack; fluids and a bland diet are the usual treatment.

The Center for Disease Control in Atlanta, Georgia reported that salmonellosis has become a major national problem, whereas a generation ago it was a medical curiosity. They state that some 20,000 cases of salmonella infection are reported each year but that the actual incidence is probably 2 million cases per year. In this decade salmonella have been traced to well water, frozen turkey, fresh chicken, eggs, smoked fish, ground beef and a contaminated batch of powdered milk.

Many varieties of salmonella may be carried by contaminated foods. Because these bacteria grow easily in moist foods of low acidity and may continue to be viable even in some dry foods, strict control of food sanitation and cooking procedures at home and in institutions, especially, is essential. The usual path of infection is from animals or animal products to man. Precautions in regard to utensils, dishwashing and food handling are outlined by Werrin and Kronick.[5] Salmonella are readily destroyed by usual cooking procedures and by pasteurization but not by freezing. Note the incident of turkey-borne multiple infection below.

The typhoid bacillus is another species of Salmonella and may be carried by contaminated water or shellfish. In the United States, however, an outbreak of typhoid fever can usually be traced to a food handler who is a "carrier" of the organism. Fortunately, the disease responds to an antibiotic, and the course is not as serious as it once was.

Shigellosis is closely related to salmonellosis. Shigella also are enteric bacteria and are the etiologic agents of bacillary dysentery in man. Young children and newborn animals are most seriously affected.

Clostridium perfringens. Perfringens poisoning which results in gastrointestinal disturbances is caused by certain strains of clostridium perfringens, a spore-forming bacteria that grows in the absence of oxygen. The spores are resistant to heat, ordinary cooking, drying, freezing, curing of meats and to irradiation. To prevent their growth meats should be cooked rapidly and refrigerated promptly below 40° F.

The symptoms of *Cl. perfringens* food infection are mild gastroenteritis, abdominal cramps and diarrhea 8 to 16 hours after eating infected food, which may be accompanied by nausea and headache. The illness is usually mild and of short duration, with recovery within 24 hours.

A report of three consecutive outbreaks of food-borne disease in one week was recently investigated and traced to turkey infected with both salmonella and *Cl. perfringens*. The turkey prepared ahead and served at three banquets in one week caused food poisoning in 23 percent of the persons present at the first, in 35 percent of those

at the second and in 69 percent of those at the third banquet. The 20- to 22-pound turkeys had been purchased frozen, thawed at room temperature, boiled for 4 hours and allowed to cool in water overnight. They were stored in a refrigerator but were probably at room temperature for some time during preparation and prior to reheating before service at each banquet. This is an example of poor food handling, if not poor sanitation.[6]

Streptococcal Infections. Hemolytic streptococcus is the type most commonly carried by food. Food and utensils may be contaminated by a carrier, from nasal discharge or skin infection. Strep sore throat, strep ear infections and scarlet fever are all caused by strains of hemolytic streptococci.

Tularemia, sometimes called rabbit fever, is caused by infection with *Pasteurella tularensis*. It is transmitted from rodents by flies, fleas and ticks and may be acquired by man from the handling of infected animals. It is characterized by an ulcer at the site of inoculation, followed by inflammation of the lymph glands and by headache, chills and fever. It is recommended that hunters use rubber gloves when dressing wild game.

Toxins Produced by Bacteria and Molds

Bacterial Exotoxins. The bacteria that produce exotoxins in foods are of two types quite different in growth habits and in the clinical symptoms of poisoning. Staphylococci and *Cl. botulinum* both produce toxins that are stable to heat, although the organisms themselves are destroyed by cooking.

STAPHYLOCOCCUS FOOD POISONING. Staphylococcus bacteria are responsible for many cases of food poisoning. Most people are sensitive to the exotoxins produced by these bacteria, and serious illness can result if enough of the toxin is present in the food. The toxin affects only the gastrointestinal tract, and the onset of symptoms occurs within 2 to 12 hours after infected food is eaten. The symptoms are severe nausea, vomiting and abdominal cramps. This kind of food poisoning is rarely fatal.

Most outbreaks of this type of food poisoning have been caused by the bacteria in prepared or unheated foods such as custard-filled pastries, cream pies, salads, precooked meats such as ham, sandwiches and creamed dishes. The bacteria get into food from boils, infected cuts, coughing, and

[5] Werrin, M., and Kronick, D.: Am. J. Nursing, 65:528, 1965.

[6] Note. Nutr. Rev., 25:94, 1967.

sneezing by food handlers followed by improper storage and inadequate reheating of foods before service. The flavor and appearance of the food may not change. Control of this type of food poisoning is largely a matter of education of food handlers.

BOTULISM.   Botulism is a rare form of food poisoning. It occurs when foods have been underprocessed. Botulin (the toxin) may also be found in some meat products such as sausage (the Latin word for sausage is botulus). Since *Cl. botulinum* is a strict anaerobe, it can grow only under conditions in which air is excluded, such as in a can or deep inside a product.

In recent years commercially processed foods have been relatively free of any poisoning caused by *Cl. botulinum.* However, in 1963 two instances of cases were caused by canned tuna fish and one by smoked fish frozen in polyethylene bags.

In 1971, two cases were reported as the result of the use of canned soup and resulted in a massive recall of all soups and sauces processed by that particular company.

The *toxin* produced is one of the most deadly biologic poisons known. On average, mortality is about 68 percent and ranges from 50 percent to 100 percent in individual outbreaks. Occasionally, entire families are killed by botulism.

The toxin is absorbed directly from the stomach and the intestinal tract. In about 12 to 24 hours it affects the nervous system, causing double vision, difficulty in swallowing, loss of speech and, when lethal, respiratory failure in from 3 to 6 days.

An antitoxin has been developed for the 5 known strains of *Cl. botulinum,* but it is of little value after advanced symptoms appear.

Toxins from Molds (Mycotoxins). Aflotoxin, a toxin produced by *Aspergillus flavus,* a fungus found in peanuts (groundnuts) which have been improperly dried, has been found to be carcinogenic for rats. No acute illness is caused in man from eating these groundnuts in countries where they are staple food, but research is being conducted to investigate the possibility of such mold-produced toxins being carcinogenic in man.[7] Research in India and other Asian countries is aimed at prevention of the damaging mold on peanuts. Commercial peanut products designed for human consumption in the United States are toxin-free, even if produced from contaminated nuts, because any trace of aflotoxin is removed in the refining process.

Naturally Occurring Toxins

It is well known that many varieties of mushrooms are poisonous and have been mistaken for edible types with disastrous results. There is no simple test which will identify edible types other than botanical characteristics.

A few plants used as foods are safe at one time and not at another. The young white shoots of pokeweed frequently are eaten with safety as greens in the early spring, but the later green shoots may cause severe illness. The green leaves of rhubarb may contain enough oxalic acid to cause illness, but the succulent leaf stems are eaten without any untoward effects. Clams and mussels on the Pacific coast may build up toxins during the summer due to an infection from certain plankton.

Viral Infections

Infectious hepatitis is the most common of viral infections spread by contaminated food. It may be spread by the consumption of contaminated water, milk or other food or by the blood of persons carrying the hepatitis virus. A food handler who is a carrier may cut his finger and thus contaminate food and this may not be discovered for some time. The incubation period is from 10 to 50 days and the virus may be in the blood 2 to 3 weeks before the onset of the disease.

Parasitic Infections

Parasitic infections are not confined to the tropics as is sometimes thought. They may be transmitted by food or drink, often by infected fish, shellfish or crustacea.

Trichinosis is the parasitic disease most likely to be encountered in the United States and is caused by improperly cooked pork from pigs that were infected with *Trichinella spiralis.* Symptoms of the infection in man include fever, muscle pain, sweating, chills, vomiting and swollen eyelids. Outbreaks have been reported from homemade sausage and other pork products improperly cured. Trichinosis can be avoided if pork is well-cooked (internal temperature of at least 137° F.) or properly cured.

Protozoan Infections

Amebic Dysentery, caused by *Entamoeba histolytica,* is another infection that may be carried by food and food handlers. It is common in the

---

[7] English, R. M.: Food and nutr. Notes and Reviews, 21:3, 1965. Abs. J. Am. Dietet. A., 47:48, 1965.

tropics. Once it is acquired, the organism remains in the tissues of the intestinal tract and causes intermittent attacks until the individual is treated. Abscesses of the liver may be a complication.

STUDY QUESTIONS AND ACTIVITIES

1. List three technics that are used in scientific farming to increase food production. How is the safety of these methods regulated to protect the consumer?

2. Name some of the activities of the FDA stemming from the Federal Food, Drug and Cosmetic Act.

3. What is meant by standards of identity? What implications are there for the nurse in relation to labeling and standards of identity?

4. What types of food additives may be considered "intentional"? Why are they used and how are they controlled?

5. How would you answer a patient who questioned the safety of the many additives foods contain today? Of the use of pesticides and the danger of traces of these being present in food?

6. What labeling procedures must be followed as a result of the "truth in packaging" law?

7. Which food-borne bacteria, carried most often in eggs or poultry, have been responsible for recent outbreaks of gastrointestinal disease?

8. What disease carried by water, milk or food is due to a virus? How long after exposure may it take to develop?

SUPPLEMENTARY READING ON SAFEGUARDING OUR FOOD SUPPLY

Eyl, T. B.: Alkyl mercury contamination of foods. JAMA, 215:287, 1971.

Food and Drug Administration: Fact Sheets (available from FDA consumer representative). U.S. Dept. H.E.W., Washington, D.C.

Hill, H. H., *et al.*: Food-borne epidemic of streptococcal pharyngitis. New Eng. J. Med., 280:917, 1969.

Hodges, R. E.: The toxicity of pesticides and their residues in food. Nutr. Rev., 23:225, 1965.

Milk-borne diseases. Nurs. Times, 62:1676, 1966.

Milstead, K. L.: Science works through law to protect consumers. J. Am. Dietet. A., 48:187, 1966.

Polk, L. D.: Nursing responsibility in a Salmonella outbreak. Nurs. Outlook, 13:56, 1965.

Public Health Service, U.S. Dept. H.E.W.: You Can Prevent Food Borne Illness. Folder, 1967. Hot Tips on Food Protection. Folder, 1966. Government Printing Office, Washington, D.C. 20201.

Pyke, M.: Food technology and society. Nutr. Rev., 28:31, 1970.

Werrin, M., and Kronick, D.: Salmonella control in hospitals. Am. J. Nursing, 65:528, 1965.

For Further References see Bibliography in Part Four.

PART TWO

Application of Nutrition to Critical Periods Throughout the Life Cycle

Growth and Development

13

Relationship of Nutrition to the Growth Process · The Growth Cycle
Nutrition and Mental Development

RELATIONSHIP OF NUTRITION TO THE GROWTH PROCESS

Introduction

The terms "growth" and "development" imply all the complex physiological changes which take place during conception (when a single-celled ovum is fertilized by a single sperm), during embryogenesis (as cells divide and differentiate to form the structures of the fetus) and during fetal life (as growth and maturation of the fetus occurs). These terms also apply to the complex physiological, psychological and sociological changes which take place during infancy, throughout childhood and adolescence into young adulthood.

Growth and development depend on both the genetic or hereditary background of the individual and the physical and cultural environment into which he is born. The food which provides the nutrients required for physical growth is one environmental factor essential for growth and development, while the feeding process itself, at least during infancy and childhood, is an integral part of psychosocial development. A poor environment—for example, inadequate nutrition—can prevent an individual from reaching his full genetic potential not only in terms of physical size and strength but also, according to all indications of contemporary research, in terms of cognitive development as well.

Growth

Growth occurs continuously from conception to full maturity, but it is not a uniform process. It consists of two periods of rapid growth separated by a period of more or less uniform but slower increase in size. The first period of rapid growth occurs in fetal life and early infancy, the second during adolescence.

Physical growth may be defined as an increase in the size of an individual as measured by changes in weight and/or height. It is an exceedingly complicated process brought about by an increase in the number of cells as a result of cell division and by the enlarging of the size of cells from increases in their protein content. Winick[1] discusses four phases of normal growth:

1. Rapid cell division with cell size remaining constant.
2. Slow-down of cell division accompanied by increase in cell size due to their increased protein content.
3. Cessation of cell division while individual cells continue to grow from increased protein content.
4. Cessation of growth itself as the protein content in the body cells remains constant.

Both animal research and limited studies of humans have shown that different organs are at various phases of growth at different times. However, during prenatal life and for variable periods into postnatal life, all organs are undergoing cell division. The human brain, for instance, reaches its maximum number of cells at about 6 months after birth (the relationship of nutrition to mental development will be discussed later in this chapter). Nerve and lymphoid tissue grow most

_____
[1] Winick, M.: Food and Nutrition News. Vol. 40, No. 7, (April) 1969.

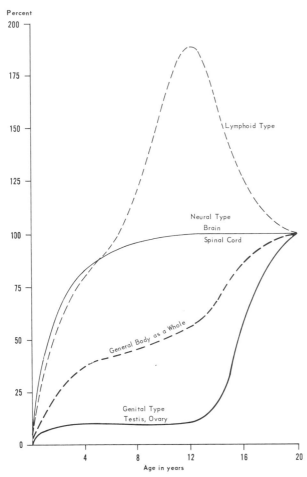

FIG. 13-1. Growth of various body tissues. (Scammon, R. E.: The Measurement of Man. Minneapolis, Univ. Minn. Press, 1930)

rapidly in the early years, the body as a whole more slowly and genital tissues remain almost dormant until puberty. Figure 13-1 shows the different rates of growth for various body tissue.

Obesity in adults may well be related to these phases of growth. There is evidence that infants who are overnourished at the stage when adipose tissue cells are rapidly increasing accumulate more fat cells in their bodies than infants whose weight gain is more carefully controlled. It is believed that this excess of adipose tissue cells persists throughout life with, of course, persistent problems of overweight.[2,3] Infant feeding is discussed in Chapter 15.

Thus the nurse should recognize, when counseling mothers, that undernutrition or overnutrition during the critical phases of growth for an organ can effect the ultimate number of cells in that organ and this in turn may have permanent effect on its function. If undernutrition or overnutrition occurs at a later phase of growth, the size of the organ may be temporarily smaller or larger but returns to normal when the nutritional needs of the individual are met. The degree of recovery seems to depend on when the damage occurred during the growth process; how long it lasted; and how severe it was. Therefore, malnutrition has the most lasting effects when it occurs early in life, persists over a long period of time and is severe enough to suggest or require hospitalization.

Development

Development or maturation refers to the progressive increase in the capacity to function both physically and mentally and is closely associated with growth. The growth process or growth cycle as it is used in this chapter, refers also to development.

THE GROWTH CYCLE

Fetal Growth During Pregnancy. During the first 2 months of pregnancy when various organ systems are developing (differentiation) the growth rate is relatively slow and the quantitative nutritional demands are small. Qualitatively, however, they are extremely important. Animal research indicates that severe malnutrition during embryonic development can produce spontaneous abortions or congenital abnormalities in the newborn. Although these findings have not been proven in humans, there remains the implication that, since this critical period occurs at an earlier stage in pregnancy than most women seek medical advice, it is most desirable for young women to acquire good dietary habits before pregnancy.

The next 7 months of pregnancy are often referred to as the growth period because the weight of the fetus increases 500-fold, from about 6 Gm. at 9 weeks to approximately 3500 Gm. at birth. Inadequate nutrition of the fetus during this time may result in stillbirths, prematurity or "small-for-date" babies. This period of growth, because of its greater nutritional demands, is more sensitive to nutritional inadequacies than the earlier period of differentiation.[4]

[2] Hirsch, J., and Knittle, J. L.: Fed. Proc., 29:1516, 1970.
[3] Eid, E. E.: Brit. Med. J., 2:74, 1970.

[4] Giroud, A.: The Nutrition of the Embryo. Springfield, Ill., Charles C Thomas, 1970.

Throughout the course of pregnancy there is also growth of the maternal tissue. About half of the weight gained during a normal pregnancy represents increases in the mother's tissues—growth of tissues in the uterus, in the breasts and the development of the placenta. Nutritional needs during pregnancy are discussed in Chapter 14.

Infancy—Growth and Development During the First Year. Rapid cell division continues into the postnatal period for varying amounts of time for different organs. During the early months of life growth is more rapid than at any other time of life. The infant will double his birth weight in about 4 months. After that the weekly gain is slower—4 to 5 ounces—for the rest of the year, but he will be likely to triple his birth weight by the end of the first year.

The infant will grow in length, from 20 to 22 inches at birth to 30 to 32 inches at the end of the year. At birth the head is large in proportion to the rest of the body and will continue to grow. This is the time when the brain and nervous system are developing rapidly and during this period a supply of essential nutrients is crucial for normal mental development.

The gastrointestinal system of a full-term infant can digest protein, emulsified fats and simple carbohydrates.

The body of the newborn infant contains a higher proportion of water than that of older children. The muscles are poorly developed and the amount of subcutaneous fat is limited but will increase during the first year. The skeleton is not fully calcified, and there is a high percentage of cartilage. A full-term infant has a store of iron and a high hemoglobin level—nature's way of providing for the early months on milk which is low in iron. The iron stores are gradually depleted, however, unless either the milk is supplemented with iron in some form or iron-rich foods are added 2 or 3 months after birth (see Chap. 15).

Preschool and School Age Growth (1 to 9 years). Growth during the second year of life slows down and a weight gain of 8 to 10 pounds is considered average. Thus the infant who tripled his weight during the first year will be approximately 4 times his birth weight at the end of 2 years. From about 2 to 9 years the average annual weight gain is about 5 pounds.

Annual increments in height gradually decrease from birth to maturity except for the period of the adolescent spurt. Birth length is usually doubled by 4 years and the average gain is about 2 inches per year until adolescence.

Body composition changes during childhood; baby fat disappears at the same time that muscles increase in size and bones harden. Body proportions also become more like the adult form as legs lengthen at a rapid rate while the head growth decelerates. Motor coordination progresses at a fast rate, as does intellectual development.

The Adolescent Growth Spurt. It is during adolescence that the second very rapid growth period occurs. This is usually between the ages of 11 and 14 for girls and 13 and 16 for boys, although it may be sooner for early-maturing children and somewhat later for late-maturing children. The growth spurts at widely different ages occur in all directions—in length and weight of bones, in muscle mass, in the laying down of body fat in the soft tissues, in the widening of the shoulders in boys and the broadening of the hips in girls, and in the accelerated growth of genital tissue. Physiologic age at this period is a much better guide to growth and development than is chronologic age. The total period of rapid growth seldom lasts more than 2 or 3 years, when adult build and stature are reached. However, growth in skeletal muscle mass continues. A further "lengthening out" may occur in both males and females up to age 30. Garn and Wagner point out that, "In a growth sense, adolescence does not terminate with college entrance but continues well beyond, to age 25 to 30 for muscle mass, to age 30 for stature, to age 30 to 40 for skeletal mass and life long for skeletal volume."[5]

Physical growth is usually measured by changes in height and weight with age. Stature is the more significant criterion because variations in build and the amount of adipose tissue may cause wide variations in weight. However, Cheek *et al.* report that the growth of adipose tissue in normal children is so predictable and uniform that weight can be a good measure of "metabolic size" in boys and girls from 5 to 17 years.[6] Development other than physical growth is more difficult

---

[5] Garn, S. M., and Wagner, B.: The adolescent growth of the skeletal mass and its implications to mineral requirements. Chap. 11. *In* Heald, F. (ed.): Adolescent Nutrition and Growth. New York, Appleton-Century-Crofts, 1969.

[6] Cheek, D. B., *et al.*: Body composition: anthropometric growth and heat production. Chap. 12. *In* Heald, F. (ed.): Adolescent Nutrition and Growth. New York, Appleton-Century-Crofts, 1969.

to measure: it deals with muscle strength and coordination, with mental health, and with adaptations and attitudes.

NUTRITION AND MENTAL DEVELOPMENT

One of the most interesting and dramatic aspects of nutrition today is its relationship to mental development in young children. Evidence clearly indicates a close association between severe protein-calorie malnutrition and impaired mental development,[7,8,9] but the degree to which malnutrition alone is the cause of mental retardation has not been clearly defined.

The brain and central nervous system grow rapidly during fetal life and early infancy, and by 6 months of age, the total number of cells in the brain has reached its maximum. By the time a child is 4 years old some 90 percent of the brain has been formed. Along with the increase in size there is a continuous complex evolution of the anatomy, biochemistry and physiology of the brain. The formation and functioning of the brain and nerve fibers and the laying down of the myelin sheaths of the nerves demands that adequate nutrients of the right type be available at this critical period.[10]

During the early formative years the brain acquires each new specific function and integrates the process into its total pattern of performance and experience. Experimental evidence suggests that the timing of this over-all procedure is of utmost importance. Each new function seems to make its appearance chronologically at a critical period of development. Therefore, any disruption of the normal sequence may result in limitation of the capacity of the brain in some specific ability. This damage may not be evident immediately but may show up at a later age.

Studies of the brains of young children who have died of malnutrition and others who died accidentally indicate that severe malnutrition during early life can result in reduced numbers of brain cells in malnourished infants as compared with normal children.[11] The significance of such reduction in the number of brain cells and its effect on brain function is not clearly understood, which leaves us without answers to several important questions. For instance, do any of us reach our total brain capacity potential? If not, to what extent can limitation in cell number be overcome by concerted efforts in intellectual stimulation?

The relationship of malnutrition and mental development in humans is extremely complicated because the environment of poverty in which we find severe malnutrition is almost always lacking in those other characteristics which are also important for an individual to reach full mental potential. The disadvantaged child is therefore at high risk not only in terms of limited physical growth but also in regard to psychosocial and cognitive development. Birch and Gussow discuss many of these problems in their recent book, *Disadvantaged Children, Health, Nutrition and School Failure.*[12]

The immediate program of action seems clear. "Every child born alive is entitled to the normal development of his or her physical and mental potentials."[13] Thus Dr. György prefaced his recommendation that a crash program for better nutrition in early childhood be followed by a long-term educational program toward this same goal. As more and more types of intervention programs for the young child are initiated, particularly in infant and child care centers, it is important that the total growth process of the child be considered by those responsible for program planning. Equal emphasis and attention must be given to the physical, emotional, social and intellectual development of the infant and child. Nurses and others who are involved in the physical care of infants should understand the intimate relationship between the various components of the developmental process. Cuddling, smiling and talking to the baby while he is being fed a nutritionally adequate diet all contribute to his total development. Good mothering with the *wrong* diet is just as devastating as poor mothering with the *right* diet. The goal is good mothering with the right diet.

STUDY QUESTIONS AND ACTIVITIES

1. What is meant by physical growth? How is it accomplished?

2. What are the phases of growth? How do these relate to brain size? to obesity?

---

[7] Cravioto, J., and Delicardie, E.: Am. J. Dis. Child., 120:404, 1970.

[8] Chase, H. P., and Martin, H. P.: New Eng. J. Med., 282:933, 1970.

[9] Yatkin, U. S., and McLaren, D. S.: J. Ment. Defic. Res., 14:25, 1970.

[10] Coursin, D. B.: Undernutrition and brain function. Borden's Rev. Nutr. Res., 26:1, 1965.

[11] Rosso, P., Hormazabal, J. and Winick, M.: Am. J. Clin. Nutr., 23:1275, 1970.

[12] Birch, H. G., and Gussow, J. D.: Disadvantaged Children: Health, Nutrition and School Failure. New York, Harcourt Brace Jovanovich, 1970.

[13] György, P.: Am. J. Clin. Nutr., 14:65, 1964.

3. When are the two periods of most rapid growth? At what age does muscle mass growth cease?

4. What are the differences in nutritional demands during the two stages of pregnancy-differentiation and growth? What are the effects if these demands are not met?

5. What effect does severe malnutrition during infancy have on brain growth?

6. What kinds of growth occur during adolescence?

SUPPLEMENTARY READING ON GROWTH AND DEVELOPMENT

Birch, H. A., and Gussow, J. D.: Disadvantaged Children—Health, Nutrition and School Failure. New York, Harcourt Brace Jovanovich, 1970.

Chase, H. P., and Martin, H. P.: Undernutrition and Child Development. New Eng. J. Med., 282:933, 1970.

Cravioto, J., and DeLicardie, E. R.: The long-term consequences of protein-calorie malnutrition. Nutr. Rev., 29:107, 1971.

Dayton, D. H.: Early malnutrition and human development. Children, 16:210, (Nov.-Dec.) 1969.

Nutrition and Cell Growth. Dairy Council Digest, Vol. 41, No. 6, (Nov.-Dec.) 1970.

Nutrition and Intellectual Growth in Children. Bull. 25A. Washington, D.C., Association for Childhood Education, 1969.

Symposium: Nutrition, Growth and Mental Development. Am. J. Dis. Child., 120:395, 1970.

Winick, M.: Nutrition and the ultimate makeup of various tissues. Food and Nutrition News, Vol. 40, No. 7, (April) 1969.

Nutrition in Pregnancy and Lactation

14

Nutritional Demands of Pregnancy • **Food Selection in Pregnancy**
Complications of Pregnancy Involving Diet • **Diet During Labor**
Diet Following Delivery • **Diet in Lactation**

NUTRITIONAL DEMANDS OF PREGNANCY

Pregnancy makes many demands on the prospective mother, not the least of which are her nutritional needs and those of the unborn infant. Although an undernourished mother may produce a healthy child, studies of nutrition of women during pregnancy have shown a definite relationship between the diet of the mother and the condition of the baby at birth. These studies have also shown that some of the complications of pregnancy, such as anemia, toxemia, and premature delivery, may result from a diet inadequate for the nutritional needs of the mother and the baby.[1] Moreover, if the mother has always eaten a diet adequate in all essentials and is in good health, she has a much better chance of bearing a healthy baby than does the mother who consistently has had a poor food intake.

The Teen-Age Mother. In the United States in 1968, there were 600,815 live babies born to teen-age mothers 19 years and younger. Of these, 9,504 were born to girls under 15 years. These young mothers represent a high risk population because there is more toxemia and an increased number of premature deliveries in this age group.[2] Their diets often consist of cola drinks, potato chips, pizza and hot dogs. It has been found that preeclampsia and essential hypertension occur more often in the white teen-age patients than in patients between 21 and 25 years of age. Weight gain over 25 pounds is

[1] Stearns, G.: JAMA, 168:1655, 1958.
[2] Hassan, H. M., and Falls, F. H.: Am. J. Obst. Gynec., 88:256, 1964.

more common in the young black girls and anemia and essential hypertension are frequent complications in this group.

The percentage of low-birth weight babies (under 2500 Gm.) born to young teen-age mothers is considerably higher than those born to more mature mothers. The highest percentage of low-birth weight infants were born to nonwhite mothers under 15 years of age. Infant mortality rates are also higher for infants born to young mothers, particularly to young girls who have had repeated pregnancies.

Many of these teen-age pregnancies occur out of wedlock and society has imposed certain stigmas upon them and has developed punitive attitudes toward them. The pregnant teen-ager often has to drop out of school; she may be shunned by her family and may find medical care difficult to obtain. Hence, many young people do not have the guidance of a physician or a prenatal clinic early in their pregnancy, and adequate counseling often comes too late for the prevention of complications.

Nutritional requirements for the adolescent during pregnancy vary widely, depending on the rate of growth and stage of maturation of the expectant mother. Early maturing girls who reach menarche at the peak of their growth spurt may conceive before their skeletal, including pelvic, maturation has been completed. Because calorie requirements parallel the growth curve (Figs. 16-1 and 16-2, p. 156), these girls have high caloric needs. Protein and calcium requirements are also high. Calorie restrictions imposed on these teen-agers may not only affect the birth weight of their infants but their own adult stature. Approximately 10 to 12 percent of pregnant teen-agers are overweight and an equal number are underweight. Even for the obese teen-ager who must meet her own nutritional demands as well as those of the fetus, some weight gain should be allowed during pregnancy.[3] The special care that should be given to the diet plans for these young girls is discussed later in this chapter.

Nutrition Studies in Pregnancy. The effect of the food intake on the condition of the newborn baby is best illustrated by the now classic studies of Burke and her coworkers[4] at the Harvard School of Public Health and the Boston Lying-In Hospital. Figure 14-1 shows the relationship of the mother's diet to the health of the baby. In a study of 284 women, it was found that those on good or excellent diets (42 mothers) had babies in good or excellent condition at birth, with only two exceptions. The mothers on fair diets (202 patients) had babies rated largely as good or fair. Those mothers on poor to very poor diets (40 patients) had babies rated as fair or poorest, with

only three exceptions. The poorest infants were those who were stillborn or born prematurely, who died within 3 days of birth, who had congenital defects or who were functionally immature.

The question sometimes is asked, what is meant by a "poor" diet? Such a diet is usually low in most necessary food nutrients; there may even be one food group, such as milk, entirely missing. An example is that of a young, pregnant mother, living in a housing development, whose husband leaves for work early. Usually she gets up and joins him in a cup of coffee and a piece of Danish pastry for breakfast. In the morning and again in the afternoon, she visits her neighbors, at which time more pastry and coffee are consumed. Often she is not hungry at lunch, nor does she enjoy preparing food only for herself, so that frequently lunch either is skipped or takes the form of a piece of fruit. Fortunately, this patient has a good dinner when her husband returns in the evening, but this is not sufficient to meet her nutritional needs, except perhaps for calories. Another patient drank up to 15 cups of tea daily, each with 2 teaspoonfuls of sugar, and consequently was seldom hungry for other food.

It will be seen from the foregoing that the importance of nutrition in pregnancy is poorly recognized by a large section of the population,

---

[3] Committee on Maternal Nutrition–Food and Nutrition Board: Maternal Nutrition and the Course of Pregnancy. National Academy of Sciences–National Research Council. Summary Report. Washington, D.C., 1970.

[4] Burke, B. S., *et al.*: J. Nutr., 38:453, 1949.

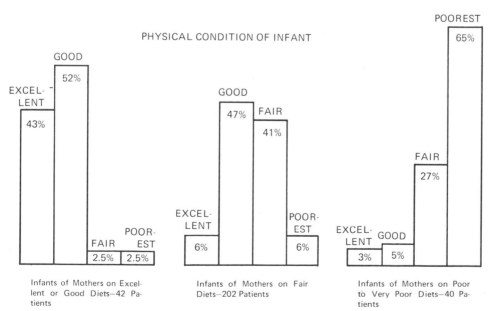

PHYSICAL CONDITION OF INFANT

Infants of Mothers on Excellent or Good Diets—42 Patients

Infants of Mothers on Fair Diets—202 Patients

Infants of Mothers on Poor to Very Poor Diets—40 Patients

FIG. 14-1. Condition of infants at birth in relation to the prenatal diet of the mother. Note the decrease in excellent and good ratings for infants and the increase in fair and poorest infants as the diet goes from good to poor. (Adapted from Burke, B. S., *et al.*: J. Nutrition, 38:453, 1949)

and that nurses, as well as many others in the medical field, must assume more responsibility for teaching this group better nutrition.

Nutritional Requirements. Table 14-1 shows the Recommended Dietary Allowances for girls and women at various ages with added allowances for pregnancy. These will vary with the weight, the age and the activity of the mother, and should be used only as a guide.

CALORIES. If the physical activity of the woman remains the same during the second and third trimesters of pregnancy, an additional 200 calories is suggested to meet the energy costs of pregnancy. The building of new tissue in the mother, the placenta and fetus, an increased work load associated with the activity of the mother and an increased basal metabolic rate contribute to increased calorie needs. However, decreased physical activity, particularly during the third trimester, may more than compensate, to the point that no additional calories may be needed. The physician, by carefully observing weight changes, is best able to recommend necessary calorie modifications. In any case the calorie increase is small, and foods must be carefully chosen if the other nutrient increases are to be met while keeping the total calories within the recommended allowance. Table 14-2 shows a suggested dietary pattern during pregnancy.

PROTEIN REQUIREMENT. The protein intake must be increased in pregnancy because of its specific contributions to growth and because, as a rule, a diet low in protein is lacking in other nutrients. An additional allowance of 10 Gm. of protein is therefore recommended to provide the protein which is accumulated by the fetus and accessory tissues during pregnancy.

Extra protein in the diet will be supplied by additional milk, meat, poultry, fish and eggs (Table 14-2). Skim milk, liquid or dried, can

TABLE 14-1. RECOMMENDED DAILY DIETARY ALLOWANCES FOR GIRLS AND WOMEN AT VARIOUS AGES, WITH ADDED ALLOWANCES FOR PREGNANCY*

	RECOMMENDED DAILY ALLOWANCES FOR NONPREGNANT WOMEN					RECOMMENDED DAILY ALLOWANCES ADDED FOR PREGNANCY
	12-14† years old	14-16‡ years old	16-18§ years old	18-22‖ years old	22-35‖ years old	
Calories (K cal)	2,300	2,400	2,300	2,000	2,000	200
Protein (Gm.)	50	55	55	55	55	10
Vitamin A (I.U.)	5,000	5,000	5,000	5,000	5,000	1,000
Vitamin D (I.U.)	400	400	400	400	. .	0††
Vitamin E (I.U.)	20	25	25	25	25	5
Ascorbic acid (mg.)	45	50	50	55	55	10
Folacin (mg.)	0.4	0.4	0.4	0.4	0.4	0.4#
Niacin (mg. equiv.)	15	16	15	13	13	2
Riboflavin (mg.)	1.4	1.4	1.5	1.5	1.5	0.3
Thiamin (mg.)	1.2	1.2	1.2	1.0	1.0	0.1
Vitamin B_6 (mg.)	1.6	1.8	2.0	2.0	2.0	0.5
Vitamin B_{12} (µg)	5	5	5	5	5	3
Calcium (Gm.)	1.3	1.3	1.3	0.8	0.8	0.4
Phosphorus (Gm.)	1.3	1.3	1.3	0.8	0.8	0.4
Iodine (µg)	115	120	115	100	100	25
Iron (mg.)	18	18	18	18	18	**
Magnesium (mg.)	350	350	350	350	300	150

* From the Committee on Maternal Nutrition—Food and Nutrition Board: Maternal Nutrition and the Course of Pregnancy. National Academy of Sciences—National Research Council. Washington, D.C., 1970.

† Body size, 44 Kg.; height, 154 cm.

‡ Body size, 52 Kg.; height, 157 cm.

§ Body size, 54 Kg.; height, 160 cm.

‖ Body size, 58 Kg.; height, 163 cm.

The diet may be supplemented with 0.2-0.4 mg. of folacin daily.

** It is recommended that the diet be supplemented with 30-60 mg. of iron per day.

†† 400 I.U. of Vitamin D are recommended for the pregnant adult woman.

be used to increase protein without adding considerably to the total calorie intake. Inexpensive dried skim milk can be used in creamed soups and casserole dishes; 1 or 2 tablespoons can also be added to regular milk to increase the protein content. Sample menus which meet the recommended dietary allowances for pregnancy are shown in Table 14-3.

CALCIUM AND PHOSPHORUS REQUIREMENTS. The pregnant woman must be supplied with calcium and phosphorus in quantities large enough for her own needs and those of the bony framework of the body of the growing fetus and for the formation of its teeth. An additional allowance of 0.4 Gm. is recommended at this time. Again, a quart of milk a day will supply a large proportion of the needed calcium and phosphorus, as well as a good proportion of the necessary protein.

MAGNESIUM REQUIREMENT. The NRC-RDA recommends an additional 150 mg. of magnesium during pregnancy. The additional milk, plus the meat, whole grain cereals, vegetables and fruit will supply the extra amount.

IRON REQUIREMENT. An adequate iron supply during pregnancy is no less important than that of calcium. Besides the mother's need for iron, the developing fetus is building its own blood supply. When the baby is born, his blood has a hemoglobin content of from 20 to 22 Gm. per 100 ml. This high level is needed in fetal life for oxygen uptake at the placenta, where oxygen is at lower pressures than it is in the lungs. Soon after birth some of the hemoglobin begins to break down until a normal level of 13 to 14 Gm. per 100 ml. of blood is reached. The iron from the hemoglobin breakdown is stored in the infant's liver to serve as a supply during the first few months of life when his diet of milk provides little iron. If the mother's intake of iron is low, this will reflect itself in the level of her own hemoglobin and, eventually, in the level of hemoglobin and available iron for storage in the infant.

Foods especially high in iron, such as livers of beef, chicken and pork, should be included frequently in the pregnant woman's diet. Other good sources are heart, kidney, tongue, all lean meats, chicken, eggs, most green, leafy vegetables, potatoes, whole-grain or enriched bread, dried fruits and dried peas and beans. It is not always easy to include sufficient iron in the daily diet, especially in the low-income group. The physician may prescribe some type of supplementary source of iron. Because of the difficulty of obtaining a sufficient intake of iron from food alone, the National Research Council's Committee on Maternal Nutrition recommends that the diet of the pregnant woman be supplemented with 30 to 60 mg. of iron per day as medication.

IODINE REQUIREMENT. Iodine is also an important element in the diet of the pregnant woman. An additional 25 mcg. of iodine is recommended during pregnancy. A deficiency of this element during pregnancy may cause goiter in the child or in the mother. The use of iodized salt is suggested for those who live in areas in which the soil and the drinking water are known to be deficient in iodine.

VITAMIN REQUIREMENTS. All vitamins are essential for the metabolism of living tissue, and doubly so in growth.

Foods rich in vitamins are those which have been discussed as essential for other nutrients: milk and milk products, eggs, meat, fish and poultry, and especially liver, whole-grain and enriched breads, green and yellow vegetables, citrus fruits, tomatoes, cabbage and potatoes. All these must be supplied liberally in the diet of the pregnant woman if she is to meet her own nutritional needs as well as those of the growing fetus.

The proper utilization of calcium and phosphorus depends on the inclusion of a certain amount of vitamin D in the diet. Most areas today offer both whole and skim fluid milk to which 400 I.U. of vitamin D per quart have been added. Some physicians order vitamin D for their patients as a medication, although not all obstetricians subscribe to this practice. Because of recent evidence indicating a relationship between abnormal calcium deposition in infants and excessive vitamin D intakes during pregnancy, the pregnant woman should be cautioned against overdosage with supplements.

Mineral oil in any form interferes with the absorption of the fat-soluble vitamins and should be avoided, if possible.

In addition to increased amounts of thiamine, riboflavin, niacin, vitamins B_6 and B_{12}, and ascorbic acid (Table 14-1), the pregnant woman may require a daily supplement of 0.2 to 0.4 mg. of folacin to prevent megaloblastic anemia (see Anemias of Pregnancy). The use of vitamin supplements (except possibly for folic acid and vitamin D) is not necessary unless, because of illness or other problems, the mother is unable to eat an adequate diet. The physician is best able to determine whether or not supplements are needed.

FOOD SELECTION IN PREGNANCY

Table 14-2 lists the foods and the quantities of each that, if consumed daily by the pregnant woman, will meet the Recommended Dietary Allowances. Such a food intake represents the so-called excellent diet found by investigators to be most likely to produce a superior infant and to maintain the mother's health at an optimum. Routine salt restriction or too rigid weight control should not be necessary if the pregnancy is proceeding normally.

Two menus based on the foregoing table, one for the adult pregnant woman and one for the pregnant adolescent girl, are presented in Table 14-3. It is assumed that both are of normal weight. Note that calories and calcium have been increased in the menu for the pregnant adolescent girl to provide for her own growth needs and those of the fetus.

Adaptations for Cost and Food Habit Patterns. It may be difficult for the mother to follow the suggested diet pattern if she has a strong dislike for a food such as milk or liver, if her food habits are culturally very different, or, most frequent of all, if the cost of the diet is higher than she can afford. However, some adaptations can be made without impairing the nutritive value of the diet too greatly. The use of dried skim milk for part or all of the whole milk will lower the cost substantially. The use of chocolate and coffee flavor, a dash of vanilla extract or of cinnamon or nutmeg may change the taste of milk sufficiently so that the mother will drink it. Some women who do not like whole milk because it makes them "sick" may be able to drink buttermilk. Milk, either fluid or dried, may be used in desserts, creamed soups and scalloped dishes. As has already been indicated, a 1-ounce slice of Cheddar (hard) cheese has approximately the same protein and calcium content as an 8-ounce glass of milk. This may be an acceptable substitute for Italian patients, who use cheese somewhat more readily than large quantities of milk. Liver, another food sometimes heartily disliked, may be eaten as liverwurst or as a liver spread in a sandwich, or it may be disguised in a variety of ways in cooked dishes.

In general, meat and eggs are expensive foods. Dried beans and peas, used by many groups in the United States as well as in many other countries, serve as a partial substitute at much lower cost. However, they must not replace the use of animal protein to too great a degree, for the legumes do not supply as good a quality of protein. Fish and eggs are excellent meat substitutes in areas and at times of year when they are cheap. Meats such as heart and tongue are less expensive than other cuts and add variety to the diet.

Fruits and vegetables, bought fresh in season, are usually least expensive. However, the frozen fruit juices, especially orange and grapefruit juice, and canned tomato juice are comparatively inexpensive sources of vitamin C all the year round. In the southeastern section of the United States, the frequent use of greens with their accompanying "pot liquor" provides a considerable source of calcium and vitamin C in the diet. Carrot sticks and celery strips, stored in the refrigerator, will provide the mother with a low-calorie snack to satisfy her craving for nibbling and at the same time help to meet her vegetable requirements.

Desserts made from milk, eggs and fruit, unsweetened or flavored with noncaloric sweetening, give a psychological "lift" to the pregnant woman.

Pica. An abnormal craving for nonfood substances (pica), such as starch and clay, has been

---

TABLE 14-2. SUGGESTED DIETARY PATTERN
DURING PREGNANCY

Whole or skimmed milk: 1 qt. (1 oz. of Cheddar cheese is equivalent to 8 ozs. milk.)

Lean meat: One liberal or 2 small servings (4 ozs.) of meat, fish or fowl; liver is desirable at least once each week.

Egg: One each day.

Fruit: Two or more servings (1 cup, 200 Gm.) each day. One serving should be citrus fruit or other good source of ascorbic acid.

Vegetables: Two or more servings of cooked or raw vegetables (1-1½ cups, 200-300 Gm.) each day; these should include dark green leafy or deep yellow vegetables; in addition, a medium potato (150 Gm.) should be eaten daily.

Bread and cereal: Whole-grain or enriched bread, at least 4 slices daily (½ cup of cereal is equivalent to 1 slice of bread).

Butter or margarine: One to 2 tablespoons.

Additional foods: Consisting of either more of the foods already listed or other foods of one's own choice adjusted to individual energy needs and in relation to desired weight gain.

Vitamin D: Some form of vitamin D to supply 400 I.U. such as 1 qt. of milk would supply.

reported by certain women during pregnancy. This practice appears to be most prevalent among black women, particularly in the south where it is often a traditional practice accepted within the immediate community. A study[5] by Edwards and associates in Alabama showed that the caloric intake of pregnant women who consumed starch and clay was reduced when these substances were omitted from the diet, indicating that they were either appetite stimulators or that deprivation of them was so emotionally upsetting as to reduce appetite. In general, the diets of these women tended to be low in protein, iron and calcium. Although the birth weight and length of the infants born to these mothers were similar to those of the control groups' infants, fewer babies born to the starch- and clay-eating mothers were rated in good condition at birth.

_____

[5] Edwards, C. H., *et al.*: J. Am. Dietet. A., 44:109, 1964.

Nutrition Education. The need of the pregnant girl or woman for nutrition information will vary with each patient. The mother having her second or third baby who feeds her family with good judgment will probably do the same for herself. All she may need is a review of dietary essentials with perhaps some suggestions for the less costly foods if her income is limited. On the other hand, a mother with a large family and a low income may need considerable guidance in wise spending. National and cultural dietary patterns will influence the choice of foods in many families and need to be reckoned with. Chapters 10 and 11 will be of help in this matter.

The most urgent nutritional problem is that of the very young pregnant woman. It has been said that "nutrition for pregnancy begins before conception," and, above all, this is true of the mother under 20. The diet of many teen-age girls is low in calcium and vitamin C. There is also a tendency to an inadequate iron intake.

TABLE 14-3. SAMPLE MENUS FOR PREGNANCY

FOR PREGNANT WOMEN OF NORMAL WEIGHT	FOR PREGNANT ADOLESCENT GIRLS OF NORMAL WEIGHT
Breakfast	*Breakfast*
Orange juice—4 oz.	Orange juice—4 oz.
Scrambled egg	Cornflakes or grits
Toast—1 slice	Scrambled egg
Butter or margarine	Toast—1 slice
Coffee	Jelly
	Milk—½ pint
Midmorning	*Midmorning*
Milk—½ pint	Milk—½ pint
Lunch	*Lunch*
Meat, cheese or peanut butter sandwich	Hamburger on a bun
Carrot sticks	Cole slaw
Oatmeal cookies	Oatmeal cookies
Milk—½ pint	Fresh fruit
	Milk—½ pint
Midafternoon	*Midafternoon*
Milk—½ pint	Frankfurter on a bun
	Milkshake or fruit juice—½ pint
Dinner	*Dinner*
Roasted or broiled beef, pork, liver or fish	Roasted or broiled beef, pork, liver or fish
Broccoli or greens	Broccoli or greens
Baked potato	Baked or French fried potatoes
Butter or margarine	Butter or margarine
Green salad with French dressing	Green salad with French dressing
Fresh or canned fruit	Fruit or ice cream
Coffee, tea or milk	Milk—½ pint
Bedtime	*Bedtime*
Milk or cocoa—½ pint	Milk shake or cocoa—½ pint

The nurse, the dietitian and the doctor will have to use patience, imagination and persistence in persuading mothers who are not doing so to follow an adequate diet. The woman who asks for calcium pills because she does not like milk needs to be taught that milk is a rich source of other needed nutrients besides calcium and be encouraged to use a variety of methods for including it in her diet. On the other hand she may be allergic to milk or lactase deficient and will require calcium pills. The young girl needs help in understanding her body's new needs, and possibly the help of the social worker or community agency in providing a good diet. The use of the attractive health literature available may aid the mother in following an improved diet, both for herself and for her family.[6] It is very possible that the foundation for good nutrition for the whole family may be laid in the obstetrician's office or the prenatal clinic.

COMPLICATIONS OF PREGNANCY INVOLVING DIET

Vomiting. During the first trimester of pregnancy the mother-to-be may be troubled with nausea. Certain foods which previously have been

---

[6] Good examples are Prenatal Care, Children's Bureau Publication No. 4, 1962, and When Your Baby is on the Way, Children's Bureau Publication No. 391, 1961, U.S. Dept. of Health, Education and Welfare. Local and state health departments also have good material available.

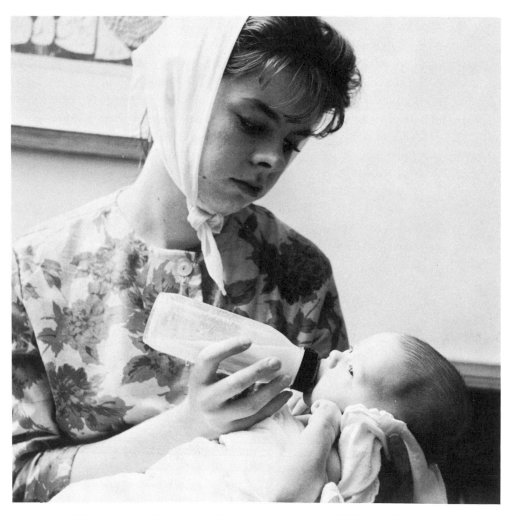

FIG. 14-2. Many of today's new mothers are teen-agers. (Children's Bureau photograph)

eaten without difficulty now may cause distress. Fats are a common cause of upset. Fluids taken with meals may also precipitate vomiting. Dry toast or a few unsalted crackers eaten before arising may be of help. Fluids should be drunk between meals, not with the meal. Skim milk may be tolerated better than whole milk. Often the nausea disappears by the middle of the day, and the mother can make up her dietary needs by increasing her food intake in the late afternoon, at dinner and before bedtime.

Vomiting, if it persists and becomes pernicious, should be treated by a physician.

Overweight in Pregnancy. Pregnancy usually is a time of well-being and often is accompanied by an excellent appetite. Most doctors guard against excessive weight gain as being detrimental to both the mother and the fetus. Figure 14-4 shows a pattern of normal prenatal gain in weight. Certain factors contribute to some variability in weight gain. Teen-age mothers tend to slightly higher

gains than more mature women; thin women gain more than obese women. Women having their first pregnancy gain more than women having second, third or fourth babies.

The Committee on Maternal Nutrition has stated the following in relation to nutrition and weight gain during pregnancy:[7]

An average weight gain during pregnancy of 24 lb. (range 20-25 lb.) is commensurate with a better than average course of pregnancy. This would be a gain of 1.5 to 3.0 lb. during the first trimester and a gain of 0.8 lb. per week during the remainder of pregnancy. There is no scientific justification for routine limitation of weight gain to lesser amounts. . . .

The pattern of weight gain is of greater importance than the total amount—a sudden sharp increase after about the 20th week of pregnancy may indicate water retention and the possible onset of pre-eclampsia. There is no evidence that the total amount of gain dur-

---

[7] Committee on Maternal Nutrition–Food and Nutrition Board: op. cit., p. 13.

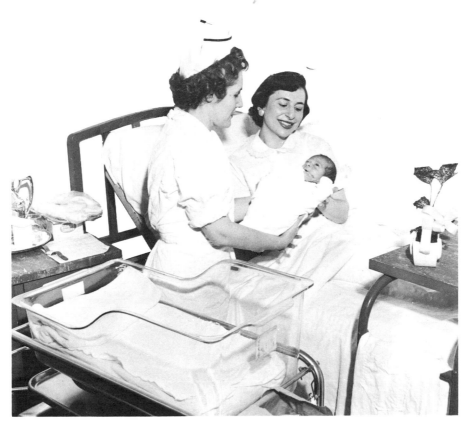

Fig. 14-3. The desirable outcome of pregnancy: a healthy, happy mother and baby. (The New York Hospital)

ing pregnancy has, per se, any causal relationship to pre-eclampsia.

Severe caloric restriction, which has been very commonly recommended, is potentially harmful to the developing fetus and to the mother, and almost inevitably restricts other nutrients essential for growth processes. Weight-reduction regimes, if needed, should be instituted only after pregnancy has terminated.

Care must be taken that any calorie-restricted diet in pregnancy is not so low in calories that the protein in the diet is used partly for energy instead of for growth. Oldham[8] has shown that this occurs when the diet is below 1,500 calories, even when the protein of the diet is adequate. Probably no diet in pregnancy should fall below 1,500 calories, and it may be more realistic to allow the mother an 1,800 calorie diet. If she adheres to this, there should be no impairment of her health or of the baby's, and her weight gain should remain at a minimum.

___

[8] Oldham, H.: Bull. Matern. Welf., 4:10, 1957.

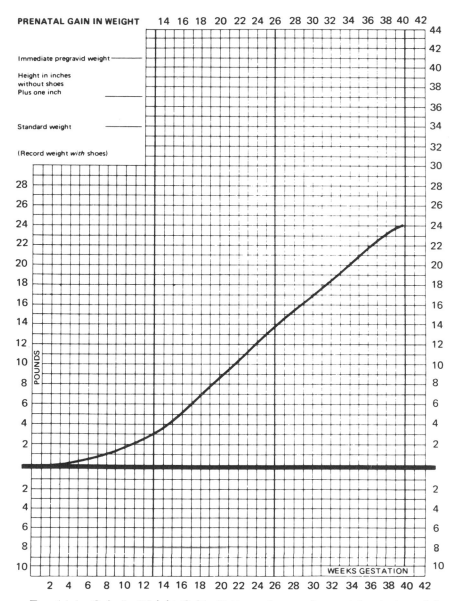

FIG. 14-4. Gain In Weight Grid. Pattern of normal prenatal gain in weight. Source: U.S. Department of Health, Education, and Welfare, Social and Rehabilitation Service, Children's Bureau.

If there is a tendency to gain too much weight, such foods as sugar, candy, jelly and other sweets, salad dressings, fried foods, fatty meats, cake, pie and desserts, and carbonated beverages should be limited or omitted entirely. It may be necessary to limit bread and potatoes; and skim milk may be substituted for whole milk (see Chap. 21).

A problem arises with the mother who believes that milk is "fattening" and reduces or omits it in her diet. As explained earlier, the substitution of calcium pills for milk markedly lowers the protein and the vitamin content of the diet and should be discouraged.

Table 14-4 shows a comparison of the recommended diet for pregnancy for a woman of normal weight, containing approximately 2,200 calories, and the restrictions necessary to bring this down to 1,800 and 1,500 calories. All these meet the Recommended Dietary Allowances for specific nutrients, except for calories (in the 1,800 and the 1,500 calorie diets) and iron. The physician may wish to prescribe folacin and iron supplementation as a precaution against the anemias of pregnancy.

Underweight in Pregnancy. The severely underweight woman and the woman who does not gain normally during her pregnancy are of as great concern as the obese mother. The reason for the underweight may be economic; this may often be discovered by the nurse, who will direct the patient to the social worker or a community agency for help. If the cause is psychological—such as a severe depression—or physical, the doctor will take the appropriate measures. Undernutrition can be as dangerous to the health of both the mother and the baby as overnutrition.

Anemias of Pregnancy. In the latter months of pregnancy there may be a slight lowering of the hemoglobin content of the mother's blood due to physiologic adjustments. By this time her total blood volume has increased considerably to provide for the placental circulation. This may not be accompanied by a corresponding increase in red blood cells; consequently, a degree of hemo-

TABLE 14-4. DIETS FOR PREGNANCY VARYING IN CALORIC CONTENT*

	2,200 CALORIES	1,800 CALORIES	1,500 CALORIES
Milk	1 qt. whole	1 qt. whole	1 qt. skimmed
Meat, fish and poultry	4 ozs.	4 ozs. lean	4 ozs. lean
Eggs	1	1	1
Fruit	2 servings citrus, 1 other	2 servings citrus, 1 other	2 servings citrus, 1 other
Vegetables	4 servings, including potato and dark green leafy or yellow vegetable	4 servings, including potato and dark green leafy or yellow vegetable	4 servings, including potato and dark green leafy or yellow vegetable
Bread and cereals	4 servings whole grain or enriched	4 servings whole grain or enriched	4 servings whole grain or enriched
Butter or margarine	3 teaspoons	3 teaspoons	3 teaspoons
Other foods	Sugar, desserts, fat for cooking; other foods to meet caloric needs	None. Saccharin may be used for sweetening.	None. Saccharin may be used for sweetening.

These diets may be restricted in sodium as follows (see Chap. 24 for details of food restriction):

1. *Moderate sodium restriction*—1,000 to 1,500 mg. sodium. Prepare all food without salt; do not add salt at table; omit all salted foods such as salt butter and bacon.

2. *Severe sodium restriction*—300 to 400 mg. sodium. Prepare all food without salt; do not add salt at table; omit all salted foods such as salted butter and bacon. Use only low sodium milk. Use only fruit for dessert.

* From the Woman's Clinic of The New York Hospital. The above diets meet the Recommended Dietary Allowances of the National Research Council for pregnancy with the exception of calories for the 1,800 and the 1,500 calorie diets and iron in all diets.

dilution occurs. However, it is of slight degree and usually is not mistaken for anemia of pregnancy.

True anemia occurring during pregnancy is due most often to an iron deficiency. Even healthy American women usually do not have iron stores large enough to meet the demands of pregnancy. Iron supplementation will aid greatly in maintaining the hemoglobin at normal levels in these patients. During the second and third trimester of pregnancy, an oral iron supplement of 30 to 60 mg. of ferrous salts is recommended. It is also essential, however, that the mother be urged to include foods rich in iron and protein in her diet, or other deficiencies may appear.

As explained earlier in this chapter, the infant's level of hemoglobin at birth and the supply of iron available for storage for use in the first few months of life are curtailed when the mother's iron intake is inadequate. The result is anemia of infancy, which is not an uncommon finding.

Megaloblastic anemia of pregnancy may be due to a poor food intake, vomiting, the fetal demands for folacin, or an unknown metabolic defect in the absorption or synthesis of folic acid coenzymes.[9] It is characterized by an extremely low

red blood cell count and an equally low hemoglobin and has some other findings associated with pernicious anemia, with which it may be confused. The administration of folic acid causes an immediate and dramatic rise in red blood cells and hemoglobin, and in appetite. Recent studies indicate that the folic acid requirement during pregnancy is greatly increased as compared with the minimum adult requirement.[10] The Committee on Maternal Nutrition suggests a supplement of 400 mcg. of folacin. If the mother does not receive treatment before the birth of the baby, the infant also will show some of the symptoms of megaloblastic anemia. It may be treated with folic acid, or, if the mother is being treated while nursing, the infant will receive enough folic acid from its mother's milk to restore its blood components to normal.

Toxemia of Pregnancy. The cause of toxemia of pregnancy is not known. It is characterized by an elevation in blood pressure, albuminuria and rapid weight gain due to edema. In the eclamptic stage there may be convulsions and coma. There is considerable controversy over the influence of nutrition on the development of toxemia. Toxemia occurs more frequently in pregnant women on

[9] Recommended Dietary Allowances, Revised. p. 35. National Academy of Sciences–National Research Council Publ. No. 1694. Washington, D.C., 1968.

[10] Alperin, J. B., *et al.*: Arch. Int. Med., 117:681, 1966. Willoughby, M. L. N., and Jewell, F. J.: Brit. Med. J., 5529:1568, 1966.

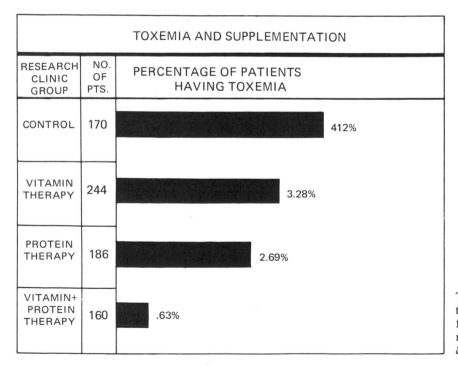

FIG. 14-5. (Tompkins, W. T., and Wiehl, D. G.: Nutritional deficiencies as a causal factor in toxemia and premature labor. Am. J. Obst. & Gynec., 62:898, 1951)

poor diets, and particularly on low protein intakes, than in corresponding groups on good diets. Epidemiologic studies show a direct relationship between the incidence of toxemia and an individual state's per capita income. The poorer the state the greater the number of cases of toxemia reported.[11]

Burke's findings[12] show that 44 percent of the women on poor or very poor diets, 8 percent on fair diets, and none on good or excellent diets developed symptoms of toxemia. Tompkins and Wiehl[13] have shown that supplementation of the diet with protein and vitamins greatly reduced the incidence of toxemia in their patients (see Fig. 14-5). Although McGanity[14] and his group in Nashville, Tenn., were not able to relate nutritional status to the health of the mother during pregnancy as clearly as other investigators, they do report an increased incidence of toxemia in mothers who ate less than 1,500 calories and 50 Gm. of protein per day during the last trimester. All these findings reinforce what was said earlier in this chapter; we have not so far provided adequate medical care, including nutrition education, for all those requiring such help during pregnancy.

Once toxemia has occurred, the dietary treatment of it varies, depending on the severity of the symptoms. In the early stages, a diet high in protein, minerals and vitamins, and low in sodium may best meet the needs of the patient. Suggestions for the restriction of sodium and calories, while maintaining the protein intake, will be found in Table 14-4 on page 133.

In the past few years a question has arisen about the relation of salt intake to toxemia. Robinson,[15] studying over 2,000 pregnant women, advised half to increase their salt intake and half to lower it. He found a lower incidence of toxemia in those having the higher salt intake. More recently, Mengert[16] placed 48 patients with proven toxemia either on a high salt intake or on a very low one. No difference in the progress of the disease was noted between the two groups of women in this study. The Committee on Maternal Nutrition dis-

courages the routine use of salt restriction and diuretics during pregnancy.

Cardiac Disease and Pregnancy. It should be remembered that the nutritional requirements of the pregnant woman with cardiac disease are the same as those of the non-cardiac pregnant patient. If it is necessary to limit the mother's salt intake, note the suggestions for moderate sodium restriction in footnote of Table 14-4. The very low sodium diet probably should be reserved for the patients being cared for in the hospital.

Diabetes and Pregnancy. Again the mother's diet must be increased to meet her larger needs and those of the growing fetus. The insulin dosage may have to be augmented accordingly. For further discussion of pregnancy and diabetes see Chapter 22.

DIET DURING LABOR

During the early part of labor, if feeding by mouth is permitted by the physician, the diet should consist mainly of carbohydrates, as they leave the stomach quickly. Protein and fat tend to remain in the stomach considerably longer, which may result in aspiration if anesthesia is given. The diet may be soft or liquid and may include white-bread toast with jelly, soda crackers, canned or cooked fruits, gelatin, fruit juices, ginger ale, broth and tea or coffee with sugar but no milk or cream. By the time the patient is in active labor, most obstetricians prefer that no food be given by mouth so as to prevent the possibility of vomiting and of aspiration of food into the trachea. Intravenous fluids are given to maintain water balance if labor is prolonged.

DIET FOLLOWING DELIVERY

A liquid diet usually is given for the first meal after delivery. After that, there is a return to the normal diet. If the mother nurses the baby, there must be an even greater allowance of food than there was during pregnancy.

DIET IN LACTATION

Lactation makes even greater demands in some respects on the maternal organism than does pregnancy. After birth the child still may be fed from the mother's body, the food now being produced by the mammary glands instead of being supplied through the blood stream, as before birth. As the baby gains in weight and becomes increasingly active, the food supply from the mother must increase.

[11] Committee on Maternal Nutrition–Food and Nutrition Board, op. cit., p. 163.
[12] Burke, B. S., and Kirkwood, B. B.: Am. J. Public Health, 40:960, 1950.
[13] Tompkins, W. T., and Wiehl, D. G.: Am. J. Obstet. Gynec., 62:898, 1951.
[14] McGanity, W. J., et al.: Am. J. Obstet. Gynec., 67:501, 1954.
[15] Robinson, M.: Am. J. Obstet. Gynec., 76:1, 1958.
[16] Mengert, W. F.: Am. J. Obstet. Gynec., 81:601, 1961.

TABLE 14-5. RECOMMENDED DIETARY ALLOWANCES FOR THE LACTATING WOMAN 22 to 35 YEARS, 58 KG., 160 CM.

NUTRIENT	AMOUNT	
Calories	3,000	
Protein	75	Gm.
Vitamin A	8,000	I.U.
Vitamin D	400	I.U.
Vitamin E	30	I.U.
Ascorbic Acid	60	mg.
Folacin	0.5	mg.
Niacin	20	mg. equiv.
Riboflavin	2.0	mg.
Thiamine	1.5	mg.
Vitamin B_6	2.5	mg.
Vitamin B_{12}	6	mcg.
Calcium	1.3	Gm.
Phosphorus	1.3	Gm.
Iodine	150	mcg.
Iron	18	mg.
Magnesium	450	mg.

Supply of Mother's Milk. A normal infant will consume daily 2½ ounces of mother's milk for each pound of his weight. An 8-pound infant will consume approximately 20 ounces, while a 15-pound baby will consume about 30 ounces. Since human milk has a caloric value of 20 calories per ounce, it will be seen readily that a nursing mother must have several hundred additional calories per day to supply food for the infant.

Dietary Requirements. The nursing woman producing approximately 850 ml. of milk daily requires 1,000 additional calories above her normal needs, not only for milk production, but also for the extra activity necessitated by the care of the baby. Besides the increase in energy requirement, there are also increases in the requirements for protein, minerals and vitamins (see Table 14-5). Fried foods and foods rich in fat generally should be avoided, as should highly seasoned foods such as sausages and pickles. Highly flavored vegetables and dried beans may also cause disturbances.

Between-meal feedings often are advisable during lactation in order to include all the necessary foods. Plenty of water as well as other liquids should be taken. A typical sample menu for a day is shown in Table 14-6.

It should be remembered that the mother must return to a normal food intake when she weans the baby from the breast or she will gain excess weight.

STUDY QUESTIONS AND ACTIVITIES

1. Even the normal healthy woman who has been eating an adequate diet will require more dietary essentials during pregnancy. Review the Recommended Dietary Allowances for women under various conditions. Which allowances increase in ratio to the caloric allowance? What other essentials should be increased during pregnancy?

2. What do nutrition studies show concerning the adequacy of diets in pregnancy of large groups of women in the United States? What is the role of the nurse in the correction of this situation?

3. Give several reasons why the adolescent may have serious nutrition problems in pregnancy. Name some of the ways in which these can be met. How can the nurse be of help?

4. Why is the nutrition of the mother previous to pregnancy so important?

5. Discuss the results of an inadequate intake of protein in pregnancy. In what forms may extra protein be added to the diet?

TABLE 14-6. SAMPLE MENU FOR A DAY FOR A LACTATING MOTHER

BREAKFAST	LUNCH	DINNER
Orange juice	Cream of mushroom soup	Green salad
Instant oatmeal or grits with milk	Cottage cheese with fruit salad	Baked ham
Scrambled eggs	Biscuit with butter or margarine	Scalloped potatoes
Toast with butter or margarine	Gingerbread with topping	Green beans
Milk. Coffee if desired	Milk. Coffee if desired	Bread with butter or margarine
		Ice cream
		Milk. Coffee if desired

MIDMORNING	MIDAFTERNOON	BEDTIME
Milk	Fruit juice	Milk

6. The mineral requirement is naturally larger during pregnancy. How may the calcium and the phosphorus requirements be fulfilled? What are the food sources of iron? How may the iodine requirements be met?

7. What danger to the infant may result from nutritional anemia in the mother? Explain.

8. List the foods and the quantity of each that must be included daily in the diet of the pregnant woman.

9. Plan a menu for a day for a healthy pregnant woman of average weight with a limited income.

10. Using Chapter 11 as a guide, write a menu for a day for a pregnant patient with a food pattern not typically American. Be sure that it is adequate for the needs of pregnancy.

11. During the first trimester there may be trouble with nausea. How may the menu be modified to relieve this?

12. If for any reason the quota of fluid milk cannot be taken each day, how may milk be used otherwise in the diet? Suggest appetizing, easily digested dishes which may be used in the menu.

13. During the third trimester toxemia may appear. Is there anything to indicate that diet may act as a preventive? If so, state the evidence.

14. How may the diet in pregnancy be restricted in sodium? Should salt be restricted routinely in pregnancy?

15. Lactation makes greater demands upon the mother than does pregnancy. What food increases should be made to provide for the supply of milk? Which foods may cause digestive disturbances? Plan a menu differing in content from the sample menu in Table 14-6, but equivalent to it in other respects.

16. What would you say to the mother who asks about substituting calcium pills for milk?

SUPPLEMENTARY READING ON NUTRITION IN PREGNANCY

Everson, G. J.: Basis for concern about teenagers diet. J. Am. Dietet. A., 36:1, 1960.

Gold, E. M.: Interconceptual care. J. Am. Dietet. A., 55:27, 1969.

Jacobson, H. N.: Nutrition and pregnancy. J. Am. Dietet. A., 60:26, 1972.

Medical News: Malnutrition during pregnancy. JAMA, 212:44, 1970.

Payton, E., *et al.*: Dietary habits of 571 pregnant southern Negro women. J. Am. Dietet. A., 37:129, 1960.

Pike, R. L.: Sodium intake during pregnancy. J. Am. Dietet. A., 44:176, 1964.

Prenatal Care. Children's Bureau Publication No. 4. U.S. Dept. H.E.W., Washington, D.C., 1962.

Rust, H.: Food habits of pregnant women. Am. J. Nursing, 60:1636, 1960.

Schram, M., and Raji, M.: The problem of underweight pregnant patients. Am. J. Obstet. Gynec., 94:595, 1966.

Seifrit, E.: Changes in belief and food practice in pregnancy. J. Am. Dietet. A., 39:455, 1961.

Semmens, J. P.: Implications of teenage pregnancy. Obstet. Gynec., 26:77, 1965.

For Further References see Bibliography in Part Four.

Nutrition During Infancy and Early Childhood — From Birth to Three Years

15

Nutritional Requirements of Infants · Breast Feeding vs. Formula Feeding
Formulas—Types and Sources · Feeding Difficulties in Infants
Introduction of Solid Foods · Nutritional Requirements of Toddlers

Because of the rapid rate of growth during the first year, infancy is one of the most critical periods in the life cycle as far as food is concerned. Nutrient needs in relationship to size are high, and optimal nutrition at this time is very important to health and vigor throughout life. Many mothers with their first babies are insecure and concerned about what and how to feed the baby. The nurse should be able to advise and help the mother develop skills in this area.

NUTRITIONAL REQUIREMENTS OF INFANTS

The energy requirement of infants is much greater per unit of body weight than it is for older children or adults. The suggested caloric allowance (Table 15-1) for the very young infant ranges from 120 calories per kilogram of body weight at birth to 100 calories per kilogram at the end of the first year. This is from 3½ to 2½ times the adult requirement.

There are several reasons for this difference in requirements. The infant is growing rapidly, but is doing so at a decreasing rate, which is reflected by the 120 calories at birth and the 100 calories at one year of age. He has more active tissue using nutrients than the adult. Also he has a greater surface area in proportion to his weight and consequently, greater heat loss. Additional calories are also needed for activity. The accompanying table (Table 15-2) shows the approximate distribution of the caloric needs of the infant at the 120 cal./Kg. level.

Both breast milk and infant formulas (normal dilution) supply approximately 20 calories per ounce (67 calories per 100 ml.); thus 24 ounces of human milk or formula will supply about 480 calories or 120 calories per kilogram for the 4-Kg. infant (120 cal. × 4 Kg. = 480 cal.)

The fluid requirement for normal healthy infants is about 150 ml. (5 oz.) per kilogram of body weight in 24 hours. This amount is usually consumed in the formula or from the breast. If extra water is lost from the skin, lungs or gastrointestinal tract, such as in hot weather, fever or diarrhea, additional water should be given. When solid foods replace formula or breast milk in the infant's diet, some extra fluids may also be necessary. This is especially true if the solid food is high in protein, sodium chloride or potassium.[1] (See Chaps. 6 and 29 for a discussion of fluid and electrolyte balance in the normal state and in the sick child.)

The protein requirement in the first year of life is greater per unit of body weight than at any other time of life. It gradually decreases from 2.2 Gm. per kilogram at birth to 1.8 Gm. per kilogram at one year of age. The RDA for protein during infancy (Table 15-1) is based on the quality of protein in human milk which is assumed to be 100 percent utilized. Most of the infants in the U.S. today, who are not breast fed, receive a modified cow's milk formula which closely simulates human milk.

Because protein provides from 9 to 20 percent of the total calories in the usual infant formulas, 1 ounce of formula will supply between approximately 0.5 and 1.0 Gm. of protein. Thus the 4 Kg. infant receiving 24 ounces of formula (20

---

[1] Fomon, S. J.: Infant Nutrition. p. 158. Philadelphia, W. B. Saunders, 1967.

TABLE 15-1. RECOMMENDED DIETARY ALLOWANCES FOR INFANTS DURING THE FIRST YEAR*

	0-2 MONTHS 4 Kg.—55 cm.		2-6 MONTHS 7 Kg.—63 cm.		6-12 MONTHS 9 Kg.—72 cm.	
Calories	120	cal/Kg. (480 cal)	110	cal/Kg. (770 cal)	100	cal/Kg. (900 cal)
Protein	2.2	Gm./Kg.† (8.8 Gm.)	2.0	Gm./Kg.† (14 Gm.)	1.8	Gm./Kg.† (16.2 Gm.)
Vitamin A	1500	I.U.	1500	I.U.	1500	I.U.
Vitamin D	400	I.U.	400	I.U.	400	I.U.
Vitamin E	5	I.U.	5	I.U.	5	I.U.
Ascorbic acid	35	mg.	35	mg.	35	mg.
Folacin	0.05	mg.	0.05	mg.	0.1	mg.
Niacin	5	mg. equiv.	7	mg. equiv.	8	mg. equiv.
Riboflavin	0.4	mg.	0.5	mg.	0.6	mg.
Thiamine	0.2	mg.	0.4	mg.	0.5	mg.
Vitamin B_6	0.2	mg.	0.3	mg.	0.4	mg.
Vitamin B_{12}	1.0	mcg.	1.5	mcg.	2.0	mcg.
Calcium	0.4	Gm.	0.5	Gm.	0.6	Gm.
Phosphorus	0.2	Gm.	0.4	Gm.	0.5	Gm.
Iodine	25	mcg.	40	mcg.	45	mcg.
Iron	6	mg.	10	mg.	15	mg.
Magnesium	40	mg.	60	mg.	70	mg.

* Adapted from Recommended Dietary Allowances. National Academy of Sciences–National Research Council Publ. No. 1694. Washington, D.C., 1968.

† Assumes protein equivalent to human milk. For protein not 100 percent utilized factors should be increased proportionately. (See text for explanation.)

calories per ounce) will get from 12 to 24 Gm. of protein per day.

As baby foods with protein sources of lower quality than milk have been introduced into the infant's diet by approximately 5 or 6 months, the recommended allowance of protein is increased. The substitution of whole cow's milk, with its greater concentration of protein per 100 Gm., for human milk (Table 15-3) accomplishes this recommendation. If, between 6 and 12 months, the infant is receiving a regular mixed diet, the amount of protein is increased from 16 Gm. for the 9 Kg. infant to about 23 Gm. (2.5 per kilogram) at one year of age.[2]

[2] Recommended Dietary Allowances. National Academy of Sciences–National Research Council Publ. No. 1694. Washington, D.C., 1968.

TABLE 15-2. DISTRIBUTION OF THE CALORIE NEEDS OF THE INFANT

	CALORIES/Kg. OF BODY WEIGHT/24 HRS.
Basal metabolism	60
Activity	25
Growth	30
Loss in stools	5
Total	120

TABLE 15-3. COMPARATIVE NUTRITIVE VALUE OF HUMAN MILK AND COW'S MILK (Nutrients per 100 grams of fluid milk)

	HUMAN	COW'S
Calories	77	65
Protein (Gm.)	1.1	3.5
Fat (Gm.)	4.0	3.5
Carbohydrate (Gm.)	9.5	4.9
Water (Gm.)	85.2	87.9
Total ash (Gm.)	0.2	0.7
Calcium (mg.)	33	118
Phosphorus (mg.)	14	93
Magnesium (mg.)*	4	12
Sodium (mg.)	16	50
Potassium (mg.)	51	114
Iron (mg.)	0.1	0.05
Vitamin A (I.U.)	240	140
Vitamin E (I.U.)†	0.2-0.5	0.02-0.25
Vitamin D (I.U.)*	2.1	1.3
Thiamine (mg.)	0.01	0.03
Riboflavin (mg.)	0.04	0.17
Niacin (mg.)	0.2	0.1
Folacin (mg.)*	0.0002	0.0003
Vitamin B_6 (mg.)*	0.01	0.064
Vitamin B_{12} (mcg.)*	0.03	0.4

Figures adapted from Watt, B. K., and Merrill, A. L., Composition of foods, raw, processed, prepared. Agr. Handbook No. 8. U.S.D.A., 1963 except as noted.

* Fomon, S. J.: Infant Nutrition. Philadelphia, W. B. Saunders, 1967.

† Recommended Dietary Allowances. National Academy of Science–National Research Council Publ. No. 1694. Washington, D.C., 1968.

Fat requirement. No specific requirement for fat can be stated, but the caloric value of fat is essential during the early months of life when energy requirements per unit of body weight are high. Human milk provides about 48 percent of its calories as fat, cow's milk—46 percent. Most commercial formulas provide 35 to 50 percent of the calories as fat. For infants to acquire adequate calories from the limited amount of formula they are able to consume, at least 15 percent of the calories must come from fat. The fat must be in an easily digestible form, preferably emulsified.

Fat is also a carrier of fat-soluble vitamins. As described in Chapter 3, the infant requires small amounts of the essential fatty acid (EFA) —linoleic acid. Human milk is an excellent source of EFA, providing 6 to 9 percent of total calories as linoleate, whereas cow's milk provides the minimum of 1 to 2 percent. Commercial formulas, by using a combination of vegetable oils, usually contain at least 3 percent, the NRC's recommended level.

Carbohydrates in Infant Feeding. Lactose, the natural carbohydrate of mammalian milks, has many advantages. It provides calories in nonirritating and easily available form. Its slow breakdown and absorption probably has a beneficial effect upon calcium absorption in the intestinal tract. Most commercial formulas use lactose as the preferred carbohydrate. However, for economy and convenience of the mother preparing a formula at home, cane sugar (sucrose) or corn syrup can be used, the amount calculated according to the caloric need.

Minerals.   Calcium—Phosporus—Magnesium. The recommended dietary allowances for calcium, phosphorus and magnesium during the first year of life apply to bottle-fed infants. These recommendations are given in Table 15-1. To prevent hypocalcemic tetany during the first week of life, a calcium-phosphorus ratio similar to that of human milk (2:1) is more desirable for the newborn than the Ca:P ratio (1.2:1) found in cow's milk. The NRC's recommendation for at least a Ca:P ratio of 1.5:1 for the first weeks of life is found in several commercial formulas. For later infancy, the cow's milk Ca:P ratio is suggested. The approximate amounts of these minerals supplied by human and cow's milk is shown in Table 15-3.

Iron. Although the normal-term infant is born with a store of iron, it is depleted by 6 months of age and hemoglobin levels fall below normal by 1 year unless an adequate source of iron is provided in the infant's diet. The RDA for infants is based on 1.5 mg. of iron per kilogram per day during the first year of life. This is a difficult recommendation to meet without the use of a supplement.

Because both human and cow's milk are poor sources of iron, breast fed infants and those receiving whole cow's milk formulas need the early introduction of a good source of iron in their diets. Commercial infant formulas fortified with iron are available and supply about 8 to 12 mg. of iron per quart. They are prescribed by many physicians as the chief source of iron during the first 2 months when the RDA is 6 mg. per day for a 4 Kg. infant.

Infant (dry) cereals, also fortified with iron, may be introduced by the second month. Because many of these supply approximately 1 mg. of iron per tablespoon, they provide the additional iron recommended for the 2 to 6 month old infant (10 mg. of iron for a 7 Kg. infant), assuming the iron-fortified formula is continued.

If the 6 to 12 months old infant is to get 15 mg. of iron as specified in the RDA, both the iron fortified formula and cereal have to be continued throughout the first year of life rather than changing at 4 to 6 months to whole cow's milk and using other forms of cereal as is the current practice. Approximately 5 to 6 mg. of iron will be supplied by the fortified formula, 5 to 6 mg. by the fortified cereal and 4 to 5 mg. by the addition of meat, egg, and vegetables and fruits carefully selected for their iron content.

Iodine. Table 15-1 gives the recommended dietary allowance for iodine during the first year. Although the amount of iodine in human milk and cow's milk varies depending on that consumed in food and water, the breast-fed infant of an adequately nourished mother is assumed to receive at least the recommended amounts. For those infants not breast-fed, Fomon points out: "The infrequency of iodine deficiency in infants in those portions of the United States in which the iodine content of the soil is low may be explained by dairy practices which result in adequate iodine content of cow's milk and/or early introduction of strained foods to which iodized salt has been added."[3]

Fluorine. In technically advanced countries the magnitude of the dental caries problem exceeds that of all other nutritional diseases. It has been dramatically demonstrated that 6-year-old chil-

---

[3] Fomon, S. J.: op. cit., p. 188.

dren born after fluoridation started in one community had significantly fewer cavities than 10- or 11-year-old children using the same water supply but born before fluoridation started.[4] These differences suggest that fluoride prophylaxis during infancy is desirable. The advisable intake tentatively proposed by Fomon,[5] 0.5 mg. per day, is approximately the amount which would be ingested by infants fed formulas diluted with equal parts of water fluoridated at the usual level of 1 p.p.m.

Other trace elements—copper, chromium, cobalt, manganese, molybdenum, selenium and zinc—are assumed to be essential for the infant in extremely small amounts which are supplied by the usual diet.

Vitamins. The recommended dietary allowances for the vitamins (Table 15-1) may be met by breast milk or cow's milk formulas consumed at a rate of approximately 800 ml. per day with the following exceptions:

VITAMIN D. The breast-fed infant should receive a supplement of 400 I.U. of vitamin D per day after about 5 days of age. If the infant is bottle-fed with the usual formula already fortified with vitamin D providing this amount, no further supplement is necessary.

VITAMIN E. "Human milk is relatively rich in tocopherol content [vitamin E] (2 to 5 I.U. of α tocopherol per liter) and would meet the infant's requirement, whereas cow's milk is relatively low (only about 1/10 to 1/2 of the amount in human milk) in vitamin E content and would not be adequate."[6] Most of the commercial infant formulas have had vitamin E added to them and supply approximately 5 I.U. per quart. Some vitamin preparations for infants also include vitamin E.

Precautions are necessary in the use of the fat-soluble vitamins, which should be given in the amounts recommended but not more than that, because an excess of these factors can be toxic (see Chap. 7).

ASCORBIC ACID. Ascorbic acid is a limiting factor for bottle-fed infants whose formulas are subjected to high heat processing. According to Guthrie,[7] infants should receive a supplementary source of ascorbic acid by the tenth day of life. A synthetic source of this vitamin rather than orange juice is frequently recommended for small infants because it minimizes any sensitizing reaction. Most commercially prepared infant formulas have had ascorbic acid added to them, and since these require no further heat processing, the vitamin C is available. When used according to the directions on the label, 1 quart of prepared formula supplies approximately 50 mg. of ascorbic acid.

FOLACIN. The recommended dietary allowance for folacin (0.05 mg. to 0.1 mg.) during the first year is not supplied by either human milk or cow's milk, both of which are relatively poor sources of this nutrient. Folic acid has been added to several of the prepared commercial formulas in amounts to supply 0.03 to 0.05 mg. of folacin per quart of formula. This may be a critical nutrient for infants born to mothers with low folic acid levels (see Chap. 14).

BREAST FEEDING VS. FORMULA FEEDING

There is much evidence that the earliest experiences of the newborn baby are of great importance to his total growth and development. This is particularly true of the way he obtains his food. Even at this early stage, he will react to the emotions of the mother, and this is of more importance than whether he is breast- or formula-fed. If the mother is relaxed and confident, the baby will respond to her and, through her, to the world about him with trust and confidence. Conversely, if the mother is tense and overanxious, or if the feeding is hurried, the baby becomes aware of discomfort. In response, there may be fretfulness or crying, which may prevent his taking the food he needs.

Certain psychological advantages have been attributed to breast-feeding. Many mothers derive satisfaction from feeling they are the source of their baby's nutriment. Also, breast-feeding permits an early establishment of an intimacy with the child that promises well for the mother-child relationship.

A mother should be encouraged to breast-feed her baby, but she should not be made to feel guilty if she prefers to bottle-feed him. If he is cuddled and made comfortable when he is being fed, whether by breast or by bottle, his feelings will be those of warmth and comfort.

According to Fomon[8] "When a young infant is breast-fed by a healthy, well-nourished mother and

[4] Dunning, J. M.: New Eng. J. Med., 272:30, 1965.

[5] Fomon, S. J.: op. cit.

[6] Recommended Dietary Allowances, op. cit., p. 28.

[7] Guthrie, H. A.: Introductory Nutrition. St. Louis, C. V. Mosby, 1967.

[8] Fomon, S. J.: op. cit., p. 42.

receives an adequate caloric intake from this source, requirements for most specific nutrients appear to be fulfilled. With the exception of iron, fluoride, vitamin D [and perhaps folacin], there would seem to be no justification for supplementation of the diet of the breast-fed infant."

While breast-feeding is nature's way to feed the baby, relatively few young mothers in the U. S. today nurse their infants for more than a few days and often not at all. In poor areas or where medical aid is not available, breast milk may be safer than a poor formula or one unhygienically prepared. Breast milk also has the advantage of freedom from contamination and of requiring no preparation. It has the advantage of immunizing the baby against certain infectious diseases through antibodies received in the mother's milk and is less likely to cause allergic reactions.

The lactating woman will find, however, that she needs more food than a non-lactating woman of her age and size and it may cost her from $2.50 to $3.00 more per week to feed herself during the time that she is sharing her nutriment with her infant.

The decision to breast-feed or bottle-feed the baby should be made during pregnancy. If the mother desires to breast-feed her infant, instructions for the preparation of her breasts prior to delivery should be given by the nurse. Some young mothers will breast-feed their infants if careful teaching and psychological as well as physical preparation is instigated early in pregnancy. Moreover, the nursing mother must be sure to have the proper diet (see Chap. 14) and get sufficient sleep and relaxation; otherwise she will not produce enough milk.

The following table shows the approximate quantity of milk consumed by an average baby under normal conditions. This shows why the mother must eat properly if she is going to produce this quantity of milk:

	Gm.	Ozs.
1st day	10	⅓
2d day	90	3
3d day	190	6⅓
4th day	310	10
5th day	350	11½
6th day	390	13
7th day	470	15⅔
3d week	500	16
4th week	600	20
8th week	800	26½
12th week	900	30
24th week	1,000	33

The thick, yellowish fluid which appears the first few days of nursing (colostrum) will nourish the baby until the milk comes a few days later. The baby should be laid beside the mother with his cheek close to her breast. He will turn his head toward the breast trying to find the nipple (rooting reflex), and the mother can help him by holding the breast so that he can get the nipple into his mouth. To express the milk and prevent nipple irritation, most of the areola should be in the infant's mouth and not just the tip of the nipple.

Nursing the baby will in itself increase the milk supply of the mother, and she will be able to satisfy his needs with an ever-increasing supply as he keeps on growing. At first the baby may be satisfied after he has emptied only one breast, but if he does not give signs that he is full, he should be given the other breast. He should be started on this breast at his next feeding so as to be sure to empty it.

If the baby is not getting enough to satisfy his hunger from the breast feeding, the doctor may prescribe an additional formula for him, to be given after he has been at the breast, or solid food such as cereal may be introduced. For one reason or another, the mother may wish to skip a breast feeding occasionally, and in such a case a formula feeding may be substituted. Beal[9] points out that in the United States today, the whole concept of breast-feeding has changed because of the tendency not only to supplement with formula but also to introduce semisolid foods early in infancy. Very few infants receive only breast milk even for the first 2 months of life.

FORMULAS—TYPES AND SOURCES

The physician usually determines the type of feeding for the newborn infant. Various factors, such as availability, ease of preparation, cost, and (most important) the infant's needs, should be considered in recommending the type and amount of feeding to be given.

Fresh Cow's Milk. Although there is a tendency toward the earlier introduction of undiluted fresh, whole homogenized or skim milk, this is rarely the form prescribed for the newborn.

Because whole cow's milk contains more protein and mineral salts and less milk sugar than human milk, it is usually modified for the newborn by dilution with water and the addition of some form of sugar. Most homogenized milk is fortified with 400 I.U. of vitamin D per quart.

9 Beal, V. A.: J. Am. Dietet. A., 55:31, 1969.

TABLE 15-4. NUTRIENTS IN SELECTED PREMODIFIED MILKS*

PRODUCT	SUGAR	FAT	AMOUNT OF NUTRIENT PER QUART (AFTER DILUTION IF INDICATED)					
			PROTEIN (Gm.)	CALCIUM (mg.)	IRON (mg.)	VITAMIN A (I.U.)	VITAMIN D (I.U.)	ASCORBIC ACID (mg.)
Baker—Infant Formula (L&P)†	lactose, dextrose, maltose, dextrins	coconut, corn, soy oil	21.4	825	7.5	2,500	400	50
Borden—Bremil (L&P)	lactose	corn, coconut, peanut oil	14.7	630	8.0	2,500	400	50
Carnation—Carnalac (L)	lactose	butterfat	26.6	804	Trace	1,035	400	80
Gerbers—Modilac (L)	lactose, dextrose, maltose, dextrins	corn oil	21.4	800	10.0	1,500	400	45
Mead-Johnson—Enfamil (L&P)	lactose	oleo, corn, coconut oil	14.7	615	1.4	1,500	400	50
Mead-Johnson—Enfamil with iron (L&P)	lactose	oleo, corn, coconut oil	14.4	615	8.0	1,500	400	50
Pet—Formil	lactose	butterfat, coconut oil, corn oil	16.0	590	Trace	2,500	400	50
Pet—Formil with iron	lactose	butterfat, coconut oil, corn oil	16.0	590	8.0	2,500	400	50
Ross—Similac (L&P)	lactose	corn, coconut oil	16.3	630 (L) 730 (P)	Trace	2,500	400	50
Ross—Similac with iron (L&P)	lactose	corn, coconut oil	16.3	630 (L) 730 (P)	12.0	2,500	400	50
Wyeth—SMA S-26 (L&P)	lactose	oleo, soy, corn, coconut oil	14.7‡	400	8.0	2,500	400	50
Recommended Daily Dietary Allowances (4.0-Kg. Infant)			8.8	400	6.0	1,500	400	35

* February, 1966, taken from published materials by the indicated company, from Baker Laboratories: Handbook of Infant Formulas. New York, Pfizer, 1964; Meyer, H. F.: Infant Foods and Feeding Practices. Springfield, Ill., Charles C Thomas, 1960.
† L&P—Liquid and powder.
‡ 40 percent casein.
From Economy in Nutrition and Feeding of Infants. Am. J. Public Health, 56:1766, 1966.

Evaporated whole milk has much to recommend it for use in infants' formulas but it is less used than formerly. Because evaporated milk is already sterilized, it is easy to prepare. The heat processing and homogenizing it undergoes results in both a soft, easily digested curd and well-distributed digestible fat. Evaporated milk contains 400 I.U. of vitamin D per reconstituted quart and is less expensive than fresh milk or commercial formula. It is available in two size cans: 5½-ounce and 13-ounce.

Condensed cow's milk with its high sugar content and **skimmed cow's milk** are considered undesirable for infant feeding. Skim milk is deficient in calories as well as in essential fatty acids.

Prepared commercial formulas are by far the most popular type of infant feeding for the newborn. They are available in a variety of forms: powdered, concentrated-liquid, ready-to-use and in feeding bottles, ready-to-feed. Their cost is related to their ease of use. Currently the two most popular forms are the concentrated-liquid, $0.01 to 0.015 per ounce (normal dilution) and the ready-to-use at approximately $0.02 to 0.025 per ounce. Several brands are marketed with and without added iron. A variety of vitamins have been added to each different brand. Almost all of them contain supplements of vitamins A and D, ascorbic acid and vitamin B_6, whereas others may also contain vitamin E, folic acid, vitamin B_{12} and other B complex vitamins.

TABLE 15-5. COMPARISON OF COSTS OF 1 QUART OF INFANT FORMULA MADE FROM DIFFERENT FORMS OF COW'S MILK

Homogenized milk	
22 ozs. milk—10 ozs. water	$0.26
1 oz. sugar	0.01
1 ml. multi-vitamins with iron	0.06
	0.33
Evaporated milk	
11 ozs. milk—21 ozs. water	0.18
1 oz. sugar	0.01
1 ml. multi-vitamins with iron	0.06
	0.25
Commercial Formulas	
(vitamins and iron added)	
Powdered form (normal dilution)	0.32
Liquid-concentrate (normal dilution)	0.42
Ready-to-feed	0.63
Nursettes—5⅓ 6-oz. bottles	1.31

Commercial formulas may also have been modified in one or more of the following ways:

Butterfat is removed and a vegetable oil or oils are added to increase the amount of unsaturated fatty acid, particularly the essential fatty acid, linoleic acid. This makes the cow's milk formula more like breast milk in essential fatty acid content, and fat in this form is better tolerated by the infant.

The protein is treated to produce a softer, more flocculent curd which is more easily digested by the infant.

The milk is diluted to reduce the calcium and, to make up for this dilution in terms of calories, sugar—usually lactose—is added. Both these modifications make the formula more like breast milk.

Dialysis may be used to reduce the sodium content of cow's milk.

Comparisons of commercial formulas are given in Table 15-4.

Only by carefully reading the labels on the individual brands can one be sure of the exact nutritive content of the formula. The nurse should urge the mothers to follow the specific directions for the form she is using. Dilution of a ready-to-use can of formula will reduce the infant's nutritive intake, whereas failure to dilute the concentrated-liquid form may result in too strong a formula which the infant may vomit. Care should also be taken to sterilize the bottles, nipples and can opener, and water if it is to be added.

If facilities for sterilizing bottles or refrigeration is unavailable such as in a home emergency or when traveling, the individual 4-, 6- or 8-ounce bottles called nursettes may be an excellent way to ensure a safe supply of milk for the infant.

Table 15-5 gives a comparison of the costs of infant formulas made from different forms of cow's milk.

Goat milk, seldom used today in the United States for infant feeding, is still used in many parts of the world. Experience shows that it is nutritionally adequate in most respects. It was formerly used to feed infants who had an allergy to cow's milk; it is still used occasionally today and is available in drug and grocery stores. Goat-milk fat differs from cow's milk in that it contains more essential fatty acids and has a greater percentage of medium- and short-chain fatty acids. These differences suggest that the fat of goat milk may be more readily digested than that of cow's milk.

Milk Substitutes. Certain infants are born with a sensitivity to the proteins of all milks. This may be mild enough to cause only irritability, or it may be severe enough to cause violent illness and even death. Several preparations have been devised as formulas to approximate human milk in carbohydrate, protein, fat, mineral and vitamin content. These contain no milk at all. Soybean preparations are used most commonly.[10] Usually, the protein in the soybean can be taken by infants allergic to the proteins of milk. A milk substitute having meat protein as a base,[11] with added vitamins and minerals, has also proved to be adequate nutritionally for such infants.

If these milk substitutes are properly supplemented, infants do as well on them as on other formula feedings. A discussion of the nutritive adequacy of milk substitutes and an excellent table of composition has been prepared by the Committee on Nutrition of the American Academy of Pediatrics.[12]

Galactosemia and lactose intolerance in infants and children is discussed in Chapter 29.

Temperature for Feeding. The formula may be given at room temperature or warmed to body temperature if desired. If the formula has been stored in the refrigerator, it should be allowed to stand long enough to reach room temperature, or the bottle may be placed in warm water until it reaches the desired temperature.

The temperature of milk should be tested by shaking a few drops on the inside of the wrist. The older infant may tolerate his formula straight from the refrigerator.

How Often to Feed. Much has been said in recent years about so-called "self-demand schedules of feeding." For many years babies were fed by the clock, regardless of whether they were hungry earlier or later than the scheduled time. Today we recognize that when a baby is hungry, that is the time to feed him, whether the interval is 2, 3, 4 or even 5 hours. The nurse, however, may need to give the inexperienced mother help in recognizing the difference between a hunger cry and a cry for something else.

A newborn baby may wake up to be fed 8 to 10 times in 24 hours. By the time he is a month old, there may be 3 hours between feedings. Most babies establish themselves on a schedule of 4-hourly feedings by the time they are between 2 and 3 months old. During this time, too, the

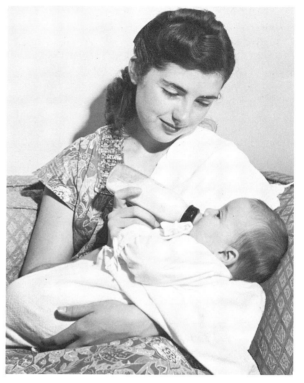

Fig. 15-1. Feeding time should be enjoyed by both mother and baby, whether he is breast- or formula-fed. (Children's Bureau photograph by Philip Bonn)

baby will begin to sleep through the night after a late evening feeding.

"Burping" the Baby. Once or twice during a feeding, the baby should be given a chance to bring up any swallowed air. Holding him up so that his stomach is against the mother's shoulder and gently patting him on the back will help to eliminate the air. An even better way is to hold the baby in a sitting position on the mother's knee, with his chin held in the palm of her hand. By leaning the baby forward and gently stroking or patting his back swallowed air is released.

Psychosocial Aspects of Infant Feeding. If the mother is feeding her baby by bottle, she should hold him as though she were breast-feeding him, cradled in her arm (Fig. 15-1), in order to give him the same sense of nearness and companionship. It is important that she feel relaxed and unhurried and that she enjoys this time with her baby. She should never allow him to eat by himself by propping the bottle up beside him. In this way his nutritional needs will be met but not his need for love and contact.

---

[10] Two such products are ProSobee made by Mead Johnson and Co.; Mull-Soy made by Borden Co.

[11] Meat Base Formula, Gerber Products Co.

[12] Pediatrics, 31:329, 1963.

By feeding on demand, the mother also eliminates the infant's frustration of hunger and helps him develop trust and security in the feeder. Talking and repeating sounds to the infant while he is being fed is an important part of the infant's learning experience and may be an important aspect of his later intellectual development.

FEEDING DIFFICULTIES IN INFANTS

Vomiting and Regurgitation. Vomiting may result from a number of causes and may or may not be a serious symptom. In regurgitation only small amounts of food are lost, while in vomiting the contractions of the stomach are sufficiently strong to empty the stomach. Regurgitation may be avoided by "burping" the infant once or twice during a feeding. Occasional vomiting is usually caused by overdistention of the stomach due to the ingestion of too large or too frequent feedings or to the swallowing of air. It may also be due to an imbalance of the food constituents, especially to an oversupply of fat, causing delayed emptying of the stomach. Persistent vomiting may be a symptom of infection, obstruction or other serious ailment and should be referred promptly to the physician. The cause should be determined and the feedings adjusted accordingly.

Colic. A baby who has hard crying spells shortly after eating is said to be "colicky." The colic, or severe abdominal cramping pain, may be caused by distention due to the swallowing of air; to gas formed by bacterial fermentation of undigested food; to overfeeding or underfeeding; to cold, excitement or only to being tired. The baby may have to be "burped" again. Making sure he is warm may help. Mothers are apt to think that his feeding is wrong, but changing the feeding usually does not help. Spock[13] says that these babies seem to grow and gain weight better than most, and that generally the condition disappears at the age of 3 to 4 months.

Diarrhea. Loose stools may be serious, and the doctor should be consulted at once. See Chapter 29 for diseases in which diarrhea is a symptom.

Constipation. Constipation in infancy is not infrequent. Many mothers are concerned when the baby has only one bowel movement per day or on alternate days. The number of movements per day is not of so much importance as the consistency of the stools. If the feces are hard and expelled with difficulty, then the child may be said to be constipated and should be treated accordingly.[14] Increasing the amount of fruit in the diet and giving additional water usually relieves the constipation. If it persists, the doctor should be consulted.

INTRODUCTION OF SOLID FOODS

The time for the addition of supplementary foods to the diet of the breast or formula fed infant has undergone marked changes in the past 20 years. Whereas earlier no solid foods were introduced until the end of the first year, the pendulum has swung all the way to offering the baby solids during the first month of life. Beal[15] has found that the average baby's willing acceptance of cereal is at 2½ to 3 months, of vegetables at 4 to 4½ months, of meat and meat soups at 5½ to 6 months, and of fruit at 2½ to 3 months. Earlier introduction of solid foods tended to meet with resistance by the infant. Beal also has shown that the age of transition from baby foods to the family diet has decreased from approximately 2 years to 13 months.

Later studies, however, indicate that most infants are fed some solid foods before they are 2 months old and that they begin to eat foods from the family diet before the end of the first year. In the following paragraphs, the authors have indicated the approximate age when new foods may be introduced.

Cereals. Cereals are usually added to the infant's diet before he is 2 months of age. Dry, precooked cereal preparations are fortified with iron, whereas the "wet-packed" jars of cereal may or may not be iron-fortified.

The dry, precooked cereals must be mixed with warm formula or whole milk, while the others may only be warmed. The cooked cereals eaten generally by the family may be prepared according to the directions on the package and given to the baby. The coarse cereals must be strained, and all of them should be thinner than those prepared for the family—thin enough to drop from a spoon. Only a small amount of cereal should be used at first, and this generally is given with the midmorning feeding. The original small amount may be increased gradually, and in a few months it may be of a thicker consistency. By

---

[13] Spock, B.: Baby and Child Care. rev. ed. New York, Hawthorn Books, 1968.

[14] Your Baby's First Year. Children's Bureau, U.S. Dept. H.E.W. Publ. No. 400. Washington, D.C., 1962.
[15] Beal, V. A.: Pediatrics, 20:448, 1957.

the 4th or the 6th month, the baby will be taking from ¼ to ½ cup twice during the day.

Fruits. Cooked, strained fruits and ripe banana may be added to the baby's diet when he is between 2 and 3 months old. Like cereals, these may be purchased in cans or jars, all ready for infant use, or they may be prepared at home. Cooked fruits should be put through a purée sieve or strainer. Strained apple sauce, prunes, peaches, pears and apricots are suitable. Ripe mashed banana may also be given. Starting with a teaspoonful once or twice a day, the baby will soon take 2 to 3 tablespoonfuls. Most babies like fruit and take it readily. This helps them to accept other solid foods, the taste of which may not appeal to them quite as much.

Vegetables. By the 3rd or 4th month, or even earlier, strained vegetables are usually introduced. Those added first are peas, string beans, spinach, carrots, beets, and squash. Fresh, frozen or canned vegetables are suitable. If prepared at home, they should be cooked in a small amount of water, as would be done for the family meal, and the baby's portion put through a purée sieve or a strainer. Again, these and other varieties of vegetables are available in cans or jars in most grocery stores, prepared and ready for serving after they are warmed. Starting with a teaspoonful at one feeding—and, later, as part of lunch—the baby will soon be taking 2 to 3 rounded tablespoonfuls. Potatoes, both sweet and white, may be added a little later, but potatoes in any form are one of the last vegetables to be accepted by most babies.

Egg Yolk. Egg yolk is a good source of iron, but since other infant foods are now fortified with iron, eggs can be deferred until other foods have been given. Eggs may be a cause of an allergic reaction, the white more so than the yolk, which is the reason for the yolk being given first. The egg may be cooked hard by placing it in boiling water, turning off the heat and letting it stand, covered, for 20 minutes. Cooking changes the protein to make it less allergenic.

Egg yolks should be crumbled and given by spoon or mixed with cereal or vegetables at first. A fourth of a yolk is a good quantity with which to start. If the baby accepts it well and there are no signs of allergy, it may be increased until he is taking a whole yolk, usually at the breakfast feeding. Whole egg may be given by the time he is a year old.

Prepared egg yolk is now available in jars ready to serve as are other infant foods.

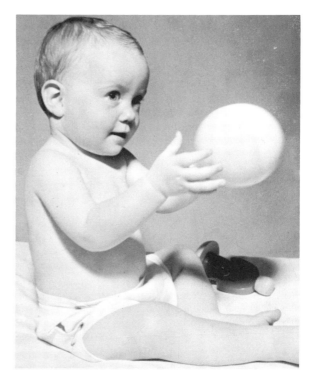

Fig. 15-2. Signs of good nutrition. Note the straight back, well-developed body, alertness and good coordination of this child. (The New York Hospital)

Meat. Meats may be added as early as 3 to 4 months or as late as 6 months, depending on the doctor's judgment about the baby's need for them. The most convenient way of serving meat to the baby is by way of the canned, strained beef, beef heart, liver, lamb, chicken, veal and pork preparations available in cans and jars at most grocery stores. To prepare meat for the baby at home, the mother should buy a lean cut of beef, pork, lamb, veal or poultry. It may be simmered or pan broiled and then put in a blender with sufficient water to achieve the desired consistency. Liver may be prepared in the same way. If a blender is not available, a fork or dull knife may be used to scrape meat off fibers from the surface of a cooked or cleaned raw piece of meat. If raw meat is used, the resulting meat pulp may be heated until it is brown in a custard cup set in a small pan of water over heat.

Meats add protein, iron and some of the B complex vitamins to the baby's diet. Again, it is best to begin slowly with a teaspoonful or less, at the evening feeding, increasing the quantity as the baby grows older.

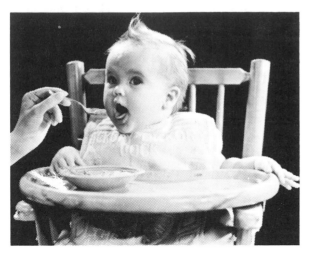

FIG. 15-3. The right start for the baby. Liking comes through learning to like. Teach the flavor of a variety of foods early. (Gesell and Ilg: Behavior of Infants. Philadelphia, J. B. Lippincott)

Widening Variety in the Infant Diet

By the time they are 6 months old, most babies will be eating some foods from each of the four food groups. They may also be starting to take some milk or fruit juice from a cup. In addition to milk a good meal plan for a baby of this age is to give him cereal and egg yolk at breakfast, vegetable and meat for lunch, and cereal and fruit for supper. The quantities will depend on his appetite. If there is a tendency to constipation, giving fruit at breakfast as well as at supper may help.

Additional Foods, 6 to 12 Months. The baby will welcome a piece of dried bread, toast or one of the infant teething biscuits to hold in his hands and chew on, particularly if his teeth are beginning to appear. If potato has not already been given, it can be added at this time, mashed fine. Puddings made mainly with milk, such as junket, cornstarch, tapioca and rice pudding, may also be added occasionally for variety. A small piece of a white, non-oily fish, such as flounder, haddock or halibut, may be substituted for meat now and then. It should be boiled gently in water to cover until it flakes, and *all bones carefully removed*.

By the time he is 9 months old, it is time to try serving some of the junior foods or foods mashed with a fork instead of baby foods or foods strained through a sieve. The change should be made gradually and should not be forced. Vegetables and fruits may be tried this way first. Meat had better be served strained until after the first year, because it is so much more difficult to swallow.

A piece of crisp bacon or a bit of raw, *peeled* apple is also often enjoyed by babies, when they are allowed to hold it in their hands and suck on it.

Mixed dishes, either junior foods or appropriate ones from the family table, may also be added. These include spaghetti with meat sauce, macaroni and cheese and tuna fish and noodles.

As the baby becomes acquainted with a variety of things, including his food, he will want to explore it with such tools as he has at his command. To quote Rabinovitch[16]: "In the second half of the first year, the baby will begin to mess with food, to feel its texture and consistency, to finger-feed himself as he recognizes his growing dexterity. Such experimentation, often difficult for the cleanliness-and-germ-conscious mother, is essential for the child as he learns to relate to food by messing, smelling and pouring. That a high degree of parental fortitude is necessary to allow for these developmental realities goes without saying."

Weaning. The weaning of a baby from milk to other food is not an abrupt transition as infants are fed today. As soon as the baby is introduced to the supplementary foods discussed earlier, he is on the way to being weaned. He will have learned to drink from a cup by the time he is 7 or 9 months old. If he still shows a desire to suck, he may have a bottle once a day. He may be drinking homogenized milk and eating a variety of foods. The proportion of calories derived from milk will decrease gradually as he obtains more of his nutrients from other foods—junior foods for a time and then simple foods from the family table.

OTHER CONSIDERATIONS IN INFANT FEEDING

Commercial Baby Foods. The widespread use of commercial baby foods by mothers in the U.S. today makes the nurse's knowledge of these foods especially important. Anderson and Fomon[17,18] in recent articles have discussed the many factors which must be considered in their use, such as the

[16] Rabinovitch, R. D., and Fischoff, J.: J. Am. Dietet. A., 28:614, 1952.
[17] Anderson, T. A., and Fomon, S. J.: J. Am. Dietet. A., 58:520, 1971.
[18] Anderson, T. A., and Fomon, S. J.: J. Pediat., 78:788, 1971.

differences and similarities between the various categories of infant foods; comparisons between the composition of the commercial infant foods and similar home-prepared foods; and the potential nutritional contribution to the diet of the infant foods.

Salt in Commercial Baby Foods. The amount of salt which is added to baby foods by the manufacturer has been of recent concern. In the report from the subcommittee of the Food and Nutrition Board concerned with food protection, it is noted that the current levels of salt in baby food, although substantially more than required by the infant, are neither harmful nor beneficial to the infant. "There is no valid scientific evidence in support of the contention that addition of salt to infant foods contributes to development of hypertension or other disease states in adult life, nor is there valid evidence that the practice is not harmful, or that salt levels now consumed by infants in the U.S. overburdens excretory mechanisms."[19] Because salt is added more for the mother's taste than the infant's, it was recommended that the amount of salt in all foods be limited to 0.25 percent, and that no additional salt be added to those foods such as fruits, currently prepared without it.

Satiety, the mechanism by which the infant is made aware that he has had enough, varies widely in babies. In some babies, the reaction is sharp and they actively resist further feeding attempts. In others, satiety is less sharply defined and interest in eating wanes gradually after a period of playfulness. Still others do not seem to know when they have had enough and will vomit what they cannot handle.

Criteria for Judging Nutritional Adequacy. The criteria for judging adequate nutrition in an infant are: a steady gain in weight; a moderate increase in subcutaneous fat; the development of firm muscles; good elimination; and a baby who is happy, sleeps well and shows normal curiosity about his surroundings.

Overnutrition. The nurse should be particularly aware of the hazards of overnutrition. She must be able to relate these to the mother who may look upon a fat baby as a healthy, happy baby and see no cause for alarm.

Infants who show an excessive weight gain from overfeeding even as early as 6 weeks of age are reported to have a greater tendency toward overweight and obesity later in childhood.[20] As

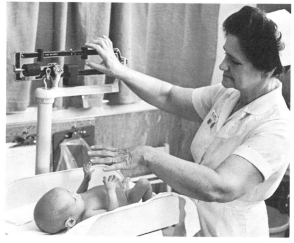

FIG. 15-4. The rate at which a child gains weight is dependent on many factors. As long as he gains weight and length steadily, and exhibits the other signs of good nutrition, there is no cause for worry. (Broadribb, V.: Foundations of Pediatric Nursing. Philadelphia, J. B. Lippincott, 1967)

previously discussed in Chapter 13, there may also be an increase in the total number of fat cells in the body of an infant who is overnourished during the phase of rapid fat cell division and this condition persists throughout his life. Although the reasons are not clear, a recent study gives evidence that obese infants also have a higher incidence of respiratory infections than those of normal weight.[21]

THE TODDLER

Nutritional Requirements of Early Childhood

The recommended dietary allowances for 1- to 3-year-olds are shown in Table 15-6.

Calories. The calorie needs from 1 to 3 years are relatively low (Table 15-6) and hence, in order to ensure a diet adequate in other nutrients, careful selection of the toddler's food is essential.

Protein. Protein needs for growth of muscles and other tissue are relatively high during this period. They are easily met, however, if the toddler consumes a pint of milk and 1 to 2 ounces of meat each day.

Minerals. *Calcium, phosphorus* and *magnesium* recommendations also depend on the inclusion

[19] Filer, L. J.: Nutr. Rev., 28:184, 1970.
[20] Nutr. Rev., 28:184, 1970.
[21] Tracey, V. V., *et al.*: Brit. Med. J., 1:16, 1971.

TABLE 15-6. RECOMMENDED DIETARY
ALLOWANCES FOR THE 1- TO 3-YEAR-OLD*

	1-2 YEARS (12 Kg.)	2-3 YEARS (14 Kg.)
Calories	1,100	1,250
Protein (Gm.)	25	25
Vitamin A (I.U.)	2,000	2,000
Vitamin D (I.U.)	400	400
Vitamin E (I.U.)	10	10
Ascorbic acid (mg.)	40	40
Folacin (mg.)	0.1	0.2
Niacin (mg. equiv.)	8	8
Riboflavin (mg.)	0.6	0.7
Thiamine (mg.)	0.6	0.6
Vitamin B_6 (mg.)	0.5	0.6
Vitamin B_{12} (mcg.)	2.0	2.5
Calcium (Gm.)	0.7	0.8
Phosphorus (Gm.)	0.7	0.8
Iodine (mcg.)	55	60
Iron (mg.)	15	15
Magnesium (mg.)	100	150

* From Recommended Dietary Allowances. National Academy of Sciences–National Research Council Publ. No. 1694. Washington, D.C., 1968.

each day of 1 pint of milk and 1 to 2 ounces of meat.

The recommended dietary allowance for *iron,* 15 mg., is not easily met with the usual diet at this age and a supplement may be necessary until increased levels of enrichment are achieved.

In areas where iodine in the soil is limited, a small amount of iodized salt in cooking and seasoning adequately provides for the recommended amounts of *iodine.*

Vitamins. A varied menu such as shown in Table 15-7 will provide an adequate intake of vitamins if the toddler's appetite permits its consumption. Foods high in ascorbic acid and vitamin A should be served each day. If fortified milk is not used, a vitamin D supplement is necessary.

Feeding the Toddler

The one-year-old begins to show a decided change in appetite and interest in food. Beal[22] has shown that, on the average, girls at 6 months and boys at 9 months decrease their milk intake markedly. For girls this persists until 2 to 3 years of age and then slowly begins to rise. In contrast, boys have a somewhat steeper decrease in milk intake than girls but recover more rapidly and by

[22] Beal, V. A.: J. Nutr., 53:499, 1954.

TABLE 15-7. SUGGESTED MEAL PLAN
FOR THE 1- TO 3-YEAR-OLD*

BREAKFAST

Fruit or juice
Cereal with milk
Toast
Butter or margarine
Milk

LUNCH OR SUPPER

Main dish—mainly meat, eggs, fish, poultry, dried beans or peas, cheese, peanut butter
Vegetable or salad
Bread
Butter or margarine
Dessert or fruit
Milk

DINNER

Meat, poultry or fish
Vegetable
Relish or salad
Bread
Butter or margarine
Fruit or pudding
Milk

SNACKS BETWEEN MEALS

Dry cereal, with milk or out of the box
Simple cookie or cracker
Raw vegetables
Canned, fresh or dried fruit
Cheese wedge
Fruit sherbet or ice cream
Toast, plain or cinnamon
Fruit juice
Fruit drinks made with milk and juice

* From Your Child from 1 to 3, Children's Bureau, U.S. Dept. H.E.W., 1966.

2½ years have reached a higher level than girls. Other foods, too, are not taken as eagerly as formerly, and some may be refused altogether. This should not be interpreted as a "poor" appetite but rather the normal appetite for that age.

All this is due in large measure to a decrease in growth rate and, therefore, to the quantitative need for food. Also, at this age, the young child is becoming increasingly intrigued by his surroundings—parents, sisters and brothers and the paraphernalia of the home, all of which vie for his attention. He wants to play with his food to feel its texture, and he tries to feed himself with his hands, refusing the same food when it is offered on a spoon.

This can become an anxious time for the inexperienced mother, accustomed to the voracious

appetite of infancy (or to the busy nurse facing a ward full of restive children). Unless the mother is guided correctly, food and eating may become a battleground between herself and the baby and may lay the groundwork for some of the anorexia and the emotional upsets related to food and eating which so often occur in the preschool years. It is important for her to understand that changes in food acceptance and the need for exploration are a part of the normal growth pattern and that all babies go through this process.

Physically, the baby is learning motor mastery of his body—eye, hand and mouth coordination, chewing, swallowing, the use of mouth and throat muscles. He "puts everything into his mouth." From his earliest days his mouth has served him as a sensory organ. He now uses it to explore whatever is within reach. Moreover, from the very beginning his feedings established his primary relationships with other people. If the mother is helped to understand and is able to enjoy her baby's developing skills and interests even when she is frustrated by the spilled milk, the dropped spoons and the gleeful contrariness, she is less likely to worry him over the food which he does or does not eat.

The diet of the 1-year-old differs only slightly from that described previously. It includes not much more than a pint of milk a day plus foods from each of the other four food groups. His vegetables and fruits are mashed or chopped instead of strained, and he has started on "finger foods." He is introduced to the family meal schedule with a midmorning and a midafternoon snack of fruit juice or milk. The cup largely supplants the bottle, and he may start to try feeding himself with a spoon.

During the second year more solid foods are added, such as chopped or sliced fruits and vegetables; ready-to-eat cereals as well as hot cereals; chopped liver, lean meat, fish and poultry instead of the strained variety. Whole egg replaces egg yolk, and a child of this age may be ready to eat 1 egg a day. Cottage cheese and other mild cheeses may be used. Butter or fortified margarine is used with toast. The 2-year-old also enjoys custard and puddings.

Food from the Family Table. By the time the infant reaches his first birthday his usual food is often from the family table. It is important that the family-food fed to the toddler is appropriate both in nutritive value and in consistency. Because caloric intake is limited, the 1-year-old cannot afford calories that do not contribute equal amounts of other nutrients. Soft drinks, candy, many types of cookies, pastries and cakes supply too many calories and not enough protein, vitamins or minerals for the toddler. The nurse should discourage mothers from feeding the toddler these foods except, perhaps, on special occasions.

When the toddler's meat comes from the family table it should be tender and cut into small pieces. Rich gravies and sauces are not appropriate for this age. Except for finger items, other foods should be cut into bite-size pieces.

Very small portions (1 to 2 tablespoonfuls) seem to encourage the toddler to eat. He should have the option of refusing certain foods as well as having additional servings of those he likes.

Making foods easy to eat for beginners helps them to develop independence in feeding themselves and will prevent accidents. Small plastic cups or tumblers are easier to handle than glass or china. If they are not filled too full, there will be less spilling.

Over-use of Milk. Earlier in this chapter it was stated that most children decrease their milk intake in favor of other foods sometime during the first year. Because milk has been the center of the diet in infancy, there is a tendency to think that it must continue to be so. When milk continues to provide the largest part of the 1- to 2-year-old's diet, nutritional anemia may result. The 1- to 2-year-old may cut his milk intake down to a pint or even less a day and, instead, eat a variety of other foods, many of which help supply his need for iron. He slowly resumes milk drinking, but it will be some years before he is able to consume a full quart and still eat a variety of other foods.

Abnormal Cravings—Pica. Pica is a craving for unnatural foods or for nonfood substances such as clay or chalk. It is most apt to occur in children between the ages of 18 and 24 months of age. Lourie *et al.*[23] found no correlation between the occurrence of pica and nutritional deficiencies. Gutelius *et al.*[24] supplemented the diet of some pica children with vitamins and minerals but failed to reduce the incidence of this craving among their subjects. These workers agree that pica is a complicated environmental, cultural and phychological problem most apt to occur among children of mothers who also practice pica themselves.

[23] Lourie, R. S., *et al.*: Children, 10:143, 1963.
[24] Gutelius, M. F., *et al.*: Am. J. Clin. Nutr., 12:388, 1963.

STUDY QUESTIONS AND ACTIVITIES

1. Why is breast feeding considered to be highly desirable for both mother and baby?

2. What should the mother's attitude be if she bottle-feeds the baby?

3. What foods in what quantity should be included in the mother's diet if she is nursing her baby? (See Chap. 14.)

4. How much iron should a 4-month-old infant get per day? How can this be supplied by food?

5. Is there evidence that fluoride in an infant's diet has any prophylactic effect during later childhood?

6. Which vitamins are most apt to be the limiting factors in bottle-fed infants?

7. Formerly there were problems in weaning an infant from formula. Why and how has this situation changed with recent methods of infant feeding?

8. Prepared commercial formulas are used generally in artificial feeding. How do they compare in composition with human milk? How do they compare in cost with either whole or evaporated cow's milk formulas?

9. Supplementary foods are introduced into the baby's diet gradually. What is the first supplement generally advised and in what amount? In what order are other foods introduced?

10. Why are we concerned today about overnutrition in infants?

11. What changes take place in the small child's food habits at about 1 year of age? Why does this occur?

12. Why do later emotional problems with food and appetite often have their origin at this period?

13. How can the nurse help to allay the mother's anxiety and sense of frustration about her child's food habits at ages 1-3 years?

14. How much milk is the 1- to 2-year-old likely to be willing to drink? What may happen if he is forced to drink a quart of milk daily?

SUPPLEMENTARY READING ON NUTRITION DURING INFANCY AND EARLY CHILDHOOD

Anderson, T. A., and Fomon, S. J.: Commercially prepared, strained, and junior foods for infants: Nutritional considerations. J. Am. Dietet. A., 58: 520, 1971.

————: Commercially prepared infant cereals: Nutritional considerations. J. Pediat., 78:788, 1971.

Beal, V. A.: Breast- and formula-feeding of infants. J. Am. Dietet. A., 55:33, 1969.

Children's Bureau: U.S. Dept. H.E.W., Washington, D.C. Breast Feeding Your Baby. C.B. No. 8, 1965; Your Baby's First Year. C.B. No. 400, 1962; Infant Care. 1966; Your Child From 1-3. 1966.

Committee on Nutrition, American Academy of Pediatrics: Vitamin D intake and the hypercalcemia syndrome. Pediatrics, 35:1022, 1965. Iron balance and requirements in infancy. Pediatrics, 43:134, 1969.

Economy in Nutrition and Feeding of Infants. Am. J. Public Health, 56:1756, 1966.

Editor's Column: Prop the baby, not the bottle. J. Pediat., 79:348, 1971.

Fomon, S. J.: Prevention of Iron-Deficiency Anemia in Infants and Children of Preschool Age. Public Health Service Publ. No. 2085. U.S. Dept. H.E.W., Washington, D.C., 1970.

Illingsworth, R. S., and Lister, J.: The critical or sensitive period, with special reference to certain feeding problems, in infants and children. J. Pediat., 65:839, 1964.

O'Grady, R.: Feeding behavior in infants. Am. J. Nursing, 71:736, 1971.

Review: Solid foods in the nutrition of infants. Nutr. Rev., 25:233, 1967.

Schmitt, M. H.: Superiority of breast-feeding—fact or fancy. Am. J. Nursing, 70:1488, 1970.

For Further References see Bibliography in Part Four.

Nutrition for Children and Youth

16

Nutritional Requirements of Children and Youth   •   Food Habits and Practices

INTRODUCTION

Children and youth comprise approximately 40 percent of the United States' total population today. The youth-oriented society of the 1970's has increasingly focused our attention on the needs of young people. New and innovative programs dealing with all aspects of childhood and adolescence, from comprehensive medical care projects for children and youth to coordinated health and educational centers for teen-age mothers and their infants, are developing in many communities; of particular concern in all of these are the needs of the disadvantaged child and the opportunities available to him. The training and experience that the nurse has in understanding the physical, psychological and social needs of individuals has made her expertise essential to all these projects, but equally important is the need to have nutritional evaluations and nutrition teaching an integral part of programs for children and youth.

This chapter will examine the nutritional requirements of the various age groups and the food habits and eating practices as these relate to nutritional requirements and developmental levels. The role and influence of school feeding programs is also discussed.

NUTRITIONAL REQUIREMENTS OF CHILDREN AND YOUTH

The Recommended Dietary Allowances, Table 16-1, for children from 3 to 10 years are the same for boys and girls. There is a gradual increase in growth and therefore, in the recommended amounts for most nutrients throughout childhood. However, because the adolescent growth spurt is markedly different between boys and girls, separate recommendations are given for boys and girls starting at age 10 years.

If the Daily Guide to Foods Needed by Children and Their Families (Table 16-2) is followed, using appropriate size servings for the different age groups, plus other foods suggested in the guide, the recommended dietary allowances for children and youth will be met.

Calories. The RDA for calories during childhood, 3 to 10 years, are based on a caloric allowance of 80 calories per kilogram of body weight. After age 10 there is a decrease in the calories per kilogram for both boys (50 calories per kilogram) and girls (35 calories per kilogram).

It is important to understand, however, that these recommendations represent average amounts for groups of children. An individual child may require more or less than the RDA, depending on his activity and rate of growth.

Adequate calories must be supplied if growth is to occur. When the caloric intake is below the requirement, protein foods will be used for energy instead of for tissue building. Macy and Hunscher[1] have shown that "a difference in intake of as few as ten calories per kilogram of body weight per day (or approximately four calories per pound) may make the difference between progress and failure in satisfactory growth."

---

[1] Macy, I. G., and Hunscher, H. A.: Nutrition, 45:189, 1951.

TABLE 16-1. RECOMMENDED DIETARY ALLOWANCES FOR CHILDREN AND YOUTH*

AGE (YEARS)	MALES AND FEMALES				MALES			FEMALES			
	3-4	4-6	6-8	8-10	10-12	12-14	14-18	10-12	12-14	14-16	16-18
Calories	1,400	1,600	2,000	2,200	2,500	2,700	3,000	2,250	2,300	2,400	2,300
Protein (Gm.)	30	30	35	40	45	50	60	50	50	55	55
Vitamin A (I.U.)	2,500	2,500	3,500	3,500	4,500	5,000	5,000	4,500	5,000	5,000	5,000
Vitamin D (I.U.)	400	400	400	400	400	400	400	400	400	400	400
Vitamin E (I.U.)	10	10	15	15	20	20	25	20	20	25	25
Ascorbic acid (mg.)	40	40	40	40	40	45	55	40	45	50	50
Folacin (mg.)	0.2	0.2	0.2	0.3	0.4	0.4	0.4	0.4	0.4	0.4	0.4
Niacin equiv. (mg.)	9	11	13	15	17	18	20	15	15	16	15
Riboflavin (mg.)	0.8	0.9	1.1	1.2	1.3	1.4	1.5	1.3	1.4	1.4	1.5
Thiamine (mg.)	0.7	0.8	1.0	1.1	1.3	1.4	1.5	1.1	1.2	1.2	1.2
Vitamin B_6 (mg.)	0.7	0.9	1.0	1.2	1.4	1.6	1.8	1.4	1.6	1.8	2.0
Vitamin B_{12} (mcg.)	3	4	4	5	5	5	5	5	5	5	5
Calcium (Gm.)	0.8	0.8	0.9	1.0	1.2	1.4	1.4	1.2	1.3	1.3	1.3
Phosphorus (Gm.)	0.8	0.8	0.9	1.0	1.2	1.4	1.4	1.2	1.3	1.3	1.3
Iodine (mcg.)	70	80	100	110	125	135	150	110	115	120	115
Iron (mg.)	10	10	10	10	10	18	18	18	18	18	18
Magnesium (mg.)	200	200	250	250	300	350	400	300	350	350	350

* From Food And Nutrition Board: Recommended Dietary Allowances. National Academy of Sciences–National Research Council, Washington, D.C., 1968.

TABLE 16-2. A DAILY GUIDE TO FOODS NEEDED BY CHILDREN AND THEIR FAMILIES*

TYPE OF FOOD	EACH DAY

Milk Group

Milk .... Children under 9 .... 2 to 3 cups
Children 9-12 .... 3 or more cups

Dairy products such as:

Cheddar cheese, cottage cheese, and ice cream .... May be used sometimes in place of milk

Vegetable-Fruit Group .... 4 or more servings

Include—

A fruit or vegetable that contains a high amount of vitamin C: Grapefruit, oranges, and tomatoes (whole or in juice), raw cabbage, green or sweet red pepper, broccoli, and fresh strawberries.

A dark green or deep yellow vegetable or fruit for vitamin A: You can judge fairly well by color—dark green and deep yellow: broccoli, spinach, greens, cantaloupe, apricots, carrots, pumpkin, sweet potatoes, winter squash.

Other vegetables and fruits, including potatoes.

Meat and Meat Substitutes .... 2 or more servings

Include—

Meat, poultry, fish, or eggs .... 1 or more servings
Dried beans or peas, peanut butter, and nuts can be used as meat substitutes.

Breads and Cereals .... 4 or more servings

Whole grain, enriched, or restored bread and cereals or other grain products such as corn meal, grits, macaroni, spaghetti, and rice.

Plus Other Foods

To round out meals and to satisfy the appetite, many children will eat more of these foods, and other foods not specified will be used, such as butter, margarine, other fats, oils, sugars, and unenriched refined grain products. These "other" foods are frequently combined with the suggested foods in mixed dishes, baked goods, desserts, and other recipe dishes. They are a part of daily meals, even though they are not stressed in the food plan.

* From Your Child from 6 to 12. Children's Bureau, U.S. Dept. H.E.W., Publ. No. 324. Washington, D.C., 1966.

Figures 16-1 and 16-2, which compare differences in increments in height and in calorie intake between early and late maturing boys and girls, are good illustrations of why the food intake of individual children must be adjusted to their specific needs.

The nurse is frequently the person responsible for keeping growth records. If a *growth chart* such as Figure 16-3 is used for recording height and weight, deviations from normal patterns can readily be seen. The chart shown is for boys from age 2 to 13. Similar charts have been constructed for girls of this age, for infants, both boys and girls, and for adolescent boys and girls. They are based on careful measurements of a selected group of children followed for the years specified and, as can be seen, show a wide range of variation.

The 50th percentile in both the height and the weight curves represents the median of all children measured. A child of stocky build is below the median for height and may be slightly above the median for weight. On the other hand, the tall, rangy child is well above the median for height and may or may not be below the median for weight.

The height and the weight recorded on such a chart at 6 month or yearly intervals show graphically how a child is progressing within his particular growth pattern. For example, a drop to a lower percentile in weight from one measuring

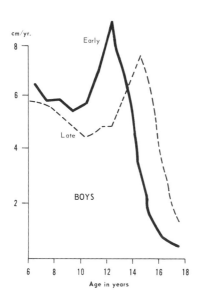

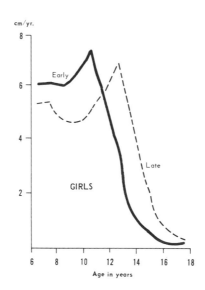

Fig. 16-1. Increments in the height of early and late maturing boys and girls (means of 20 in each group). Mitchell, H. S., *et al.*: The Adolescent Growth Spurt and Nutrient Intake. Presented at the International Congress of Nutrition, Hamburg, Germany, August 8, 1966)

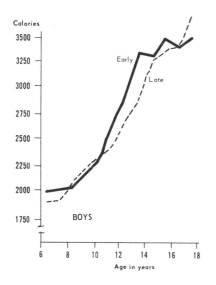

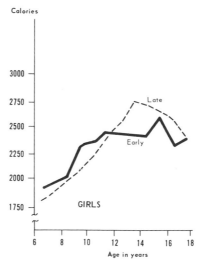

Fig. 16-2. Total caloric intakes of early and late maturing boys and girls (means of 20 in each group). Mitchell, H. S., *et al.*: The Adolescent Growth Spurt and Nutrient Intake, Presented at the International Congress of Nutrition, Hamburg, Germany, August 8, 1966)

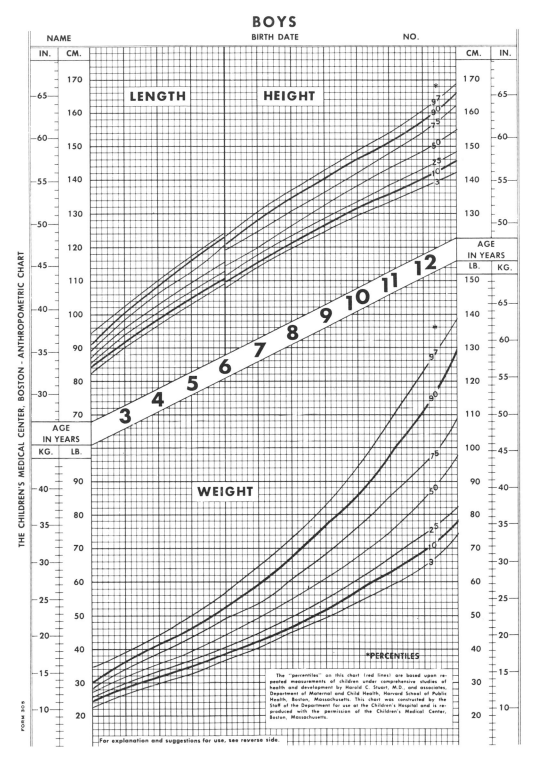

FIG. 16-3. Anthropometric Height = Weight Chart for Boys. For explanation of use see text. The break in height at the 6 year level occurs because up to that time the length of the child has been measured as he lay recumbent, while after this age the standing height is measured. The 50th percentile is the median range. Most children will fall somewhere between the 10th and the 90th percentile. From Children's Medical Center, Boston, Mass.

period to the next may indicate inadequate caloric intake, particularly if the height trend is in the same direction. The nurse will wish to determine the reason for this deviation. Likewise, a shift in weight to a higher percentile, if not accompanied by a similar height increase, should also alert the nurse to possible overnutrition.

The basic foods listed in Table 16-2 need to be supplemented by varying amounts of butter or margarine, salad dressings, jams, jellies, desserts and occasionally other sweets to meet the calorie needs of the different age groups.

Protein. Protein needs to be increased with growth, and protein intake should rise as calories are increased if a variety of foods is eaten. The milk and meat groups, including fish, eggs, cheese and peanut butter, meet the protein needs adequately. However, if the calories are obtained largely from carbohydrates, including candy and soft drinks in excess, both the quantity and the quality of the protein intake suffers.

Minerals. Milk in the amounts recommended is the main source of *calcium* and *phosphorus* and together with meat contributes significant amounts of magnesium. *Iron* needs for children can be met by an adequate intake of meat, eggs, green leafy vegetables, whole grain and enriched breads and cereals and potatoes. Dried beans, peas and peanut butter contribute a share of iron if these products form a staple article of the diet. Adolescent boys may be able to meet the RDA for iron because of the large quantities of these foods which they consume to meet caloric needs. The adolescent girl, however, probably needs an iron supplement, particularly after menstruation begins and iron is lost from the body. The necessary iodine is supplied by the use of iodized salt in cooking or as seasoning.

Vitamins. Vitamin needs are more likely to be met when a variety of foods is included in the diet. Milk, butter, fortified margarine and green and yellow vegetables and fruits will provide vitamin A. Milk fortified with vitamin D will ensure a sufficient intake of this vitamin. The B-complex vitamins will be included if good-quality protein foods, as well as enriched bread and cereals, appear frequently in the diet. In our Southern states, where cornmeal rather than wheat flour is frequently used, it is important to obtain enriched cornmeal when this is possible. In at least one Southern state, rice must be enriched by law. Vitamin C needs are not met as easily as other nutritional requirements.

Poor children especially do not always receive adequate amounts of ascorbic acid. Citrus fruits and tomatoes may be expensive items when not in season. Many of the fruit-flavored juices which are popular drinks with children do not supply significant amounts of ascorbic acid. If these are used to any extent by the young child to replace citrus juices, it is well to check on their vitamin C content. Raw potatoes are a good source of this vitamin but lose a large percentage of it in commercial processing, and the processed form of potato is the one most frequently found in the diets of children and adolescents. Cabbage and other leafy vegetables, particularly raw, contribute some of this vitamin to the diet whenever these foods are served.

FOOD HABITS AND EATING PRACTICES

The Preschool Child—3 to 5 years

The daily food guide (Table 16-2) serves as the basis of the diet for the 3- to 5-year-old child, although the size of servings is about half the average size used for older children and adults. A good estimate for size of a serving of a food served at a meal is approximately 3 tablespoons for the 3-year-old and 4 tablespoons for the 4-year-old. The 3- to 5-year-old should be encouraged to drink 1 to 1½ pints of milk a day. Some of this milk requirement may be provided in creamed soups and custards or other desserts included in his meals. Helping prepare and serve "instant puddings" is real fun for the preschooler and an excellent way to increase milk consumption in this age group.

Whole fruits and vegetables, both cooked and raw, should begin to appear in his menu. Meat should be cut in small pieces rather than ground. Remember that often at this age, a child will gladly eat such foods as raw carrots and lettuce with his fingers but refuse them if he has to use a fork or a spoon, because it is too difficult to manage the food with them.

It is usually desirable for the preschool child to have a midmorning, midafternoon and bedtime snack in addition to his regular meals. Some pediatricians feel that there is room for further study and research on the question of the number of meals best suited to the needs of the preschool child. Stitt[2] wonders "whether good nutrients dis-

---

[2] Stitt, P. G.: Nutrition Education Conf. Jan. 29, 1962. Washington, D.C.

tributed fairly evenly over the waking hours may not be what many children seem to reach toward." Milk, if not consumed at a regular meal, or fruit juice accompanied by bread, crackers or plain cookies, may form a good light meal or snack. Desserts, to be appropriate for the 3- to 5-year-old child, should furnish essential protein, minerals or vitamins as well as calories. They should not be given as rewards for finishing a meal or withheld as punishment for not doing so, but perhaps even offered with the meal if the child so prefers.

Children differ greatly in their natural preferences for food, but some patterns emerge clearly. "Finicky" food habits and food jags are characteristic of this age group. They may want to eat nothing except peanut butter sandwiches and fruit juice, or two to three hard cooked eggs at a sitting, but these patterns usually do not persist for very long, and soon they will settle down again to normal meals. The overall pattern of food intake from week to week and month to month is more important than the occasional food binge or refusal.

Project Head Start, serving children ages 3 to 5, has offered an opportunity of studying the food preferences of children from low-income families. These children usually lack experience with a wide variety of foods. Thus any program for the disadvantaged child should include experience with a variety of foods at the same time as it includes culturally familiar foods.

Preschool Day Care Centers. As a result of the intensive demand for adequate child-care facilities more and more day care centers are opening in our communities. The Child Development Center, a term currently being used for some of these, indicates their focus on the total development of the child—physical, psychosocial and intellectual. Many of these centers not only serve meals as part of the physical care of the child but also use food and mealtimes as an integral part of the learning and socializing process. They afford excellent opportunities for developing good food habits in children.

The breakfast and/or lunch served in the day care centers is a good chance to introduce children to fruit juices, fruits in season, and raw vegetables. They are pretty sure to like the familiar and simple main dishes, bread and butter and milk. Eating in company with other children, perhaps for the first time, often encourages the less venturesome to try something new. A story about a new

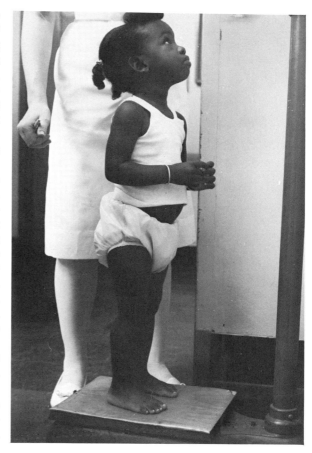

FIG. 16-4. A healthy child at the Pediatric Clinic, The New York Hospital. Note sturdy build, straight back, and alert interest in being weighed. (Children's Bureau photograph)

food and a small sample served attractively may make the difference between rejection and acceptance. Parent involvement in the programs of the center provides a chance for nutrition education for the entire family.

The nurse in a day care center plays an important role in evaluating the development of the child. In her parent conferences, she can discuss the child's growth progress, his food pattern and his mealtime behavior. She can function as a link between home and center by receiving and giving suggestions for the child's care. When the mother visits the center, the nurse may help her to observe and understand the eating behavior of the child.

The School Age Child—5 to 10 years

The basic food plan (Table 16-2) is the same for the school age child except that serving sizes increase until they are equal to or greater than the average adult serving.

The meal patterns for the school age child may vary depending on what the school provides and to what extent these services are used by the family. In any case the mother needs to plan the family's meals around the school situation.

Breakfast for the child going off to school is an important meal. Because many mothers today have a variety of responsibilities, the preparation of this meal is often shared with the whole family. The school age child with a minimum of help can prepare a simple breakfast. Many schools in low-income areas have introduced a breakfast program to provide disadvantaged children with a good start for the school day.

Under certain circumstances, especially if the school does not have a school lunch program, a bag lunch has to be carried from home. The bag lunch should be planned to supplement breakfast and dinner in terms of the foods selected from the food guide. Many children still need and enjoy snacks during this period. The after-school snack particularly is important and should be planned so as not to interfere with the evening meal.

Children's food habits develop along with other aspects of their growth. The 5- to 7-year-olds prefer plain foods such as meat, potatoes, raw vegetables, milk and fruits. Although most casserole dishes, mixtures of all kinds, fat meats and gravies are not liked, spaghetti and meat sauce, pizza, and macaroni and cheese are notable exceptions. By 6 or 7 they are willing to try new foods and to accept foods previously disliked. By 8 there is a ravenous appetite with few refusals but strong preferences. Food may be judged by odor or color, and food served attractively makes an impression. By 9 the child usually has a keen interest in food, likes to help prepare it and is positive in his likes and dislikes. Some eat everything at this age, but plain foods still are preferred.

One of the best methods for developing good food habits in children is for the whole family to eat wisely. If the mother and the father, knowing that they can expect certain variations in food acceptance by their children, can maintain a reasonably firm stand about over-all behavior, mealtimes can and should be one of the pleasant times of day for the whole family.

Children are great imitators. Although they may object, on the one hand, to being asked to conform, on the other they may be heard to say proudly to some friend, "My mother won't let me eat that."

Role of the Elementary School. For many children, elementary school is their introduction to group feeding. This can be difficult if the school does not make special provisions for the first and, perhaps, second graders. The hurry and confusion of most school cafeterias is not a conducive atmosphere for the average 6-year-old to eat and enjoy his lunch. A smaller group in a quieter place, such as the classroom, is a more satisfactory arrangement for this age. This arrangement also affords the opportunity to use the luncheon meal as an educational tool to develop the child's interest in food.

The nutritional contributions of the school lunch are particularly important to those children who do not receive adequate food at home. However, all children can share the social aspects of group feeding, and this in itself may be the incentive for a child to. try an unfamiliar food or to drink all his milk because the other children do.

The Challenges of Youth—10 to 18 years

Because the growth spurts for girls and boys usually occur at different ages (11 to 13 or 14 years for girls and 12 to 15 years for boys), their nutritional requirements during adolescence also vary. Before the spurt, the recommendations are only slightly higher than for the 8- to 10-year-olds and after the growth spurt taper off to the adult level.

All the foods included in the Daily Guide to Foods Needed by Children and Their Families (Table 16-2) are essential in the diet of the adolescent but in markedly increased quantities. A rapidly growing boy will need a quart or more of milk or its equivalent a day to meet his calcium requirement, and girls during their period of rapid growth also need a quart of milk daily. Skim milk may be substituted for whole milk if excess weight, real or imaginary, is a factor. The increased milk intake will provide good-quality protein for growth as well. All the other foods listed, eaten in sufficient quantity, will provide for the greatly increased physiologic needs during this period of growth and stabilization.

Besides adequate calcium, protein and calories, girls need an iron supplement when menses begin. An adequate amount of foods high in iron, such as lean meats, liver, eggs, green leafy vegetables, enriched breads and cereals and potatoes, should also be included in the daily food intake. This is

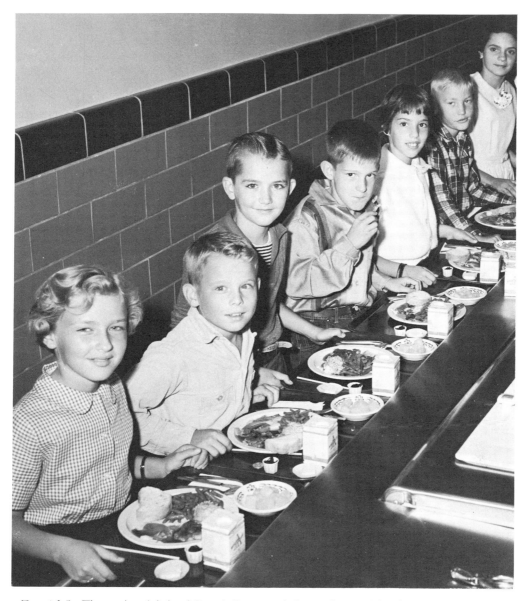

Fig. 16-5. The national School Lunch Program helps make good lunches available to school children. (U.S. Department of Agriculture photograph)

a period when the young girl, beginning to look forward to eventual marriage and motherhood, should be helped to realize that good nutrition is an important factor in the bearing of healthy babies.

During this period of rapid physical growth and sexual development, there is a concurrent maturing of the whole personality, with its attendant strains and stresses. The identity crisis of the teen-ager results in a drive for independence from parental restriction, coupled with an increased need for guidance and reassurance. There is a tremendous need for peer group approval, and following fads in food habits is common. The adolescent must be given the opportunity to make his own decisions, and parents must be understanding of this urge for independence, yet be willing to help when needed.

Because boys and girls differ in their response to this growth period, they are discussed separately.

Boys. As shown in Figure 16-6, the diets of adolescent boys at all ages were generally found to be adequate for protein, vitamin A, riboflavin and ascorbic acid; however, iron, calcium and thiamine were low in the diets of certain age groups.

The adolescent spurt stimulates appetite, as is well recognized. The energy and nutrient requirement for this spurt in any one boy is not known. If the increments of height gained as shown in Figure 16-1 are compared with the caloric intake for the same boys (Fig. 16-2), it is not surprising that the early maturers experienced an earlier increase in food intake than the late maturers.[3]

That serious undernutrition in boys still exists is known from the number of army recruits rejected as being physically unfit, but, on the whole, the nutritional outlook for boys is good.

Girls. With many girls the story is different. Despite the abundance of food in the United States and the inclusion of nutrition education in most elementary and high schools, the USDA Food Consumption Survey (Fig. 16-6) shows that teen-age girls, at all ages, comprise one of the most poorly fed groups in our population. The most serious deficits were in iron and calcium

[3] Mitchell, H. S., *et al.*: Proc. VII Int. Cong. Nutrition, 1967.

SEX—AGE (YEARS)	PROTEIN	CALCIUM	IRON	VITAMIN A VALUE	THIAMINE	RIBO-FLAVIN	ASCORBIC ACID
MALE AND FEMALE:							
Under 1			x x x x				
1-2			x x x x				
3-5			x x				
6-8							
MALE:							
9-11		x					
12-14		x x	x x x		x		
15-17		x	x				
18-19							
20-34							
35-54		x					
55-64		x x					
65-74		x x					
75 & over		x x x		x		x x	x
FEMALE:							
9-11		x x x	x x x x		x		
12-14		x x x	x x x x	x	x		
15-17		x x x x	x x x x		x x		
18-19		x x x	x x x x	x	x		
20-34		x x x	x x x x		x	x	
35-54		x x x x	x x x x		x	x x	
55-64		x x x x			x	x	
65-74		x x x x	x	x	x x	x x	
75 & over		x x x x	x	x x	x x	x x x	

x—1 through 10%   xx—11 through 20%   xxx—21 through 29%   xxxx—30% or more

Fig. 16-6. Nutrients Less Than the Recommended Dietary Allowances. (National Academy of Sciences–National Research Council, 1968) (From Food Intake and Nutritive Value of Diets of Men, Women and Children in the U.S., Spring, 1965. Agr. Res. Serv. U.S.D.A., Washington, D.C., 1969.)

with smaller numbers in vitamin A and thiamine. This finding is particularly critical in view of today's early marriage and childbearing ages (see Chap. 14), with the additional nutritional demands being made on the young mother's body.

The caloric intake of adolescent girls shows quite a different picture from that of the boys (see Figs. 16-1 and 16-2). One can almost read into these graphs the psychology of the early-maturing girls who were concerned about their rapid growth and increase in height ahead of the boys their age. Thus they curtailed their total food and often chose unwisely with respect to essential nutrients. The late-maturing girls did not make as drastic a reduction in caloric intake until much later.

The concern of teen-age girls often centers on weight reduction, whether necessary or not. There is probably no great harm in this, if the essential foods to meet nutritional needs are included in the diet. However, if soft drinks, candy and other sweets are substituted for milk, fruits and vegetables, as is often the case, there may be a reduction in essential minerals and vitamins but not in calories.

Adolescent Obesity. A word of warning concerning adolescent obesity is necessary in any discussion of nutritional needs of this age group. Although the basic cause of juvenile-onset obesity is not well-understood, the fact that most fat children remain fat adults indicates an urgent need to prevent its development when possible and also to treat it when it occurs.

A minority of both boys and girls have the habit of consuming more calories than they can use for energy and growth and thus become overweight for their height and age. Whether this is due to underactivity or to overeating or to a combination of the two, adolescent obesity presents a real problem to the teen-ager's social and emotional adjustments as well as to his future health. Obese adolescents are discriminated against in many ways. They are rejected by their peer group, harassed by their parents, set apart from the average by the fashion industry, laughed at in movies and television, and generally excluded from the mainstream of teen-age life.[4]

Improving the poor self-image that the obese adolescent frequently has of himself is usually the first step in his treatment. As his self-confidence is developed, his determination to effect change can often be depended on to motivate him through the long and difficult struggle with weight control. Although adolescent weight control is more successful with parental understanding and cooperation, the teen-ager must be the one responsible for his food intake. Weight control is discussed in Chapter 21.

STUDY QUESTIONS AND ACTIVITIES

1. What are some food preferences and prejudices of children at various ages?
2. What is the probable effect of a poor breakfast on the total food intake? Why do American families so often eat an inadequate breakfast?
3. Why do you think adolescent girls eat so much more poorly than boys in the same age group? Have you had experience with this problem yourself?
4. What are the food needs of the teen-ager? Do girls have additional nutritional needs compared with boys? What are these, why do they occur and how may they be met?
5. How is the Daily Guide to Foods Needed by Children and Their Families adapted to meet the nutritional needs of the various age groups?
6. Why is adolescent obesity of particular concern to the nurse?
7. Observe a preschool child during mealtime either in the hospital or a day care center. What was the menu served to the child? What were the portion sizes? Approximately how much of the various items did the child eat? Describe his eating technics. Were there any opportunities for socializing during the meal?

SUPPLEMENTARY READING ON NUTRITION OF CHILDREN AND YOUTH

Beal, V. A.: Dietary intake of individuals followed through infancy and childhood. Am. J. Public Health, 51:1107, 1961.
————: Iron nutriture from infancy to adolescence. Am. J. Public Health, 60:666, 1970.
Bettelheim, B.: Food to Nurture the Mind. The Children's Foundation, 1026 17th St., N.W. Washington, D.C., 1970.
Children's Bureau: Your Child from 6 to 12. 1966. Moving into Adolescence. 1966. U.S. Dept. H.E.W., Washington, D.C.
Dairy Council Digests: Nutritional status of the teen-ager. D.C.D. 35: No. 1, (Jan.-Feb.) 1964. Nutrition and physical fitness. D.C.D. 36: No. 5 (Sept.-Oct.) 1965. The effect of nutrition on body composition. D.C.D. 37: No. 1, (Jan.-Feb.) 1966.

---

[4] Peckos, P. S.: Food and Nutrition News (Dec.-Jan.), 1970-71.

Daniels, A. M.: Training school nurses to work with groups of adolescents. Children, 13:210, (Nov.-Dec.) 1966.

Everson, G. L.: Bases for concern about teen-agers diets. J. Am. Dietet. A., 36:17, 1960.

Hammar, S. L.: The role of the nutritionist in an adolescent clinic. Children, 13:217, (Nov.-Dec.) 1966.

Hill, M. M.: Food Choices: The Teen-age Girl. Brochure. Nutrition Foundation. New York. 1966.

Obert, J. C.: When the bell rings. Am. J. Nursing, 61:89, 1961.

Peckos, P. S., and Heald, F. P.: Nutrition of adolescents. Children, 11:27, (Jan.-Feb.) 1964.

For Further References see Bibliography in Part Four.

Geriatric Nutrition

17

Nutrition of Older People · Food Requirements Change With Age
Planning Meals For Older People
Community Food and Nutrition Programs For the Older-age Adult

INTRODUCTION

Nutritional requirements for the mature person and the older adult are not fundamentally different from those of the young adult. However, because the aging process gives each age group unique characteristics, geriatric nutrition is worthy of special consideration.

The difference between the terms aged and aging should be clearly defined: the aged are people; aging is a continuous process. Aging begins at conception and terminates at death. Thus birth, growth, maturation and senescence are all part of the normal aging process. Aging proceeds more rapidly during the growing years because change is more rapid at that time. In the adult, the aging process slows down and the rate of this change may be further retarded; the active period of life may be extended by good health practices.

The figure of 20 million persons over 65 years of age in the United States in 1971 is about double the number of that age group 31 years earlier in 1940. Of these, over 60 percent are widowed or unmarried, and many live alone. One-half of the women and ⅓ of the men over 65 years living alone had annual incomes under $1,000. Medical science, which is largely responsible for this increase in the number of senior citizens today, is also challenged to learn more about the degenerative and chronic diseases common in this group. The social sciences also have a responsibility to help make later years of life more livable.

Besides the obvious changes of aging, there are invisible changes within the body that may develop as gradually as the hair turns gray. Therefore, authorities emphasize that an adult's nutrition must be considered in terms of the past, the present and the future. The nutritional state of a person at 70 or 80 reflects not only his current food practices but all of his previous dietary history as well. This can be observed by anyone with a close and long association with older persons. As Dr. Swanson[1] comments:

> The older a person grows, the longer and more complex is his dietary history. The variations in nutritional status and dietary needs of a group of adults thus are bound to be greater than corresponding variations in a group of young people. Recommendations for the food needs of this age group must be pointed especially to the needs of individuals.
>
> The same nutritional principles that describe adequate diets for earlier periods of life apply to the diets of adults. Even though the adult has grown up —matured—his basic food supply still must provide all the nutrients necessary for maintaining body structure and for operating its machinery.

Good nutrition is only one of the practices which help to maintain strength and vigor, but it can be practiced three times a day—and it is abused more frequently than any other.

It has been demonstrated repeatedly that older people can adjust to circumstances, learn new skills and adopt new food habits. We cite a few examples: the 80-year-old man who learned to eat salads when a thoughtful housekeeper chopped them to make them easier to eat yet kept them colorful and attractive; the two women in Figure 17-1 serving as volunteers in the hospital, feeling useful and adapting themselves to needed tasks;

---

[1] Swanson, P.: Nutrition Needs After 25. Food. The Yearbook of Agriculture. Chap. 28. U.S.D.A., Washington, D.C., 1959.

165

the elderly homemaker who still liked to try new gadgets and ready-prepared foods to make work easier and yet provide interest and variety in meals for two. "Never too old to learn" is a far truer adage than "You can't teach an old dog new tricks."

None of us is too young to begin thinking about improving the health of later years. People buy annuities and life insurance for the future; why not consider other steps which may give even greater security and comfort?

NUTRITION OF OLDER PEOPLE

Food Habits and the Consequences

Food habits of older people do not always coincide with their food needs. Several surveys of the food choices of older people have been made in different localities; all report much the same trends. In a Boston survey of 104 geriatric patients, most of them over 70, Davidson[2] found a marked decrease in consumption of meat and milk and an increased use of eggs, but no caloric deficit. In fact, 84 percent of the men and 71 percent of the women were above desirable weight. He observed factors that seemed to affect the food habits of these elderly retired people: social situation (over half of them lived alone), reduced income, limited cooking and refrigeration facilities,

_____
[2] Davidson, C. S.: Am. J. Clin. Nutr., 10:181, 1962.

marketing difficulties, condition of the teeth, sense of smell, problems of swallowing, food faddism and long-standing misconceptions concerning what constituted good nutrition.

Susceptibility to Fads. Unfortunately, many adults in late middle age, or older, are misled in their search for "eternal youth" or relief from their aches and pains. They hear and believe the glamorous TV and radio promotions of various panaceas—elixirs or multivitamin and mineral mixtures claimed to be remedies for all sorts of ills. They read and believe the faddy health books, especially those that have been flooding the book market during the past decade. It is well-known that food and nutrition quackery thrives in areas where middle income retired people congregate. So-called health food stores may carry many desirable food items, but they also stock a variety of items ("health foods") promoted by the faddists.

Food Requirements Change with Age

The dietary requirements of later life are influenced by a number of factors such as general health, degree of physical activity, changes in ability to chew, digest and absorb food, efficiency in the use of nutrients by the tissues, alteration in the endocrine system, emotional state and mental health. The nutrient and calorie allowances that maintain one person in optimum health may be inadequate or more than adequate to meet the needs of another apparently similar individual.

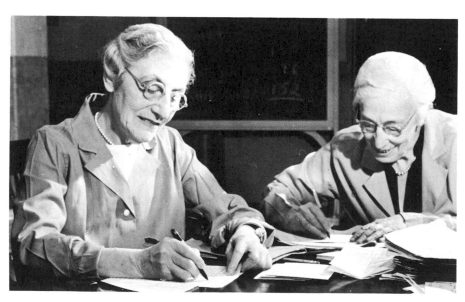

FIG. 17-1. Two long-faithful volunteers happy doing a needed job. (The New York Hospital)

Dr. Swanson's comment is especially pertinent:[3]

A person at 70 is an historical record of all that has happened to him—his injuries, infections, nutritional imbalances, fatigues and emotional upsets. Old people, therefore, differ from each other much more than do younger folk. All this needs to be considered in food planning for any old person. Each one is an individual, quite unlike anyone else.

Calorie Needs

As age advances there is a progressive decrease in metabolism coincident with less physical activity; thus, the calorie need is some 16 percent lower at 65 than at 22 years of age. For example a woman of 65 weighing 128 pounds may need only 1,700 calories, whereas she needed 2,000 or more at age 22, when she weighed the same but was more active. If she does not reduce her caloric intake to conform to her needs, she will store the excess as fat—so common in older people, particularly women.

WHEN CALORIES NEED TO BE REDUCED

The food sources of these reduced calories must be chosen with care to include all essential factors and in higher proportion than in former years because the total food consumed is less. There is an obvious need for foods which carry a full quota of proteins, minerals and vitamins. The day is past when a reduction in the amount of all foods was a satisfactory solution. It is essential to reduce consumption of empty calories—sugar, rich desserts, cakes, candies, fats and alcohol.

Reduction in total calories involves a most difficult task of alteration of food habits. For the majority of persons, habit is perhaps one of the greatest obstacles in the path of an optimal diet. The longer the habits are continued, the more fixed they become. The food habits of older people are apt to be so fixed that it is difficult to change them unless the way is made easy.

Whoever is planning or preparing the meals for *overweight* persons—the homemaker herself, a health aide or housekeeper—can eliminate some calories behind the scenes (if necessary) while still keeping meals attractive and in the familiar pattern. If people do not see the high calorie foods, one psychological barrier has been overcome. By substituting for rich cakes and pastries such items as puddings and custards made with skim milk, angel food cake and more fruit desserts, gelatins, whips, etc., calories are saved without sacrificing flavor. Also low-calorie salad dressings, less butter or margarine on vegetables,

and gravies made with a minimum of fat are devices for the cook to use before the food reaches the table.

When appropriate, the nurse concerned with the continuing education of the patient may make specific suggestions along this line in keeping with the socioeconomic status of the patient and his cultural pattern of eating.

Surplus calories are not the only reason for curtailing the carbohydrates and the fats in the diets of older people. Some of them seem to have a reduced capacity for metabolizing sugars, and this may result in a fluctuating blood sugar level. When this is true, fewer sweets are advisable. Other foods in moderation, such as potatoes, cereals and bread, are better tolerated to meet the caloric needs.

Fats are the most concentrated source of calories and often the invisible component of common foods. For those who eat out, foods fried in deep fat are apt to be popular, since fats give flavor and satiety value to meals, but too much fat may result in indigestion or discomfort for some elderly people. The most serious problem for the middle aged and past middle aged group concerns the type and amount of fat in the diet and their relation to the blood cholesterol level and to the incidence of atherosclerosis. There are still many uncertainties and misconceptions concerning this problem, which is discussed in Chapters 3 and 23.

WHEN CALORIES NEED TO BE INCREASED

Quite another problem exists for the really elderly, or the disabled and shut-in who may not get enough food to meet his caloric or other nutritional requirements. If he lives alone or has poor cooking facilities, there is little incentive or opportunity to market and cook for himself.

Sometimes appetite fails to tempt the very elderly to eat enough food or the right kind of food. The reduced calories in such cases seldom carry enough of the essential nutrients.

The undernutrition which may occur can often be relieved by attention to foods with low bulk and concentrated calories, high in protective values and prepared in a way which the person enjoys. This may not be easy for the person living alone or as a member of a large family where attention to the younger members of the family seems more important to the homemaker than tempting the appetite of an elderly grandmother. For others the same problem may stem from the necessity of eating in hotels or restaurants where food does not appeal to the appetite or may be too expensive.

---

[3] Swanson, P.: op. cit.

Protein Requirements

Apparently, protein needs are not reduced appreciably with age, and yet many older people eat less protein than when they were younger. This is most likely to happen when marketing is difficult, cooking facilities are poor or the money for food is limited. It can also happen among those of better economic status when denture troubles, lack of appetite or too little energy prevent the preparing or the eating of meats or other protein foods.

Some good-quality protein is essential at each meal regardless of age. The Recommended Dietary Allowances suggest no reduction in protein with age, as they do in calories. Thus, the proportion of protein making up the total calories is increased.

The requirement for certain amino acids may even be increased to meet changes in body function with age. Bigwood[4] found the methionine and lysine requirements of six male subjects 50 to 70 years of age to be substantially greater than for younger males.

Special attention may need to be given to meeting the protein requirements of the older person if he is sharing in the family meals planned to meet the higher caloric food habits of the younger members of the family. An extra glass of milk (perhaps reconstituted dry skim milk) at meals or between meals may be the answer. If the person lives alone, milk, cheese and eggs are often used as alternates for meat, fish or poultry because of ease in preparation. Adequate calories tend to spare protein, so that the total food intake should always be taken into account.

Mineral Requirements

The calcium needs of older people seem to be as great as the needs of younger adults.

Inadequate calcium intake along with some endocrine disturbance may cause the loss of calcium from the bones and lead to osteoporosis and resulting fragility, so frequently responsible for fractures. Lowered gastric acidity and hepatic and pancreatic insufficiency may contribute by impairing calcium absorption. Increased excretion of calcium due to impaired kidney function or to reduced physical activity may also play a role in osteoporosis.

Dr. Swanson's comments are pertinent[5]:

We cannot consider bony tissue in the adult as static material. It is a dynamic substance, which constantly remodels itself. Formation of new bone and destruction of old bone go on simultaneously. These processes approximately balance each other in the healthy adult. . . . As a person grows older, however, the process of bone destruction may overbalance that of bone building. That this occurs is suggested by observations that the average weight of the skeleton decreases gradually after age 35. The extent to which such decalcification may proceed without injury is not known. We do know that it does not always occur in all individuals.

But we cannot ignore the fact that osteoporosis, or deficient bone substance, certainly is not uncommon in later life. . . . It is commoner among older women than among men. Persons with marked osteoporosis tend to eat food poor in a number of nutrients, including calcium. They also tend to improve in health and to store calcium when the diet is improved.

Osteoporosis is prevalent among older people around the world and especially so in countries where calcium intakes are relatively high. The reasons for poor calcium absorption or utilization in older people is still subject to speculation. There is a possibility that traces of fluorine in drinking water may improve calcium utilization and thus decrease the incidence of osteoporosis. A survey of people living in high- and low-fluoride areas of North Dakota[6] showed osteoporosis more common in the low-fluoride areas than in the higher fluoride areas. This finding served to confirm earlier suggestions of the benefit of fluoride for older people.

At present the best suggestion is to provide liberal amounts of milk and milk products. These may be used in cooking, creamed soups, milk desserts, etc. The use of nonfat dry milk is to be encouraged in cooking as an inexpensive source of good protein and calcium. Present evidence favors about 0.8 Gm. of calcium per day.

Needs for other minerals are apparently similar to those for all adults, as discussed in Chapter 6.

Vitamin Requirements

Unfortunately, little is known regarding the vitamin requirements of older people and whether there is a change with age or association with

---

[4] Bigwood, E. J.: Nutritio et Dieta, 8:226, 1966.

[5] Swanson, P.: op. cit.
[6] Bernstein, D. S.: JAMA, 198:499, 1966.

chronic disease. However, there is no evidence that vitamin requirements are reduced with advancing years, and it is safe to assume that older people need all the vitamins that they did in earlier years.

If there has been merely a marginal supply of any of the vitamins in the diet for many years, then a reduction in total food eaten may be sufficient to precipitate minor nutritional deficiencies. The time factor which is inevitable with advancing age may permit cumulative effects to show up.

PLANNING MEALS FOR OLDER PEOPLE

The planning of food to meet the needs of the older age group presents many problems, which are as varied as the circumstances in which such people live. They may be living alone, or with one or two other older people, and marketing and preparing meals for themselves; they may be the older member in a younger family; they may be cared for by a practical nurse or a housekeeper.

Whoever is responsible for planning and preparing food should be aware of likes and dislikes, special needs and limitations. There are numerous factors, such as ignorance of nutritional facts, food prejudices, fear of new foods, lack of money, limited cooking facilities and poor appetite, which should be considered. The Daily Food Guide described in Chapter 10 is as important for meeting the nutritional needs of older people as it is for younger ones. The public health nurse may be able to advise or help with the planning where such problems seem to interfere with obtaining adequate food.

The elderly person, too often a forgotten member of the household, may require some special foods or food preparation, but so far as possible he or she should be a member of the family at mealtime and eat foods prepared for the family. If digestive ability is limited, the family meals should be so planned that the older person may avoid fried foods, rich sauces, pastries and other foods that disagree with him. When lack of meal-

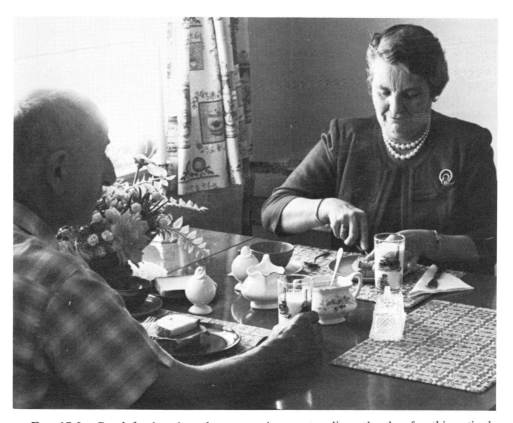

FIG. 17-2. Good food and a pleasant environment enliven the day for this retired couple. (Administration on Aging, U.S. Dept. H.E.W., Washington, D.C.)

time appetite makes an adequate food intake difficult, a midmorning and a midafternoon lunch of something light, such as hot malted milk or orange juice, may be offered. A hot drink at bedtime may be welcomed by an older person and may help to induce sleep.

The older handicapped person, living alone, may encounter real difficulties in preparing meals for himself. *Homemaking for the Handicapped* offers many suggestions to those with physical limitations to assist them in homemaking skills.[7]

When groups of older people are confined in institutions or nursing homes, they sometimes become depressed. Volpe and Kastenbaum[8] reported on a ward of 34 confused and deteriorated older men who were agitated and hostile and had poor appetites. They were transferred to a larger ward where a record player was installed and games provided and with large tables for meals. They dressed in white shirts and ties and had an afternoon snack of beer, crackers and cheese. Within a month the atmosphere changed and behavior improved.

Bulletins and pamphlets published by national and state agencies and by insurance companies give simple information about food for older people.

One publication reminds us that making simple food attractive and appropriate to the specific needs of an elderly person is appreciated far out of proportion to the effort involved. An example of good planning occurred at the golden wedding of the parents of one of the authors. One parent was a partial invalid and had a denture problem. The dinner menu of fruit cocktail, turkey croquettes, mashed potatoes, peas, aspic salad, ice cream and a beautiful anniversary cake was a meal that all guests could enjoy, including the guests of honor, who would have been embarrassed by a different menu. Senior members of most families enjoy the young folks at family parties, but they do not want to be conspicuous because of their infirmities. With a little preliminary planning of an appropriate menu, the party can be fun for young and old.

[7] May, E. E., Waggoner, N. R., and Boettke, E. M.: Homemaking for the Handicapped. New York, Dodd, Mead & Co., 1966.

[8] Volpe, A., and Kastenbaum, R.: Am. J. Nursing, 67: 100, 1967.

COMMUNITY FOOD AND NUTRITION PROGRAMS FOR THE OLDER-AGE ADULT

Many communities have programs which provide services especially appropriate for the older-age adult. The following discussion indicates the variety of different types of opportunities which may be available for the senior citizen in his community. The nurse should become knowledgeable about the resources in her local area.

Food Stamps and Donated Commodities. The local community may have a food stamp or donated commodities program to aid all low-income persons in obtaining an adequate diet. Many older age adults, living on very limited incomes, are eligible for assistance from whichever one of these programs the local community provides. The welfare department determines eligibility, depending on the size and income of the family unit.

In the *food stamp* program, those eligible to participate must purchase food stamps at a bank or other authorized agency. The actual purchasing power of these stamps is greater than the amount which the consumer pays for them. The stamps or coupons may be used to buy food in any cooperating retail store. Although they represent a real saving in terms of food dollars, many older citizens with very little cash to spend hesitate to make the proportionately large monthly or semimonthly investment which is necessary to purchase the coupons. This aspect of food budgeting is an area where the nurse may be able to help the older client understand the long-term advantages of such a program.

The local welfare department also certifies eligibility for *donated commodities* depending on the family size and income. In this program, certain donated foods are made available to be picked up by the eligible recipients at specific times and places. This system, although supplying a variety of different kinds of foods at no cost to the recipient, is often difficult for the elderly person: the place and time may be inconvenient as far as transportation is concerned; the packaging may be too large for the one- or two-member family; or the food processing may not be appropriate for modified diets, as in the case of sodium restriction. Foods may also be included that are unfamiliar to the older person. By understanding the various aspects of the problem, the nurse may be able to assist the senior citizen to plan for the economical use of donated foods.

Home Health or Neighborhood Aides. For the person capable of remaining in the home where assistance in meal management can be furnished, home health or neighborhood aides have been made available by certain community agencies. These aides are trained to go into homes to "provide advice, nutrition counseling, education, information services and moral support on such matters as marketing, food preparation, handling and storage, uses of equipment and budgeting."[9] Nurses together with other members of the home care team such as dietitians, nutritionists or home economists, help train and supervise home health aides. The provision of these services enables many an elderly person to continue to maintain himself for longer periods of time in his own home than could be possible otherwise.

Portable Meals Programs. Often referred to as meals-on-wheels, portable meals programs have been initiated in many cities by various community groups. They are for the home-bound person who cannot prepare his own meals. They often provide 2 meals a day (one hot and one cold) for 5 days a week. Because breakfasts and weekend meals are usually not included, participants in these programs must have some additional resource for providing meals in the home.

Community Group Feeding Programs. In recent years a variety of group-feeding projects have been started in communities to provide the older adult with good nutrition in a sociable atmosphere. Federal grants have helped sponsor many of these in different locations throughout the country. All sorts of facilities have been used, from churches and schools to housing projects and senior citizen day care centers. For the older person who is able to go to the center and is interested in meeting people, these programs offer recreational as well as nutritional benefits to the participants. Many of these also include nutrition or consumer education programs.

The senior citizen is often hesitant about searching for and requesting help; so it is especially important for the nurse to know the opportunities available and how to take advantage of them.

STUDY QUESTIONS AND ACTIVITIES

1. Surveys have shown that older people are apt to omit certain foods from their diets. Which ones are these and which nutrients are deficient as a result?

2. Why is the caloric requirement of older people reduced? How much reduction in caloric intake is recommended between age 22 and 65?

3. What advice would you give an older person who should reduce his calorie intake? How may calories be increased for the underweight older person?

4. What disease in older people may result from failure to absorb or utilize calcium? What suggestions are offered that may help to improve calcium utilization?

5. If an elderly person shares the family fare but eats less of everything than younger members, which nutrients may be lower than recommended? How can this be remedied?

6. In what circumstances may the use of vitamin concentrates be justified?

7. If an older person with whom you are associated is a food faddist or a follower of some of the quack books, how would you attempt to correct his false ideas? What reliable sources of information would you recommend? (See Chap. 10.)

8. What nutrition services for older people are available in your community?

SUPPLEMENTARY READING ON GERIATRIC NUTRITION

Alvarez, W. C.: Osteoporosis, a disease that attacks millions. Geriatrics, 25:77, 1970.

Current Comment: Nutrition and eating problems of the elderly. J. Am. Dietet. A., 58:43, 1971.

Jalso, S., Burns, M., and Rivers, J. M.: Nutrition beliefs and practices. J. Am. Dietet. A., 47:263, 1965.

Lane, M. M.: The ideal geriatric diet. Nursing Homes, 16:27, (Jan.) 1967.

LeBovit, C.: The food of older people living at home. J. Am. Dietet. A., 46:285, 1965.

Pelcovits, J.: Nutrition for older Americans. J. Am. Dietet. A., 58:17, 1971.

Piper, G. M.: Nutrition in coordinated home care. J. Am. Dietet. A., 39:198, 1961.

Piper, G. M., and Smith, E. M.: Geriatric nutrition. Nurs. Outlook, 12:51, 1964.

Review: Fluoride, bony structure, and aortic calcification. Nutrition Rev., 25:100, 1967.

Stare, F. J.: Good nutrition from food, not pills. Am. J. Nursing, 65:86, 1965.

Stone, V.: Give the older person time. Am. J. Nursing, 69:2124, (Oct.) 1969.

Volpe, A., and Kastenbaum, R.: Beer and TLC. Am. J. Nursing, 67:100, 1967.

For Further References see Bibliography in Part Four.

---

[9] Howell, S. C., and Loeb, M. B.: Nutrition and aging —a monograph for practitioners. The Gerontologist, 9:77, (Autumn) 1969.

PART THREE

Diet in Disease

Introduction to Part Three

Setting the Climate • **Interpretation of the Diet Plan** • **Patient Education**
Knowledge • **Patient-Centered Care** • **Communication Skills**

Under the guidance of the physician and the diet order which he devises, the nurse and dietitian share with him the responsibility for the dietary component of patient care. Each brings to this responsibility his own professional orientation and functions, but for each the focus is the patient.

It is helpful to consider dietary care under three major headings: (1) setting a climate in which it is possible for the patient to eat; (2) interpreting or reinforcing the physician's explanation of the purpose of the dietary plan of care; and (3) assisting the patient through education to accept and to carry out a modification of his food practices. Patient education is not limited to those requiring therapeutic diets; it includes those individuals who are faced for any reason with modifying food practices to ensure an appropriate intake of nutrients.

SETTING THE CLIMATE

For the nurse, setting the climate means the skillful application of those comfort, hygiene, and safety measures she is taught early in her educational experience with patients—for example, positioning the bed patient so that he may feed himself or be fed comfortably, or scheduling treatments and medications so that he is ready to eat when food is served. Whether the nurse herself sets the climate or directs those who assist her, she influences, to a great degree, the acceptance of food by the patient.

For the dietitian, setting the climate includes the establishing of food service schedules for the convenience of the patient, and the planning of the menus and the preparation of foods that are acceptable to him. It is well to recognize that individuals under stress of illness may not be able to accept new and unfamiliar foods or methods of food preparation. The dietitian's creativity is not to be denied but it should be creativity acceptable to the patient by virtue of his past experiences with food.

Setting the climate for patients is a joint responsibility of the administrative personnel in the nursing and dietary departments. Providing a climate for the acceptance of food requires careful planning of nursing and dietary routines and procedures, based on a mutual appreciation of each other's day-to-day responsibilities and pressures. But, with service to the patient as the major goal, coordination of functions often results in both effective nursing and dietary care.

INTERPRETATION OF THE DIET PLAN

In her continuous and close contact with the patient the nurse is often the first to become aware of a patient's anxiety or confusion about his physician's diet order, be it a "normal" or a therapeutic one. Many of the expressions of concern which may come to the nurse's attention are of the moment, and a simple explanation or answer to a question often reassures the patient at that time.

When the dietitian is in the patient area at mealtime and at other times during the day she will also become aware of patients' concerns and will need to help them understand the "whys" of their doctors' diet orders.

To reduce, rather than add to, a patient's anxieties or confusion, close communication among physician, nurse, and dietitian is essential. Also, it is important to recognize that reassurances of the moment to relieve anxiety should not be equated necessarily with education. In a stressful situation, what the patient hears today may be forgotten tomorrow.

PATIENT EDUCATION

When a patient needs instruction in normal nutrition, or in a minor modification of his diet, it is expected that physician, nurse or dietitian are all able to do this. When, for therapeutic reasons, the diet of a patient is complex, it is expected that the dietitian will assume the major responsibility for educating the patient. She alone is the member of the health team qualified by education and training to assume this function. For example, a patient with renal disease, who requires a diet modified in protein, sodium and potassium, will need to be instructed by a highly skilled dietitian if he is to manage this complicated diet successfully at home. And, just as important, his diet instruction cannot be done satisfactorily on the day he is discharged from the hospital.

Diet instruction for any patient must be anticipated by physician, nurse, and dietitian and done well in advance of his discharge from the hospital. Education to change behavior takes time; the patient needs time to learn how to cope with a diet he may have to use for many years to come. The nurse, in many situations, coordinates the planning for discharge. She may also be the one who knows and shares with the physician and the dietitian how the patient feels about his diet, what his problems will be when he goes home, and what he needs to be taught.

Sharing the responsibility for dietary care and patient education implies that both the nurse and the dietitian will possess: (1) knowledge of the science and art of foods and nutrition; (2) personal attitudes which will be reflected in patient-centered care; and (3) equal skill in communicating with the patient, and with each other.

KNOWLEDGE

Knowledge of the science and art of foods and nutrition is basic to creating a climate for the acceptance of food, interpreting the physician's diet plan, and educating the patient. The way in which the nurse and the dietitian use their knowledge will vary. The effect of a cerebral vascular accident on the swallowing reflex of a patient will be viewed differently by each: the nurse will consider the effect when positioning the patient for feeding; the dietitian, when selecting food of the right consistency for this same patient.

The degree to which both will apply their knowledge of foods and nutrition will also vary. The nurse applies her knowledge of the diet modification in chronic renal disease to interpret the diet plan to the patient correctly and to reinforce the dietitian's instructions when necessary. The dietitian will apply the same principles in devising the diet plan and in educating the patient. Both nurse and dietitian need to understand the metabolic aberrations in renal disease. At the same time both need to know the nutrient composition of foods at the per serving level—the dietitian, however, in more detail than the nurse.

PATIENT-CENTERED CARE

A true commitment to patient-centered care is required of both nurse and dietitian. Chapter 11 explains how the food habits of an individual will reflect his social and cultural heritage, and how one patient's food habits will be different than another's. The nurse and dietitian will demonstrate their acceptance of these individual differences when they take the time to discover what a patient usually eats, and use this information properly in meeting his nutritional needs. Also, if the nurse or dietitian is to gain the confidence of the patient, each must question the patient and listen to his answers in a way that makes it possible for him to tell them what he really eats.

COMMUNICATION SKILLS

Nurses and dietitians use the same communication skills. Both learn about the patient by reading his record, by observing him and listening to him, and by interviewing him. Both are committed to sharing their knowledge of the patient through appropriate notations in his record, through team conferences in the clinical unit, and through a variety of other institutional routines. Without communication with the patient and with each other in behalf of the patient, patient-centered care is not achieved.

Assessment of Patient Needs

18

Introduction · **Cultural Factors** · **Psychological Influences** · **Physical Condition**
Potential for Learning

Some of the modifications of the normal diet that are commonly made in the treatment of disease will be described in the chapters in this section of the book. To achieve their purpose these modified diets must be followed as accurately and carefully as the physician's orders for medication and other treatment. However, unlike a medication, food is a part of everyday life. It is not primarily associated with illness, and it has many meanings besides that of satisfying hunger. For this reason there may be severe stumbling blocks to the patient's acceptance of a therapeutic diet, whereas he will accept a distasteful medication or a painful treatment without question.

The dietary modification prescribed for the patient must be translated successfully into foods with which he is already familiar, and into a meal pattern similar to that of his family. When this is done there is a far greater probability of the diet being followed and thus being successful in regard to its therapeutic goal. At the same time, both the nurse and the dietitian must recognize that they may encounter a patient whose previous food practices may need to be drastically changed, not modified, to meet the therapeutic goal of his diet. A patient facing this problem requires special support and understanding as he struggles to change his food habits.

As one seeks to help a patient to accept a therapeutic modification of his food practices as part of the treatment of his disease, it must be kept in mind that his food habits are part of his social and cultural heritage. In addition, certain psychological factors and his physical condition will influence his acceptance of food during his illness. The following sections of this chapter discuss some of the factors which one needs to consider in assessing a patient's needs, and in planning his diet with him.

CULTURAL FACTORS

Cultural heritage, family background and status, religious customs, family patterns of food preparation and service, emotional experiences with food, as well as exposure to nutrition education, food fads, and superstitions all contribute to the individual's food habits. A variety of ethnic patterns may be encountered in the hospital (see Chap. 11). The Orthodox Jewish, the Puerto Rican, the Mexican, the Polish and the Italian patient may have food habits different from each other's and from those of other Americans. Even in the United States food patterns may vary widely by region. A patient from the South who finds himself in a Northern hospital may feel that, because of the way vegetables are cooked, they are insipid and uninteresting and he may flatly refuse to eat them. These differences may well be the first problem confronting the nurse and the dietitian when they are helping the patient to adjust to needed diet modifications in the hospital.

Most people's lives are set in families, and to eat in bed and by one's self may accentuate the patient's illness in his mind. Some hospitals try to meet this problem by having as many patients eat together as possible, and here the hospital ward, with several patients in a room, may actually be a better setting than a single room with its lone private patient. Even a low-sodium diet may be accepted when its restrictions are shared with a fellow patient.

PSYCHOLOGICAL INFLUENCES

Illness may change a person's psychological orientation to everyday occurrences and personal relationships; the need for the familiar and the customary is immeasurably increased. Because what, how and with whom we eat is an everyday occurrence, illness, which interrupts this pattern, may have serious psychological repercussions. The fear, the worry, the insecurity and the frustration that possess the patient as he changes from an independent, healthy individual to one dependent on others in illness is often expressed through regressive behavior. Fussiness, anorexia or demands for extra attention are traits that may be exhibited by the worried patient. Babcock says that "it is easier to show discouragement through anorexia than it is to explain that one is feeling inadequate and depressed in the presence of a frightening disease or a disheartening experience."[1]

The apparent apathy or uncooperativeness of a patient may mean not that he does not want to eat, but that the food offered to him is unacceptable because of its emotional connotations. His food habits have developed slowly through the years and have become a personal and guarded part of himself, so that many foods may be associated with specific feelings and emotions separate from their nutritional significance. Such foods as milk, cocoa, custards, junket, creamed and strained foods, first met with in infancy, become associated with the dependency and the security of that period. Some adults will refuse such foods despite their apparent nutritional value simply because they resent the dependency of illness. Because of the sense of security they convey, others may cling to using these same foods, even though they may not be desirable nutritionally or psychologically.

Desserts, sweets and delicacies have become reward foods to many people because they first were received as a reward for cleaning one's plate or being a good child. It is not surprising that adolescents, and older people too, indulge in excessive intake of such foods when they are under stress and in need of psychological reward.

In the United States some foods have gained special status. Steaks, chops, green salads and butter are four examples of these foods. Patients may resent suggestions to reduce the cost of food by substituting ground meat for steaks and chops, or margarine for butter. On the other hand the young homemaker who is well aware of the cost of food uses ground meat and margarine.

Tea, coffee and alcoholic beverages may be thought of as adult foods by some patients because they were forbidden to them as children. Excessive use of these beverages, to the exclusion of milk, may be an expression of a desire to seem mature. On the other hand, some cultural groups use tea, coffee and alcoholic beverages regularly as part of the daily diet for the whole family, including the children.

It must not be forgotten that the appearance of the food and the tray also will produce a psychological effect which may determine acceptance or rejection of the meal. Hot food must be served *hot* and cold food *cold*. A pot of *hot* coffee or tea may make the remainder of a restricted diet acceptable. It tells the patient, as no words can, that those about him really care about him and are making every effort to make his food as palatable as possible.

The therapeutic diet itself may have meaning for the patient that is not evident to the professional staff. Everyone rejoices with the patient who progresses from a liquid diet to one containing solid food as concrete evidence that he is getting better. But, should that patient ask if he must follow a sodium-restricted diet for the rest of his life, are we aware that he may be inquiring in reality if he is going to have cardiac disease permanently, with all that this implies? The therapeutic diet which must be of long duration may give to the patient a real sense of deprivation, with depressing overtones that are difficult to resolve.

All those concerned with the nutrition of people need to be cognizant of what food means to people under various circumstances. Attempts to change long-established and deeply ingrained patterns may be met with resistance. The overzealous nurse, dietitian or physician who is trying to teach a patient "what is good for him, nutritionally," may interpret the patient's response as "ignorance" or "lack of cooperation." Pumpian-Mindlin writes[2]: "To accomplish the prime purpose of regulating and guiding what goes into a patient's mouth, one must learn to listen carefully to what first comes out of the same mouth. . . . Otherwise one may find himself in the position of having more than mere words thrown in one's face." We must be able to interpret what the patient says or does not say about food, what he

---

[1] Babcock, C. G.: J. Am. Dietet. A., 28:222, 1952.

[2] Pumpian-Mindlin, E. J.: J. Am. Dietet. A., 30:576, 1954.

does with food, and how he reacts to food service in the light of his emotional as well as his metabolic needs. Whatever dietary changes may be necessary for his therapy must be made within this framework if they are to be successful.

PHYSICAL CONDITION

Through observation the physical characteristics of the patient which may influence his acceptance of food or ability to feed himself may be identified. Because of her constant contact the nurse, more readily than the dietitian or even the doctor, will often be the one to make these observations.

Older patients may have lost some of their teeth, making chewing difficult if they are placed on a general house diet. Some individuals will use poor fitting dentures for cosmetic reasons and remove them at meal time. The adolescent boy with a fractured jaw may complain bitterly of hunger because his liquid house diet has not been modified sufficiently in calorie content or frequency of feeding to satisfy his needs. Patients recovering from oral surgery will not be appreciative of the effects of citrus juices on a sore mouth. Assessment of the ability to swallow is critical for certain patients if aspiration and its adverse effects are to be avoided.

Patients with emphysema and other respiratory difficulties may be forced to eat and drink slowly and, therefore, may need their trays for a longer period of time than other patients. Providing adequate nutrients and fluids for these individuals may require four or five meals per day.

Many individuals with sight problems, including the blind, can and prefer to feed themselves. They will need to be oriented to the placement of dishes and other articles on their trays. They may need help in pouring beverages, in opening milk cartons, and in removing protective coverings from foods. Individuals with poor manipulative skills such as the arthritic or the multiple sclerosis patient may need the same kind of assistance. Assessing the ability of any handicapped individual and providing the proper assistance not only will reduce his frustrations and promote his independence but also may help him to achieve a reasonable nutrient intake.

Every patient does not require the same size serving of food. A nursing note which states "appetite poor" may really mean that the patient was served too much food not, as this note is usually interpreted, that the patient did not eat enough food. A high-calorie diet for an 82-year-old, 5-foot 1-inch chronically ill woman may be 2,000 calories and for a 27-year-old, 6-foot 2-inch man after an hemorrhoidectomy, 3,500 calories.

The long-term or chronically ill patient presents a special challenge to both the nurse and the dietitian. The scheduling of treatments and nursing care are often critical factors in obtaining a proper

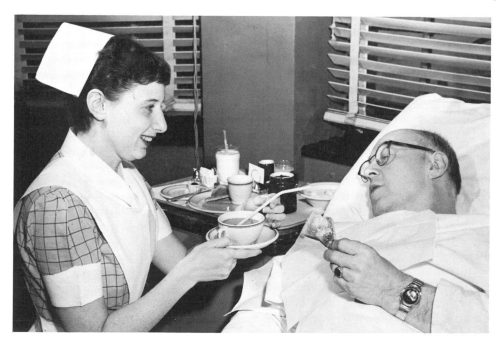

FIG. 18-1. The patient who must be fed is more likely to eat and enjoy his meal if the person assisting him is cheerful and unhurried. (The New York Hospital)

food intake. The best meal of the day for some of these patients is breakfast because they are rested or, for some of the older patients, because breakfast has always been an important meal. As the day progresses they may become increasingly tired and tend to eat less. Therefore, treatments should be planned so that the patient may rest before the noon and evening meals. Some of these patients may require only minimal assistance at breakfast and considerably more at the evening meal.

Interval nourishments for the chronically ill patient need to be carefully planned. A 400-calorie milkshake at 10:30 A.M. may result in the patient's refusal of an 800-calorie meal at 12:00 noon. Four meals, with the last one served at 8:00 or 9:00 P.M., may be a more effective plan for providing for his nutrient needs, especially if he is accustomed to an evening snack at home.

The patient restricted to prolonged bed rest benefits from nursing care procedures which promote the maximum movement by, or of, himself. Research has shown us that immobilization, even with adequate food intake, promotes negative nitrogen and calcium balance which may result in progressive muscular weakness. Turning and positioning the patient as ordered by the physician and providing passive exercise during personal care will help to prevent the adverse metabolic effects of immobility.

Cycle menus which repeat the same menus every four to six weeks are used in many hospitals. The long-term or chronically ill patient presents real problems to the dietitian, especially if he experiences two or three periods of a cycle menu plan, even though the menu items are familiar and acceptable to him. For some patients this will not be a problem; for others, it will. Family members or friends can often be helpful when a patient becomes bored with the hospital's food by occasionally providing a favorite dish from home, although they will need direction from the dietitian so that their contribution will fit his diet plan.

The wife of a patient who will require a sodium-restricted diet for the years ahead may demonstrate her understanding of the dietitian's instructions and her skill in adjusting her methods of food preparation by bringing her husband the "fruits" of her labors. At the same time she may feel a certain satisfaction from participating in her husband's care.

POTENTIAL FOR LEARNING

The nurse and the dietitian in their roles as educators will begin by discovering, through observation, listening, and interview, what the patient knows about nutrition and diet; his attitudes toward his illness and diet; and his readiness for learning, when necessary, how to manage a complex therapeutic diet.

Studies tell us that, as our nutrition education programs in elementary and secondary schools have been improved, we have a better educated young adult population today than in the past. If we are to avoid boring patients by giving them nutrition information they already have, we need to find out what they know and how they use it. In this way we can discover the problem, if any, and focus our teaching on the patient's real need.

As we listen to the patient his vocabulary will give us numerous clues as to the words and kinds of explanations we will need to use in teaching him. For example, if the patient is a newly diagnosed diabetic who is an organic chemist he may expect the nurse or dietitian to use the word "carbohydrate"; whereas, the mother of six children who reads and understands at the 6th grade level will need to be approached quite differently. In helping her to understand diabetes and her diet we would more likely use the word "sugar."

With the increasing use of programmed instruction both the nurse and the dietitian will want to watch for clues as to whether or not a patient is literate, in English or any other language. We have not always been aware of this in the past as we used printed instructions, since children, friends, or other patients may have interpreted such instructions for the patient.

The dietitian who begins diet instruction as early as possible during the patient's hospitalization can use the trays served each day to demonstrate to him the kinds and amounts of food he will be eating at home. At the same time, she can involve him or a member of his family in the planning of his daily menu. This approach to patient education not only prepares the individual and his family for his discharge but also, in many instances, stimulates the patient's interest in learning about his diet.

STUDY QUESTIONS AND ACTIVITIES

1. Select a patient who has been identified as a "feeding" problem. With the assistance of your instructor determine what the patient's problem

really is. Either through your nursing care plan or communication with the appropriate individual(s) how can you work toward a solution to the problem?

2. With a classmate and with the help of your nursing instructor choose two patients with whom neither of you has had previous contact. The patients should be the same sex, about the same age, and, if possible, from the same socioeconomic class. Each student should select and study one patient's chart. Using the information gained from your study of Part One of this book and from courses in the social sciences, list the food practices you expect of your patient. Through observation and interview discover what his practices actually are. In clinical conference you and your classmate will report how each of these patients met your individual expectations and how each one differed from these expectations.

SUPPLEMENTARY READING ON ASSESSMENT OF PATIENT NEEDS

Aiken, L. H.: Patient problems are problems in learning. Am. J. Nursing, 70:1916, 1970.

Babcock, C. G.: Attitudes and the use of food. J. Am. Dietet. A., 38:546, 1961.

Bermosk, L. S.: Interviewing: a key to therapeutic communication in nursing practice. Nurs. Clin. of N. Am., 1:205-214, 1966.

Cantoni, M.: Adapting therapeutic diets to the eating patterns of Italian-Americans. Am. J. Clin. Nutr., 6:548, 1958.

Fathauer, G. H.: Food habits—an anthropologist's view. J. Am. Dietet. A., 37:335, 1960.

Guidelines for the therapeutic dietitian in making notations on the medical record. J. Am. Dietet. A., 49:215-216, 1966.

Hacker, D. B., and Miller, E. D.: Food patterns of the Southwest. Am. J. Clin. Nutr., 7:224, 1959.

Jernigan, A. K.: Discharge diets versus patient education. Hospitals, 45:100-101, (Feb. 16) 1970.

Johnson, D.: Effective diet counseling begins early in hospitalization. Hospitals, 41:94, (Jan. 16) 1967.

Kaufman, N.: Adapting therapeutic diets to Jewish food customs. Am. J. Clin. Nutr., 5:676, 1957.

Levine, M. E.: The intransigent patient. Am. J. Nursing, 70:2106, 1970.

Morris, E.: How does a nurse teach nutrition to a patient? Am. J. Nursing, 60:67, 1960.

Outpatient diets match cultural backgrounds. Hospitals, 45:70, (June 16) 1971.

Paynich, M. L.: Cultural barriers to communication. Am. J. Nursing, 64:87, 1964.

Simon, J.: Psychologic factors in dietary restriction. J. Am. Dietet. A., 37:109, 1960.

Stitt, P. G.: Helping medical students find the strength in people. Children, 13:104, (May-June) 1966.

Stone, V.: Give the older person time. Am. J. Nursing, 69:2124, 1969.

Torres, R. M.: Dietary patterns of the Puerto Rican people. Am. J. Clin. Nutr., 7:349, 1959.

Valassi, K. V.: Food habits of Greek-Americans. Am. J. Clin. Nutr., 11:240, 1962.

Vargas, J. S.: Teaching as changing behavior. J. Am. Dietet. A., 58:512, 1971.

Wilson, N. L., *et al.*: Nutrition in pulmonary emphysema. J. Am. Dietet. A., 45:530, 1964.

For Further References see Bibliography in Part Four.

Progressive Hospital Diets

19

The Diet Order • The Diet Manual • Management of Patient Food Service
Progressive Hospital Diets • Fluid Intake

INTRODUCTION

The Diet Order. A patient's diet prescription is ordered by the physician, and will be found in the orders written by him at the time the patient is admitted to the hospital. The order will depend on the patient's condition and may vary from nothing-by-mouth to a normal or regular diet. The diet order is changed as the patient's condition changes. If he is known to have a disease which requires the modification of the normal diet as part of his treatment, or if diagnostic procedures during hospitalization discover this, a therapeutic diet will be ordered.

The Diet Manual. The diet manual is a compilation of routine and therapeutic diet plans and is used for ease of communication among the physician, the nurse, and the dietitian. The manual serves as a guide to the kinds and amounts of food the dietary department will serve to a patient to fulfill his physician's diet order. Under Medicare in the Conditions of Participation for Hospitals,[1] the dietary department is required to have an up-to-date manual which has been approved jointly by the medical and dietary staffs. A copy of the manual used by a hospital is usually available in the Ward Office or at the head nurse's desk for the convenience of physicians and nurses.

In teaching hospitals and in many large hospitals, physicians and dietitians, working together in committee, frequently compile a diet manual for use in their institutions. Some of these manuals are used only by the hospital in which they were written, while others have been published and are used by a variety of institutions. Diet manuals

have also been compiled by the combined efforts of a State Department of Health and the State Dietetic Association, for use by small hospitals and nursing homes in a particular state. (See partial list of diet manuals at the end of this chapter.)

As a general rule the first section of a manual will describe routine or standard diets for infants, children and adults, including soft and liquid diets; the following sections will describe a variety of therapeutic diets used in the treatment of disease. Diet manuals often differ in the terms used to describe diets, and in the recommendations for the foods to be used in a diet plan. The nurse should become thoroughly familiar with the diet manual used by the hospital in which she is located.

This chapter discusses the management of patient food service, the general principles used in setting up the routine diet plans—sometimes referred to as house diets or progressive diets—and meeting fluid needs of patients.

MANAGEMENT OF PATIENT FOOD SERVICE

In acute care hospitals, menu planning, food buying and preparation, and the delivery of meals to the patient area are directed by a qualified administrative dietitian. A qualified clinical dietitian, in conjunction with the administrative dietitian, is responsible for planning daily menus and therapeutic regimens with the patients. In some hospitals the patient's tray is delivered to his bedside by a dietary department employee; in others by an employee of the nursing service. In either situation, nursing and dietary services are concerned with the needs of the patient, his comfort and satisfaction. Communication and cooperation between the two services are achieved most

---

[1] Health Insurance for the Aged: Conditions of Participation for Hospitals, p. 20. Soc. Sec. Adm. HEW HIM—1, 1966.

effectively by a joint dietary-nursing service committee with the responsibility for establishing and reviewing routines which best serve the patient.

Food Service Management. Two management systems are used in hospitals today. Under one system the hospital administers all aspects of the dietary department including patient and employee food service and the nutritional care of patients. Under another system the hospital contracts with a food service or catering company to manage all aspects of the dietary department. Either system, properly managed, can provide quality food service for patients and employees.

Food Service Systems. Two types of food service systems, centralized and decentralized, are used to deliver food to the patient area. In centralized service, a patient's tray is completely assembled in or near the food production area and delivered to the patient area in a specially designed cart or by a conveyor system or dumbwaiter. The tray is delivered to the patient directly from the cart or from a service pantry.

Decentralized service refers to the method by which bulk food is transported from the production area to a service kitchen in the patient area. The patient's tray is assembled in the service kitchen and delivered to the bedside. Either system requires that nursing and dietary departments carefully coordinate their schedules so that patients receive palatable, attractive food.

Cost analysis of these two systems have generally shown that the centralized one is the most economical method for serving adult patients. However, decentralized service is to be preferred in pediatric units caring for children ages 2 to 12. Portion size varies by age and appetite in this group to such an extent that tray service in or close to the patient area is desirable in order to avoid overwhelming children with more food than they can eat. The needs of the adolescent can be met, where necessary, with double adult size servings.

Meal Service Schedules. Traditionally hospital dietary departments have served patients three meals a day—morning, noon, and night. When necessary, beverages and snacks have been available between meals. This schedule is used by many hospitals and appears to reflect the habits of the patients it serves.

Recently, due to labor costs and problems of staffing in the dietary department, new meal service schedules have been adopted. In some hospitals food is served four times a day: a continental breakfast, usually coffee and a roll, at 7:00 a.m.; brunch or lunch at 10:30 a.m.; dinner at 3:30 or 4:00 p.m.; and a snack, usually a sandwich and beverage at 8:00 or 8:30 p.m. The continental breakfast and the evening snack is frequently served on disposable materials and, with the exception of coffee, prepared by the food service workers at low work load periods during the day. Within an 8-hour work day one group of highly skilled cooks can prepare both the brunch and the dinner. Some hospitals use a five- rather than a four-meal plan which includes the brunch and dinner meal plus three snack-type meals.

Where patient acceptance of the four-meal plan has been evaluated it has been discovered that they like the plan. Nursing personnel have also accepted this revised meal schedule. They point out that on busy medical units fewer patients miss a major meal due to delayed breakfasts for tests or treatments, and the patients enjoy the snack served in the evening at the end of visiting hours. The four- or five-meal plan has been successful in those extended care facilities and nursing homes which serve geriatric patients who often may need frequent, small meals.

Selective Menus. The hospital patient is offered a daily menu from which he can select his meals. Two or more items in each section of the menu are usually offered; for example, at dinner there may be a choice of roast beef or fried chicken, mashed or baked potato, etc. In some, but not all hospitals, the patient requiring a therapeutic diet is also offered a selective menu. The printed menus are marked by the patient each day usually for service the next day.

Selective menus, even when alternatives are limited, have improved patient food acceptance. Patients with poor vision or who cannot read need assistance. All selective menus need to be evaluated daily to insure adequate nutrient intake by the patient. The individual who consistently selects a less than adequate diet needs professional guidance.

When selective menus are used by patients requiring therapeutic diets, diet instruction must be given so that his selections will fulfill his diet plan. The selective menu can serve as a "paper and pencil test" of a patient's knowledge of his therapeutic diet and serve to identify, as instruction progresses, areas where reinforcement of instruction is needed.

PROGRESSIVE HOSPITAL DIETS

Regular, Standard, General. A variety of terms are in current use to describe the normal hospital diet which will provide a patient with the calories and nutrients he needs. It is intended for ambulatory patients and for those whose condition does not require a therapeutic diet.

The foods chosen for the regular diet menu will reflect the preferences characteristic of the cultural background and the economic status of the majority of those served by the institution. The choice of food will be further determined by its suitability for quality and quantity preparation, seasonal availability and local market costs and conditions. It is not surprising, therefore, that patients and staff members coming from backgrounds different from that of the local area may find some unfamiliar items on the menu.

The pattern dietary, Table 19-1, reproduced on the following page for the convenience of the reader (see Chap. 10), constitutes the basic pattern on which the regular hospital diet is planned. This pattern furnishes the nutrients recommended by the National Research Council for an adult, with the exception of calories and iron. It is assumed that when the menu for the regular diet is planned, "other foods" as desired and as required by a patient will be added. For example, cream or milk and sugar will be served with the breakfast cereal and coffee; or other beverages may be served with the three meals, either with or without sugar and cream. Jelly with the toast may add pleasure to the meal as well as additional calories. Soup and crackers are desirable additions. Two more vegetables may be added, one of them raw, if the patient's condition permits. If not, additional citrus fruit, such as orange or grapefruit juice, is desirable. Desserts also furnish not only calories but other important nutrients as well. It is well to remember that some patients may require fewer calories than usual, since even ambulatory patients are less active during hospitalization than they are at home or at work.

The nutritional adequacy of a regular diet depends not only on the selection of foods and the amounts served but also on the protection of the nutrients in food during preparation and cooking, including the time and temperature of these processes.

The regular diet may be modified by food selection and methods of food preparation and in consistency for patients who cannot tolerate it but do not require a therapeutic diet. These modifications of the regular diet are the light or convalescent diet; the soft diet, including the surgical soft, medical soft, and dental soft diets; and the full liquid and clear liquid diets. Foods Used in Progressive Hospital Diets (Table 19-2) illustrates the types of food used in planning regular, light, soft and full liquid diets; and Table 19-3, Typical Menus for Progressive Hospital Diets, illustrates how these foods are used in menu plans.

Light or Convalescent Diet. A light, or convalescent, diet is intended for convalescent patients not yet able to tolerate the regular diet and for those with minor illnesses. It must be appetizing and readily digested. The chief difference between this diet and the regular diet is the method of preparation. The foods are cooked simply, and fried foods and rich pastries are omitted. Other fat-rich foods, such as pork (except bacon) and salad dressing, are avoided. Bran and strong or gas-forming vegetables are avoided, as well as most raw vegetables and fruits. All foods included in the soft and the liquid diets may be served on the light diet. In some hospitals this classification is omitted.

Soft Diet. The soft diet is soft in texture and consists of liquids and semisolid foods. It is an intermediate step between the liquid and the light diets. It is indicated in certain postoperative cases, in acute infections and in some gastrointestinal conditions; also, it may be ordered for the debilitated patient for ease of eating.

It is low in residue and is readily digested. Little or no spices or condiments are used in the preparation. It is somewhat more restricted than the light diet in fruit, meat and vegetables.

The foods used in the medical soft diet are generally the same as those used in the soft diet in Table 19-2. In the surgical soft diet less tender meats and certain vegetables and fruits may be puréed or blenderized.

Dental or Mechanical Soft Diet. The regular diet may need modification for patients with poor teeth or none, or with dentures which they are unable or unwilling to wear. The nurse can be of help by seeing that the term "dental soft" is included in the diet order. Additional cooked vegetables or juices should be substituted for salads, and no whole meats should be served, unless the physician approves of the patient eating whole tender meats. Otherwise the diet should follow the foods used in the Light Diet.

The Full Liquid Diet. Liquid diets are usually prescribed for the postoperative patient, or the patient acutely ill with an infection, gastrointestinal tract disturbances, or a myocardial infarction. (See Table 19-2 for the kinds of fluids used and Table 19-3 for a suggested menu.)

Clear Liquid Diet. If the patient's condition requires it, only clear fluids may be offered him. In addition to water, clear broth, fruit juices, thin

TABLE 19-1. EVALUATION OF A PATTERN DIETARY FOR ITS NUTRITIVE CONTENT[1]

FOOD GROUP	AMT. IN GM.	HOUSEHOLD MEASURE	CALORIES	PROTEIN Gm.	FAT Gm.	CARBOHYDRATE Gm.	MINERALS				VITAMINS				
							CALCIUM Mg.	PHOSPHORUS Mg.	MAGNESIUM Mg.	IRON Mg.	A I.U.	THIAMINE Mg.	RIBOFLAVIN Mg.	NIACIN Mg.	ASCORBIC ACID Mg.
Milk or equivalent[2]	488	2 c. (1 pint)	320	17	17	24	576	452	63	.2	700	.16	.84	.3	5
Egg	50	1 medium	81	7	6	..	27	102	5	1.2	590	.06	.15	Tr.	..
Meat, fish or fowl[3]	120	4 ozs., cooked	376	30	31	..	13	212	104	3.3	280	.14	.23	6.1	..
Vegetables:															
Potato, cooked	100	1 medium	65	2	..	15	6	48	22	.5	..	.09	.03	1.2	16
Deep green or yellow, cooked[4]	75	½ c.	21	2	..	6	44	28	29	.9	4,700	.05	.10	.5	25
Other, raw or cooked[5]	75	½ c.	45	2	..	10	16	41	18	.9	300	.08	.06	.6	12
Fruits:															
Citrus[6]	100	1 serving	44	1	..	10	18	16	12	.3	140	.06	.02	.3	43
Other[7]	100	1 serving	85	..	..	22	10	21	16	.8	365	.03	.04	.5	4
Bread, white, enriched	70	3 slices	189	6	2	35	59	68	15	1.7	..	.17	.15	1.7	..
Cereal, whole grain or enriched[8]	130 30	⅔ c. cooked or 1 oz. dry	89	3	1	18	12	95	34	.9	..	.08	.03	.7	..
Butter or margarine	14	1 tablespoon	100	..	11	..	3	2	2	..	460	..	..	..	..
Totals			1,415	70	68	140	784	1,085	320	10.7	7,535	.92	1.65	11.9[9]	105
Compare with recommended allowances[10]													NIACIN EQUIV.		
Reference man (70 Kg., 22 yrs. old)			2,800	65	..	..	800	800	350	10.0	5,000	1.40	1.70	18	60
Reference woman (58 Kg., 22 yrs. old)			2,000	55	..	..	800	800	300	18.0	5,000	1.00	1.50	13	55

[1] Calculations from Composition of Foods. Handbook No. 8. U.S. Department of Agriculture, Rev. 1963.
[2] Milk equivalent means evaporated milk and dried milk in amounts equivalent to fluid milk in nutritive content; cheese, if water-soluble minerals and vitamins have not been lost in whey; and food items made with milk.
[3] Evaluation based on the use of 700 Gm. of beef (chuck, cooked), 200 Gm. of pork (medium fat, roasted), 200 Gm. of chicken (roaster, cooked, roasted) and 100 Gm. of fish (halibut, cooked, broiled) per 10-day period.
[4] Evaluation based on figures for cooked broccoli, carrots, spinach and squash (all varieties).
[5] Evaluation based on figures for raw tomatoes and lettuce, and cooked peas, beets, lima beans, and fresh corn.
[6] Evaluation based on figures for whole orange and grapefruit, and orange and grapefruit juices.
[7] Evaluation based on figures for banana, apple, unsweetened cooked prunes and sweetened canned peaches.
[8] Evaluation based on figures for shredded wheat biscuit and oatmeal.
[9] The average diet in the United States, which contains a generous amount of protein, provides enough tryptophan to increase the niacin value by about a third.
[10] From the National Research Council Recommended Dietary Allowances, revised 1968.

TABLE 19-2. FOODS USED IN PROGRESSIVE HOSPITAL DIETS

TYPE OF FOOD	REGULAR DIET	LIGHT DIET	SOFT DIET	FULL LIQUID DIET
Fruits	All	All cooked and canned fruits, citrus fruits, bananas	Fruit juices, cooked and canned fruits (without seeds, coarse skins or fiber), bananas	Fruit juices, strained
Cereals and cereal products	All	Cereals: dry or well-cooked, spaghetti and macaroni, not highly seasoned	Same as light diet	Gruels, strained or blended
Breads	All	Enriched and whole-wheat bread, crackers	Same as light diet	
Soups and broths	All	All	Broth, strained cream soups	Same as soft diet, or blended
Meat, fish and poultry	All	Tender steaks and chops, lamb, veal, ground or tender beef, bacon, chicken, sweetbreads, liver, fish	Tender chicken, fish and sweetbreads; ground beef and lamb	
Eggs	Eggs cooked all ways	Soft-cooked eggs	Same as light diet	Eggnogs*
Dairy products	Milk or buttermilk; cream; butter; cheese, all kinds	Milk or buttermilk; cream, butter; cottage and cream cheese, Cheddar cheese used in cooking	Same as light diet	Milk or buttermilk, cream
Vegetables	All, including salads	Cooked vegetables: asparagus, peas, string beans, spinach, carrots, beets, squash Salads: tomato and lettuce Potatoes: boiled, mashed, creamed, scalloped, baked	Cooked vegetables: same as light diet Salads: none Potatoes: same as light diet	Vegetable juices
Desserts	All	Ices, ice cream, junket, cereal puddings, custard, gelatin, simple cakes, plain cookies	Same as light diet	Ices, ice cream, gelatin, junket and custard
Beverages	All	Tea, coffee, cocoa; coffee substitutes; milk and milk beverages; carbonated beverages	Same as light diet	Same as light diet

* Because of the danger of salmonella infection when raw egg is used, a pasteurized commercial eggnog preparation is recommended.

TABLE 19-3. TYPICAL MENUS FOR PROGRESSIVE HOSPITAL DIETS

REGULAR DIET	LIGHT DIET	SOFT DIET	FULL LIQUID DIET
		BREAKFAST	
Fresh pear	Orange	Orange juice	Orange juice, strained
Oatmeal with milk or cream	Oatmeal with milk or cream	Oatmeal with milk or cream	Strained oatmeal gruel with milk or cream
Scrambled eggs	Soft scrambled eggs	Soft scrambled eggs	Coffee with cream and sugar
Buttered whole-wheat toast	Buttered whole-wheat toast	Buttered whole-wheat or white toast	10 A.M.
Coffee with cream and sugar	Coffee with cream and sugar	Coffee with cream and sugar	Eggnog*
		DINNER	
Vegetable soup	Vegetable soup	Strained vegetable soup	Broth
Roast veal	Roast veal	Ground beef	Ginger ale with ice cream
Mashed potato	Mashed potato	Mashed potato	Coffee with cream and sugar
Buttered broccoli	Buttered carrots	Buttered carrots	
Tomato salad with French dressing	Tomato salad with French dressing	Bread: whole-wheat or white	
Bread: whole-wheat, rye or white	Bread: whole-wheat, rye or white	Butter	
Butter	Butter	Vanilla ice cream with chocolate sauce	3 P.M.
Peppermint stick ice cream	Peppermint stick ice cream		Malted milk or buttermilk
Milk	Milk	Milk	
		SUPPER	
Cream of pea soup with crackers	Cream of pea soup with crackers	Cream of pea soup with crackers	Strained cream of pea soup
Macaroni au gratin	Macaroni au gratin	Macaroni au gratin	Plain gelatin with whipped topping
Head lettuce salad with Russian dressing	Head lettuce salad with French dressing	Buttered beets	Tea with cream and sugar
Bread	Bread	Bread	
Butter	Butter	Butter	
Fruit gelatin	Fruit gelatin	Plain gelatin with whipped topping	9 P.M.
Tea with cream and sugar	Tea with cream and sugar	Tea with cream and sugar	Hot cocoa

* See note, Table 19-2.

gruels made with water, plain gelatin, and tea and coffee are generally used. Carbonated beverages may or may not be used, depending on the policy set by the physicians and dietitians.

Both the clear and the full liquid diet are low in nutritive value. The clear liquid diet is used for only limited periods of time, usually no longer than 24 to 36 hours. When the full liquid diet must be used for a period of time special attention must be given to improving its nutritive value. Skim milk powder, protein supplements, cream, and sugar may be used to increase its protein and calorie content.

Patients receiving liquid diets will require a feeding every 2 to 3 hours during the day and evening. When it is not possible for the dietary department personnel to serve these patients other than at regularly scheduled meal times, nurses have found it helpful to remind themselves of a patient's need for an interval feeding by noting this at the proper time interval in the nursing care plan. Also, when the nurse observes that a patient is ready for more than a liquid diet, she can often tactfully suggest this to the physician so that he will revise the patient's diet order.

FLUID INTAKE

A basic nursing responsibility is the provision of appropriate oral fluid intake for each patient—normally 1500 to 2500 ml. per day for adults. In situations where fluid intake is critical and the daily amount of oral fluid intake is defined in the physician's orders, for example, for the patient in renal failure or the patient with an elevated temperature due to infection, close communication between dietary and nursing services is required to carry out the order for fluids and satisfy the patient. In this chapter the fluid needs of the patient with an elevated temperature due to infection is reviewed. Other critical problems of fluid intake are discussed in succeeding chapters.

In patients with acute infection, excessive fluid loss may occur through the skin and lungs and through the gastrointestinal tract (diarrhea) which, without the replacement of fluid, can result in dehydration. Electrolyte depletion or retention can also occur. Severe dehydration with electrolyte imbalance can lead to death. Asiatic cholera is a dramatic example: this infection produces a sudden, massive diarrhea which within a few hours leads to shock and death.

Severe dehydration due to infection is usually treated by intravenous fluids (dextrose and water and/or electrolyte solutions). At this stage many individuals will not tolerate fluids by mouth. When oral fluids are tolerated, not only water but broth, tea, coffee, carbonated beverages, fruit and vegetable juices, and milk should be offered. These beverages, in addition to adding variety, also contribute to the patient's electrolyte intake (3 ounces canned tomato juice contains approximately 200 mg. sodium and 227 mg. potassium, Table 4, p. 355). Most of the fluids listed will also contribute to the patient's carbohydrate intake.

In addition to fluid and electrolyte loss, an elevation in body temperature is always accompanied by an increase in metabolism. In most febrile conditions (acute or chronic) the metabolism rate is increased 7 percent for each degree Fahrenheit

rise in temperature (12 percent for each degree Centigrade). As a result, the carbohydrate stores are quickly exhausted, and body protein and fat are used for energy if insufficient food is eaten. As soon as the patient with an infection can tolerate food, as well as fluids, he should be assisted in selecting food which will meet his energy and other nutrient needs.

STUDY QUESTIONS AND ACTIVITIES

1. Compare the menu selections of a patient on a regular diet with the pattern dietary. Will his selections provide adequately for his nutrient needs?

2. Record the 24-hour intake of a patient on a clear liquid diet. Using the food tables in Part Four, estimate his calorie and nutrient intake. How adequate was this diet for him?

3. Compare the soft diet in the diet manual your hospital uses with the soft diet in Table 19-2. Are there any differences in the foods used in the two plans? With the help of your instructor, determine the reasons for these differences.

SUPPLEMENTARY READING ON PROGRESSIVE HOSPITAL DIETS AND FLUID INTAKE

Doyon, P. R.: Automated food delivery systems. Hospitals, J.A.H.A., 44:109, (Feb. 1) 1970.

Erlander, D.: Dietetics—a look at the profession. Am. J. Nursing, 70:2402, 1970.

Fenton, M.: What to do about thirst. Am. J. Nursing, 69:1014, 1969.

Mumma, W. R.: Four meals a day. Hospitals, J.A.H.A., 44:77, (Apr. 16) 1970.

Newton, M. E., and Folta, J.: Hospital food can help or hinder care. Am. J. Nursing, 67:112, 1967.

DIET MANUALS

Diet Therapy in Patient Care, Boston, Massachusetts Dietetic Assoc., 1969.

Mayo Clinic Diet Manual, ed. 4, Philadelphia, W. B. Saunders, 1971.

Turner, D.: Handbook of Diet Therapy, ed. 5. Chicago, University of Chicago Press, 1971.

For Further References see Bibliography in Part Four.

Food Composition as a Basic Tool in Diet Therapy

20

Dietary Modifications · Nutrient Composition of Foods
Generalizations About Nutrient Composition · Effects of Processing on Nutrient Composition
Dietetic Food · Exchange System of Diet Calculation

INTRODUCTION

In diet therapy the food intake is modified as a part of the treatment of disease and is used when the kinds and amounts of foods provided by the progressive hospital diets are not appropriate. The patient's disease or disability determines the specific modification he needs. The nurse and dietitian must understand the reason for modifying the diet that a patient is served. However, the practical aspects of diet therapy, planning and serving the proper food and fluids acceptable to the patient, are the responsibility of the dietitian and the nurse.

In this chapter, a summary of dietary modification is given, and the basic tool of diet therapy—foods as sources of calories and nutrients per serving—and a method commonly used to calculate therapeutic diets the Exchange System is discussed. Application to specific problems is given in detail in succeeding chapters.

Dietary Modifications

Therapeutic diets are prescribed as part of the treatment in the following situations:

1. Need for Modification of Caloric Intake. The calorie content of the diet is modified for overweight and underweight patients. Calorie modification is also used as a preventive measure, in the treatment for patients of normal weight, especially those individuals for whom hospitalization has greatly reduced their usual energy expenditure.

2. Problems of Utilization of Nutrients by the Cells and Organs of the Body. The treatment of a variety of diseases requires a specific modification of the intake of one or more nutrients—for example, primarily carbohydrate in diabetes mellitus; protein, sodium and potassium in severe renal disease; protein and sodium in cirrhosis of the liver; fatty acids, type of carbohydrate, cholesterol and sodium in heart disease; and a specific amino acid, phenylalanine, in phenlketonuria.

3. Abnormalities of Digestion and Absorption. Foods offered are modified in texture and consistency in the treatment of diseases of the gastrointestinal tract such as peptic ulcer and diarrhea. Also, food may be modified because of the lack of a digestive enzyme(s) such as lactase; the lack of bile to emulsify fat as in gall bladder disease; or because the end product of digestion cannot be absorbed.

4. Nutritional Rehabilitation. The nutritionally debilitated patient needs special attention to help him reestablish proper food intake, especially the patient who has eaten poorly before surgery or the emotionally disturbed patient who comes to treatment dehydrated and malnourished.

Whatever the modification, care must be taken to ensure the nutritional adequacy of the therapeutic diet and also to teach the patient how his particular diet order may be met from his family's food. When the therapeutic diet plan cannot for any reason provide an adequate intake of vitamins and minerals, the physician should be informed so that he can supplement the diet with vitamin and mineral preparations.

FOOD COMPOSITION AS THE BASIC TOOL OF DIET THERAPY

The basic tool of diet therapy is the knowledge of the proximate energy and nutrient composition of food—calories, protein, fat, carobohydrate, minerals and vitamins. In addition, special constituents of food must be identified such as lactose, a specific carbohydrate; gluten, a specific protein; and cholesterol (a lipid), a special class of fat. The nutrients in foods are discussed in Part One of this book and an extensive table of the nutrient composition of common foods is found in Part Four, Table 1.

Food Composition Tables. Food composition tables give the calorie, protein, fat, carbohydrate, mineral and vitamin content of a defined amount of a food. The defined amount of a food is given in grams, usually 100 Gm. The household measure of the gram weight may or may not be stated. Table 1, page 315 gives the nutrient composition of 100 Gm. and of the common household measure of each food listed.

Protein, fat and carbohydrate values are given in grams in all tables. The values for minerals are given in milligrams with the exception of calcium which may be given in grams. Vitamins are given in International Units for A and D and in milligrams or micrograms for the other vitamins (1 mcg. equals 0.001 mg.). When figures are used from more than one food composition table to estimate the nutrient composition of a meal or a day's intake, care must be taken to see that the units of measure are the same in each table. If not, the units from one table will need to be converted to correspond to the other. If the primary table used gives calcium in grams and the secondary table in milligrams, all figures should be converted to grams (1 mg. of calcium equals 0.001 Gm.). For example: Table 1 in Part Four gives thiamine values in milligrams while the tables in Food Values of Portions Commonly Used[1] by Church and Church give thiamine values in micrograms.

Food composition tables are as essential to diet therapy as the drug formulary from the pharmacy

is to prescribing the dose of a medication. However, the figures in the food tables are not as accurate for the nutrients in food as the formulary is for drugs. For example, the ascorbic acid in the orange juice on Mr. A's breakfast tray may vary from day to day while the amount of digitoxin in the dose Mr. A is given will remain the same from day to day. If Mr. A drinks 7 ounces of orange juice, from the figure for ascorbic acid in reconstituted frozen orange juice in Table 1, one might conclude that he receives exactly 90 mg. Actually, if the frozen orange juice Mr. A is served is reconstituted correctly and served within a reasonable period of time after being reconstituted, Mr. A receives *approximately* 90 mg. of ascorbic acid.

The food composition tables are not inaccurate in the sense that they are wrong, but rather, that the nutrient values given in them reflect certain conditions and problems which must be taken into consideration when we use them.

Food composition tables are derived from research in numerous food technology laboratories. The figures for one food may be derived from the analysis of many samples; therefore, the nutrient composition of the food consumed today is apt to be like the values given in the table. Whole milk is a good example of a food which has often been analyzed. However, the figures for another food may represent only one or two analyses and the food consumed today could vary to some extent from the one or two samples analyzed in the laboratory.

The nutrient composition of fruits and vegetables can vary due to differences in variety, stage of maturity or growing conditions. Also new methods or modification of old methods of food processing may affect nutrient composition.

However, the food composition tables or a method derived from them (that is discussed later in this chapter) are used in calculating modified diets when a specific limit is set on nutrient(s) intake. The therapeutic successes that result demonstrate that the tables are accurate enough to serve this purpose. A list of commonly used food composition tables is found at the end of this chapter for those who wish to supplement Table 1, in Part Four.

Average Servings. An average serving of a food is used in dietetics to describe an amount of food in a household measure by weight or volume or in a common unit which can be readily recognized, such as 3 ounces of cooked roast meat; ½

---

[1] Church, C. F., and Church, H. N.: Food Values of Portions Commonly Used. ed. 11. Philadelphia, J. B. Lippincott, 1970.

pint or one 8-ounce cup of milk; ½ cup of cooked carrots or one slice of bread. Average servings were developed as an aid in calculating diet plans and in patient education.

An average serving may or may not be a 100 Gm. serving. One-half cup of cooked carrots is approximately 100 Gm. while 8 ounces of milk is 244 Gm., almost 2½ times 100 Gm.

Patients may describe their food intake in average size portions. However, when gathering information about an individual's food intake as one aspect of nutritional assessment, care must be taken to be sure that the patient does describe an "average" serving. A strawberry tart for one man may be a 9-inch strawberry pie. An ounce of cream in one woman's coffee may be 1 ounce of whipping cream, not coffee cream. One pat of butter for one man may be 15 Gm., not 5 Gm., the "average" serving.

SOME GENERALIZATIONS ABOUT THE NUTRIENT COMPOSITION OF FOODS

The complexity of food composition tables may "turn off" the uninitiated. The health counselor at the patient's bedside or in the ambulatory care clinic cannot carry a food composition table or textbook with her at all times, although she should have one readily accessible to her. The Daily Food Guide (page 93) can be used to assess an individual's usual food intake but this guide may not be adequate in all situations. Life styles vary in our society and food practices which differ from the Food Guide can supply adequate nutrient intakes. Some generalizations about food composition are offered in this section to assist the counselor to answer on-the-spot questions about food or cope with the assessment of intake in the individual whose food practices are "different."

Energy. The major American food problem today seems to be calories. We have become a society of weight-watchers without, in many instances, knowing what we are watching. *Fat* is the nutrient which most directly affects the energy value of a food. One Gm. of fat yields 9 calories while 1 Gm. of protein or carbohydrate yields 4 calories.

Varying amounts of fat may occur naturally in foods. This variation is illustrated in Table 20-1, Calories, Protein and Fat in 100 Grams of Selected Meat, Fish and Poultry (Cooked Without the

TABLE 20-1. CALORIES, PROTEIN AND FAT IN 100 GRAMS OF SELECTED MEAT, FISH AND POULTRY*
(Cooked Without the Addition of Fat)

FOOD—100 Gm.	CALORIES	PROTEIN (Gm.)	FAT (Gm.)
Chicken, light meat, without skin	166	32	3
Cod, broiled	170	29	5
Beef, steak broiled			
lean and fat	387	23	32
lean meat	200	32	8
Pork, roast loin or shoulder			
lean and fat	373	23	31
lean meat	283	29	13

* See Part Four, Table 1.

Addition of Fat). It will be noted that if one eats 100 Gm. of broiled steak, including both the lean and fat parts, he consumes significantly more calories than if he eats 100 Gm. of the cooked lean part only. These figures also illustrate why only lean meat is used in planning fat-controlled diets (see Chap. 23).

The effect of the addition of fat to food during preparation is illustrated in Table 20-2, Calories and Fat in 100 Grams of Boiled, Mashed and French Fried Potatoes. Note that a potato, in and of itself, is not a high calorie food but the addition of fat markedly increases its calorie value. In the same manner, if the cod in Table 20-1 is breaded and fried the calorie value of the 100 Gm. serving will be increased. Another example of the effect of the quantity of fat on the calorie value of a food

TABLE 20-2. CALORIES AND FAT IN 100 GRAMS OF BOILED, MASHED AND FRENCH FRIED POTATOES*

FOOD	CALORIES	FAT
Boiled†	65	Tr.
Mashed‡	94	4
French Fried	274	13

* See Part Four, Table 1.
† Pared before cooking.
‡ Milk and table fat added.

TABLE 20-3. CALORIES AND FAT IN ONE CUP
OF WHOLE MILK,* SKIMMED MILK* AND
PARTIALLY SKIMMED MILK†

FOOD	WEIGHT (Gm.)	CALORIES	FAT
Milk, whole	244 (1 c.)	160	8.5
Milk, skim	246 (1 c.)	80	Tr.
Milk, partly skimmed‡	246 (1 c.)	145	5

* See Part Four, Table 1.
† U.S.D.A. Home and Garden Bulletin No. 72.
‡ 2% nonfat milk solids added.

TABLE 20-4. WATER, CALORIES, AND
CARBOHYDRATE IN 100 GRAMS OF SELECTED
FRUITS AND VEGETABLES*

FOOD	WATER (percent)	CALORIES	CARBO-HYDRATE (Gm.)
Broccoli, cooked	91	26	5
Tomatoes, raw	94	22	5
Pears, raw	83	61	15
Potato, cooked	83	65	15
Banana, raw	76	85	22
Corn, fresh on cob	74	91	21

* See Part Four, Table 1.

is shown in Table 20-3, Calories and Fat in One Cup of Whole Milk, Skimmed Milk, and Partly Skimmed Milk.

Gravies and sauces may or may not be a significant source of calories. One cup of gravy made with 2 tablespoons of flour and pan drippings from which *all* fat has been removed contains approximately 60 calories while 1 cup of gravy made with 2 tablespoons of flour and pan drippings from which the fat has *not* been removed may contain as much as 500 calories. Therefore, ¼ cup of the gravy (an average serving) without fat will contain 15 calories while ¼ cup with fat may contain as much as 125 calories.

The energy value of fruits and vegetables varies directly with the water and carbohydrate content. Table 20-4, Water, Calories, and Carbohydrate in 100 Grams of Selected Fruits and Vegetables, illustrates this variation. In general the flowers, leaves and stems of vegetables and certain fruits have a high water and low carbohydrate content while seeds, tubers and roots, and certain fruits, have less water and more carbohydrate. Fat added

to season cooked vegetables and sugar added to fruits increases the calorie content of a serving.

Sugar and flour combined with fats in desserts account for the calorie value of these foods. This is illustrated in Table 20-5, Calories, Fat and Carbohydrate in Average Servings of Selected Desserts. Snack foods, an increasingly important source of calories in the diets of both children and adults, are discussed in Chapter 21.

The size of the portion of a food consumed in a meal also affects total calorie intake. Three ounces (100 Gm.) roast pork, lean and fat, contains approximately 370 calories; 6 ounces, approximately 740 calories. A serving of apple pie, which is ⅛ of a 9-inch pie, is 410 calories; ¼ of the same 9-inch pie is 600 calories.

Protein. The Milk Group and the Meat Group in the Daily Food Guide (page 93) if consumed in the recommended amounts, contribute the great-

TABLE 20-5. CALORIES, FAT AND CARBOHYDRATE IN AVERAGE SERVINGS OF SELECTED DESSERTS*

FOOD	WEIGHT (Gm.)	CALORIES	FAT (Gm.)	CARBOHYDRATE (Gm.)
Brownies	50 (1 bar)	242	16	25
Ice Cream	100 (¾ c.)	207	13	21
Chocolate Cake (with frosting)	100 (1 piece)	369	16	56
Apple Pie	160 (⅛ of 9″ pie)	410	18	61

* See Part Four, Table 1.

est total quantity of protein to the usual diet. In our country, many people do not consider dried beans or peas or nuts a significant source of protein, even though these foods are listed as alternates for meat in the Daily Food Guide. Many people classify dried beans or peas as primarily starchy (carbohydrate) foods. However, in situations where either money for food purchasing is limited or the individual prefers to use dried beans and peas rather than meat, the protein content of these foods must also be considered when appraising the adequacy of the intake of protein. The protein content of bread and cereals should also be considered as well as dried beans and peas.

Minerals. The major source of calcium in the American diet is milk or milk products, except butter, cream and cottage cheese. The Daily Food Guide recommends for adults 2 or more cups of milk. This amount contains approximately 576 mg. (.57 Gm.) of calcium—a significant contribution to the 0.8 Gm. recommended by the National Research Council. When less than the recommended amount of milk is consumed, before one concludes that an individual's daily calcium intake is less than adequate, it must be remembered that the usual selection of foods from the other groups will contribute 0.2 to 0.3 Gm. of calcium per day (see Table 19-1, p. 185). Also, one must always consider the kinds and amounts of processed foods with nonfat skim milk solids added that are used daily; or to discover the amount of milk or cheese that is used in food preparation in the home.

The evidence presently available appears to indicate that adequate iron intake is a problem. Our best food source of iron—liver—is not a popular food. Careful study is being given to the amount and availability of the iron in food and it can be anticipated that a higher level of iron enrichment of cereals and flours may be used in the future.

Vitamins. The fat-soluble vitamins require special attention. An adequate intake of vitamin A can be derived from *deep* green and *dark* yellow fruits and vegetables and milk fats and fortified margarine. The plant form of vitamin A is beta-carotene and requires an adequate fat intake for absorption.

Milk, meat and whole or enriched grain products (cereals, breads and flours) are important contributors to an adequate intake of the B vitamins. Consumed in amounts recommended in the Daily Food Guide these three foods will supply from ½ to ⅔ of the Daily Recommended Allowances of these nutrients. The recommended amounts of fruits and vegetables will supply the remainder. Special care must be taken to insure an adequate thiamine intake. As with iron, it can also be anticipated that the level and extent of thiamine enrichment of refined cereals and flours or meals may be increased in the future.

A daily serving of citrus fruit or tomatoes will provide adequate vitamin C intake. If liberal servings of fresh potatoes, other fresh vegetables and fresh fruits are consumed daily the diet will also be adequate in vitamin C (ascorbic acid).

EFFECTS OF FOOD PROCESSING ON NUTRIENT COMPOSITION

Canning. Properly canned fruits and vegetables have approximately the same nutrient composition as fresh ones. It is possible that the canned products might be better than the fresh if the latter are not protected in shipment from farm to market or stored and cooked correctly by the homemaker. The calorie value of most canned fruits is greater than fresh due to the addition of sugar during processing. The majority of canned vegetables will differ in sodium composition compared with fresh ones because salt (NaCl) is added during processing.

Meat, fish and poultry canned without the addition of items other than salt and spices will have approximately the same nutritive composition as the fresh products.

Freezing. Frozen fruits, vegetables, meat, fish and poultry will be comparable in nutrient composition to the fresh products if other food items are not added. Plain frozen vegetables, without the addition of butter or sauces for seasoning, are equal to fresh or canned ones. Salt, and in some instances monosodium glutamate, may be added to plain frozen vegetables. When salt is added it is listed on the label. Frozen fruits may or may not have sugar added during processing. Frozen orange juice concentrate does not have sugar added, but most of the orange-flavored breakfast drinks do have sugar added. The calorie value of frozen meat, fish or poultry can be greater than fresh if a gravy or sauce has been added or if the product is breaded and fried before freezing, such as frozen fish sticks.

Enrichment and Fortification. Most, but not all, grain products—cereals, flour and bread—are enriched with thiamine, riboflavin, niacin and iron. There are standards for the levels of enrichment for grain products. These standards are presently being reviewed and may be revised in the near future.

Skimmed milk, both fluid and nonfat dry milk solids, may or may not be fortified with vitamins A and D. The labels on these products must be read in order to identify whether or not they are fortified. The standard of identity of margarine requires fortification with vitamin A.

Convenience Foods. Convenience foods have come onto the retail market in volume in the past 10 years and the information needed to compare the nutritive value of these products with comparable products made in the home is not readily available.

Table 20-6, Nutrient Composition of Homemade and Convenience-Packaged Macaroni and Cheese, shows the calorie and nutrient variation in only one product—macaroni and cheese. For two of the items in the table—Brand B-1 and Brand B-2—all of the data are not available. Brand A is a canned product; B-1 a dry mix; and B-2 and Brand C are frozen products. It will be noted that the convenience-packaged products vary significantly in calorie, protein, and calcium content from the product made from a commonly used home recipe.

Table 20-7, Nutrient Composition of Homemade and Homebaked Sugar Cookies, illustrates the variation in a product when enriched and unenriched flour is used. The nutrient composition of the homemade cookies was calculated from a recipe using enriched flour. From the nutrient values provided by the manufacturer for the chilled cookie dough to be baked in the home, it appears that unenriched flour is used in this convenience product. The caloric values are similar.

Because our information is limited it is difficult to evaluate the effect of convenience foods on the nutritive quality of an individual's diet. The White House Conference on Food, Nutrition and Health studied this problem, and as a result the manufacturers of convenience foods are carefully reevaluating the nutrient composition of their products. Also, a committee of the National Research Council is presently studying this problem (see Chap. 12).

One problem in therapeutic dietetics is the addition of unanticipated ingredients to convenience foods. Wheat flour, that contains gluten, and nonfat dry milk solids, that contain lactose, are commonly used in manufacturers' recipes when they may not be included in a home recipe. Patients with gluten-induced enteropathy (celiac disease) or lactase deficiency may not be able to consume commonly used convenience foods. Also, the type and amount of fats in convenience foods may prohibit individuals on fat-restricted or fat-controlled diets from using these products.

Additives, Seasonings and Flavor Enhancers. Food additives, seasonings and flavor enhancers containing sodium are frequently added to processed foods. The most common items are salt and monosodium glutamate (Accent). When an individual must restrict his sodium intake (Chap. 23), many processed food items cannot be included in his diet plan.

DIETETIC FOODS

Cyclamate, a nonnutritive sweetening agent, was widely used prior to the 1969 ruling of the Food and Drug Administration prohibiting its use in beverages, foods or as a sugar substitute. Before the ban went into effect, approximately ½ of the carbonated beverages sold in the United States were artificially sweetened with cyclamate. Canned fruits, flavored gelatins, pudding mixes, jellies, candies and other products sweetened with cyclamate were also available in the average supermarket.

Sodium saccharin may still be used as a nonnutritive sweetener but the products in which it is used do not have the same taste acceptance as those sweetened with cyclamate. Other nonnutritive sweeteners presently on the market contain saccharin and small amounts of a carbohydrate.

Canned fruits packed in water without any sweetening agent or sweetened with a minimum of sugar are available today. Flavored gelatin with sodium saccharin and a limited number of other products are also available in the supermarkets for individuals who must restrict their intake of calories or calories and carbohydrate (either total carbohydrate or carbohydrate supplied by simple sugars). The labels on these products will state the nutritive values of a specific serving of the contents of the container as required by the Food

TABLE 20-6. NUTRIENT COMPOSITION OF HOMEMADE AND CONVENIENCE-PACKAGED MACARONI AND CHEESE

FOOD	WEIGHT IN (Gm.)	HOUSEHOLD MEASURE	CALORIES	PROTEIN (Gm.)	FAT (Gm.)	CARBOHYDRATE (Gm.)	CALCIUM (mg.)	IRON (mg.)	VITAMIN A (I.U.)	THIAMINE (mg.)	RIBOFLAVIN (mg.)	NIACIN (mg.)
Macaroni and Cheese*	100	½ c.	215	8	11	20	181	0.9	430	0.10	0.20	0.9
Brand A†	100	½ c.	97	3.7	4.2	11.0	56	0.6	230	0.09	0.09	1.2
Brand B-1‡	100	½ c.	179	5.8	7.1	23.0	81	NA	NA	NA	NA	NA
Brand B-2‡	100	½ c.	170	7.8	8.4	15.5	224	NA	NA	NA	NA	NA
Brand C§	100	½ c.	134	5.9	6.0	13.9	127	0.4	237	0.03	0.11	0.32

(Figures courtesy Preschool Nutrition Survey).
* See Part Four, Table 1. Values calculated from a recipe.
† Canned.
‡ Same manufacturer: B-1 dry mix; B-2 frozen.
§ Frozen.
NA—Figures not available.

TABLE 20-7. NUTRIENT COMPOSITION OF HOMEMADE AND HOMEBAKED SUGAR COOKIES

FOOD	WEIGHT IN (Gm.)	HOUSEHOLD MEASURE	CALORIES	PROTEIN (Gm.)	FAT (Gm.)	CARBOHYDRATE (Gm.)	CALCIUM (mg.)	IRON (mg.)	VITAMIN A (I.U.)	THIAMINE (mg.)	RIBOFLAVIN (mg.)	NIACIN (mg.)
Homemade sugar cookies*	20	2″ diam.	89	1.2	3.3	16	15	0.3	22	.03	.03	0.2
Homebaked sugar cookies†	20	2″ diam.	90	0.7	4.5	12	6	0.06	14	.004	.006	0.04

(Figures courtesy Preschool Nutrition Survey).
* Handbook #8 Values calculated from a recipe using enriched flour.
† Dough, chilled unbaked, commercial.

and Drug Administration regulations. It is strongly advised that the student inspect the labels of the dietetic foods in a supermarket and note the calorie value and carbohydrate content of a serving of a variety of canned fruits and nonnutritive sweeteners.

Many patients are confused about dietetic foods. They think that any food labeled dietetic may or must be used on their diets. For example, a woman who was restricting her calories because she was obese used salt-free canned vegetables even though she did not have to restrict her salt (sodium) intake. The vegetables were labeled "dietetic," therefore, she thought she must use them on her low calorie diet. When counseling an individual about his therapeutic diet, care must be taken to point out the dietetic foods he might use.

EXCHANGE SYSTEM OF DIET CALCULATION

By the 1940's, dietitians and physicians were aware that the use of food composition tables to calculate therapeutic diets, especially diets for the diabetic patients, was cumbersome, time consuming, and needlessly precise. Also, they realized that an individual does not have the time or inclination to calculate for each day the energy and nutrient composition of the food required by his therapeutic diet. (Even nursing and dietetic students take a dim view of an assignment that requires them to calculate the energy and nutrient composition of the food they have consumed in only *one* day.)

TABLE 20-8. DAILY FOOD GUIDE COMPARED WITH EXCHANGE SYSTEM

Daily Food Guide	Exchange System
MILK GROUP	MILK EXCHANGE
MEAT GROUP	MEAT EXCHANGE
VEGETABLE FRUIT GROUP	VEGETABLE EXCHANGES
	Group A
	Group B
	FRUIT EXCHANGES
BREAD CEREAL GROUP	BREAD EXCHANGES
	FAT EXCHANGES

After careful study, a committee of The American Dietetic Association, working cooperatively with the Committee on Education of the American Diabetes Association and representatives of the Diabetes Branch of the United States Public Health Service, published a simplified system of diet calculation for diabetic patients.[1] This system, widely used today, is known as the Exchange System of diet calculation. Although originally planned for the calculation of diabetic diets, the system or modifications of it are widely used to calculate other therapeutic diets; for example, calorie-restricted or fat-restricted diets.

In the exchange system, foods with similar con-

[1] J. Am. Dietet. A., 26:575, 1950.

TABLE 20-9. NUTRIENT COMPOSITION OF FOOD EXCHANGES*

GROUP†	AMOUNT	WEIGHT (Gm.)	PROTEIN (Gm.)	FAT (Gm.)	CARBOHYDRATE (Gm.)	CALORIES
Milk, whole	½ pt. (8 oz.)	240	8	10	12	170
Vegetables, Group A	as desired	..	..	..	..	..
Vegetable, Group B	½ cup	100	2	..	7	35
Fruit Exchanges	varies	..	..	..	10	40
Bread Exchanges	varies	..	2	..	15	70
Meat Exchanges	1 oz.	30	7	5	..	75
Fat Exchanges	1 tsp.	5	..	5	..	45

* Table 20-9 and 20-11 modified from Caso, E. K.: J. Am. Dietet. A., 26:575, 1950.
† For lists of foods in each exchange, see Table 20-11.

TABLE 20-10. DATA USED TO CALCULATE THE
COMPOSITION OF VEGETABLES—GROUP B

FOOD	CARBOHYDRATE CONTENT (Starch and sugar) Gm./100 Gm.	WEIGHTINGS (Based on usual rate of consumption)
Beets	8.0	3
Carrots	7.5	4
Onions	7.2	1
Peas, green (medium)	9.0	4
Pumpkin	5.1	—
Rutabaga	6.7	½
Squash, winter	4.9	2
Turnip	4.6	1
Weighted Average	7.0	

tent of protein, fat and/or carbohydrate per serving are grouped together; milk, vegetables, fruit, bread, meat and fat. Table 20-8, Daily Food Guide Compared with Exchange System of Diet Calculation, illustrates the similarities and differences in food classification between the Daily Food Guide (see p. 93) and the Exchange System of Diet Calculation. The Milk, Meat and Bread-Cereal Groups of the Daily Food Guide are also in the Exchange System. The Vegetable Fruit-Group of the Daily Food Guide becomes two items in the Exchange System, Vegetable Exchanges and Fruit Exchanges. The Vegetable Exchanges are subdivided into two groups, Group A and Group B. Fat Exchanges are included in the Exchange System but not in the Daily Food Guide (see *Other Foods* in Food Guide. p. 93).

Table 20-9, Nutrient Composition of Food Exchanges, gives the average protein, fat, carbohydrate and energy composition of each exchange. With the exception of the meat serving which is 1 ounce, the size servings of the items within each exchange are average servings. The average size serving of meat for an adult is approximately 3 or 4 ounces or 3 or 4 times the protein, fat and calorie figures given in Table 20-9. Whenever the term cup is used to define a serving, it means the standard 8-ounce measuring cup and a teaspoon or tablespoon refers to standard measuring spoons.

The nutrient values for the foods in the exchanges in Table 20-9 are not the same as those in Part Four, Table 1, page 315. The nutrient composition of the exchanges are average values that have been rounded off to the nearest whole number. Table 20-10, Data Used to Calculate the Composition of Vegetables—Group B, is adapted from the original committee report to show how the carbohydrate value (7 Gm. in ½ cup) for vegetables in Group B was derived.

Table 20-11, Exchange Lists, gives the foods included in each group. Each list should be read and studied carefully and any special directions should be carefully checked such as: the notation that when skim milk is substituted for whole milk, two fat exchanges should be added to replace the fat in whole milk; and the notation about the Vegetable Exchanges—Group A, that are not assigned any calorie or carbohydrate values in Table 20-9. The nutrient values of each exchange apply only to the serving size of the food as described, not for example, to fruits canned or frozen with sugar added or cooked meat served with gravy. It will also be noted that certain vegetables are listed with the Bread Exchanges. These contain 15 Gm. of carbohydrate per serving as listed, such as ⅓ cup of corn. The items in the Fruit Exchanges are listed by serving size that yields 10 Gm. of carbohydrate. Bacon and nuts are listed in the Fat Exchanges, not in the Meat Exchanges as might be expected. Their primary contribution is fat rather than protein.

Average values for minerals and vitamins have not been calculated for the Exchange System because of the wide variations within each Exchange. For example, whole milk contains vitamin A while skim milk unless fortified with vitamin A, does not. Therefore, giving a vitamin A value to a milk exchange would imply that all items listed in the Exchange contain vitamin A. When a diet pattern is calculated by the Exchange System, care must be taken to insure proper mineral and vitamin composition.

The dietitian uses the Exchange System to calculate a diet pattern which translates the physician's diet order into the kinds and number of servings of food (exchanges) to be consumed by the patient each day. She uses the nutrient values in Table 20-9 to calculate the pattern. The patient then selects the specific foods he wants to eat at each meal using the foods listed in Table 20-11. An example of the use of the Exchange System in diet calculation is shown in Chapter 21 in Table 21-3, Composition of a 1,200-Calorie Diet. The

TABLE 20-11. EXCHANGE LISTS

(Adapted from Meal Planning with Exchange Lists, The American Dietetic Association,
620 N. Michigan Ave., Chicago, Ill. 60611)

FOODS THAT NEED NOT BE MEASURED

(Insignificant carbohydrate or calories)

Coffee	Cranberries (unsweetened)
Tea	Mustard (dry)
Clear broth	Pickle (unsweetened)
Bouillon (fat free)	Saccharin
Lemon	Pepper and other spices
Gelatin (unsweetened)	Vinegar
Rennet tablets	Seasonings

Chopped parsley, mint, garlic, onion, celery salt, nutmeg, mustard, cinnamon, pepper and other spices, lemon, saccharin and vinegar may be used freely.

LIST 1. MILK EXCHANGES

One exchange of milk contains 8 Gm. of protein, 10 Gm. of fat, 12 Gm. of carbohydrate and 170 calories.

This list shows the different types of milk to use for one exchange:

TYPE OF MILK	AMOUNT TO USE
Whole milk (plain or homogenized)..	1 c.
*Skim milk	1 c.
Evaporated milk	½ c.
Powdered whole milk	¼ c.
*Powdered skim milk (nonfat dried milk)	¼ c.
Buttermilk (made from whole milk)..	1 c.
*Buttermilk (made from skim milk)...	1 c.

One type of milk may be used instead of another, for example, ½ cup of evaporated milk in place of 1 cup of whole milk.

* Skim milk and buttermilk have the same food values as whole milk, except that they contain less fat. Two fat exchanges are added when 1 cup of skim milk or buttermilk made from skim milk is used in place of whole milk.

LIST 2. VEGETABLE EXCHANGES: GROUP A

Group A contains little protein, carbohydrate or calories. You may use as much as 1 cup at a time without counting it.

Asparagus	Cauliflower
*Broccoli	Celery
Brussels sprouts	*Chicory
Cabbage	Cucumbers

LIST 2 (*Continued*)

*Escarole	Lettuce
Eggplant	Mushrooms
*Greens	Okra
Beet greens	*Pepper
Chard	Radishes
Collard	Sauerkraut
Dandelion	String beans, young
Kale	Summer squash
Mustard	*Tomatoes
Spinach	*Watercress
Turnip greens	

* These vegetables contain a lot of vitamin A.

LIST 2. VEGETABLE EXCHANGES: GROUP B

Each exchange contains 2 Gm. of protein, 7 Gm. of carbohydrate and 35 calories.

½ cup of vegetable equals 1 exchange:

Beets	Pumpkin
*Carrots	Rutabagas
Onions	*Squash, winter
Peas, green	Turnip

* These vegetables contain a lot of vitamin A.

LIST 3. FRUIT EXCHANGES

One exchange of fruit contains 10 Gm. of carbohydrate and 40 calories.

This list shows the different amounts of fruits to use for one fruit exchange:

FRUIT	AMOUNT TO USE
Apple (2″ diam.)	1 small
Applesauce	½ c.
Apricots, fresh	2 medium
Apricots, dried	4 halves
Banana	½ small
Blackberries	1 c.
Raspberries	1 c.
*Strawberries	1 c.
Blueberries	⅔ c.
*Cantaloupe (6″ diam.)	¼
Cherries	10 large
Dates	2
Figs, fresh	2 large
Figs, dried	1 small
*Grapefruit	½ small
*Grapefruit juice	½ c.
Grapes	12

TABLE 20-11 (*Continued*)

LIST 3 (*Continued*)

FRUIT	AMOUNT TO USE
Grape juice	¼ c.
Honeydew melon	⅛ medium
Mango	½ small
*Orange	1 small
*Orange juice	½ c.
Papaya	⅓ medium
Peach	1 medium
Pear	1 small
Pineapple	½ c.
Pineapple juice	⅓ c.
Plums	2 medium
Prunes, dried	2 medium
Raisins	2 tbsp.
*Tangerine	1 large
Watermelon	1 c.

* These fruits are rich sources of vitamin C. Try to use one of them each day.

LIST 4. BREAD EXCHANGES

One exchange contains 2 Gm. of protein, 15 Gm. of carbohydrate and 70 calories.

This list shows the different amounts of foods to use for one bread exchange:

BREAD, CEREAL, ETC.:	AMOUNT TO USE
Bread	1 slice
Biscuit, roll (2″ diam.)	1
Muffin (2″ diam.)	1
Cornbread (1½″ cube)	1
Cereals, cooked	½ c.
Dry, flake and puff types	¾ c.
Rice, grits, cooked	½ c.
Spaghetti, noodles, cooked	½ c.
Macaroni, etc., cooked	½ c.
Crackers, graham (2½″ sq.)	2
Oyster (½ c.)	20
Saltines (2″ sq.)	5
Soda (2½″ sq.)	3
Round, thin (1½″)	6
Flour	2½ tbsp.
Vegetables:	
Beans and peas, dried, cooked	½ c.
(Lima, navy, split pea, cowpeas, etc.)	
Baked beans, no pork	¼ c.
Corn	⅓ c.
Popcorn	1 c.
Parsnips	⅔ c.
Potatoes, white	1 small
Potatoes, white, mashed	½ c.

LIST 4 (*Continued*)

BREAD, CEREAL, ETC:	AMOUNT TO USE
Potatoes, sweet, or yams	¼ c.
Sponge cake, plain (1½″ cube)	1
Ice cream (omit 2 fat exchanges)	½ c.

These foods are measured carefully because they have a lot of carbohydrate.

LIST 5. MEAT EXCHANGES

One meat exchange contains 7 Gm. of protein, 5 Gm. of fat and 75 calories.

This list shows the different amounts of foods to use for one meat exchange:

MEAT	AMOUNT TO USE
Meat and poultry (medium fat)	1 oz.
beef, lamb, pork, liver, chicken, etc.	cooked
Cold cuts (4½″ x ⅛″)	1 slice
salami, minced ham, bologna, liver- wurst, luncheon loaf	
Frankfurter (8-9 per lb.)	1
Egg	1
Fish: haddock, etc.	1 oz.
Salmon, tuna, crab, lobster	¼ c.
Shrimp, clams, oysters, etc.	5 small
Sardines	3 medium
Cheese: Cheddar type	1 oz.
Cottage	¼ c.
*Peanut butter	2 tbsp.

* Peanut butter is limited to 1 exchange a day unless the carbohydrate in it is allowed for in the meal plan.

LIST 6. FAT EXCHANGES

One fat exchange contains 5 Gm. of fat and 45 calories.

This list shows the different foods to use for one fat exchange:

FAT	AMOUNT TO USE
Butter or margarine	1 tsp.
Bacon, crisp	1 slice
Cream, light	2 tbsp.
Cream, heavy	1 tbsp.
Cream cheese	1 tbsp.
Avocado (4″ diam.)	⅛
French dressing	1 tbsp.
Mayonnaise	1 tsp.
Oil or cooking fat	1 tsp.
Nuts	6 small
Olives	5 small

specific food selections for one day are shown in Table 21-4, Suggested Menu, 1,200-Calorie Diet.

STUDY QUESTIONS AND ACTIVITIES

1. In clinical conference discuss your analysis of a patient's one-day intake of calories and nutrients.

2. List five foods which you think are starchy or fattening. Using Table 1 in Part Four calculate the calories, protein, fat and carbohydrate in the size serving you would eat. What percent of your Recommended Dietary Allowances (see Table 10-1, p. 91) for calories does each serving provide?

3. Survey the dietetic foods, beverages and nonnutritive sweeteners in a supermarket in your community. Make a list of the items you can add to the Exchange Lists in Table 20-11.

4. List the ingredients on the labels of five different TV dinners available in your supermarket with which you are not familiar.

SUPPLEMENTARY READING

Toward the New. Agriculture Information Bulletin No. 341. U.S.D.A., 1970.

Watt, B. K., and Murphy, E. W.: Tables of food composition: scope and needed research. Food Technology, 42:50, 1970.

FOOD COMPOSITION TABLES

Church, C. F., and Church, H. N.: Food Values of Portions Commonly Used. ed. 11. Philadelphia, J. B. Lippincott, 1970.

Nutritive Value of Foods. Home and Garden Bulletin No. 72. U.S.D.A., Rev. 1970.

Watt, B. K., and Merrill, A. L.: Composition of Foods: Raw, Processed and Prepared. Agriculture Handbook No. 8. U.S.D.A., Rev. 1963.

For Further References see Bibliography in Part Four.

Weight Control

21

**Health Implications of Weight Status • Obesity • Causes • Prevention
Dietary Treatment • The Calorie-Restricted Pattern Dietary • Treatment Other Than Diet
Patient Education • Underweight**

INTRODUCTION

The concept of what constitutes correct weight has undergone marked revision in recent years. Even today the definition of the terms *normal* or *desirable* weight is sharply debated. To assess the weight status of individuals we have traditionally used height-weight tables derived from experience with life insurance policyholders. The first tables for adults were based on the heights and weights of men and women at various ages. The figures in these tables were averages and reflected the actual weights of the individuals. Since the data showed an increase in weight with age the recommended weight for height in the tables increased with each age group. For example: it was recommended that a woman 5 feet 4 inches tall weigh 131 pounds at age 30, and 144 pounds at age 55.[1]

In recent years the height-weight tables have been reevaluated and revised. It is recognized that, when growth in height has been achieved, there is no biological need to gain weight in excess of that which is satisfactory for the individual. Also the best health prognosis is found in individuals of average or less than average weight in their early 20's who maintain this weight throughout their adult years. Studies indicate that certain diseases in adults are associated with excessive weight, and that fat people are more likely to die at a younger age than people of normal weight (see Fig. 21-1).

It must be remembered that body weight is made up of a number of components: fat, muscle, organs, bone and fluid. At the same time as height and weight data have been reevaluated, body build and body fatness have been studied. As yet there is no method for estimating body build easily. Given two men of the same height, the one with a large frame will normally weigh more than the one with a small frame.

The revised weight tables in current use reflect the concern for maintaining over the life span the weight appropriate for an individual at age 25 and, at the same time, take into consideration body build. The Metropolitan Life Insurance Company's Desirable Weight Tables, published in 1960, give desirable weight ranges for heights for men and women 25 years of age and over, and allow for differences in body frame, which is designated as small, medium, and large. The range for a 5'4" woman with a small frame is 108 to 116 pounds; with a medium frame, 113 to 126 pounds; and with a large frame, 121 to 138 pounds (see Part Four, Table 8).

Overweight—Obesity. Although there is not as yet general agreement, the following descriptions of overweight and obesity are being used. *Overweight* is "over-heaviness" and the term does not carry any direct implications with regard to fatness. *Obesity* is described as a bodily condition marked by excessive generalized deposition and storage of fat or adipose tissue. Until we are able to estimate with some degree of accuracy an individual's fatness, it will continue to be difficult to identify the obese individual, except for those individuals who are obviously obese.

Underweight. In the United States in recent years the problem of *underweight* in the popula-

---

[1] Cooper, Barber and Mitchell, 7th ed., 1940.

tion other than in children has received little attention. We continue to regard 20 percent or more below desirable weight to be dangerous.

Health Implications of Weight Status

The adverse effects on health of excessive body fatness have been mentioned in the preceding paragraphs. The evidence from mortality and morbidity data presently available to us indicates that certain hazards to health are associated with obesity. These hazards can be classified as follows: (1) changes in normal body functions; (2) increased risk of developing certain diseases; (3) detrimental effects on established diseases; and (4) adverse psychological reactions.

The changes in normal body function most fre-

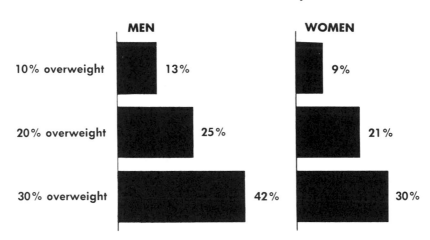

OVERWEIGHT SHORTENS LIFE

Excess Mortality*

	MEN	WOMEN
10% overweight	13%	9%
20% overweight	25%	21%
30% overweight	42%	30%

EXCESS MORTALITY DUE CHIEFLY TO HEART AND CIRCULATORY DISEASES

Excess* for Principal Diseases Among Persons About 20% or More Overweight

	Men	Women
Heart disease	43%	51%
Cerebral hemorrhage	53%	29%
Malignant neoplasms	16%	13%
Diabetes	133%	83%
Digestive system diseases (gall stones, cirrhosis, etc.)	68%	39%

*Compared with mortality of Standard risks

(Mortality ratio of Standard risks = 100%)

FIG. 21-1. (From Overweight—Its Significance and Prevention. Metropolitan Life Insurance Company. Derived from The Build and Blood Pressure Study, Society of Actuaries, 1959)

quently observed in the obese are respiratory difficulties; cardiovascular dysfunction and elevated blood pressure; menstrual abnormalities; and impaired carbohydrate tolerance that may be severe enough to classify as diabetes mellitus (see Chap. 22).

In the obese, both men and women, an increase in mortality over the expected has been associated with diabetes, heart and circulatory diseases and digestive diseases. The markedly obese experience a higher mortality than individuals who are slightly obese. Obese pregnant women are more prone than nonobese women to toxemia and to complications during delivery, including stillbirths.

Loss of excessive fat benefits the individual who has had a myocardial infarction, or who has circulatory problems, diabetes mellitus, or problems of the skeletal system, including osteoarthritis, ruptured intervertebral discs and many other varieties of bone and joint disease.

Some, though not all, obese patients have psychological disturbances. It is difficult to determine whether the obesity is the cause or result of the disturbance. For some, the problem may result from a conflict with the standards of society—for example, the acceptance of the standards for weight set by models, entertainers and other public figures.

The health hazards of underweight are less well understood. Underweight people often suffer from nonspecific symptoms such as fatigue and mild infections. Statistics indicate that tuberculosis is found more frequently in underweight persons than those of normal weight.

OBESITY

Prevalence and Incidence. Obesity is considered a major public health problem today although there are limited statistics for the general prevalence and incidence in the total population. However, the available data indicate a substantial prevalence of obesity at every age in both sexes. Excessive weight gain occurs more frequently at certain ages or periods in the life cycle. In women it occurs after the completion of growth, during pregnancies, and after the menopause. In men there is no one period when they are apt to be obese. They tend to gain weight between 25 to 40 years of age with some acceleration after age 40.[2] Individuals who become obese as children or adolescents are apt to be obese adults and have more

difficulty losing fat and maintaining the loss than those who become obese as adults.

Causes

FOOD INTAKE

Obesity is the result of a positive energy balance and can be due to a calorie intake which exceeds the energy need. While excessive food intake does account for most obesity, not every obese person necessarily eats large quantities of food. Based on the fact that a pound of body fat contains approximately 3,500 calories, an intake in excess of even 100 calories a day will add up to 3,000 calories a month, or almost a pound of body weight. Over a year this will amount to a weight gain of 10 pounds.

PHYSICAL ACTIVITY

Energy expenditure is as important as food intake in the development of obesity. In the past 25 to 50 years life in the highly developed areas of the world has undergone great changes. Work hours have been shortened, labor-saving machinery has been installed in homes and factories, transportation is easier, homes are well-heated, and even our leisure-time occupations are sedentary rather than active. This has reduced the energy needs of the body markedly, but, by and large, food habits have not changed sufficiently to offset the decreased need. Although the American breakfast is considerably smaller today than that which our forefathers were accustomed to eating, the coffee break, morning and afternoon, the increased use of sugar, the ubiquitous candy bar and the TV "snack" have more than compensated for the change in breakfast patterns. (See Table 21-1, Caloric Values for Common "Snack" Foods.)

A number of investigators have observed that the obese person, and particularly the obese child and adolescent, is less active than his counterpart of the same age. Whether this is due to his inability to keep pace with other children or to apathy born of emotional conflict, the inactivity lowers the energy need of the body and in this way contributes to the overweight. The above is also true of obese women as compared to women of normal weight. In obese men the difference in activity is less striking but still of significance.

FAMILY PATTERNS

Studies show that overweight and obesity tend to exist as a family pattern. Mayer[3] found that 8

---

[2] Obesity and Health. U.S. Dept. H.E.W.-U.S. P.H.S. Publ. No. 1485, 1966.

[3] Mayer, J.: Am. J. Clin. Nutr., 9:530, 1961.

TABLE 21-1. CALORIC VALUES FOR COMMON "SNACK" FOODS

	AMOUNT OR AVERAGE SERVING	CALORIE COUNT
"Just a Little Sandwich"		
Hamburger on bun	3-in. patty	330
Peanut butter	1 tbsp. P.B.	330
Cheese	1-oz. cheese	280
Ham	1-oz. ham	320
TV Snack		
Pizza (cheese)	⅛ of 14-in. diam. pie	185
Popcorn with oil and salt	1 c.	40
Pretzel, thin, twisted	1	25
Cheese fondue	½ c.	265
Dips (sour cream)	½ c.	248
Chippers	10	150
Beverages		
Carbonated drinks, soda, root beer, etc.	6-oz. glass	80
Cola beverages	12-oz. glass (Pepsi)	150
Club soda	8-oz. glass	5
Chocolate malted milk	10-oz. glass (1¾ c.)	500
Ginger ale	6-oz. glass	60
Tea or coffee, straight	1 c.	0
Tea or coffee, with 2 tablespoons cream and 2 teaspoons sugar	1 c.	90
Alcoholic Drinks		
Ale	8-oz. glass	155
Beer	8-oz. glass	110
Highball (with ginger ale—ladies' style)	8-oz. glass	185
Manhattan	Average	165
Martini	Average	140
Wine, Muscatel or Port	2-oz. glass	95
Sherry	2-oz. glass	75
Scotch, bourbon, rye	1½-oz. jigger	130
Fruits		
Apple	1 3-in.	75
Banana	1 6-in.	130
Grapes	30 medium	75
Orange	1 2¾-in.	70
Pear	1	65
Salted Nuts		
Almonds, filberts, hazelnuts	12-15	95
Cashews	6-8	90
Peanuts	15-17	85
Pecans, walnuts	10-15 halves	100
Candies		
Chocolate bars,		
Plain, sweet milk	1 bar (1 oz.)	155
With almonds	1 bar (1 oz.)	140
Chocolate-covered bar	1 bar	270
Chocolate cream, bon bon, fudge	1 piece 1-in. square	90-120
Caramels, plain	2 medium	85
Hard candies, Lifesaver type	1 roll	95
Peanut brittle	1 piece 2½ x 2½ x ⅜ in.	110

(Adapted from Smith Kline and French Laboratories)

TABLE 21-1. CALORIC VALUES FOR COMMON "SNACK" FOODS (*Continued*)

	AMOUNT OR AVERAGE SERVING	CALORIE COUNT
Desserts		
Pie:		
Fruit—apple, etc.	1/6 pie 1 average serving	410
Custard	1/6 pie 1 average serving	265
Mince	1/6 pie 1 average serving	400
Pumpkin pie with whipped cream	1/6 pie 1 average serving	460
Cake:		
Chocolate layer	3-in. section	350
Doughnut, sugared	1 average	150
Sweets		
Ice Cream:		
Plain vanilla	1/6 qt. serving	200
Chocolate and other flavors	1/6 qt., 2/3 c.	260
Orange sherbet	1/2 c.	120
Sundaes, small chocolate nut with whipped cream	Average	400
Ice-cream sodas, chocolate	10-oz. glass	270
Midnight Snacks for Icebox Raiders		
Cold potato	1/2 medium	65
Chicken leg	1 average	88
Glass milk	7-oz. glass	140
Mouthful of roast	1/2 in. x 2 in. x 3 in.	130
Piece of cheese	1/4 in. x 2 in. x 3 in.	120
Leftover beans	1/2 c.	105
Brownie	3/4 in. x 1 3/4 in. x 2 1/4 in.	140
Cream puff	4 in. diam.	450

to 9 percent of children of normal weight parents became obese. When one parent is obese, the likelihood of the child becoming obese is 40 percent, and this proportion rises to 80 percent when both parents are obese. There may be a genetic component, since this distribution is not true for adopted children. However, in such families the pattern of food intake tends to be excessive and the body image of a "well-fed person" is the preferred one. Such families may eat because plenty of food denotes prosperity or success in life, or because increased food intake has become an established pattern for relieving tension, boredom or emotional stress.

EMOTIONAL PROBLEMS

Many people who are overweight eat because they have nothing else to do. They may eat when they are under strain or when they feel unappreciated or lonely. Food now becomes a symbol of love, of satisfaction, or security. Stunkard and his co-workers[4] have described a so-called *night-eating syndrome* in some gravely obese patients. Such a patient eats little during the day, but in the evening and in the early night hours he consumes large quantities of food. Some of these patients exhibited symptoms of severe emotional stress when an attempt was made to reduce their weight. The investigators concluded that it might be wiser to allow such patients to remain obese than to precipitate an emotional illness with a weight reduction program.

ENDOCRINE GLANDS

In a small percentage of patients obesity is caused by a disturbance of function of one or more of the endocrine glands, such as the thyroid (hypothyroidism) or the pituitary. In hypothyroidism part of the excess weight is due to fluid retention. Obesity should not be attributed to glandular abnormalities unless this is determined by specific diagnostic tests.

BALANCE BETWEEN HUNGER AND SATIETY

In recent years there has been renewed interest in the physiologic control of hunger and satiety.

[4] Stunkard, A. J., *et al.*: Am. J. Med., 19:78, 1955.

Many individuals maintain a balance between food intake and energy expenditure which keeps their weight comparatively stable over a period of many years. The work of Schachter[5] indicates that eating is triggered by a different set of signals in the obese than in those individuals of normal weight. His experience seems to indicate that in the obese there is no relationship between the state of hunger and eating behavior. Instead such external factors as smell, sight, taste and other people's actions determine what and when the obese eats.

Prevention of Obesity

Successful weight reduction and the maintenance of weight loss are not easily achieved. It is hoped that, as we learn more about the causes of obesity, health workers will focus their attention on the prevention of obesity at all stages in the life cycle.

INFANTS AND CHILDREN

Studies indicate that many obese adults were obese children. Prevention of obesity begins with the careful supervision of the feeding of infants and children. The nurse in the pediatrician's office, the public health nurse in the clinic and home, and the school nurse can all play a role in prevention. Accurate weighing and measuring of infants and young children combined with a diet interview with the mother will give the physician clues to the development of a weight problem. Effective nutrition counseling of the mother may correct the problem in its earliest stages. At the same time it must be remembered that the weight status of a child may reflect a problem of mother-child relationships, not solely a nutrition problem (see Chap. 15).

For the school-age child the physical education programs in elementary and secondary schools should be directed to helping all boys and girls develop a lifetime pattern of physical activity. The present emphasis on team sports, which provide activity for only a few students, does not always help the individual to be active in his adult years (see Chap. 16).

ADULTS

As adults settle into a routine of daily living in their late twenties and early thirties, and if physical activity is limited because of the demands of their employment, a conscious effort should be made to limit calorie intake. For many of these adults this means decreasing their intake of such foods as sugar, high-calorie desserts and snacks, cream and other fats. The Pattern Dietary (Chap. 19, p. 185) with reasonable additions of food to maintain weight provides a guide for these individuals. For example: a man who maintained his normal weight at age 20 with a calorie intake of 3,000 calories may find at age 30 he will maintain his weight on 2,500 calories. Both the activity and the time devoted to it must be taken into consideration when exercise is combined with food intake to control body weight. It is the daily increase in physical activity rather than the occasional vigorous activity which is effective in controlling weight. Table 21-2 shows the calories expended by the 70 Kg. man (154 pounds) or the 58 Kg. woman (128 pounds) in a few activities. It must be noted that these figures are for a full hour of continuous activity. For many adults in our society it is difficult to devote 1 hour every day to walking or swimming. A conscious effort to increase activity throughout the day may be possible—for example, walking to the second bus stop instead of the first, walking to the nearby grocery store or newsstand in place of driving the car, or walking up one flight of stairs instead of taking the elevator. In our society today finding a place to walk is often the real problem: many of our suburban areas have no sidewalks.

Controlling weight by diet and exercise is a family affair. The homemaker is often the one who bears the major responsibility for food. If her family has a tendency to gain weight easily she will have to pass up the recipes on the women's page of the newspaper which require ½ pint of whipping cream, 1 pint of sour cream, 6 ounces of cream cheese or ½ to ¾ pound of butter. She can, on the other hand, control calories behind the scene by reducing the fat she uses in food prepara-

TABLE 21-2. CALORIE EXPENDITURE FOR SOME TYPES OF ACTIVITY*

	70 KG. MAN Cals./hour	58 KG. WOMAN Cals./hour
Painting furniture	200	160
Walking (3 ml./hr.)	240	190
Skating	340	285
Swimming (2 mi./hr.)	685	570

* Calculated from the table *Energy Expenditures for Everyday Activities* in Chapter 5.

5 Schachter, S.: Science, 161:751, 1968.

tion by substituting skim milk for whole milk in sauces and puddings and by broiling rather than pan frying meat.

Dietary Treatment

Since an abnormal amount of adipose tissue is a storage of energy in excess of need, the calorie intake must be less than the actual daily energy need if the body is to draw upon and reduce its surplus of fat.

Determination of Present Practices. The first step in helping the obese patient is to determine, through individual interview, how he usually has lived his day and, specifically, his food and beverage intake and physical activity. An appraisal of his habitual food intake will give an indication of his daily calorie intake and the kinds of food he eats; an appraisal of his activity pattern will give an indication of his energy expenditure. From this information one can estimate a reduced calorie intake for him which should promote weight loss.

Calories. Considerable difficulty may be encountered in determining the level of reduced calorie intake for an individual. His previous intake may have been underestimated, or his energy expenditure overestimated. In theory, without increasing activity a deficit in intake of 500 calories per day, compared with previous intake, should promote a weight loss of approximately 1 pound per week. (500 calories × 7 = 3,500 calories = 1 pound of fat.) A relatively sedentary obese woman 55 years old and 5 feet, 4 inches tall, who has been consuming approximately 1,700 calories per day, should lose weight on a 1,200-calorie diet, while a moderately active obese business executive 35 years old and 6 feet tall, who has been consuming 2,500 to 3,000 calories, should lose weight on a 2,000-calorie diet.

A deficit of 1,000 calories per day should promote a loss of 2 pounds per week. It is considered unwise for an individual to lose more than 2 pounds per week unless he is under the close supervision of his physician. It is generally considered unwise for a patient to be given a diet of less than 1,000 calories unless he is hospitalized.

Regardless of the level of calorie restriction prescribed by the physician, it must be recognized that, through variations in daily food selection and serving size, the actual calorie intake at home will not be exactly the number of calories ordered. For example a 1,200-calorie diet may vary by chance from 1,000 to 1,400 calories. Also, physical activity will vary from day to day. To be successful in carrying out a calorie restriction the patient needs careful diet instruction. Patient education is discussed later in this chapter.

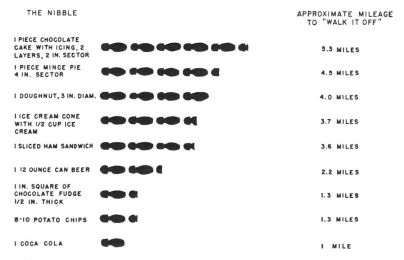

MILEAGE TO WALK OFF THAT NIBBLE

THE NIBBLE		APPROXIMATE MILEAGE TO "WALK IT OFF"
I PIECE CHOCOLATE CAKE WITH ICING, 2 LAYERS, 2 IN. SECTOR		5.3 MILES
I PIECE MINCE PIE 4 IN. SECTOR		4.5 MILES
I DOUGHNUT, 3 IN. DIAM.		4.0 MILES
I ICE CREAM CONE WITH 1/2 CUP ICE CREAM		3.7 MILES
I SLICED HAM SANDWICH		3.6 MILES
I 12 OUNCE CAN BEER		2.2 MILES
I IN. SQUARE OF CHOCOLATE FUDGE 1/2 IN. THICK		1.3 MILES
8-10 POTATO CHIPS		1.3 MILES
I COCA COLA		I MILE

FIG. 21-2. Mileage to walk off that nibble (from Peyton, A. B.: Practical Nutrition. ed. 2, p. 178. Philadelphia, J. B. Lippincott, 1962; adapted from Hauck, H. M.: How to control your weight. Ithaca, N. Y., New York State College of Home Economics).

Protein. At least 1 Gm. of protein per kilogram of desirable body weight for adults is used to supply the body's needs for this nutrient. Some doctors will prescribe a higher intake, 1½ Gm. of protein per kilogram. This allows for a more liberal use of meat, fish, eggs, and cottage cheese in the diet plan. At a very restricted level of calories (1,000 calories) this requires the careful selection of lean meat and fish.

Fat and Carbohydrate. Since these two nutrients constitute the greatest source of calories in the diet, they must be reduced. However, there is considerable difference of opinion as to whether carbohydrate or fat should be cut to a minimum. The usual calorie-restricted diet will derive approximately half its calories from carbohydrate, as in the normal diet, and the calories from fat will be considerably reduced. One advantage of this division is that it permits the use of commonly accepted foods such as bread.

On the other hand, both Young[6] and Cederquist[7] and her co-workers advocate a diet with less carbohydrate and more fat than is usually included in the diet plan. They claim that patients find that such a diet has greater satiety value and, therefore, it is easier for the patient to follow.

Minerals and Vitamins. Care should be taken to see that the calorie-restricted diet plan provides all the other essentials of a normal diet, such as minerals and vitamins, in quantities at least equivalent to the Recommended Dietary Allowances. If the calorie intake is very restricted (less than 1,000 Cal.) vitamin and mineral supplements may be needed.

Alcohol. One Gm. of alcohol provides 7 calories. Also, in some alcoholic beverages carbohy-

---

[6] Young, C. M.: J. Am. Dietet. A., 45:134, 1963.
[7] Cederquist, D. C.: J. Am. Dietet. A., 40:535, 1962.

drate contributes calories. If these beverages are to be used, their calorie value must be calculated in the Calorie Restricted Pattern Dietary. For some patients the calories from the alcoholic beverages they consume may be the difference between losing and not losing weight (see Table 5, Part Four).

Water. Water and other nonnutritive fluids are not restricted unless there is some heart or kidney complication. Sometimes there is fluid retention in women prior to menstruation, which may temporarily mask the real loss of body fat. Early weight loss in some patients may be fluid loss rather than loss of adipose tissue.

PLANNING THE CALORIE-RESTRICTED
PATTERN DIETARY

1,200-Calorie Diet. Table 21-3, Composition of a 1,200-Calorie Diet demonstrates the calculation of one level of calorie restriction using the Exchange System. (See Chap. 20, pp. 196 to 200 for explanation of the use of Exchange System in calculating diet patterns and the lists of foods in each exchange group.) The foods used to carry out this calculated diet plan may be distributed among three meals, three meals and an evening snack, or five or six small meals a day. The suggested menu in Table 21-4 shows how the amounts of food might be used in three meals. The reader is urged to check to see if the total number of exchanges in Table 21-3 have been used in 21-4.

It must be stressed that no food other than noncalorie beverages and seasonings may be added to the 1,200-Calorie Diet. For example, if fat is added to a serving of cooked vegetables, it has to be part of the fat calculated in the pattern. When canned fruits are used, they must be those canned without sugar. Also, care must be taken to use

TABLE 21-3. COMPOSITION OF A 1,200-CALORIE DIET

FOOD EXCHANGE	AMOUNT		CALORIES	PROTEIN (Gm.)	FAT (Gm.)	CARBOHYDRATE (Gm.)
	NUMBER	HOUSEHOLD MEASURE				
Milk, skim	2	2 c. (1 pt.)	160	16	—	24
Vegetables, Group A		as desired				
Vegetables, Group B	1	½ c.	35	2	—	7
Fruit	3	varies	120	—	—	30
Bread	3	varies	210	6	—	45
Meat	6	6 oz.	450	42	30	—
Fat	3	3 tsp.	225	—	15	—
Totals			1200	66	45	106

the size serving defined in the exchange lists (see Chap. 20).

1,800-Calorie Diet. Table 21-5, Composition of an 1,800-Calorie Diet demonstrates the calculation of a more liberal calorie restricted diet. It will be noted that in this 1,800-Calorie Diet whole milk is used in place of the skim milk in the 1,200-Calorie Diet. Also, 1 tablespoon of sugar and 6, rather than 3, teaspoons of fat are included in this plan. These two items may be used to flavor other foods or provide for calories in a simple dessert. The reader is urged to plan a suggested menu using the amounts of foods listed in Table 21-5. (See Table 20-11 in Chap. 20 for foods in the Exchange Lists.)

Other Approaches to Weight Loss

Starvation Regimens. Recently, workers in metabolic research have used this method to study obesity.[8] Water and other noncaloric fluids together with vitamin and mineral supplements have been allowed. Hospitalized patients appear to tolerate this approach for periods of 30 days or more. During fasting, weight loss is rapid, averaging 1 to 3 pounds per day. Long-term follow-up reports of this regimen show that it is no more effective than other approaches to the treatment of obesity. Because of the potential hazards of this method of weight reduction—e.g., anemia and gout—it is used only with closely supervised hospitalized patients. It should never be self-administered.

Formula Diets. Liquid formula diets fortified with vitamins and minerals are now available in

---

[8] Drenick, E. J., *et al.*: JAMA, 187:100, 1964.

most supermarkets. They contain approximately 225 calories per 8-ounce serving; and four 8-ounce servings per day yield 900 calories. Their advantage lies in the fact that they provide a specific number of calories per serving: their disadvantage is the monotony of a bland liquid diet. Some people have found it helpful to use the formula diet for one meal a day and eat a calorie-restricted diet at other mealtimes. These formulas generally made from nonfat dry skim milk with vitamins and minerals added are relatively expensive.

TABLE 21-4. SUGGESTED MENU
1,200-CALORIE DIET

BREAKFAST

4 oz. orange juice
1 egg
1 slice toast
1 tsp. butter
Coffee without cream or sugar

NOON MEAL

2 oz. ham
Tomato and lettuce
2 slices of bread
1 tsp. mayonnaise
8 oz. skim milk
1 small apple

EVENING MEAL

3 oz. lean roast beef
½ cup carrots with 1 tsp. butter
Cucumber and lettuce with vinegar
8 oz. skim milk
½ small grapefruit

TABLE 21-5. COMPOSITION OF A 1,800-CALORIE DIET

FOOD EXCHANGE	AMOUNT		CALO-RIES	PROTEIN (Gm.)	FAT (Gm.)	CARBO-HYDRATE (Gm.)
	NUMBER	HOUSEHOLD MEASURE				
Milk, whole	2	2 c. (1 pt.)	340	16	20	24
Vegetables, Group A		as desired				
Vegetables, Group B	1	½ c.	35	2	—	7
Fruit	3	varies	120	—	—	30
Bread	6	varies	420	12	—	90
Meat	8	8 oz.	600	56	40	—
Fat	6	6 tsp.	270	—	30	—
Sugar		1 tbsp.	46	—	—	12
Totals			1831	86	90	163

Maintenance of Weight Loss

Once the patient has achieved his weight loss, he should be warned not to return to his previous dietary practices. He will need assistance in establishing a pattern dietary that suits his situation. Unless he has increased his physical activity significantly, most adults will discover that the calorie-restricted diet, especially if it was a moderate and not a drastic restriction, is his basic normal diet with only minor modifications for weight maintenance.

Treatment Other Than Diet

Drugs. Drugs or proprietary preparations to decrease weight should be taken only under the supervision of the physician. Anorexigenic agents —the amphetamines and other drugs—have been used to promote weight loss. They depress appetite but it has been observed that their effectiveness decreases after about 6 weeks. In increasing doses they have unpleasant side effects. For the obese person who also has cardiac disease these drugs are dangerous.

Thyroid hormone has been used as an adjunct to diet therapy on the grounds that obese patients are in a hypometabolic state and need this metabolic stimulant if weight loss is to be accomplished. When an individual has hypothyroidism, hormone preparations are required to achieve a weight loss. For obese individuals with normal thyroid function—the majority of patients—thyroid hormone is dangerous.

Diuretics and Laxatives. The indiscriminate use of diuretics and laxatives, which promote a fluid loss, may give the patient a false sense of accomplishment when he weighs himself. His weight loss will reflect a water loss, not a decrease in adipose tissue. Only when the physician observes an abnormal fluid retention in a patient will a diuretic be part of the patient's therapy.

Patient Education

Diet Instruction. The nurse and the dietitian must have an extensive knowledge of the calorie content of average servings of commonly used foods before participating in the diet instruction of the obese patient. One problem confronting the nurse and the dietitian is the average lay person's lack of this knowledge. On the other hand, individuals who have tried a variety of reducing diets may be highly expert at counting calories.

The lay person who lacks any specific information about the calorie value of foods at the per serving level often incorrectly classifies a food or food group as "fattening." For example, many people classify bread as "fattening." One regular-sized slice of bread weighing about 23 Gm. contains 60 to 70 calories. "Diet" bread, weighing about 18 Gm. per slice, contains 45 to 50 calories. For an individual, bread will be "fattening" when his excessive daily calorie intake can be attributed to an excessive intake of calories from bread.

Obese patients may also need considerable assistance with food selection and methods of food preparation. The monotony of the diet is often a problem and suggestions on how to prepare meals may help a patient enjoy his meals. Each meal served to the hospitalized patient should be planned to show him the variety possible in his diet.

Predicting Success. Since it can be said by many obese patients that "it is easy to lose weight, I have done it ten times," attempts have been made to identify the characteristics of those persons who can lose and maintain a weight loss. From the evidence available today the person who is most likely to lose weight successfully[9]:

1. Is slightly or moderately above a desirable weight for him, due to excess adipose tissue.
2. Gained weight as an adult.
3. Never attempted to lose weight as an adult.
4. Is well-adjusted emotionally.
5. Accepts weight reduction as a realistic goal.

Bruch[10] indicates from her experiences that there are those patients who prefer to be obese and who meet the stresses of daily living more successfully when they are obese. Young[11] has shown in a series of studies that the reasonably stable individual is the most likely to achieve weight reduction, the anxious, tense or insecure person is less successful, and those who have little or no success present deep emotional problems.

UNDERWEIGHT

Leanness or underweight may be due to an inadequate caloric intake, to excessive bodily activity or to both. Physical disease such as malignancy, gastrointestinal disorders, chronic, infectious disease or endocrine disturbances such as hyperthyroidism may be a cause of progressive weight loss.

Underweight due to an inadequate caloric intake may be a serious condition, especially in the

9 Health and Obesity. P.H.S. Publ. No. 1485, 1966.
10 Bruch, H.: Am. J. Clin. Nutr., 5:192, 1957.
11 Young, C. M., *et al.*: J. Am. Dietet. A., 31:1111, 1955.

young. Resistance to infection, particularly to tuberculosis, may be lowered; and the occurrence of the complications of pregnancy in young women may result from malnutrition due to an inadequate caloric intake.

Underweight, like overweight, is a relative term, being based on the ideal weight for a given height, build and sex. More than 10 percent below the ideal usually is considered to be abnormal, especially in persons under 25, and is worthy of medical investigation.

Diet for Underweight

Table 21-6 shows the kinds of foods used to increase calorie intake. Reasonable goals that take into consideration the individual's age, height and previous weight status must be set with each underweight patient. In one clinical setting the doctors, nurses and dietitians were concerned because Mrs. P., age 59 and 5 feet 2 inches tall, weighed 62 pounds. Mrs. P. was underweight and needed to increase her usual calorie intake of 1,200 to 1,400 calories per day. The staff set a goal for Mrs. P. of a weight gain of 50 pounds Assessment of Mrs. P.'s weight status over her total life span revealed that she had never weighed more than 80 pounds and that weighing 112 pounds did not appeal to her at all. In time Mrs. P. did gain 20 pounds on a 2,000-calorie diet. She felt better and, needless to say so did the staff.

Some guidelines for assisting the underweight patient are:

1. An adequate diet as described in Chapter 19.

2. Adequate calorie intake that may be obtained by: (a) increasing the quantity of food eaten at each meal, (b) increasing the carbohydrate and, to some extent, the fat intake, and (c) adjusting the frequency of feedings. For some patients this last recommendation may be achieved by offering nourishments between meals, for others it may be more appropriate to offer a hearty bedtime snack of a sandwich or a dessert plus a beverage.

3. One to 1½ Gm. of protein per kilogram of body weight to combat any previous inadequate intake.

4. Adequate intake of vitamins and minerals, especially thiamine.

5. A reduction in bulk from excessive servings of fruits and vegetables in favor of foods with more concentrated calorie value.

6. Easily digested foods. Carbohydrate-rich foods are especially indicated, since carbohydrate

TABLE 21-6. KINDS OF FOODS USED FOR INCREASED CALORIES

PRINCIPLES

1. High in caloric value: 25-50 percent above normal
2. High in protein: 90-100 Gm. for adults
3. High in vitamins, especially in the vitamin B complex
4. Nourishment may be served between meals and before retiring

FOODS USED

Milk
Milk and cream

Cheese
All kinds

Fats
Butter and margarine; all other fats

Eggs
Cooked in all ways

Meats, fish and fowl
All varieties; bacon and fat meats are indicated if the patient tolerates them

Soups
Preferably creamed or thick soups

Bread, cereals, macaroni products
All kinds; preferably whole grain or enriched

Vegetables
All vegetables, including potatoes

Salads
All kinds; oil dressings especially desirable

Fruits
All fresh and cooked fruits and juices, jellies, jams and marmalades

Desserts
Ice cream, custards, tapioca and rice puddings, cake, fruit desserts, other desserts

Beverages
Tea, coffee, cocoa, served with cream and sugar; fruit juices; malted preparations

Vitamin concentrates
If ordered by the physician

is both easily digested and quickly converted into body fat. Foods rich in fat may be used to increase the fuel value without unduly increasing the bulk, but they must be used with discretion. Fat-rich foods lessen the appetite of many patients, and too much fat in any form is frequently distasteful unless cleverly disguised. The uncooked fats, such as cream, butter, and salad oils are usually better tolerated than the fat in fried foods.

It will be noted that the diet described in Table 21-6 is a house, or regular, diet supplemented with cream, extra butter, high caloric desserts and nourishment between meals.

Nursing Problems

The diet must be built up gradually, otherwise the patient may not be able to tolerate the sudden increase. Care must be taken to ascertain the likes and the dislikes of the patient and to prepare the food as appetizingly as possible, both as to methods of cooking and appearance when served. Above all, the patient must be encouraged to accept the necessity for his cooperating by consuming all food served to him. Low caloric soups, salads and beverages should not be eaten at the beginning of a meal, as they tend to give temporary satiety and to diminish appetite for the more substantial part of the meal.

Anorexia Nervosa

A very severe form of underweight is occasionally found in young people, most frequently young women, which is due to mental illness. Although these patients may seem to be physically well, and may protest that they eat sufficient amounts of food, they are often 30 percent or more underweight, and their actual food intake is negligible. Since rejection of food is part of their illness, it is best not to press the need for calories on such patients but to serve pleasing meals without comment, in the hope that, as they recover, their food intake will increase.

STUDY QUESTIONS AND ACTIVITIES

1. In conversation with the adult patients to whom you give nursing care this week ask each patient to recall what he or she weighed at age 12, 18, 25, 35, 45, and 55. For some patients it will be easier for them to relate weight to some event in their lives—e.g., graduation from high school, the time of marriage, induction into the armed forces, or, for women, their weight at the time of the birth of their first baby. Do any of these patients illustrate: (1) normal weight over their life span thus far; (2) obesity throughout their life span; (3) obesity which developed during their adult years?

2. In conversation with adult patients discover what foods they consider "fattening." In clinical conference with your classmates and instructor discuss these ideas.

3. Calculate a 1,500-calorie pattern dietary for yourself. For 3 days, use this pattern to select your food in the hospital dining room, at your favorite snack bar, and any meal you might eat at home or in a restaurant. Record all food and beverages you consume each day. Appraise the calorie value of each day's intake. In clinical conference with your instructor discuss the problems you met and your feelings about "counting" calories each day.

4. With the assistance of your instructor make appointments to accompany the dietitian when she does the diet interview and when she gives diet instruction to an obese patient. Observe and talk with this patient at one meal time for at least 3 days and report your observations to the dietitian. Summarize this experience and with the dietitian report to your classmates in clinical conference.

5. How can the nurse help in the prevention of obesity?

6. Why might an obese physician, nurse or dietitian be ineffective in helping a patient lose weight?

SUPPLEMENTARY READING ON WEIGHT CONTROL

Dally, P.: Anorexia Nervosa. New York, Grune & Stratton, 1969.

Dwyer, J. T., and Mayer, J.: Potential dieters: who are they? J. Am. Dietet. A., 56:510, 1970.

Mayer, J.: Overweight: Causes, Cost, and Control. Englewood Cliffs, N.J., Prentice-Hall, 1968.

Monello, L. F., and Mayer, J.: Obese adolescent girls, an unrecognized "minority" group. Am. J. Clin. Nutr., 13:35-39, 1963.

Moore, M. E., Stunkard, A., and Srole, L.: Obesity, social class, and mental illness. JAMA, 181:962, 1962.

Obesity and Health: U.S. Dept. H.E.W.-U.S.P.H.S. Publ. No. 1485, 1966.

Seltzer, C. C., and Mayer, J.: Body build and obesity: who are the obese? JAMA, 189:677, 1964.

For Further References see Bibliography in Part Four.

Diet in Diabetes Mellitus

22

Metabolic Aberrations · **Symptoms** · **Goal of Therapy** · **Diet Therapy**
Teaching the Patient · **Special Concerns**

INTRODUCTION

Diabetes mellitus, a disorder of glucose metabolism, is one of the common chronic diseases in the United States today. Diet therapy is a part of the treatment of all diabetic patients. For some individuals, usually the older obese ones (maturity-onset), the disease can be controlled by dietary modification alone. Other individuals, usually the young, nonobese ones (growth-onset), require both dietary modification and the hormone, insulin, to control the blood glucose level.

Oral hypoglycemic agents, such as Orinase or Diabinase, may be used in place of insulin in maturity-onset patients. A recent study,[1] however, indicates that patients using oral agents appear to have a greater number of deaths from cardiovascular disease than patients treated with insulin. Although the evidence from this study is not conclusive, some clinicians hesitate to use oral hypoglycemic agents in the treatment of maturity-onset diabetes.

The daily intake of carbohydrate in food, which becomes glucose in the body (see Chap. 2) is the prime concern in diet therapy for patients with diabetes mellitus. However, dietary protein and fat must also be considered because of the complex interrelationships of protein, fat and carbohydrate in the intermediary metabolism in the body (see Chap. 9). Because cardiovascular disease may accompany diabetes, especially in older patients, it may be necessary to consider the type and amount of dietary fat and/or the restriction of sodium when planning the diabetic diet (see Chap. 23).

Metabolic Aberrations. The disorders in intermediary metabolism that occur in untreated diabetes mellitus are presented in Figure 22-1. With the decrease in the entry of glucose into the cell, the amount of glucose circulating in the blood increases. The normal level of fasting blood glucose (FBS, fasting blood sugar) ranges from 60 to 100 mg. percent. The untreated diabetic will have a fasting blood glucose greater than 100 mg. percent (hyperglycemia). When the blood glucose exceeds approximately 160 mg. percent the excess is excreted in the urine (glycosuria). Thus the potential energy of the glucose, which is not available to the cell, is lost to the body. At the same time water is lost from the body because it is required for the excretion of the glucose.

This sequence of events—hyperglycemia followed by glycosuria—accounts for the excessive thirst (polydypsia), copious urination (polyuria), and hunger (polyphagia) accompanied by weight loss which many untreated diabetics experience. As Figure 22-1 indicates, sodium is also lost with the water. If the water and sodium loss is great enough, dehydration results. There is an increased excretion of potassium and of nitrogen, as urea, from the increase in breakdown of protein. These products of catabolism require water for excretion and, therefore, this aberration also contributes to the dehydration which can occur in untreated diabetes.

The increase in fatty acid breakdown in untreated diabetes results in the production of an abnormal amount of ketone bodies which appear in the blood (ketonemia). Two of the three com-

---

[1] Diabetes (Supplement 2), 19:747-830, 1970.

pounds classified as ketone bodies—acetoacetic acid and betahydroxybutyric acid—are organic acids. The accumulation of these acids in the blood leads to diabetic acidosis or ketosis. At the same time, the kidney excretes these acids in the urine (ketonuria) which, like the excretion of glucose in the urine, increases the loss of water from the body. The third ketone body, acetone, is volatile and is excreted by the lungs, giving a "fruity" odor to the breath of the individual in diabetic acidosis. If severe enough the acidosis leads to diabetic coma and, if untreated, ultimately to death.

Symptoms. In the adult diabetic the onset of symptoms is usually slow. Acidosis will not de-velop unless the individual is under stress from an overwhelming infection or an acute vascular episode such as a myocardial infarct. There will be mild hyperglycemia and some glycosuria. With-out an annual physical examination the disease may go undetected for a number of years. When medical care is finally sought, the presenting symptoms are usually fatigue, thirst, increased urination, and weight loss despite increased food intake. Sometimes skin infections, such as fu-runcles, or impaired vision may be the reason for seeking medical care.

With growth-onset diabetes in children and younger adults the individual will usually experi-ence all the classical symptoms of diabetes: poly-

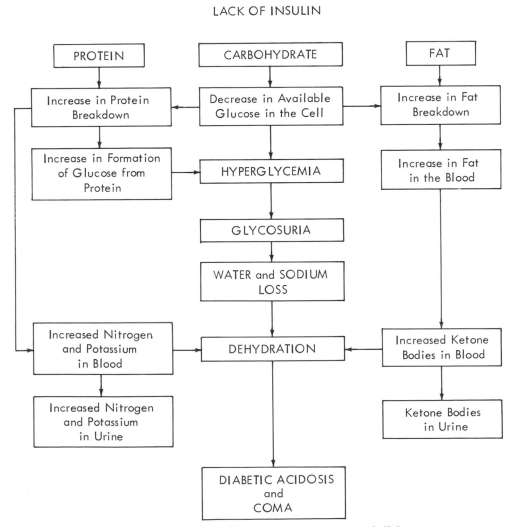

FIG. 22-1. Metabolic aberrations in untreated diabetes.

dypsia, polyphagia, polyuria and weight loss. Soon after the onset of these symptoms diabetic acidosis may occur. Mothers of children young enough to need help in getting a drink of water can often recall when the polydypsia first began.

Goal of Therapy. The basic goal of therapy in the treatment of diabetes mellitus is to help the patient achieve and maintain a normal blood sugar level with the hope of delaying the onset of associated vascular disease. The basic elements of this therapy are: (1) diet; (2) insulin or oral hypoglycemic agents if needed; (3) physical activity appropriate to the individual; (4) personal hygiene, and (5) constant medical supervision. Only diet therapy will be discussed in detail in this book.

Approaches to Therapy. There is a sharp controversy among physicians in the United States as to the best method of treating the patient with diabetes mellitus. The disagreement centers on the control of blood sugar levels. A group of conservative physicians believe that blood sugar levels higher than normal, resulting in the presence of sugar in the urine, contribute to the onset and the severity of vascular disease in diabetes. Hence diet and insulin therapy are regulated carefully so that the blood sugar levels will be kept within normal limits and no sugar will be found in the urine. This careful treatment of diabetes is known as chemical regulation; it is achieved by the use of a weighed diet.

A group of liberal physicians believe, from the evidence available to them, that careful regulation does not delay the onset of vascular disease. They treat their patients with insulin, if needed, and a liberal diet as long as no symptoms of diabetes other than glycosuria, without ketonuria and weight loss, are present. The physicians who advocate this approach to treatment claim that the patient lives a more nearly normal and satisfying life. This regimen is called the clinical method of regulation, and the patient is placed on an unmeasured or "free" diet, restricting only sugar and foods high in sugar.

A third group, the majority of physicians who treat diabetic patients, have adopted a middle-of-the-road approach. Their treatment plan is neither as limiting as the chemical method nor as liberal as the clinical method. They use the Exchange Lists for diet planning, a somewhat liberal yet moderately accurate method, which is based on standard household measures (see Chap. 20).

Regardless of the method used, the nurse and the dietitian must be aware that diet is an integral part of the treatment of any patient with diabetes mellitus. Mild diabetes, especially if the patient is obese and his diagnosis and treatment are not delayed, may be controlled by diet alone, whereas the severe diabetic will require diet plus insulin or an oral hypoglycemic agent to control his disease. In either case the diet, in addition to helping to control the disease, must meet the individual's nutritional needs.

DIET THERAPY

The Diet Prescription. CALORIES. The calorie requirement for the nonobese adult diabetic is the same as for normal individuals of the same sex, age, height, and activity. However, the diabetic is cautioned to maintain his weight at a level slightly below his desirable weight. Therefore, his calorie prescription may be somewhat less than for a normal individual. It is usually based on 30 to 35 calories per kilogram (2.2 pounds) of ideal body weight (1,750 to 2,000 calories for a woman whose ideal weight is 58 Kg.). The calorie requirement for a child or adolescent diabetic, neither of whom is usually obese, is the same as others of his age group.

The calorie prescription for an obese adult diabetic is designed to promote a weight loss. It is based on 20 to 25 calories per kilogram of ideal body weight, depending on his activity (1,150 to 1,450 calories for an obese woman whose ideal weight is 58 Kg.).

CARBOHYDRATE. Forty to 50 percent of the calorie prescription is usually derived from carbohydrate. For example: at 40 percent a 1,200-calorie diet will contain 120 Gm. of carbohydrate, and a 2,000-calorie diet will contain 200 Gm. of carbohydrate.

The distribution of the carbohydrate in the day's diet is equally as important as the total quantity. For patients who do not require insulin, the day's carbohydrate is divided equally between his three meals, or four if he is accustomed to a bedtime snack. This distribution is used to promote, in so far as possible, a constant level of blood sugar throughout the day. Such division also applies to patients using oral hypoglycemic agents.

For patients using moderate-acting insulins (Lente and NPH), the distribution of carbohydrate in the day's diet is usually ordered by the physician. As a general rule about ½ of the total carbohydrate is given prior to the time of peak action, about 8 hours after injection, and ½ of the carbohydrate is given after this time. One example of dividing the day's carbohydrate by this method is 1/6 for breakfast, 2/6 for the noon meal, 2/6 for the evening meal, and 1/6 at bedtime. The bedtime snack is used to protect the patient against insulin reactions during the night.

Another method commonly used to distribute the day's carbohydrate is to subtract 10 to 30 Gm. from the total. This amount of carbohydrate is used for a bedtime snack. The remaining grams of carbohydrate in the diet prescription may be distributed equally among three meals (see Calculation of Diabetic Pattern Dietary, p. 217); or by some other division required to regulate the patient's blood sugar level. It is expected that there will be a reasonable distribution of protein and fat and, therefore, total calories, throughout the day's meal plan. Some physicians require that protein and fat as well as carbohydrate be distributed in the day's diet according to the figures for distribution in the diet orders. For example: an order for 1/6 at breakfast means 1/6 of the day's carbohydrate, protein and fat for breakfast.

PROTEIN. The protein allowance for the adult diabetic is the same as for the normal person—0.9 Gm. per kilogram of body weight. For the child or adolescent the allowance is the same as for his age group. In practice the amount of protein in a diabetic diet prescription is usually greater than the amount in a normal one because the amount of carbohydrate and, therefore, of calories from carbohydrate, is restricted. The amount of protein in a diabetic diet for an adult will usually not exceed 1½ Gm. per kilogram of body weight. Larger amounts of protein are not needed and, as they are expensive, they add to the cost of the diet plan. If severe renal or liver disease is present the protein will be restricted.

FAT. After establishing the protein and carbohydrate of the diet, fat is used to supply the remainder of the calories. This will vary from 35 to 45 percent of calories from fat. Since the kind of fat in the diet—i.e., the quantity of saturated vs. polyunsaturated fatty acids—may have a relationship to the development of atherosclerosis, the physicians may modify the type of fat included in the diet of the diabetic (see Chap. 23).

Planning the Pattern Dietary With the Diabetic Patient

The first step in translating a physician's diet prescription into a pattern dietary for a newly diagnosed diabetic patient is to discover where he lives and works and with whom and what he eats each day. The foods he likes, accepts, and can afford should be used whenever possible in setting up his diet, because this or a similar diet will be the way he will eat for the rest of his life. In the following pages the three methods of diet planning—the exchange method, weighed diets and unmeasured diets—will be presented, with the major emphasis on the most commonly used one: the exchange method.

Meal Planning With Exchange Lists. This method for planning diabetic pattern dietaries is presented in Chapter 20, pages 196 to 200. The reader is advised to study this section before proceeding to the following discussion of the calculation of an 1,800-Calorie Diabetic Diet.

Table 22-1, Calculation of a Diabetic Pattern Dietary, illustrates a way in which a diet prescription for an 1,800-calorie diet with 180 Gm. of carbohydrate, 80 Gm. of protein, and 80 Gm. of fat might be translated into a diabetic pattern dietary for a patient. It will be noted that part of the prescription is used for a bedtime snack and the rest distributed in three approximately equal meals. Daily menu choices are selected by the patient from the Exchange Lists, pages 198 to 199 (see Table 22-2, Suggested Menu).

For those learning how to calculate a diabetic diet the first step is to distribute those exchanges—milk, vegetables, fruit, and bread—that will fulfill the carbohydrate prescription in the physician's diet order. As previously explained (p. 215), the amount of carbohydrate for each meal, and snack if included, will be indicated by the diet order. The second step is to distribute the protein, primarily the meat exchanges; the last step is to distribute the fat exchanges.

The totals of the grams of protein, fat and carbohydrate in the pattern dietary calculations may vary by approximately 5 Gm. from the figures in the diet prescription. Some protein and fat should be included in each meal and in the evening snack. Parts of exchanges should not be used in calculating the diet unless they reflect the patient's preference. For example, a patient may want only ½ of a milk exchange (4 ounces) at breakfast for his cereal. This is practical only if he usually eats his breakfast at home. In a restaurant he would use only part of a 6 to 8 ounce serving of milk yet would pay for the whole serving.

When a patient customarily uses a food that does not appear in one of the Exchange Lists, for instance pinto beans which are not listed in the Bread Exchanges, the size serving that gives the same nutritive value as the exchange can be calculated from a food table. (See Table 1 in Part Four, or Handbook 8, U.S.D.A.) Exchange Lists modified for various cultural food patterns are available from state and city health agencies, social

TABLE 22-1. CALCULATION OF DIABETIC PATTERN DIETARY
Diet Prescription: Protein, 80 Gm.; Fat, 80 Gm.; Carbohydrate, 180 Gm.; Calories, 1,800

MEAL		PROTEIN (Gm.)	FAT (Gm.)	CARBOHYDRATE (Gm.)	CALORIES
Breakfast	1 Fruit Exchange	..	..	10	40
	2 Bread Exchanges	4	..	30	136
	1 Meat Exchange	7	5	..	73
	1 Milk Exchange	8	10	12	170
	2 Fat Exchanges	..	10	..	90
	Total for Meal	19	25	52	509
Noon meal	2 Meat Exchanges	14	10	..	146
	2 Bread Exchanges	4	..	30	136
	Any A Vegetable	..	..	..	..
	2 Fruit Exchanges	..	..	20	80
	2 Fat Exchanges	..	10	..	90
	Total for Meal	18	20	50	452
Evening meal	3 Meat Exchanges	21	15	..	219
	3 Bread Exchanges	6	..	45	204
	Any A Vegetable	..	..	..	..
	1 B Vegetable	2	..	7	36
	2 Fat Exchanges	..	10	..	90
	Total for Meal	29	25	52	549
Bedtime snack	1 Bread Exchange	8	10	12	68
	1 Milk Exchange	2	..	15	170
	Total for Meal	10	10	27	238
	Total for Day	76	80	181	1,748

welfare agencies, and the visiting nurse services in large cities; or the dietitian can set up Exchange Lists to meet a patient's cultural food practices.

When a patient's preferences or limited income is a factor, the number of fruit and vegetable exchanges included in the diabetic pattern dietary need not exceed the quantity required for an adequate daily intake of ascorbic acid and other vitamins. The remainder of the carbohydrate may then be distributed among bread, spaghetti, potatoes, etc., which are lower in cost, and which may be preferred to large quantities of vegetables and fruits.

Exchanges may be used in the preparation of "mixed" dishes. These can be prepared for the whole family, with the patient receiving his correct portion. The patient or his family may also find *A Cookbook for Diabetics*[2] useful in adding variety to the diabetic diet.

Weighed Diets. The physician who uses the chemical method to treat the diabetic will require his patients to purchase a scale which weighs in grams. The patient will weigh each serving of food at each meal. The instruction materials for

[2] Behrman, D. M.: Am. Diabetes A., 1959. 18 E. 45th Street, New York, N.Y. 10017. Price $1.00.

TABLE 22-2. SUGGESTED MENU FOR 1,800 CALORIE DIABETIC PATTERN DIETARY

BREAKFAST
½ small grapefruit
1 poached egg on 1 slice of toast
1 slice of toast with 1 tsp. butter
8 ounces of milk
2 cups of coffee with 2 tbsp. coffee cream

NOON MEAL
2 ounce hamburger pattie
1 hamburger roll (large)
1 tsp. mayonnaise
1 thin slice bermuda onion
lettuce and mustard
1 medium apple
1 cup coffee with 1 tbsp. coffee cream

EVENING MEAL
3 ounces sliced turkey
1 cup mashed potato
½ cup peas
tossed salad with vinegar and 1 tsp. oil
1 dinner roll and 1 tsp. butter
coffee without cream

BEDTIME SNACK
8 ounces milk
1 piece of sponge cake

the patient will give the gram weight of each serving of food. The equivalent household measure may also be included. Many physicians have adapted the exchange system or constructed a similar system for this method of diet instruction. The nutrient values of foods used by some physicians may vary to some degree from those used in the exchange system, therefore the nurse or dietitian will need to use the nutrient values used by the physician when calculating the pattern dietary for a patient. As the patient acquires experience in weighing his food he becomes expert in judging serving size and may be advised by his physician to weigh his food only one day a week to check his practices. Even some physicians who use the exchange system have their newly diagnosed patients weigh foods for a short time in order to learn to judge serving size.

The Unmeasured or "Free" Diet. The physician who uses this method usually guides his patients to establish daily food practices very similar to the Pattern Dietary (Chap. 19, p. 185) at the calorie level required by the individual. The patient actually sets up his own diet pattern and the physician adjusts the insulin to the intake. Concentrated sweets such as sugar, jelly, honey, candy, sweetened fruits, frosted cakes, pies, and sweetened fruit juices and sweetened carbonated beverages are omitted. Concentrated sweets are excluded because they are quickly absorbed, raise the blood sugar level above the kidney threshold and are then excreted in the urine. The patient derives no benefit from the calories so lost.

Special Diet Foods. At present the regulations of the Federal Food and Drug Administration covering Foods for Special Dietary Purposes are under revision. Diabetic patients should be warned that those foods advertised as low or reduced in sugar may still contain too much carbohydrate from sources other than sucrose to be used in their diets.

Diet Planning and Associated Diseases. The diabetic diet may need to be modified if other disease is also present. In the case of an elderly, debilitated patient, the diet may have to be Soft as outlined in Chapter 19. If there is disease of the intestinal tract a low residue or a bland diet (see Chap. 25) may be indicated. In cardiac disease sodium may need to be restricted (see Chap. 23). The American Dietetic Association has available supplements to the exchange lists which are modified in texture for bland, low fiber diets, and low in sodium for those patients who require a sodium-restricted diet.[3]

The amount and kind of fat in the American diet as it relates to cardiovascular disease, particularly coronary heart disease, is under careful study (see Chap. 23). Diabetic diets containing 1,800 calories or more tend to have the same percent of calories from fat as the ordinary American diet (40 to 45 percent). In the diabetic diet this amount of fat is used to compensate for the restriction of carbohydrate to 40 percent of total calories. Because it has been observed that coronary artery and other vascular disease is associated with diabetes, the kind and amount of fat included in the diabetic diet is also being studied. Some physicians are modifying the kind of fat in the diabetic diet from primarily saturated fats to a greater use of polyunsaturated fat. A modified fat exchange list which reflects this trend is available from the American Dietetic Association.

TEACHING THE PATIENT

The diabetic patient must be helped to face the fact that his disease cannot be cured but that, with proper dietary care, and the use of insulin or one of the oral drugs if necessary, he can live a comfortable and productive life. Teaching the patient in simple terms what his disease is and why his dietary restrictions are necessary is often a responsibility shared by the physician and the nurse. As soon as the patient's diabetes is stabilized, actual dietary instruction should begin, with the doctor, the nurse and the dietitian working closely together. Stone has demonstrated that given adequate instruction and time to learn, the majority of diabetic patients can manage their diets successfully.[4]

The patient's trays are an important first step in teaching. From them he will learn the size of food portions and the foods which have approximately the same composition and, therefore, may be exchanged for each other. The foods that do not appear on the tray, such as sugar, jelly, canned or cooked sweetened fruits and desserts with sugar added, are also points to be emphasized in teaching. The approximate quantity of food served at each meal, particularly if the patient is receiving insulin or one of the oral drugs, needs to be pointed out.

When a specific plan for the patient's diet is constructed, care must be taken that it fits into

---

[3] Caso, E. K.: J. Am. Dietet. A., 32:929, 1956.
[4] Stone, D. B.: Am. J. Med. Sci., 241:436, 1961.

his life situation. The diet for a small child will differ from that of an active adolescent; both will differ from the diet of the man who works. Again, adjustments must be made for the older man or woman, often with other serious disease as well, who lives alone, perhaps on a very small income. The dietary pattern should be fitted to the person for whom it is designed, not the person fitted to the pattern. Economic necessity, cultural preferences and personal likes and dislikes must all be incorporated insofar as possible. There is no reason why an Italian patient may not have "pasta" and the Chinese or Arabic patient rice in place of bread and potatoes. Fortunately, the exchange system allows for a considerable amount of choice.

Also available to help the diabetic adjust to the new demands being made on him is the bimonthly magazine published for patients by the American Diabetes Association.[5] It contains information about the disease, stories of patients and recipes based on the Exchange Lists. It has a fine section for children with diabetes.

The family, too, may need encouragement and support in the adjustment to the diagnosis of diabetes in one of its members. This is particularly true for parents when one of their children develops the disease.

In all this the nurse, the dietitian and the physician, as well, must work as a team. The nurse will often elicit questions and information from the patient which will help to fit his diet restrictions to his need. And, most of all, those who teach the diabetic patient must realize that it is not only difficult to change one's dietary pattern, but also difficult to adhere to the new pattern. Patience, support and encouragement are needed until the diabetic has accepted the restrictions of his disease and has learned to live comfortably with them.

SPECIAL CONCERNS

Diabetic Acidosis and Coma. Diabetic acidosis and coma require emergency treatment by the physician and the nurse to reestablish fluid and electrolyte balance and normal metabolism. If the patient is in coma, or if he is nauseated and vomiting, insulin and intravenous fluids will be used to treat him. As his hyperglycemia and ketonemia decrease, and when he can tolerate it, he will be offered a variety of fluids by mouth. When his

condition is stabilized he will be given a diabetic diet and insulin.

Replacements. It is expected that diabetic patients receiving insulin or an oral hypoglycemic agent will consume all the food served at each meal to prevent the possibility of insulin shock. When a patient refuses a food, especially one which is primarily carbohydrate, he should be provided with a substitute equal in carbohydrate to the food refused.

If a patient refuses the major portion of a meal for any reason, the physician may require that the total available glucose of the meal be replaced. To calculate the total available glucose in a meal, the number of grams of carbohydrate calculated in the patient's pattern dietary are added to the number of grams of carbohydrate equal to 58 percent of the grams of protein and 10 percent of the grams of fat. It is estimated that 58 percent of the protein and 10 percent of the fat in a diet give rise to glucose. For example: a meal calculated to provide 30 Gm. of protein, 30 Gm. of fat and 60 Gm. of carbohydrate has 80 Gm. of available glucose (30 Gm. of protein × 0.58 = 17.4 Gm. of glucose; 30 Gm. of fat × 0.1 = 3 Gm. of glucose; and 60 Gm. of carbohydrate = 60 Gm. of glucose). This amount of carbohydrate may have to be given in several small feedings within the next 2 or 3 hours to prevent insulin shock.

Surgery. Today diabetic individuals undergo surgery with comparative safety. In emergencies, such as an acute appendix, there is usually no reason to delay surgery because of diabetes. In these situations the patient is given insulin and intravenous fluids and glucose.

When there is time to prepare for surgery the status of the patient's diabetes is carefully evaluated and, if his disease is not well-controlled, the proper diet and insulin treatment is instituted before he undergoes surgery. On the day of surgery, breakfast is withheld. A small dose of regular or the usual dose of moderate acting insulin may be given before surgery. After the operation glucose and fluids with sufficient insulin are given intravenously. Oral feedings of liquids such as fruit juices, broth, tea and ginger ale are started as early as possible. Later the patient's usual diet is resumed.

Diabetes in Pregnancy. Diabetes in the mother has always been a special hazard in pregnancy. There is increased fetal loss in the course of the pregnancy as well as an increased loss of infants carried to term as compared with the nondiabetic

---

[5] ADA Forecast, Amer. Diab. A., 1 E. 45th Street, New York, N.Y. 10017.

patient. In the past few years, however, by keeping close watch on the mother, obstetricians have been able to secure a far greater number of successful pregnancies than formerly.

Early prenatal care is an important factor in the salvage of these babies as well as in the maintenance of the health of the mother. Again there is a difference of opinion about the type of dietary control, but all physicians agree that the nutritional needs of pregnancy must be adequately met (see Chap. 14), with sufficient insulin to cover the increased food intake.

Diabetes in Children. Although it is estimated that children under 14 years of age make up approximately only 5 percent of the known diabetics, they present the most serious problems in the management of the disease. Their disease is more severe and less stable than the maturity-onset type.

The outlook for children who develop diabetes has changed markedly from the preinsulin days when the disease invariably was fatal. White[6] reported on 1,072 patients whose onset of diabetes occurred before the age of 15 and who had had the disease 20 years or more. Of these, 879 were living at the time of the study. Of the 879 patients, 71 percent had had diabetes from 20 to 29 years, 24 percent had had diabetes from 30 to 34 years and 5 percent had had the disease for more than 35 years.

However, in a large percentage of such patients, complications develop after 15 to 20 years or more of diabetes. These include diminished vision and heart and kidney disease, all attributable to blood-vessel changes. In a later paper[7] White states that 90 percent of patients who developed diabetes before the age of 15 and had had the disease for 30 years or more could be shown to have such blood-vessel changes. Thus, although much has been gained in lifespan for the young diabetic, much remains to be done.

The controversy over the best approach to treatment applies particularly to young patients (see p. 215). Those physicians who advocate chemical control direct the parents and children to weigh food; and those advocating clinical control have the children share the family meals. Some physicians use Meal Planning with Exchange Lists.

Whatever the school of thought is in regard to control of the diet, all physicians agree that the nutritional needs of the diabetic child are the same as those of the nondiabetic (see Chaps. 15 and 16).

If there has been any marked weight loss before the disease is discovered, which is usually the case, the diet prescribed should be such as to allow the child to recover this loss. As he grows and develops, there must be periodic adjustment of the diet and the dosage of insulin. Strenuous physical activity may be compensated for by small amounts of food before the exercise.

Particularly in the adolescent years, when girls and boys grow very rapidly, it is essential that the diet keep pace with the nutritional needs, and that insulin be increased accordingly.

Both the diabetic child and his parents will require long-term and constant instruction and support if the disease is to be kept under control. Tact, sympathy and understanding will do much to help them in the acceptance and the adjustments which will be necessary over the years.

STUDY QUESTIONS AND ACTIVITIES

1. Find out the total number of adult diabetic patients in your hospital today. The therapeutic dietitian's records of diet orders will give you this information most readily. How many of these diets are also calorie restricted? (1,500 calories or less) How many are also restricted in sodium? Do any diet orders for these diabetics also require modification of fatty acid composition?

2. Using the patient's chart and the physician's daily orders, summarize and present to your classmates in clinical conference the insulin and diet changes in a post-partum woman who is a diabetic. Include the pediatrician's progress notes and orders for her infant, especially feeding changes.

3. Through observation and interview discover how a patient with well-controlled diabetes, who has been admitted for elective surgery, has managed his activities of daily living including his diet prior to admission to the hospital. What resources has he used in the past for guidance and counseling? If indicated, what further help does he need, and who should help him, during his convalescence from surgery?

4. Record the 24-hour food and nutrient beverage intake of a patient with diabetes. Using the appropriate food value system appraise his calorie and nutrient intake. Compare his actual intake of calories, protein, fat, and carbohydrate with the diet order prescribed by his physician. Compare his mineral and vitamin intake with guidelines appropriate for him. If there is any significant discrepancy between intake and order, seek the assistance of your instructors in identifying the reason and in solving the problem.

[6] White, P.: Diabetes, 5:445, 1956.
[7] White, P.: Diabetes, 9:345, 1960.

5. What percentage of carbohydrate is metabolized as glucose in the body? Of protein? Of fat? How much glucose will the body obtain from the Pattern Dietary which contains 90 Gm. of protein, 100 Gm. of fat and 200 Gm. of carbohydrate?

6. The carbohydrate allowance for a diabetic patient is 150 Gm. He is receiving insulin. How will the carbohydrate of his diet probably be divided for the day?

7. Plan a diabetic diet with the following diet order: protein 75, fat 110, carbohydrate 200, carbohydrate divided for insulin, using the Exchange Lists in Chapter 20. The patient is a man with a large appetite.

8. Give five substitutions that a diabetic can make for a slice of bread.

9. What is meant by the chemical regulation of diabetes? The clinical regulation? Why is there controversy over these two methods of regulation?

10. What is meant by a "free" diabetic diet? What advantages are claimed for it?

SUPPLEMENTARY READING ON DIABETES

Caso, E. K.: Supplements to diabetic diet material. J. Am. Dietet. A., 32:929, 1956.

Collier, B. N., and Etzwiler, D. D.: Comparative study of diabetes knowledge among juvenile diabetics and their parents. Diabetes, 20:51, 1970.

Felig, P., and Bondy, P. K. (eds.): Symposium on diabetes mellitus. Med. Clin. N. Am., 55:877, 1971.

Garnet, J. D.: Pregnancy in women with diabetes. Am. J. Nursing, 69:1900, 1969.

Hinkle, L. E.: Customs, emotions and behavior in the dietary treatment of diabetes. J. Am. Dietet. A., 41:341, 1962.

Jernigan, A. K.: Diabetic patients require education and understanding. Hospitals, 44:77, (Nov. 1) 1970.

Krysan, G. S.: How do we teach four million diabetics. Am. J. Nursing, 65:105, 1965.

Moore, M. L.: Diabetes in children. Am. J. Nursing, 67:104, 1967.

Murawski, B. J., et al.: Personality patterns in patients with diabetes mellitus of long duration. Diabetes, 19:259, 1970.

Podolsky, S.: Special needs of the diabetic undergoing surgery. Postgrad. Med., 45:128, (Feb.) 1969.

Sharkey, T. P.: Diabetes mellitus: present problems and new research. J. Am. Dietet. A., 58:201, 336, 422, 528, 1971.

Stone, D. B.: A rational approach to diet and diabetes. J. Am. Dietet. A., 46:30, 1965.

Watkins, J. D., et al.: A study of diabetic patients at home. Am. J. Public Health, 57:452, 1967.

PATIENT RESOURCES

Danowski, T. S.: Diabetes as a Way of Life, ed. 2. New York, Coward-McCann, 1970.

Gormican, A.: Controlling Diabetes with Diet. Springfield, Ill., Charles C Thomas, 1971.

Rosenthal, H., and Rosenthal, J.: Diabetic Care in Pictures, ed. 4. Philadelphia, J. B. Lippincott, 1968.

For Further References see Bibliography in Part Four.

Diet in Cardiovascular Disease

23

Introduction · The Sodium-Restricted Diet · The Fat-Controlled Diet

INTRODUCTION

Diseases of the heart and the vascular system—cardiovascular disease—account for much of the illness in the adult population in our society. Most of the patients who are hospitalized for the treatment of cardiovascular disease require some type of modified diet. If any of these patients are overweight due to overfatness, their diets are restricted in calories to promote weight reduction (Chap. 21). Cardiac patients with edema (Chap. 6) due to congestive failure, hypertension or mild renal failure, a complication of cardiovascular disease, require a sodium-restricted diet as well as a diuretic.

The patient with coronary artery disease due to atherosclerosis—a specific type of cardiovascular disease—requires very complex dietary treatment. The extensive research of the past 25 years indicates that food habits are one risk factor in the development of atherosclerosis. Other risk factors are genetic tendency, elevated blood lipids, diseases such as hypertension and diabetes, and personal health habits such as cigarette smoking and inactivity. It has been demonstrated that modification of the intake of dietary lipids—fats, fatty acids, and cholesterol—can modify the elevated blood lipids in individuals with atherosclerosis. For some individuals the carbohydrate content of the diet may also need to be modified because in intermediary metabolism, blood glucose can contribute to total blood lipids (Chap. 9).

Patients with myocardial infarcts, the acute phase of coronary heart disease are usually offered a liquid diet when first admitted to the intensive coronary care unit, and then, as they recover, progress to a soft diet (Chap. 19). Neither the liquid nor the soft diet should contain excessive amounts of fat. When these patients are moved from the coronary care unit to a general medical unit they are usually given a fat-controlled diet. If necessary, the fat-controlled diet may also be restricted in sodium and calories.

The sodium-restricted diet and the fat-controlled or modified fat diet are discussed in the following sections of this chapter.

THE SODIUM-RESTRICTED DIET

Sodium in Foods and Beverages

Salt. Salt or sodium chloride, commonly used in cooking and preserving food, is approximately 40 percent sodium. Thus, 1 Gm. of salt (1,000 mg.) contains 0.4 Gm. or 400 mg. of sodium. It can readily be seen why salt, added to foods during cooking or at the table, must be omitted or used only in very limited amounts on sodium-restricted diets. Also foods that have had sodium added during processing or preservation are avoided.

Food. With few exceptions all of our food, by nature, contains sodium but the amounts vary by food groups. Animal foods are our most important sources of sodium; plant foods usually contain the least sodium. Milk, meat, fish, fowl, and eggs, processed or cooked without the addition of salt or any other sodium compound, contribute the greatest amount of sodium in the restricted diet. (See Table 23-3, Sodium Content of Food Exchanges.)

Animal fats and vegetable oils naturally contain only very little or no sodium. Therefore, at certain levels of sodium restriction salt-free butter and unsalted margarine are used. Vegetable oils and cooking fats made from vegetable oils do not have salt added in processing and may be used in the sodium-restricted diet.

Cereals, breads, fruits, and vegetables, processed and cooked without the addition of salt or other sodium compounds, contribute the least amount of sodium to the restricted diet. There are exceptions in the vegetable group: artichokes; beets, carrots, white turnips; celery; spinach, kale, beet greens, chard, dandelion greens and mustard greens—these contain more sodium per serving than other commonly used vegetables. For example, ½ cup of carrots (100 Gm.) cooked without salt contains about 50 mg. of sodium, whereas ½ cup of broccoli (100 Gm.) cooked without salt contains about 10 mg. of sodium.

Food Processing. The greatest source of the sodium in our food is the sodium added in food processing and preservation. Easily recognized examples of this are bacon and ham; salted crackers, potato chips, popcorn and other snack foods; and olives, pickles and sauerkraut.

The cereals and bread and other bakery products in our markets have salt and other sodium compounds added in processing or preparation. Bread made without salt or other sodium compounds is now available in many areas because of the great demand by individuals needing sodium-restricted diets. One slice of bread made with salt contains about 150 mg. of sodium (see Fig. 23-1); 1 slice made without salt contains about 5 mg. Unsalted melba toast is also generally available.

Canned foods, packaged mixes and other convenience foods such as frozen dinners, frozen vegetables with sauces and seasonings added, and frozen waffles and pizza all have sodium added. The same applies to canned soups, gravies and soup mixes; mayonnaise and salad dressings; and condiments such as chili sauce, ketchup, and meat sauces. Sodium is not added to canned fruits; also vegetables naturally low in sodium, and canned without the addition of salt, are generally available in our markets.

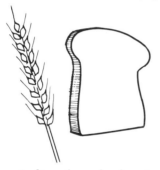

A slice of regular bread contains about 150 milligrams of sodium.

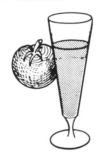

A half cup of canned tomato juice contains about 275 milligrams of sodium.

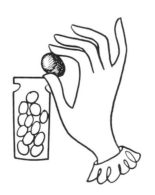

Just one large olive will add 130 milligrams of sodium to the diet.

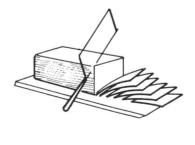

One ounce of processed cheddar cheese contains about 420 milligrams of sodium.

Fig. 23-1. A few examples of foods high in sodium content.

Sodium may also be added in food processing where we do not expect it. Fresh peas and lima beans contain very little sodium and are used in the sodium-restricted diet. But frozen peas and lima beans are omitted because they are sorted in salt solution in the processing plant and pick up significant amounts of sodium. One half cup of fresh peas cooked without salt has about 1 mg. of sodium; ½ cup of frozen peas cooked without salt has about 115 mg. of sodium. This is only one example of an unexpected addition of salt in food processing and illustrates why patients who require a sodium-restricted diet need careful instruction.

Sodium compounds other than salt which may be used in food processing are: disodium phosphate in quick-cooking cereals; monosodium glutamate in a variety of foods, to enhance the flavor; sodium alginate in chocolate milk and ice creams for smooth textures; sodium benzoate as a preservative in jams, jellies, relishes, sauces and salad dressings; sodium hydroxide to soften skins of certain fruits, olives and hominy; sodium propionate to inhibit mold growth in cheese and bread; and sodium sulfite to bleach certain fruits before coloring such as maraschino cherries.

Baking powder and baking soda (sodium bicarbonate) are also important sources of sodium. A sodium-free baking powder for home use is available in some of our markets.

Labels and Label Reading. Although the booklets and other materials which may be used in patient education will warn him to "read labels," this may not be as helpful as it sounds. The Food and Drug Administration (see Chap. 12) allows many processed foods such as mayonnaise and ketchup to be sold without listing the ingredients on the label. These and other foods are prepared under a standard of identity which specifies the kind and the minimum content of each ingredient and, therefore, in such cases the listing of sodium on the label is not required.

On many packages and containers, even when properly labeled, the salt content of the food is listed by a variety of terms such as salt, sodium chloride, sodium, Na, or soda. The patient must be cautioned that these terms are synonymous and that foods containing them must be avoided (see Fig. 23-2).

Low-Sodium Dietetic Foods. Products offered as low-sodium dietetic foods come under the regulations of Food for Special Dietary Uses of the Food and Drug Administration. These regulations are presently under revision (1972) but it appears that those which apply to sodium content of food will not be changed. Under the regulations the label must clearly show the content of sodium, in mg. per 100 Gm. of food, and the number of milligrams of sodium in a specified serving of such food. It is helpful to remember that 100 Gm. is approximately 3 ounces.

Some of the foods labeled "low sodium" may not be usable on a sodium-restricted diet because, although reduced in sodium as compared with the regular food, they still contain too much sodium per serving. Low-sodium soups, for instance, may still contain too much sodium to be included in the diet. Vegetables, such as those previously listed as having a high natural sodium content, even when canned without salt, should not be used if they are not listed on the sodium-restricted diet.

Seasonings. A variety of spices and herbs which can be used to make the diet more palatable are listed in Table 23-1. Fortunately, most of these are low in sodium. It must be remembered that some commonly used seasonings and condiments contain salt. These are celery, garlic and onion salt; dried parsley and onion flakes; prepared mustard, Worcestershire and soy sauce; and sodium glutamate and meat tenderizers. Patients who have not previously used a variety of spices and herbs should be cautioned to use them sparingly until they are sure they enjoy the new flavors.

SALT SUBSTITUTES. Salt substitutes are available at drugstores and some food markets. They usually contain potassium or ammonium in place of sodium. The potassium substitute may be contraindicated if there is kidney damage and the ammonium ones if there is extensive liver damage. In the hospital they may be offered to patients on sodium-restricted diets routinely or only by order of the physician. Those patients who use a salt substitute need to be advised to use it sparingly because in excessive amounts some individuals find the taste unpleasant. One of the substitutes, labeled "seasoned," has a variety of spices added and is very palatable.

"Koshering" of Food. Jewish patients who follow the orthodox dietary laws salt their freshly slaughtered meat and fowl to extract the blood, allowing it to stand for an hour or so, then washing it thoroughly before cooking. Although this will remove some of the added salt, a good deal will have penetrated the inner portion of the meat. Kaufman[1] states that meat so treated has from 334 to 375 mg. of sodium per 100 Gm., depending on the manner of cooking. She suggests that Jewish patients be taught to salt their meat lightly and allow it to stand for the minimal amount of time;

[1] Kaufman, M.: Am. J. Clin. Nutr., 5:676, 1957.

after it has been rinsed and soaked in water, it should be boiled in a generous amount of water and the broth should be discarded. Meat so treated was found to contain 63 mg. of sodium per 100 Gm. As an alternative, she suggests the use of ammonium chloride salt in place of sodium chloride for drawing out the blood.

The Drinking Water. In some areas of the country drinking water may present a special hazard because of its high sodium content. This may

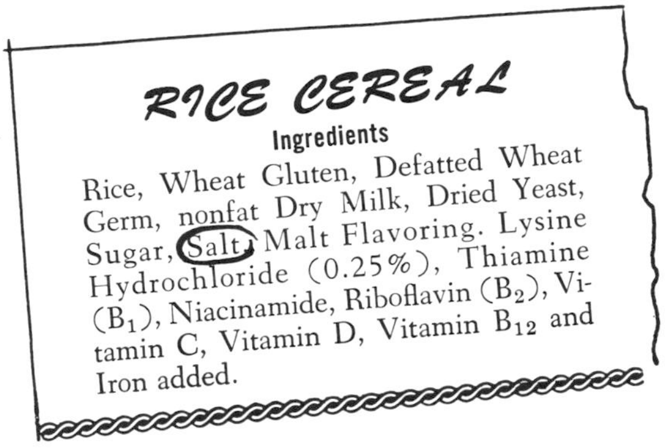

RICE CEREAL
Ingredients
Rice, Wheat Gluten, Defatted Wheat Germ, nonfat Dry Milk, Dried Yeast, Sugar, Salt, Malt Flavoring. Lysine Hydrochloride (0.25%), Thiamine (B₁), Niacinamide, Riboflavin (B₂), Vitamin C, Vitamin D, Vitamin B₁₂ and Iron added.

Some cereals have salt added.

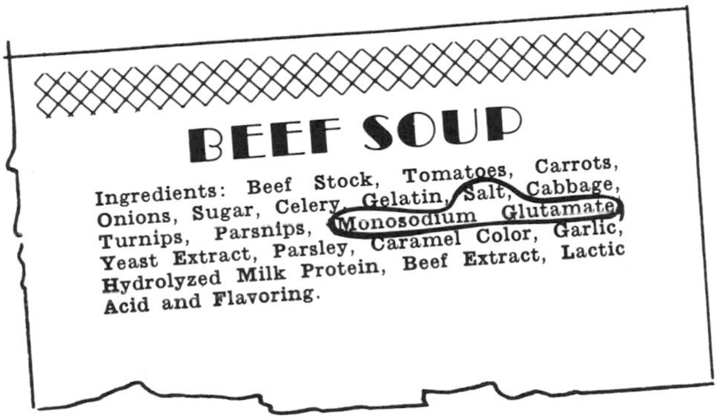

BEEF SOUP
Ingredients: Beef Stock, Tomatoes, Carrots, Onions, Sugar, Celery, Gelatin, Salt, Cabbage, Turnips, Parsnips, Monosodium Glutamate, Yeast Extract, Parsley, Caramel Color, Garlic, Hydrolyzed Milk Protein, Beef Extract, Lactic Acid and Flavoring.

Even if this can of soup did not contain salt it should not be used because of the monosodium glutamate.

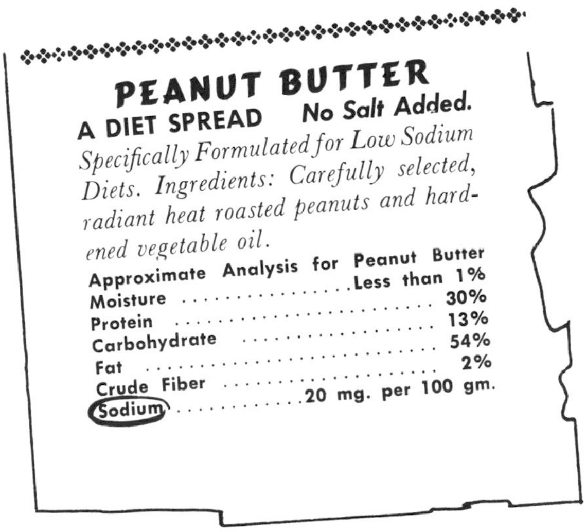

PEANUT BUTTER
A DIET SPREAD   No Salt Added.
Specifically Formulated for Low Sodium Diets. Ingredients: Carefully selected, radiant heat roasted peanuts and hardened vegetable oil.

Approximate Analysis for Peanut Butter
Moisture .... Less than 1%
Protein 30%
Carbohydrate 13%
Fat 54%
Crude Fiber 2%
Sodium .... 20 mg. per 100 gm.

Dietetic foods must be labeled carefully.

FIG. 23-2. Examples of labeling.

TABLE 23-1. SEASONINGS, EXTRACTS, HERBS AND SPICES

LOW IN SODIUM MAY BE USED FREELY		HIGH IN SODIUM DO NOT USE
Allspice	Mint	Bouillon cubes, regular
Almond extract	Mustard, dry, or mustard seed	Catsup
Anise seed	Nutmeg	Celery flakes, seed, salt
Basil	Onion, onion juice, or onion	Chili sauce
Bay leaf	powder	Garlic salt
Bouillon cube, low-sodium	Orange extract	Horseradish, prepared with salt
dietetic if less than 5 mg.	Oregano	Instant vegetable broth
of sodium per cube	Paprika	Meat extracts
Caraway seed	Parsley	Meat sauces
Cardamon	Pepper, fresh green or red	Meat tenderizers
Catsup, dietetic	Pepper, black, red, or white	Monosodium glutamate
Chili powder	Peppermint extract	Mustard, prepared
Chives	Pimiento peppers for garnish	Olives
Cinnamon	Poppy seed	Onion salt
Cloves	Poultry seasoning	Parsley flakes
Cocoa (1 to 2 teaspoons)	Purslane	Pickles
Coconut	Rosemary	Relishes
Cumin	Saccharin, calcium (sugar	Saccharin, sodium (sugar
Curry	substitute)	substitute)
Dill	Saffron	SALT
Fennel	Sage	Salt substitutes, unless recom-
Garlic, garlic juice, or garlic	Salt substitutes, if recommended	mended by the physician
powder	by your physician	Soy sauce
Ginger	Savory	Tomato paste
Horseradish root or horseradish	Sesame seeds	Worcestershire sauce
prepared without salt	Sorrel	
Juniper	Sugar	
Lemon juice or extract	Tarragon	
Mace	Thyme	
Maple extract	Turmeric	
Marjoram	Vanilla extract	
Meat extract, low-sodium	Vinegar	
dietetic	Wine if allowed	
Meat tenderizers, low-sodium	Walnut extract	
dietetic		

Adapted from "Your 1,000 milligram Sodium Diet," The American Heart Association, New York, N.Y. 10010.

be due either to the sodium content of the soil from which the water is drawn or to the use of water softeners.

In a recent study of over 2,000 local water supplies,[2] widely distributed throughout the United States and covering approximately 50 percent of the population, great variation in sodium content was found, as shown in Table 23-2.

It will be noted that only 58 percent or a little over a half the water supply was within the range of none to 20 mg. of sodium per liter (approximately a quart). Water used for coffee and tea, for drinking and for food preparation is estimated at 2½ to 3 quarts per person a day. When water contains more than 20 mg. of sodium per quart,

it quickly begins to affect the sodium content of the diet. The patient should obtain information about his community's water by contacting the department of health.

"Soft Drinks." Bottled "soft drinks" may be high in sodium due to the sodium content of the water in the area where they are manufactured. Low caloric beverages may have their sodium content increased still further by the substitution of sodium saccharin, an artificial sweetener, for sugar. They are therefore omitted when careful sodium restriction must be maintained.

Sodium in Medications

The physician will avoid prescribing medications which contain sodium. The patient should be cautioned to take no medication, "patent" medicine

2 White, J. M., *et al.*: J. Am. Dietet. A., 50:32, 1967.

or home remedy without consulting his physician. Baking soda (sodium bicarbonate) is a popular home remedy for indigestion or "heart-burn"; and many alkalizers, antacids, headache remedies, sedatives and cathartics are high in sodium and should not be used.

The Diet Prescription

Depending on the condition of the patient, the physician's diet order will state in milligrams the specific amount of sodium he wants the patient to have each day. The order for sodium restriction may also be combined with one for calorie restriction (Chap. 21) or for diabetes (Chap. 22). In the past there was considerable confusion because the diet order restricting sodium intake tended to be general, rather than specific. Such terms as salt-poor, low-salt, or salt-free diet gave little indication of the amount of sodium desired. This confusion has disappeared as we have learned how the body uses sodium, and how to analyze foods for their sodium content. The most commonly used levels of sodium restriction are 1,000 and 2,000 mg. The 2,000 mg. diet is considered a mild restriction of sodium. If required a 500-mg. restriction may be ordered.

500-Milligram Sodium Diet. A diet order for 500 mg. of sodium or less is considered a severe restriction and will be used only in special situations. Planning the 500-milligram sodium pattern dietary is discussed in the next section of this chapter. The water used for drinking or in cooking must contain no more than 20 mg. of sodium per quart, or distilled water must be used.

When less than 500 mg. of sodium (200 to 300 mg.) is required, special low-sodium milk—either Lonalac or dialyzed whole milk, fresh or canned—will be used to ensure an adequate intake of protein, calcium and the other nutrients usually supplied by milk. Dialyzed milk, which contains more potassium than regular milk, may be contraindicated if there is kidney damage, or other reason for restricting potassium. On the other hand if the diuretic being used promotes potassium loss, the dialyzed milk can help replace potassium. Sometimes 600-, 700-, or 800-milligram sodium diets will be ordered.[3] The 500-milligram pattern dietary can be modified in various ways to fulfill these orders.

1,000-Milligram Sodium Diet. Diet orders for 1,000 mg. of sodium are used for patients who require only a moderate restriction of sodium

intake. Some of these patients may tolerate 1,200- to 1,500-milligram sodium diets, and diets in this range may be ordered. Planning the pattern dietary for the 1,000-milligram sodium-restricted diet is discussed in the following section of this chapter.

2,000-Milligram or Mild Sodium-Restricted Diet. The sodium content of this diet is usually 2,000 mg. but it may range from 2,000 to 3,000 mg. No salt is added to food at the table, limited amounts are used in food preparation, and foods obviously high in salt are omitted. The average house diet will contain 3,000 to 6,000 mg. or more of sodium.

Planning the Sodium-Restricted Pattern Dietary

SODIUM-RESTRICTED FOOD EXCHANGE METHOD

A widely used method for planning the sodium-restricted pattern dietary is based on the Exchange System. Table 23-3, Sodium Content of Food Exchanges, gives the average sodium values of the Exchanges. These are values for foods produced,

TABLE 23-2. RANGE OF SODIUM ION IN DRINKING WATER FOR A SAMPLING PERIOD*

RANGE OF SODIUM ION CONCENTRATION	NUMBER OF SAMPLES	PERCENT OF TOTAL SAMPLES
mg./L.		
0- 19.9	1,194	58.2
20- 49.9	391	19.0
50- 99.9	190	9.3
100-249.9	178	8.7
250-399.9	74	3.6
400-499.9	10	0.5
500-999.9	14	0.7
Over 1000	2	0.1

* From White, J. M., *et al.*: Sodium ion in drinking water. J. Am. Dietet. A., 50:32, 1967.

TABLE 23-3. SODIUM CONTENT OF FOOD EXCHANGES*

FOOD	HOUSEHOLD MEASURE	GM.	MILLIGRAMS OF SODIUM
Milk Exchanges	8 ounces (½ pint)	240	120
Meat Exchanges	1 ounce	30	25
Vegetable Exchanges	½ cup	100	9
Fruit Exchanges	1 serving	varies	2
Bread Exchanges	varies	varies	5
Fat Exchanges	1 tsp.	5	negligible

* Foods produced, processed or prepared without the addition of any sodium compound.

[3] Johns Hopkins Hospital, Manual of Applied Nutrition. ed. 5, p. 126.

TABLE 23-4. SODIUM-RESTRICTED DIET EXCHANGE LISTS

MILK EXCHANGES
One cup (8 ounces) contains 120 mg. of sodium

USE	DO NOT USE	
Regular (whole) milk	Ice cream	Chocolate milk
Skim milk (liquid or reconstituted according to directions on the package)	Sherbet	Condensed milk
	Malted milk	Fountain drinks
Unsalted buttermilk (ask the dairy)	Milk shakes	Junket tablets
Evaporated milk (½ cup = 1 cup whole milk)	Instant cocoa mixes	

If skim milk, either fresh or powdered, or buttermilk is used, add 2 teaspoons of fat for each glass unless calories are restricted.

Milk used in cooking must be counted in the day's allowance.

Substitutes for not more than 1 glass of milk a day: 2 ounces of meat, poultry or fish *or* 6 ounces (¾ container) of plain yogurt.

MEAT EXCHANGES
Each ounce, cooked, contains 25 mg. of sodium

USE

Meat or poultry, fresh, frozen or dietetic canned

Beef	Tongue, fresh	Turkey
Lamb	Liver	Rabbit
Pork	Chicken	
Veal	Duck	

Fish, fresh* or dietetic canned, all except those listed under Do Not Use.

An average serving of cooked meat, poultry or fish is 3 ounces. Allow an extra ounce or two for shrinkage, bone and fat when shopping.

One egg contains 70 mg. of sodium. Egg should not be substituted for meat.

Substitutes for 1 ounce of meat, poultry or fish: ¼ cup unsalted cottage cheese, 1 ounce low-sodium dietetic cheese, or 2 tablespoons low-sodium dietetic peanut butter.

* Fresh fish must be rinsed thoroughly in clear water because it is sometimes kept in salt water or temporarily frozen with salt before it reaches the market.

DO NOT USE

Brains, kidneys

Canned, salted or smoked meat:

Bacon	Meats, koshered by salting
Bologna	
Chipped beef	Luncheon meats
Corned beef	Sausage
Frankfurters	Smoked tongue
Ham	

Frozen fish fillets

Canned, salted or smoked fish:

Anchovies	Herring
Caviar	Sardines
Salted cod	

Canned tuna or salmon unless low-sodium

Shellfish:

Clams	Oysters
Crabs	Scallops
Lobster	Shrimp

VEGETABLE EXCHANGES
One serving—½ cup—contains about 9 mg. of sodium

USE

Any fresh, frozen* or low-sodium dietetic canned vegetables or vegetable juices except those listed under Do Not Use.

Some patients may not tolerate strong-flavored vegetables.

Restaurants usually add salt and monosodium glutamate to vegetables.

* A few frozen vegetables, such as peas and lima beans, have had salt or other sodium compound added during processing. Read labels.

DO NOT USE

Canned vegetables and vegetable juices unless low-sodium dietetic.

Frozen vegetables if processed with salt.

These vegetables in any form:

Artichokes	Whole hominy
Beet greens	Kale
Beets	Mustard greens
Carrots	Sauerkraut
Celery	Spinach
Chard	White turnips
Collards	
Dandelion greens	

TABLE 23-4. SODIUM-RESTRICTED DIET EXCHANGE LISTS (*Continued*)

FRUIT EXCHANGES
Each serving contains about 2 mg. of sodium

USE	DO NOT USE
Any kind of fruit or fruit juice—fresh, frozen, canned or dried.*	Fruit flavored beverage mixes and powders. Commercial gelatin dessert.
The size of a serving of fruit varies, depending on the fruit. Examples of 1 serving: a small apple, ½ cup fruit cup, 2 medium plums.	
Substitute for fruit juice: low-sodium dietetic tomato juice.	
* See Table 20-11 for complete listing.	

LOW-SODIUM BREAD EXCHANGES
Each serving contains about 5 mg. of sodium

USE	DO NOT USE
Low-sodium bread and rolls, unsalted Melba toast, plain unsalted Matzo	Regular breads, crackers, rolls, muffins
	Commercial mixes
Unsalted cooked cereals:	Cooked cereals containing a sodium compound (read label)
Farina Rolled wheat Hominy grits Wheat meal Oatmeal	Dry cereals other than those listed or those that have no more than 6 mg. of sodium in 100 Gm. of cereal (read label)
Dry cereals:	Pizza
Puffed rice Shredded wheat Puffed wheat	Self-rising cornmeal
	Self-rising flour
Macaroni products and cereals:	Potato chips
Macaroni Barley Noodles Unsalted popcorn Spaghetti Flour Rice	Pretzels
	Salted popcorn

Count as 1 serving 1 slice of bread, 1 roll or muffin, 4 pieces of Melba toast; ½ cup cooked cereal, ¾ cup dry cereal; ½ cup cooked noodles, rice, etc.; 1½ cup popcorn; 2½ tablespoons flour.

Low-sodium bread, rolls, etc., are made without salt and with yeast or sodium-free baking powder or potassium bicarbonate.

Substitute for a serving of bread or cereal *one* of the following:

Dried beans or peas—½ cup cooked

Corn ⅓ cup or ½ small ear

Potato, white—1 small

Potato, mashed—½ cup

Sweet potato—¼ cup or ½ small

TABLE 23-4. SODIUM-RESTRICTED DIET EXCHANGE LISTS (*Continued*)

FAT EXCHANGES
Contain practically no sodium

USE	DO NOT USE
Butter, unsalted	Regular butter
Margarine, unsalted	Regular margarine
Fat or oil for cooking, unsalted	Commercial salad dressings or mayonnaise unless
French dressing, unsalted	low-sodium dietetic
Mayonnaise, unsalted	Bacon, bacon fat
Cream, light or heavy, sweet or sour (see limitation below)	Salt pork
	Olives
Nuts, unsalted	Salted nuts
One serving equals 1 level teaspoon of butter, margarine, fat, oil or mayonnaise; 1 tablespoon French dressing; 1 tablespoon heavy cream*; 2 tablespoons light cream*; 6 small nuts.	Party spreads and dips

* Cream contains more sodium than other fats and is limited to 2 tablespoons a day.

MISCELLANEOUS FOODS
The following foods contain no sodium

USE		DO NOT USE
Coffee	Limes	Beverage mixes, including instant cocoa and fruit flavored powders
Coffee substitutes	Plain, unflavored	
Tea	gelatin	Fountain beverages, including malted milk
Cocoa powder	Vinegar	Soft drinks, both regular and low caloric
Sugar, brown and white	Cream of tartar	Bouillon cubes, powders or liquids
Honey	Potassium bicarbonate	Sodium saccharin
Sugar substitute:	Sodium-free baking	Commercial candies
Calcium saccharin	powder	Commercial gelatin desserts
Lemons	Yeast	Instant vegetable broth
		Regular baking powder
		Baking soda (sodium bicarbonate)
		Rennet tablets
		Molasses
		Pudding mixes

processed and prepared without the addition of salt or any other sodium compound.

The Exchange Lists for the sodium-restricted diet are in Table 23-4. If they are compared with the Exchange Lists in Chapter 20, it will be seen that there is only one Vegetable Exchange List in the sodium-restricted Exchange Lists. The sodium value, 9 mg. per ½ cup serving cooked without salt, applies to both Vegetable Exchanges—Groups A and B—in the exchanges. It will be remembered that certain vegetables in both Groups, A and B, may not be used on sodium-restricted diets because of their high natural sodium content (for example, spinach, kale, carrots, etc.). Although 1 ounce of meat and one egg are interchangeable for protein and calories, this is not true for sodium. One egg contains 70 mg. of sodium while 1 ounce

of meat, cooked without salt, contains only 25 mg. of sodium. Therefore, 1 egg cannot be substituted for 1 ounce of meat in a sodium-restricted diet. Careful study of the Sodium Exchange Lists on the preceding pages point out these and other variations between the Sodium Restricted Exchange Lists and the Exchange Lists in Chapter 20.

500-Milligram Sodium-Restricted Diet Pattern. Table 23-5 shows how the sodium-restricted Exchanges can be combined to provide a 500-mg. sodium pattern dietary and, at the same time, provide the nutrients needed by an adult. It will be seen that milk, meat, fish, fowl and eggs account for ⅖ of the sodium intake each day. The remainder of the sodium comes from the foods naturally low in sodium, and from the water used in drinking and cooking. To reduce this pattern dietary

TABLE 23-5. A 500-MILLIGRAM SODIUM-RESTRICTED DIET PATTERN

FOOD	AMOUNT	SODIUM (Approximate mg.)	CALORIES (Approximate)
Milk	1 pint	240	340
Meat, poultry, fish	4 ounces, cooked	100	300
Egg	1	70	75
Vegetables	4 ½-cup servings	36	100
Fruit	3 servings	6	120
Bread, unsalted	6 exchanges	30	420
Fat, unsalted	3 exchanges	—	135
Totals		482	1,490

to about 250 mg. of sodium one pint of Lonalac or dialyzed whole milk (about 12 mg. of sodium) is substituted for one pint of regular milk (240 mg. of sodium).

The foods in the quantities listed in the 500-Milligram Sodium-Restricted Diet will provide the Recommended Dietary Allowances, with the exception of iron for women. Using the Exchange System for calculating the calorie value, this is a 1,500-calorie diet. Some patients, those who need to lose weight, will have to omit some of the bread and potato and possibly use skim in place of whole milk. Other patients will need additional food to meet their caloric requirement. Foods which will supply calories without adding to the sodium content of the diet are sugar, honey, jams, jellies and marmalades (if made without sodium benzoate), cream for coffee, an increased use of unsalted fats, and desserts made with the allowed ingredients.

Adjustment of the diet will also have to be made for individual preferences and needs. Two additional ounces of meat may be more acceptable to a patient in place of one of the 8-ounce glasses of milk, particularly if he dislikes milk. The remainder of the milk may be used with coffee and on cereal.

The 500-milligram sodium pattern dietary can serve as the foundation for diets of 600, 700, or 800 mg. of sodium. The patient's preferences, the amount of money he can spend for food, and the ease with which he can buy low-sodium diet foods should be taken into consideration. For example, if a patient who requires a 600 mg. sodium diet is using only 2 teaspoons of margarine per day,

he could substitute 2 teaspoons of salted margarine. Two teaspoons of unsalted margarine have little or no sodium, and 2 teaspoons "with salt added" contain 100 mg. of sodium. The salted margarine is cheaper and generally more readily available.

The 1,000-Milligram Sodium-Restricted Diet Pattern. An example of a 1,000-milligram sodium-restricted diet pattern is shown in Table 23-6. It will be noted that the only difference in this pattern compared with the 500-milligram one is the use of Bread Exchanges made with salt. In the 500-milligram pattern there are six unsalted Bread Exchanges and in the 1,000-milligram pattern there are three unsalted and three Bread Exchanges with salt. Another possible variation would be the use of salted margarine or butter in place of the unsalted kind. One slice of salted bread of the usual size, about 3½ inches by 4 inches and no more than ½ inch thick, contains approximately 150 mg. of sodium. One level teaspoon (One Exchange) of salted butter or margarine contains about 50 mg. of sodium. Therefore, two slices of salted bread and 3 teaspoons of salted margarine or butter have approximately the same sodium content as three slices of salted bread. Otherwise all food used in the 1,000-milligram sodium diet is unsalted.

The addition of ¼ *scant* teaspoon of salt to the 500-milligram sodium-restricted diet pattern is another method of adding 500-mg. of sodium to the diet. This method of converting a 500-milligram sodium-restricted diet to 1,000-mg. has been rec-

TABLE 23-6. A 1,000-MILLIGRAM SODIUM-RESTRICTED DIET PATTERN

FOOD	AMOUNT	SODIUM (Approximate mg.)	CALORIES (Approximate)
Milk	1 pint	240	340
Meat, poultry, fish	4 ounces, cooked	100	300
Egg	1	70	75
Vegetables	4 ½-cup servings	36	100
Fruit	3 servings	6	120
Bread, unsalted	3 exchanges	15	210
Bread, salted	3 slices	450	210
Fat, unsalted	3 exchanges	—	135
Totals		917	1,490

ommended but some physicians are strongly opposed to it. They feel that it makes it difficult for the patient, should his condition require it at some future time, to reduce his sodium intake to less than 1,000-mg. Also, patients who accept foods without added salt and become used to omitting salt report that they have "lost their taste" for salt and do not enjoy it. For the patient who cannot tolerate food without salt, and if his physician agrees, the ¼ *scant* teaspoon of salt may make it possible for him to have an adequate diet, which he would not have without the salt.

Mild Sodium-Restricted Diet Pattern, 2,000 mg. of Sodium. This diet permits the use of foods processed and cooked with moderate amounts of salt and other sodium compounds. Highly salted foods are not used. Table 23-7, the Mild Sodium-Restricted Diet, illustrates the additions which can be made to a 500-milligram sodium diet to provide a reasonably mild sodium-restricted diet. When a 2,000-milligram sodium-restricted diet is ordered it should be carefully calculated to provide 2,000 mg. of sodium, not more or less.

TABLE 23-7. THE MILD SODIUM-RESTRICTED
DIET PATTERN

This diet should follow the 500-Milligram Sodium-Restricted Diet, with the following additions:

Salt

A moderate amount of salt may be used for cooking, but none may be added at the table. Garlic, onion and celery salt may be used if they replace salt in cooking

Meat, poultry, fish, eggs

Brains, kidneys, frozen fish fillets, regular canned tuna and salmon and all shellfish are permitted

Vegetables

All vegetables, fresh, frozen or canned, except sauerkraut, are allowed

Bread and cereals

Regular bread and rolls, but none with salt topping, are permitted. All cereals are allowed

Fats

Salted butter and margarine and commercial salad dressings are allowed

All other restrictions as listed on the 500-Milligram Sodium-Restricted Diet must be observed.

Teaching the Patient

Teaching Materials. Three excellent booklets are available for helping the patient to understand his sodium-restricted diet. These were prepared by the American Heart Association in conjunction with the American Dietetic Association, the Council on Foods and Nutrition of the American Medical Association, the Nutrition Foundation and the Public Health Service of the Department of Health, Education, and Welfare. The diets are constructed on the Exchange system presented in this chapter. The three booklets are entitled "Your 500 Milligram Sodium Restricted Diet"; "Your 1,000 Milligram Sodium Restricted Diet"; and "Your Mild Sodium-Restricted Diet." The first two booklets have also been issued as a simplified leaflet. They are available to the patient through his physician, who may obtain them from his local heart association, or, where there is no local association, from the American Heart Association.[4]

The Patient's Problems. Learning to omit salt from his diet is not an easy process for most patients. Not only do foods taste flat, but they serve as a continual reminder that something is wrong with him. When a patient newly placed on sodium restriction asks the nurse "How long will I be on this diet?" he may be asking in reality if he will have heart disease the rest of his life. Unless he is carefully instructed throughout his stay in the hospital, the cardiac patient may think that, although his diet was instrumental in his improvement, now that he is better he does not need to continue to restrict his sodium intake at home.

Depending on the degree of sodium restriction ordered by the physician, one of the three booklets from the American Heart Association, or one of the two leaflets described above, may be of help to the patient in learning how to adapt his food to the prescribed restrictions, but it must be implemented with specific suggestions to meet his own needs. The nurse and the dietitian must be ready to answer questions, to direct the patient's thinking, to give concrete suggestions, and to be ever ready with encouragement and support. Again, the teaching should be begun early in the patient's hospital stay, so that he has a chance to think through the needed adjustments for sodium restriction before he has to adapt to them at home.

In teaching the patient on a sodium-restricted diet it is especially important to find out something

---

[4] American Heart Association, 44 East 23rd Street, New York, N.Y. 10010.

about his home circumstances and his cultural background. Both the wife and the husband should be taught what is required if the husband is the patient. Since an older patient may live with a son or a daughter, whoever is the homemaker should receive instruction along with the patient.

Patients who do not have adequate cooking facilities and are accustomed to eating their meals in restaurants will need help in adjusting to the demands made by sodium restriction. Southern patients in the habit of cooking with bacon or salt pork must be warned about this. This is also true for people who eat "soul" foods. Jewish patients, following their dietary laws of heavily salting their meats before cooking (koshering) will need help in readjusting their deeply ingrained convictions. (See earlier in this chapter.) Italian patients should be warned not to use commercial tomato paste, olives, Italian cheese and Italian bread. Tomato paste can be made at home, omitting salt and spices containing sodium. Occasionally an Italian bakery will make low-sodium bread if there is sufficient demand for it. Japanese and Chinese patients must be cautioned particularly to omit monosodium glutamate and soy sauce, both of which are used commonly in the seasoning of their food. Greek patients and those coming from the Near East frequently use heavily salted olives as an accompaniment to meals. When counseling a patient it is essential not only to obtain information on his food habits from him, but also to look up the foods common to his culture which may interfere with his ability to maintain a sodium-restricted regimen. (See Chap. 11 for descriptions of varying food patterns, and also the Supplementary Readings following Chaps. 11 and 18.)

THE FAT-CONTROLLED AND MODIFIED-FAT, CARBOHYDRATE-CONTROLLED DIETS

Role of Diet in Atherosclerosis

Our present knowledge of the role of diet in the development of coronary heart disease has been derived from two types of studies. Groups of investigators have studied the diet and the incidence of the disease in numerous population groups around the world while others have studied individuals in metabolic research centers. Both types of studies have focused on the relation of dietary lipids to blood lipids, specifically the amount of cholesterol and the amount and type of fat in the diet and the serum cholesterol and other lipids in the blood. Recently one group of investigators have identified familial types of lipid abnormalities called hyperlipoproteinemias.

Population Studies. The information gathered after World War II from the study of food intake and the incidence of coronary heart disease in a number of countries showed that the incidence of disease in the populations studied seemed to be related to the amount of fat in the national diet. For example, the Japanese, who at that time consumed about 10 percent of their total calories as fat (see Fig. 23-3), had a low incidence of coronary heart disease compared with Americans who were consuming about 40 percent of their total calories as fat. At the same time it was observed that in populations with low fat intakes the serum cholesterol levels were appreciably lower than in Americans with high fat intakes.

These observations of the relationship of the amount and type of fat in the diet to coronary heart disease did not apply equally to all the groups studied. For example, certain pastoral tribes in Africa who have a high milk intake and, therefore, a high saturated fat intake have a relatively low serum cholesterol level and incidence of coronary heart disease. It is suspected that physical activity may explain this difference, since the members of these tribes are more active than the other populations which were observed.

Diet Studies. Following these population studies, extensive research was done to determine the effect of polyunsaturated fat on serum cholesterol levels in man and animals. The results of these investigations indicate that saturated fats tend to increase serum cholesterol, while fats containing primarily polyunsaturated fatty acids tend to decrease serum cholesterol.[5] Monounsaturated fats appear to have no effect on serum cholesterol levels. Formula diets were used in these studies. There is, as yet, no agreement on the mechanism(s) by which the degree of saturation of fats affects serum cholesterol levels.

As a result of the population studies and the research on fatty acids, other research workers have studied the effect of modified diets on serum cholesterol levels. A number of investigators have studied individuals, primarily men, under metabolic research conditions, while other investigators have studied groups of men living and eating at

---

[5] Ahrens, E. H., Jr., *et al.*: JAMA, 164:1905, 1957.

home with their families. (See Chap. 3 for explanation and food sources of saturated and unsaturated fatty acids.)

The work of Page and Brown and their coworkers in Cleveland is one example of the first type of research. These investigators have determined critical limits for the fat and cholesterol composition of a diet effective in reducing serum cholesterol. Their research involved 134 normal, free-living, active subjects who were served test diets prepared in a research kitchen. All but 15 of the subjects were men between the ages of 20 and

55 years.[6] Table 23-8, based on their work, shows that there are critical limits in the fatty acid and cholesterol composition of diets which had a significant effect on lowering the serum cholesterol levels of their subjects. A diet with 36 to 40 percent of calories from fat was effective in lowering serum cholesterol when less than 14 percent of total calories were provided by saturated fatty acids, more than 14 percent of total calories were

_____

[6] Brown, H. B., and Farrand, M. E.: J. Am. Dietet. A., 49:303, 1966.

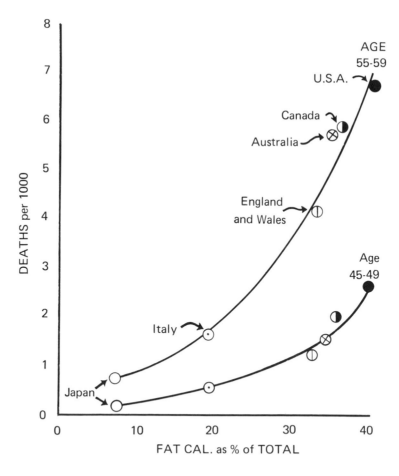

DEGENERATIVE HEART DISEASE IN MEN

Fig. 23-3. Mortality from degenerative heart disease in two age groups, as related to percentage of fat calories in total calories of the national diet. (From Keys, A.: Atherosclerosis: a problem in newer public health. J. Mt. Sinai Hosp., 20:118)

TABLE 23-8. CRITICAL LIMITS OF DIETARY FAT COMPOSITION FOR
SERUM CHOLESTEROL REDUCTION*

COMPONENT	DIET WITH 36-40 PERCENT FAT CALORIES	DIET WITH 25-30 PERCENT FAT CALORIES
Saturated fatty acids	less than 14% calories	less than 11% calories
Polyunsaturated fatty acids (linoleic)	more than 14% calories	more than 13% calories
Cholesterol	less than 350 mg.	less than 300 mg.

* Brown, H. B., and Farrand, M. E.: J. Am. Dietet. A., 49:303, 1966.

from polyunsaturated fatty acids (linoleic), and the diet contained less than 350 mg. of cholesterol. A diet containing 25 to 30 percent of calories from fat was effective when less than 11 percent of total calories were provided by saturated fatty acids, more than 13 percent by polyunsaturated fatty acids, and the diet contained less than 300 mg. of cholesterol.

Christakis[7] and his group in New York have studied 814 men, living at home and eating with their families, ages 40 to 59 years who were placed on a diet relatively rich in polyunsaturated fatty acids. This diet resulted in a significant decrease in serum cholesterol levels, and maintained the decrease for as long as 5 years. A control group of 463 men was also studied. Compared with the control group the diet group had less morbidity from new coronary disease.

Hyperlipoproteinemia

Frederickson and his co-workers at the National Heart Institute, National Institutes of Health, using very sophisticated research methods have shown that there are: (1) familial or primary types of abnormalities in blood lipids, and (2) secondary abnormalities in blood lipids due to diseases such as diabetes mellitus and hypothyroidism. His group has also demonstrated how the diet should be modified according to the familial or primary types of abnormalities in blood lipids.

The term hyperlipoproteinemia is used to describe Frederickson's types of lipid abnormalities. Lipids, which are not water-soluble, are transported in the blood by protein therefore, the term hyperlipo-, elevated lipids, and -proteinemia, excess blood proteins. The blood lipids are primarily cholesterol and triglycerides. The proteins that transport the lipids are of a special type.

Frederickson has identified five types of hyperlipoproteinemias and five types of dietary modifications. These diets reflect the previous work on the effect of polyunsaturated fatty acids on blood cholesterol and other lipid levels and add newer work on the effect of dietary carbohydrate.

Type I Hyperlipoproteinemia is characterized by elevated amounts of cholesterol and an excessive increase of triglycerides in the blood. This problem is related to fat intake and is treated by a diet restricted to 25 to 35 Gm. of fat per day.

Type II Hyperlipoproteinemia, a common inheritable disorder, is characterized by elevated blood cholesterol levels in the range of 300 to 600 mg. per 100 ml. and is treated by a diet as low as possible in cholesterol and high in polyunsaturated fatty acids.

Type III Hyperlipoproteinemia, a relatively uncommon problem characterized by a moderate elevation of cholesterol and other lipids is treated by a diet controlled in carbohydrate—approximately 40 percent of total calories; controlled in fat—40 percent of total calories with high polyunsaturated fatty acids; and cholesterol restricted to less than 300 mg. per day. If the individual is overweight, it is essential that total calories are restricted to promote weight loss.

Type IV Hyperlipoproteinemia, the most common type of abnormality and often associated with diabetes mellitus and, probably, premature atherosclerosis, is characterized by elevated cholesterol and normal or elevated triglycerides. This type is treated by a diet controlled in carbohydrate, not to exceed 3½ to 4 Gm. per kilogram of body weight; higher than the average American diet in polyunsaturated fatty acids but not as high as Types II and III; and restricted in cholesterol to 300 to 500 mg. per day. If the individual is overweight, total calories are restricted to promote weight loss.

[7] Christakis, G., *et al.*: JAMA, 198:129, 1966.

Type V Hyperlipoproteinemia, which may be familial but is often seen secondary to diabetic acidosis, pancreatitis, alcoholism and nephrosis, is characterized by elevated cholesterol and triglycerides. This type is treated by a diet restricted in fat to 50 to 85 Gm. per day, in cholesterol to 300 to 500 mg. per day and in carbohydrate to 5 Gm. or less per kilogram of body weight per day.

Alcohol is not recommended for individuals with Type I and V Hyperlipoproteinemia and is recommended only at the physician's discretion with the other types.

Diet Prescription

Prior to the work of Frederickson the diet used in the treatment of coronary heart disease was the Fat-Controlled Diet. This diet is planned to provide an excess of polyunsaturated fatty acid and less than 300 mg. of cholesterol. The Fat-Controlled Diet is still ordered for patients with coronary heart disease. However, in major medical centers Frederickson's Type I through V diets are being used in the treatment of these patients. In some hospitals the diets are ordered by type while in others the order identifies the modifications desired. For example, a Type IV diet may be ordered as follows: modified fat, controlled carbohydrate, moderately restricted cholesterol. If required, a calorie restriction may also be stated in the order.

In the following section planning the Fat-Controlled Diet is presented. In addition the Type IV and the Cholesterol-Restricted Diets are discussed.

PLANNING THE FAT-CONTROLLED PATTERN DIETARY

Foods for the Fat-Controlled Diet. It is well to recognize that this is a therapeutic diet which requires significant changes in an individual's food practices. The most critical changes in food selection required by this diet occur in the following groups: (1) milk and other dairy products; (2) meat, fish and poultry; (3) eggs; and (4) fats. Table 23-9, Nutrient Composition of Food Exchanges for Fat-Controlled Diet, is a modification of Table 20-9, Nutrient Composition of Food Exchanges (Chap. 20).

It will be observed that there are major differences between the two tables in the nutrient values of the milk, meat and fat exchanges, and that values are given for saturated fat and linoleic fatty acid in addition to values for total fat. Adding the

TABLE 23-9. NUTRIENT COMPOSITION OF EXCHANGES FOR FAT-CONTROLLED DIET*

FOOD GROUP	AMOUNT	Gm.	PROTEIN Gm.	FAT Total Fat Gm.	FAT Satu- rated Fat Gm.	FAT Linoleic Fatty Acid Gm.	CHOLES- TEROL mg.	CARBO- HYDRATE Gm.	CALORIES
Milk, skim	½ pt. (8 ozs.)	240	8	tr.	. .	. .	7	12	80
Vegetables Group A	as desired	. .	. .	. .	. .	. .	. .	. .	. .
Group B	½ cup	100	2	. .	. .	. .	. .	7	35
Fruit	varies	. .	. .	. .	. .	. .	. .	10	40
Bread and Cereal	varies	. .	2	0.5	. .	. .	. .	15	70
Meat, lean only	1 oz.	30	8	2	0.6	0.1	21	. .	50
Egg (3/week)	3/7	21	3	3	0.9	0.2	118	. .	35
Fat (Veg. oil)[1]	1 tablespoon	14	. .	14	2.0	8.0	. .	. .	125
Fat ("Special" Margarine Corn oil, etc.)	1 tablespoon	14	. .	11	2.5	3.7	. .	. .	100
Fat ("Special" Margarine Safflower oil)	1 tablespoon	14	. .	11	1.9	6.3	. .	. .	100

* Compiled with the assistance of M. C. Zukel.
[1] Corn, cottonseed, safflower, soybean oil.

figure for saturated fat to the figure for linoleic fatty acid in an Exchange will not give the same figure as the one in the fat column because the figure for monounsaturated fat is not given. (See Part Four, Table 2.) Linoleic fatty acid is used to calculate the polyunsaturated fat in a diet because it is the one which occurs in food in significant amounts. The cholesterol values are given for those foods which contain this nutrient.

The nutritive composition of the Vegetable and Fruit Exchanges and the foods in these two Exchanges are the same as those in Table 20-11. These Exchange lists will not be reproduced in this chapter (see Chap. 20). The Milk, Bread, Meat and Fat Exchange Lists for the Fat-Controlled Diet are given in Table 23-10. A Sugar and Dessert Exchange List is also included in this Table for those individuals who do not require any calorie restriction.

Milk Exchanges. The only item in this list in the Fat-Controlled Diet is skim milk. This may be fluid skim milk, nonfat dried milk or buttermilk made from skim milk. Milk fat contains a significant amount of saturated fat. (See Part Four, Table 2.) Therefore, milk fat in any form—whole milk, cream, butter, cheese made from whole milk, or ice cream—is not used in this diet plan. There is no vitamin A in skim milk, since it is in the milk fat. Vitamin A has been added to some skim milks and it is wise to use these products to ensure an adequate vitamin A intake. Also the cholesterol in skim milk is much less than the amount in whole milk. Eight ounces of skim milk contains approximately seven mg. of cholesterol while 8 ounces of whole milk contains approximately 26 mg.

Bread Exchanges. The major modification in the items in this list compared with the Bread Exchanges in Table 20-11 is in the type of fat used in making hot breads, e.g., biscuits, muffins and cornbread. Only the fats and oils in the Fat Exchange list in Table 23-10 are used in the recipes for these breads. The amount of fat in a serving of these products is counted as part of the fat planned in a diet pattern. The 0.5 Gm. of fat for Bread Exchanges is included to account for the fat in cereals.

Plain cake and ice cream which are included in the Bread Exchanges in Table 20-11 are omitted from the Bread Exchanges for fat-controlled diets. Because of the egg and milk fat in cake and the milk fat in ice cream these foods are not included

in this exchange list. It will be noted that only crackers made without fat such as pretzels and bread sticks are included in these lists. Bread crumbs, flour and cornmeal have been added for use in food preparation, especially for cooking meat and fish.

Meat Exchanges. There is considerable difference between the nutrient values and the items in this Exchange list compared with the Meat Exchanges in Table 20-11. If a Fat-Controlled pattern dietary is to provide the amount of the polyunsaturated fatty acid, linoleic, required by the physician's diet prescription, careful selection of the kinds and amounts of meat must be made. Only lean cuts of those items listed in the Meat Exchange in Table 23-10 can be used in order to avoid an intake of saturated fats in excess of the prescribed amount.

The calorie and nutrient values for one Meat Exchange in Table 23-9 were derived from weighted averages of the values for the meat, fish and poultry items in the Meat Exchange list. All the items in this list contain less than 13 Gm. of total fat per 100-Gm. portion.* Lean beef, lamb, pork and ham contain more saturated fat than poultry, fish and veal. Therefore, beef, lamb, pork and ham are limited to three meals and poultry, fish and veal are used for the other eleven main meals in a week. If beef, lamb, pork and ham are used more frequently, the weighted values for one meat exchange will not apply and the intake of saturated fat will be in excess of that calculated in the diet plan.

Liver and shellfish are not included in the Meat Exchanges due to their high cholesterol content. Poultry without skin is used since the major amount of the fat in poultry is in the skin. Eggs are limited to three per week not only because of the saturated fat content but also because of the cholesterol content. When cholesterol is limited to 200 mg. or less per day eggs will be omitted from the diet plan entirely, with adequate protein provided by the Milk and Meat Exchanges.

Fat Exchanges. Together with the Meat Exchanges these are critical factors in achieving a fat-controlled intake. The items in the Fat Exchange list (Table 23-10) are certain vegetable oils; French dressing and mayonnaise made with these oils; and special margarines. The oils are limited to cottonseed, soy, corn, and safflower.

* Handbook No. 8, 1963 revision. U.S.D.A.

TABLE 23-10. FOOD EXCHANGE LIST FOR FAT-CONTROLLED DIETS*

MILK EXCHANGES

(One serving contains 8 Gm. of protein, 12 Gm. of carbohydrate, 7 mg. of cholesterol, and 80 calories)

Skim milk	1 c.
Non-fat dried milk	¼ c.
Buttermilk (made from skim milk)	1 c.

VEGETABLE EXCHANGES

See Exchange Lists, Chapter 20, Table 20-11.

FRUIT EXCHANGES

See Exchange Lists, Chapter 20, Table 20-11.

BREAD EXCHANGES

(One serving contains 2 Gm. of protein, 0.5 Gm. of fat, 15 Gm. of carbohydrate and 70 calories)

Bread (white, whole wheat, raisin, rye, pumpernickel, French, Italian or Boston brown bread)	1 slice
Roll (2 to 3 inches across)	1
*Biscuit, muffin (2″ diam.)	1
*Cornbread (1½″ cube)	1
Melba toast (3½″ x 1½″ x ⅛″)	4
Matzo (5″ x 5″)	1
Bread sticks, rye wafers	¾ oz.
Cereal, cooked	⅓ c.
dry, flake or puffed	¾ c.
Rice, grits, cooked	½ c.
Spaghetti, noodles, cooked	½ c.
Macaroni, cooked	½ c.
Dry bread crumbs	¼ c.
Flour	3 tablespoons
Cornmeal	2½ tablespoons
Beans, peas, dried, cooked	½ c.
Corn, kernels or creamstyle	⅓ c.
Corn on the cob, medium ear	½ c.
Potatoes, white (2″ diam.)	1
Potatoes, sweet	¼ c.

MEAT, FISH AND POULTRY EXCHANGES

(One ounce contains 8 Gm. of protein, 2 Gm. of fat, 0.6 Gm. of saturated fat, 0.1 Gm. of linoleic fatty acid, 21 mg. of cholesterol, and 50 calories)

Meat selections from the following list are limited to 3 meals a week and to 3 ounces per serving

Beef—lean	1 oz.
Hamburger—ground round or chuck	

* Made with Fat Exchanges only.

Roasts, pot roasts, stew meats—
sirloin tip, round, rump,
chuck, arm
Steaks—flank, sirloin, T-bone,
porterhouse, tenderloin,
round, cube
Soup meat—shank or shin
Other—dried chipped beef

Lamb	1 oz.
Roast or steak—leg	
Chops—loin, rib, shoulder	
Pork	1 oz.
Roast—loin, center cut ham	
Chops—loin	
Tenderloin	
Ham	1 oz.
Baked, center cut steaks, picnic, butt, Canadian bacon	

Meat selections for 11 of the 14 main meals each week are made from the following list:

Poultry (without skin)	1 oz.
Chicken, turkey, cornish hen, squab	
Fish—any kind (not shellfish)	1 oz.
Veal—any lean cut	1 oz.
Cottage cheese, preferably uncreamed	¼ c.
Peanut butter	2 tablespoons

Eggs—limit to 3 per week (3/7 of an egg contains 3 Gm. of protein, 3 Gm. of fat, 0.9 Gm. of saturated fat, 0.2 Gm. of linoleic fatty acid, 118 mg. of cholesterol, and 35 calories).†

FAT EXCHANGES

(One tablespoon of vegetable oil contains 14 Gm. of fat, 2.0 Gm. of saturated fat, 8.0 Gm. of linoleic fatty acid, and 125 calories.)

Corn oil	1 tablespoon
Cottonseed oil	1 tablespoon
Safflower oil	1 tablespoon
Soybean oil	1 tablespoon
French dressing (made with any of the oils listed above)	1½ tablespoons
Mayonnaise (made with any of the oils listed above)	1 tablespoon
Special margarine	1 tablespoon

(One tablespoon of special margarine, corn oil, contains 11 Gm. of fat, 2.5 Gm. of saturated fat, 3.7 Gm. of linoleic fatty acid, and 100 calories.)

(One tablespoon of special margarine, safflower, contains 11 Gm. of fat, 1.9 Gm. of saturated fat, 6.3 Gm. of linoleic fatty acid, and 100 calories.)

† If the cholesterol in the diet is limited to 200 mg. per day, eggs cannot be used.

TABLE 23-10. FOOD EXCHANGE LIST FOR FAT-CONTROLLED DIETS* (*Continued*)

SUGAR AND DESSERT EXCHANGES		
(One serving contains about 50 calories)		

Sugars

White, brown or maple	1 tablespoon
Corn syrup or maple syrup	1 tablespoon
Honey	1 tablespoon
Molasses	1 tablespoon
Jelly, jam or marmalade	1 tablespoon

Desserts

Tapioca or cornstarch pudding ¼ c.
(Made with fruit and fruit juice
or with skim milk from milk calculated in diet plan)

Gelatin dessert	⅓ c.

Fruit whip	¼ c.

(Made with egg whites,
no cream)

Water ice	¼ c.
Sweetened canned or frozen fruit	⅓ c.

(Equals 1 fruit exchange and
1 tablespoon sugar)

Angel cake, plain	1 small piece

Sweetened carbonated

beverages	6 ounces

Candies

Gumdrops	3 medium or 14 small
Marshmallows	3 large
Hard fruit drops	4

* Adapted from Zukel, M. C.: Fat-controlled diets. Am. J. Clin. Nutr., 16:270, (Feb.) 1965.

These are the vegetable oils with the most significant amount of linoleic fatty acid (see Table 23-11).

Commercial French dressings and mayonnaise can be used because they are made with cottonseed, soy or corn oils. The amount of cholesterol from eggs in commercial mayonnaise is not significant (8 mg. per 1 tablespoon) but if used in excessive amounts could add to the total cholesterol in a diet, especially if cholesterol is limited to 200 mg. per day. Salad dressing, mayonnaise type, should not be used as its composition differs markedly from regular mayonnaise.

The "special" margarines are those made either from corn or safflower oil. It will be observed that Table 23-9 gives separate values for corn oil and safflower oil margarines, and shows that the safflower oil margarine contains more linoleic fatty acid than the kind made with corn oil. These margarines are usually soft and are packaged in a tub. The first ingredient named on the label of the package will state either liquid corn or safflower oil. Unfortunately, this does not necessarily, under present labeling regulations, ensure that the margarine will contain the amount of linoleic fatty acid given in Table 23-9. As a general rule, the best guide to purchasing margarine with a significant amount of linoleic fatty acid is to look for the soft type in a tub, with safflower oil as an ingredient listed on the label. Whipped toppings and coffee creamers are also omitted because the type of fat used in these products varies.

Sugar and Dessert Exchanges. This exchange provides calories from sugars and simple desserts, and is useful in planning diets containing 1,800 calories or more. It must also be remembered that milk fat in any form cannot be used in the desserts listed.

TABLE 23-11. APPROXIMATE FATTY ACID COMPOSITION OF VEGETABLE OILS*

VEGETABLE OIL	SATURATED FATTY ACIDS†	MONOUNSATURATED FATTY ACIDS†	POLYUNSATURATED FATTY ACIDS†
Coconut	86	7	—
Cocoa butter	56	37	2
Olive	11	76	7
Peanut	22	43	29
Cottonseed	25	21	50
Soy	15	20	59
Corn	10	28	54
Safflower	8	15	72

* From USDA Home Economics Report No. 7.
† Grams per 100 Gm. ether extract or crude fat.
Brown, H. B., and Farrand, M. G.: J. Am. Dietet. A., 49:303, 1966.

CALCULATION OF FAT-CONTROLLED DIET

Table 23-12, Nutrient Composition of a 1,500-Calorie Fat-Controlled Diet, illustrates the calculation of a fat-controlled pattern dietary. Approximately 22 percent of the total calories are provided by protein, 46 percent by carbohydrate, and 30 percent by fat. About 13 percent of the total calories are provided by linoleic fatty acid, and less than 11 percent by saturated fats. It will be observed that this diet contains approximately 260 mg. of cholesterol and, if eggs are not used three times per week, the cholesterol in the diet would be less than 200 mg. per day. Table 23-13 offers a suggested menu for a 1,500-Calorie Fat-Controlled Diet.

PLANNING THE TYPE IV DIET

The exchanges used in planning the Type IV diet pattern are very much like those used to plan the Fat-Controlled Diet. However, there are *two* important differences. The Sugar and Dessert Exchanges in Table 23-10 are excluded from the Type IV Diet because the carbohydrate in this diet is restricted to 36 to 40 percent of the total calories and also because some physicians exclude

TABLE 23-13. SUGGESTED MENU FOR 1,500-CALORIE FAT-CONTROLLED DIET

BREAKFAST

8 ounces orange juice
1 cup cooked oatmeal
8 ounces skim milk

NOON MEAL

Chicken sandwich
  2 slices bread
  2 ounces chicken
  1 tbsp. mayonnaise
  Lettuce
Fresh peach
8 ounces skim milk

EVENING MEAL

4 ounces roast veal
½ cup peas
½ cup winter squash
Sliced tomato with 1 tsp. French dressing
2 biscuits (made with allowed fat)
½ tbsp. safflower margarine
¼ cup fruit whip (made with egg white)

TABLE 23-12. NUTRIENT COMPOSITION OF A 1,500-CALORIE FAT-CONTROLLED DIET

Food	Amount	Weight Gm.	Protein Gm.	Total Fat Gm.	Saturated Fat Gm.	Linoleic Fatty Acid Gm.	Cholesterol mg.	Carbohydrate Gm.	Calories
Milk, skim	1 pt. (2 c.)	480	16	tr.	..	..	14	24	160
Vegetables, Group A	as desired	varies	..	..	..	..	..	..	..
Group B	1 cup	200	4	..	..	..	..	14	70
Fruit	3 servings	varies	..	..	..	..	..	30	120
Bread and cereal	6 servings	varies	12	3.0	0.6	..	..	90	420
Meat, lean	6 ounces	180	48	12	3.6	0.6	126	..	300
Egg	3/wk. (3/7)	21	3	3	0.9	0.2	118	..	35
Fat (veg. oil)[1]	2 tablespoons	28	..	28	4.0	16.0	..	..	250
Fat (Special margarine safflower)	½ tablespoon	7	..	5.5	1.0	3.1	..	..	50
Sugar (dessert)	1 tablespoon	12	..	..	..	..	..	12	50
Totals			83	51.5	10.1	19.9	258	170	1,455

[1] Corn, cottonseed, safflower, soybean oil.

TABLE 23-14. NUTRIENT COMPOSITION OF EXCHANGES FOR CARBOHYDRATE-CONTROLLED, MODIFIED FAT, MODERATELY-RESTRICTED CHOLESTEROL DIET (TYPE IV)*

FOOD	AMOUNT	WEIGHT Gm.	PROTEIN Gm.	TOTAL FAT Gm.	CHOLES-TEROL mg.	CARBO-HYDRATE Gm.	CALORIES
Milk, skim ....½ pt. (8 oz.)		240	8	Tr.	7	12	80
Vegetables							
Group A ....as desired		..	..	..	..	..	..
Group B ....½ cup		100	2	..	..	7	35
Fruit ....varies		..	..	..	..	10	40
Bread and Cereal ......varies		..	2	..	..	15	70
Meat, Lean ....1 oz.		30	8	3	21	..	60
Egg 3/wk (3/7)		21	3	3	118	..	35
Fat† ....1 tablespoon		14	..	11	..	..	100

* Adapted from The Dietary Management Of Hyperlipoproteinemia, A Handbook for Physicians. Bethesda, Maryland, National Heart and Lung Institute, 1970.

† Vegetable oils and special margarines only.

all sucrose from the diet of a patient with Type IV hyperlipoproteinemia.

The nutrient values for the Meat Exchanges and the Meat Exchange List for the Type IV Diet differ from the Fat-Controlled Diet. The nutrient values of the Meat Exchange in the Type IV Diet are 8 Gm. of protein, 3 Gm. of fat and 60 calories for 1 ounce of lean meat (see Table 23-14). The nutrient values of the Meat Exchange in the Fat-Controlled Diet are 8 Gm. of protein, 2 Gm. of fat and 50 calories (see Table 23-9). The ratio of polyunsaturated to saturated fatty acids

is not as critical in the Type IV Diet as in the Fat-Controlled Diet; therefore, no figures are given for linoleic acid in Table 23-14. The Fat Exchanges used to plan the Fat-Controlled Diet are used in planning the Type IV Diet to insure adequate amounts of polyunsaturated fatty acids. The number of weekly servings of lean beef, lamb, pork and ham are not limited in the Type IV Meat Exchange List (see Table 23-15). However, it is advisable to select poultry, fish and veal as often as lean beef, lamb, pork and ham to avoid an excessive intake of saturated fatty acids.

TABLE 23-15. FOOD EXCHANGE LISTS FOR CARBOHYDRATE-CONTROLLED, MODIFIED FAT, MODERATELY-RESTRICTED CHOLESTEROL DIET (TYPE IV)*

MILK EXCHANGES
See Exchange Lists, Chapter 23, Table 23-10

VEGETABLE EXCHANGES
See Exchange Lists, Chapter 20, Table 20-11

FRUIT EXCHANGES
See Exchange Lists, Chapter 20, Table 20-11

BREAD EXCHANGES
See Exchange List, Chapter 23, Table 23-10

FAT EXCHANGES
See Exchange List, Chapter 23, Table 23-10

MEAT EXCHANGES
(One ounce contains 8 Gm. of protein, 3 Gm. of fat, 21 mg. of cholesterol, and 60 calories.)

Select *lean,* well-trimmed cuts of meat, fresh or frozen.

Beef	Veal
Lamb	Poultry (without skin)
Pork	Fish (if canned, drain well)
Ham	Creamed cottage cheese

EGGS—limit to 3 per week
(Substitutions for 1 egg: *2 ounces* of *one* of the following

Shellfish—oysters, lobster, shrimp, clams, crab.
Liver, sweetbreads, heart.
Cheddar cheese—once a week *only*).

* Adapted from The Dietary Management of Hyperlipoproteinemia, A Handbook for Physicians. Bethesda, Maryland, National Heart and Lung Institute, 1970.

Table 23-16 illustrates the calculation of a Type IV, 1,500-Calorie Diet since many of these patients also require a calorie-restricted diet. This 1,500-Calorie Diet plan should be compared with the Fat-Controlled, 1,500-Calorie Diet in Table 23-12. The differences in the carbohydrate in the diets should be carefully noted.

For the hospitalized patient careful precautions must be taken to insure that the patient who requires a Fat-Controlled or Type IV Diet is not served vegetables that have been seasoned with butter, meat that is well marbled with fat or meat from which the visible fat has not been removed, or hot breads made with other than vegetable oil shortening. At the same time, relatives and friends should be instructed to avoid offering the patient chocolate candies and ice cream or beverages made with whole milk and ice cream.

PATIENT EDUCATION

The patient who requires a Fat-Controlled or a Type IV diet will need careful, detailed diet instruction. The first step is a complete diet history to determine his previous food practices. Since these diets require extensive changes in the average American diet, a comprehensive diet history helps to identify more readily those food practices of a patient that can be continued as well as identify those that will of necessity be changed.

It is also important to discover where and with whom the patient eats his meals. These patients are not able to adhere to their diets if they eat all or most of their meals in restaurants. With careful selection an occasional meal in a restaurant is possible. For example: a possible restaurant meal might be roasted or broiled lean meat, green salad with vinegar and oil dressing, fruit and skim milk.

Since the majority of patients who experience heart attacks are men, it is essential that the wife be present for the diet history and all diet instruction. It is possible that many of her food-buying practices and methods of food preparation will need to be changed. For example, if she has always made fruit whip with whipped cream, she will need to be instructed to make it with egg whites. Or if she has found it convenient to use frozen dinners frequently, she may need help in planning the preparation of meals which require more of her time in the kitchen.

Many of these patients and their wives will be well-motivated to learn how to cope with the fat-controlled diet. The press, popular magazines and television, have all helped to make the middle-aged American conscious of the need for "poly-unsaturates" in their diets. Unfortunately, some of these media have oversimplified the problem by emphasizing only one food—for example, changing from butter to "special" margarines without considering the need also to change to skim milk and lean meat.

A very useful teaching aid is the booklet, Planning Fat-Controlled Meals for 1,200 and 1,800 Calories (revised 1966). This booklet, prepared in cooperation with the American Dietetic Association and the Heart Disease Control Program, U.S. Public Health Service, is published by the

TABLE 23-16. NUTRIENT COMPOSITION OF A 1,500-CALORIE CARBOHYDRATE-CONTROLLED, MODIFIED FAT, MODERATELY-RESTRICTED CHOLESTEROL DIET (TYPE IV)

FOOD	AMOUNT	WEIGHT Gm.	PROTEIN Gm.	TOTAL FAT Gm.	CHOLES- TEROL mg.	CARBO- HYDRATE Gm.	CALORIES
Milk, skim ....1 pt. (2c)		480	16	Tr.	14	24	160
Vegetables							
Group A ....as desired		varies	..	..	..	..	..
Group B ....½ cup		100	2	..	..	7	35
Fruit ....3 servings		varies	..	..	..	30	120
Bread and Cereal ......5 servings		varies	10	1.0	..	75	350
Meat, Lean ....7 ounces		210	56	21.0	147	..	413
Egg 3/wk (3/7)		21	21	3.0	118	..	35
Fat* ....3½ tablespoons		49	..	38.5	..	..	350
Totals			105	63.5	279	136	1,463

* Vegetable oils and special margarines only.

American Heart Association.* Copies are available to the patient on a physician's prescription only. They are available to physicians, dietitians, and other professional persons on request.

Instruction booklets for Dietary Management of Hyperlipoproteinemia Type I through Type V are available free of charge to physicians from the National Institutes of Health.†

PLANNING THE CHOLESTEROL-RESTRICTED PATTERN DIETARY

Cholesterol in Food. Meat, organ meat, shellfish, eggs, and dairy products are the major sources of cholesterol in the American dietary. Plant foods generally do not contain cholesterol.

Table 23-17, Cholesterol Content of Food (per Exchange-size serving), lists the average number of milligrams of cholesterol in the meat, milk and fat exchanges. It can be seen that egg, liver, shellfish and butter are the most significant contributors of cholesterol at the per serving level. The substitution of two eggs (550 mg. of cholesterol) for 2 ounces of meat (42 mg. of cholesterol) in a day's menu plan significantly increases the total cholesterol intake.

The Pattern Dietary. The Pattern Dietary (p. 185, Chap. 19) contains approximately 500 mg. of cholesterol per day provided that liver is not selected as a serving of meat, and the selection of other foods to meet an adult's allowance for calories does not contain additional eggs, butter, or whole milk. This means that cakes, cream pies, milk puddings, ice cream and whipped cream cannot be used for dessert in the daily menu plan for a diet restricted in cholesterol.

A significant reduction in cholesterol in the Pattern Dietary can be achieved by omitting the egg each day (minus 275 mg. of cholesterol) and adding one ounce of meat (plus 21 mg. of cholesterol). Egg white, which does not contain cholesterol, can be used. All organ meats and shellfish contain a greater amount of cholesterol than muscle meat and fish and, therefore, cannot be used. The use of margarine in place of butter also reduces the amount of cholesterol in the Pattern Dietary. To increase the polyunsaturated fatty acid content of the cholesterol-restricted diet, corn oil or safflower oil is used or margarine made with these.

---

* A.H.A., East 23rd Street, New York, N.Y. 10010.
† National Heart and Lung Institute, Bldg. 31, Room 4A10, National Institutes of Health, Bethesda, Maryland 20014.

TABLE 23-17. CHOLESTEROL CONTENT
OF FOODS*
(per Exchange-size serving)

FOOD	HOUSEHOLD MEASURE	WEIGHT (Gm.)	CHOLES-TEROL (mg.)
Whole milk	8 oz.	240	24
Egg	1	50	275
Meat, fish	1 oz.	30	21
Chicken (with skin)	1 oz.	30	18
Liver	1 oz.	30	90
Sweetbreads	1 oz.	30	75
Shrimp, crab	1 oz.	30	38
Lobster, oysters	1 oz.	30	60
Cheese, cheddar	1 oz.	30	30
Butter	1 tbsp.	14	35
Margarine (all veg. fat)	1 tbsp.	14	0

* Calculated from Table 4, Handbook No. 8, U.S.D.A., 1963.

STUDY QUESTIONS AND ACTIVITIES

1. Make out a menu for a day for a patient with congestive heart failure whose diet order is: 1,000 mg. sodium, soft diet, five meals.

2. Will your menu in 1 above meet all the patient's nutrient needs including calories?

3. Which foods used in planning a sodium-restricted diet contain the most sodium? Which, the least?

4. What warning must be given a patient about the use of salt substitutes?

5. Is low-sodium bread available in your community? How does its price compare with regular bread?

6. Which cooking ingredients and seasonings must a patient on a sodium-restricted diet be warned not to use?

7. Which seasonings, spices and condiments may be used to make a sodium-restricted diet more palatable?

8. What should the cardiac patient be taught about labeling?

9. What are some of the regional and cultural food patterns which may make it difficult for a patient to adhere to a sodium-restricted diet?

10. List the foods that contain the greatest percentage of linoleic fatty acid.

11. Is it correct to say that all plant oils contain only linoleic fatty acid and that all animal fats contain only saturated fat? (See Chap. 3 and Table 2, Part Four.)

12. List some of the foods commonly used in the American diet that are omitted on the fat-controlled diet.

13. Accompany the dietitian when she takes the diet history and instructs a patient who requires a fat-controlled or modified fat diet. While giving nursing care to this patient, discover how well he understands his diet instructions. Share your observations with the dietitian before her next appointment with this patient. Report this experience to your classmates in clinical conference with them, your nursing instructor and the dietitian.

14. Which food, if any, did the patient on the fat-controlled diet miss most?

15. Calculate a 2,000 calorie, Type IV diet containing 195 Gm. carbohydrate, modified fat, and 300 to 500 mg. cholesterol.

16. What food must be restricted in a diet plan limited to 300 to 500 mg. cholesterol? What food is omitted?

17. Why should whipped toppings and coffee creamers not be used on a fat-controlled diet?

18. Can a diet without eggs be adequate in all nutrients?

SUPPLEMENTARY READING ON CARDIOVASCULAR DISEASE

Brown, H. B.: Food patterns that lower blood lipids in man. J. Am. Dietet. A., 58:303, 1971.

Brown, H. B., and Farrand, M. E.: Pitfalls in constructing a fat-controlled diet. J. Am. Dietet. A., 49:303, 1966.

Christakis, G., et al.: Effect of the anti-coronary club program on coronary heart disease risk-factor status. JAMA, 198:129, 1966.

Edit. Prevention of CHD (coronary heart disease). JAMA, 215:1813, 1971.

Heap, B.: Sodium-restricted diets. Am. J. Nursing, 60:206, 1960.

Heap, B., et al.: Simplifying sodium-restricted diets. J. Am. Dietet. A., 49:327, 1966.

Hovath, R. A.: Variation in the fatty acid distribution of filled milk products. Am. J. Clin. Nutr., 24:397, 1971.

Levy, R. I., et al.: Dietary management of hyperlipoproteinemia. J. Am. Dietet. A., 58:406, 1971.

Mijanich, P., and Ostwald, R.: Fatty acids in newer brands of margarine. J. Am. Dietet. A., 56:29, 1970.

Newborg, B.: Sodium-restricted diets: sodium content of wines and other alcoholic beverages. Arch. Internal Medicine, 123:692, 1969.

Planning Fat-Controlled Meals at 1,200 and 1,800 Calories, Revised 1966. New York, American Heart Association.

Pye, O. F., et al.: Developing a program of learning on the fat-controlled diet. Am. J. Dietet. A., 57:428, 1970.

————: Programmed Instruction for Fat-Controlled Diet, 1,800 Calories. New York, American Heart Association, 1969.

Rimer, D. G., and Frankland, M.: Sodium content of antacids. JAMA, 173:995, 1960.

Standal, B. R., et al.: Fatty acids, cholesterol, and proximate analysis of some ready-to-eat foods. J. Am. Dietet. A., 56:392, 1970.

Wiesman, C. K.: The art of seasoning low-sodium diets. Nursing Homes, 20:12, (Feb.) 1971.

Your 500 Milligram Sodium-Restricted Diet (booklet and leaflet); Your 1,000 Milligram Sodium-Restricted Diet (booklet and leaflet); Your Mild Sodium-Restricted Diet (booklet); American Heart Association, New York, N.Y.

Zukel, M. C.: Fat-controlled diets. Am. J. Clin. Nutr., 16:270, 1965.

RESOURCES FOR PATIENTS

American Heart Association: Recipes for Fat-Controlled, Low-Cholesterol Meals, from local Heart Associations or American Heart Association, 43 East 23rd Street, New York, N.Y. 10010.

Bond, C. B. Y., et al.: The Low Fat, Low Cholesterol Diet. rev. ed. Garden City, N.Y., Doubleday & Co., 1971.

Payne, A. S., and Callahan, D.: Fat and Sodium Control Cookbook. ed. 3. Boston, Little, Brown & Co., 1966.

For further references see Bibliography in Part Four.

Diet in Renal Disease; Kidney Stones

24

Principles of Diet Modification · Potassium in Foods · Protein in Foods
Exchange System for the Protein-Sodium-Potassium-Restricted Diet · Kidney Stones

INTRODUCTION

The kidneys, along with the lungs, are the chief excretory organs of metabolic end products from the body. Practically all the waste materials resulting from catabolism, except carbon dioxide which is eliminated by the lungs, are carried by the blood to the kidneys where they are filtered and the waste products excreted in the urine.

Water is the chief constituent of the urine, the quantity varying mainly with the amount taken into the body and the amount excreted by means of the skin and lungs. Normal urine contains about 5 percent of solids, consisting of a variety of electrolytes, both basic and acid, and the end products of protein metabolism, of which the largest constituent is urea nitrogen (see Chap. 6).

The kidneys are subject to disease, as are other organs of the body. There may be congenital malformation and a decreased number of nephrons, or cysts may be present, occluding some of the functioning nephrons. Infection may occur, as in pyelonephritis; there may be inflammation of kidney tissue as in nephritis and nephrosis; kidney damage may result from long continued hypertension, or from decreased blood flow in severe cardiac disease or trauma; or the kidney pathways may be blocked by the formation of kidney stones.

In kidney disease the filtering mechanism is usually affected, and substances not normally found in the urine, such as albumin, one of the proteins in the blood, may then be present. Conversely, substances normally cleared from the blood by the healthy kidney may not be fully eliminated. Two of these are urea, and, in very severe disease, potassium. They are found in increased quantities in the blood.

Kidney disease may be acute, followed by healing; or it may be recurrent and eventually become chronic, with an ever decreasing number of functioning nephrons. When the kidney no longer is able to maintain the normal composition of the blood by excreting all of the waste products, the patient is said to have uremia (referring to the retention of urea nitrogen in the blood) and to be in kidney failure. Eventually there is oliguria (diminished secretion of urine), or even anuria (complete suppression of urine). Death intervenes unless hemodialysis or a kidney transplant is available.

The diet order for a patient with kidney disease is determined by the state of his kidney function. However, the orders for most patients will include modification of fluid and electrolyte intake—water, sodium and, in renal failure, potassium—and modification of protein intake. Caloric intake is also important because without adequate calories body protein is metabolized for energy, thus, increasing the amount of urea to be excreted by the kidneys. In addition, especially for those patients with kidney stones, calcium intake may be modified.

The principles of diet modification in kidney disease, planning diets of varying protein, sodium, and potassium content, and the calcium-restricted diet are discussed in this chapter. (Review sodium-restriction in Chap. 23.)

PRINCIPLES OF DIET MODIFICATION

Fluids and Electrolytes. Total fluid intake may be increased or decreased compared with the normal intake of approximately 2,000 to 2,500 ml. for adults. When the kidney is unable to concentrate the urine resulting in excessive amounts of water lost from the body, the fluid order increases to compensate for this loss. When the filtration ability (glomerular filtration rate, GFR) of the kidney is reduced, fluid intake is decreased. In acute renal failure or in the terminal phase of renal disease (uremia) the total 24-hour fluid intake is reduced to equal urine output. This could be as low as 200 ml.

Whether the fluid intake is increased or decreased, the sodium intake from food may be decreased. Patients with excessive water loss also lose sodium and other electrolytes required for acid-base balance. These electrolytes are replaced by medications. With fluid restriction due to decreasing glomerular filtration rate there is some restriction of sodium intake. In acute renal failure with a very limited glomerular filtration rate the intake of both sodium and potassium is restricted.

Careful communication between dietary and nursing services is required to carry out the fluid orders for any patient with renal disease. Other than water which may or may not be a significant source of sodium and potassium, many fluids commonly offered to hospitalized patients contain significant amounts of sodium and/or potassium. For example: orange juice and tea contain potassium; and tomato juice canned with salt contains sodium and potassium. If a diet is severely restricted in electrolytes a 4- to 8-ounce serving of any one of these beverages could contribute to a serious error in therapy.

Severe fluid restrictions present special problems. The nurse needs water to give with medications and the dietitian needs fluids to enhance the palatability of the diet. These patients are usually nauseated and vomit frequently. Hourly communication between nursing personnel and the dietitian is needed to help these patients.

Protein. When kidney function is intact the protein content of the diet should be normal—0.9 Gm. per kilogram for adults. When albumin is lost in the urine the dietary protein intake may be increased in an effort to compensate for this loss. Usually the adult allowance is increased to 1½ to 2 Gm. per kilogram of body weight. Moderate increases in foods containing protein—meat, fish, poultry, eggs, milk, and cheese—achieve the desirable level of intake. If edema is present, sodium is restricted.

The protein in the diet is restricted with increasing renal failure to reduce the amount of urea to be excreted. The diet is restricted to 30 to 50 Gm. (approximately 0.5 Gm. per kilogram) or less per day for the terminal renal failure patient, the one on hemodialysis at home, or the hospitalized patient on hemodialysis in preparation for kidney transplant. Careful attention is given not only to the total quantity of protein in the diet but also to the quality of the protein—the essential amino acid content (see Chap. 4).

Concern for the essential amino acid content of the diet used with patients in renal failure (uremia) derives from a variety of studies. In 1963, in Italy, Giordano[1] showed that uremic subjects were able to use the nitrogen in their excessive amounts of blood urea nitrogen to synthesize nonessential amino acids when the diet contained adequate amounts of the essential amino acids and calories. This regimen resulted in marked clinical improvement and a decrease in blood urea nitrogen.

Giordano used pure amino acids. Subsequent investigators, using proteins of high biological value (egg and milk) to provide adequate amounts of essential amino acids and adequate calories from fat and carbohydrate, achieved the same clinical success. In this country the first protein-restricted, high-biological-value diets contained approximately 20 Gm. of protein. Today a more liberal diet, 30 to 50 Gm. of protein and adequate calories, is used successfully in conjunction with hemodialysis.[2] Also this diet is usually restricted in sodium and potassium. An exchange system for calculating protein-, sodium- and potassium-restricted diets is given in Table 24-1 and the exchange lists in Table 24-2.

Calories. All patients with renal disease require an adequate caloric intake. Most patients with primary renal disease are rarely obese. Some

---

[1] Giordano, C.: J. Lab. Clin. Med., 62:231, 1963.
[2] Berlyne, G. M.: Nutrition Rev. 27:219, 1969.

patients with renal failure secondary to trauma, hypertension and cardiac disease may be obese. These latter patients may be given moderately calorie-restricted diets.

In acute renal failure when all protein is excluded from the diet, calories from carbohydrate and/or fat are required. Epstein[3] recommends 100 to 150 Gm. of glucose consumed over a 24-hour period to minimize protein catabolism. He has had clinical success with a solution of 50 Gm. of lactose, 25 Gm. of sucrose and 25 Gm. of glucose dissolved in the water allowed and flavored with lemon juice to reduce the sweetness. This solution is to be sipped throughout the day. Medications can be given with this beverage. It is possible that the lactose in this solution could cause diarrhea. For this reason, Dr. Epstein recommends that the solution be sipped, not taken in quantity at any one time. (See Lactose Intolerance, Chap. 25, Diet in Gastrointestinal Disease.) Also, there may be problems with keeping this amount of lactose in solution in 300 ml. or less of water. Crystals of lactose may form at the end of a day: reboiling and cooling the mixture may be required to put the lactose back into solution. Dr. Epstein feels that the 400 calories from glucose in his formula are adequate and that a higher calorie intake with a mixture of carbohydrate and fat is not required.

In an emergency such as acute renal failure, 8 ounces of a mixture made from 4 ounces of water and 4 ounces of light Karo syrup flavored with 1 teaspoon of lemon juice can be used to provide calories. Eight ounces of this solution contains approximately 340 calories, 85 Gm. of carbohydrate, 65 mg. of sodium, and 8 mg. of potassium.

A commercial product, Controlyte,* free of protein, with minimal electrolytes, can be used to provide calories. This product contains 233 calories in 100 Gm. of powder that may be dissolved in water, or fruit juice, depending on the amount of potassium allowed. Vitamins have been added to this product. Another product is Cal-Power,† a lemon flavored beverage that contains 575 calories per 8 fluid ounces, approximately 2 calories per milliliter, 30 mg. of sodium and 3 mg. of potassium. It is packaged in 8-fluid-ounce cartons. It is relatively sweet to taste but has a pleasant flavor when frozen. A nasogastric feeding of glucose and a vegetable oil in emulsified form (Lipomul‡) has been recommended. Earlier, Kolff suggested butter and sugar mixtures[4] to be taken by mouth. Most patients find these butter mixtures distasteful.

PLANNING DIETS OF VARYING PROTEIN, SODIUM AND POTASSIUM CONTENT

Potassium in Food. Potassium is in the cells of all living tissue and is, therefore, widely distributed in all foods with the exception of pure fats and oils. The average adult intake of potassium varies from 2000 to 6000 mg. per day. In terminal renal failure the potassium in the diet may be restricted to 2500 to 1500 mg. or less per day.

Because potassium is in the cell, it cannot be easily removed from the food. The potassium in vegetables can be reduced to some extent by cooking in water. For example, Louis and Dolan[5] report that soaking raw potatoes before cooking for 30 minutes results in a loss of approximately 75 percent of the potassium—from 387 mg. to 86 mg. per 100 Gm. The water the potatoes are soaked in is discarded and fresh water is used to boil the potatoes.

Canned vegetables and fruits also appear to lose some potassium in processing. For example 100 Gm. fresh apricots have 281 mg. of potassium and canned apricots, 246 mg.; 100 Gm. of frozen peas (cooked) have 152 mg. of potassium and canned peas, 95 mg. (see Table 4, Part Four). Canned vegetables and fruit are drained carefully when served to a patient whose diet is restricted in potassium because the potassium is in the juice. Also, when fluids are restricted the juice would add to total fluid intake.

The bran layer of grains has a higher concentration of potassium than the endosperm. A 25

[3] Epstein, F. H.: In Harrison, T. R., *et al.*: Principles of Internal Medicine. Chapter 300. New York, McGraw-Hill, 1970.
  * D. M. Doyle Pharmaceutical Co., Minneapolis, Minn.
  † General Mills Chemical Co., Minneapolis, Minn.

‡ Upjohn Company, Kalamazoo, Michigan.
[4] Kolff, W. J.: Am. J. Med., 12:667, 1952.
[5] Louis, C. J., and Dolan, E. M.: J. Am. Dietet. A., 57:42, 1970.

Gm. slice of regular white bread contains 25 mg. of potassium, and a 25 Gm. slice of whole wheat, 65 mg. of potassium. Highly milled grains, especially cornstarch and wheat starch, are practically free of potassium. The starch of certain roots, arrowroot and tapioca, are also practically free of potassium. Therefore, these starches—corn, wheat, arrowroot and tapioca starch—are used in baked products or as thickening agents in puddings in planning renal diets. (See section on special starch for renal diets.)

Tea and coffee, either regular or instant, are significant sources of potassium and, therefore, are excluded or served in very limited amounts on potassium-restricted diets. In 1 level teaspoon of instant coffee there are approximately 45 mg. of potassium, and 63.4 mg. in 1 level teaspoon of instant tea. At a restriction of 1500 mg. or less per day of potassium, it is difficult to use more than 4 fluid ounces (120 ml.) of coffee or tea and plan a diet pattern that meets the nutrient needs of an individual.

Water may also be a significant source of potassium. In areas where the water is high in potassium, the renal failure patient may need to use distilled water for cooking and drinking. The local health department has information about the potassium content of the water supply.

Neither salt substitutes nor sodium-free baking powder can be used because of the potassium content. Depending on the level of sodium restriction, an alum type baking powder (Calumet) may be used to make bread and cakes with wheat starch. This baking powder, compared with other types, is relatively free of potassium. (See footnote, Part Four, Table 4, page 353.)

Protein in Foods. It is shown in Table 24-1 Protein, Sodium and Potassium Content of Food Exchanges (p. 249), that a value for protein is given for each exchange or each subdivision within each exchange except for fat. In Chapter 20, Table 20-9, Nutrient Composition of Food Exchanges, figures for protein content were given for only the milk, meat, bread and vegetable B exchanges because in calculating most modified diets the concern is with those foods which contribute the most significant amounts of protein.

In calculating the protein-sodium-potassium-restricted diet pattern for renal failure patients, the quality of the protein—the essential amino acids and the total amount of nonessential amino acids (actually total nitrogen to be excreted by

the kidney)—is also taken into consideration. The major portion of the protein in the renal diet pattern is contributed by a limited amount of high quality protein from meat, egg and milk. Care is taken that only a limited amount of protein (nitrogen) is provided by bread and cereals, vegetables and fruits. Therefore, the protein in all fruit and vegetable exchanges is calculated.

Special Starch for Renal Diets. Because the protein in the renal diet is limited, those foods such as cereals, breads, and desserts made with regular flour, which are good sources of calories, cannot be used in quantity to meet the patient's energy needs.

Two wheat starch products that are relatively free of nitrogen and lower in potassium compared with regular wheat flour are available for making bread, muffins, biscuits, cookies and pie crust for renal patients. These products are: Dietetic Paygel-P, General Mills,* Cellu Wheat Starch and Cellu Low Protein Baking Mix.† Each company provides recipes for using its product. The directions for making bread with these wheat starches must be followed carefully because the protein (gluten) of regular flour that gives the structure to yeast bread, has been removed from the wheat starch. The structure, texture and flavor of breads made from these wheat starches differ from bread made with regular flour. Some patients readily accept the product while others do not. Besides the calories in the wheat starch bread, the butter, jelly or jam served with the bread can make significant contributions to total calorie intake. The pies and cookies made from wheat starch are usually well-accepted. The manufacturer's materials give the caloric and nutrient composition per serving of their recipes. (See end of this chapter for directions for securing recipes using wheat starches.)

Patient Acceptance of the Protein-Sodium-Potassium-Restricted Diet. The patient being prepared for kidney transplant or the patient in terminal renal failure often finds this drastic change in his usual food practices difficult to accept. Also, many of these patients, especially prior to hemodialysis, are anorexic and nauseated. They present a special challenge to both the nurse

---

* General Mills, Minneapolis, Minn.

† Cellu-Featherweight, Chicago Dietetic Supply House, LaGrange, Ill.

and dietitian. It is the responsibility of the dietitian to calculate the complex diet pattern, plan the daily meals, and with the nurse help the patient accept his diet.

Exchange System for the Protein-Sodium-Potassium-Restricted Diet

Table 24-1 gives the nutrient composition of the exchanges used to calculate the diet pattern. It will be noted that calorie values are not given. Careful inspection of Table 24-2, Protein, Sodium and Potassium Exchange Lists, shows that the items in many of these lists vary widely in calorie value. For example, in the Milk Exchanges there is whole milk, light and heavy cream and ice cream. Also it is shown that potatoes are a vegetable, not a bread exchange. The potassium

content and to some extent the protein, accounts for the placement of potatoes with vegetables, not bread.

The canned fruits listed in the fruit exchanges are those canned with sugar while the vegetables are those canned or cooked without salt. If the sodium restriction is moderate (1500 to 2000 mg.) a small amount of salt may be added in cooking.

The fat exchanges are those with salt added. Because those foods that are the major contributors of sodium to the diet—milk, meat, and eggs—must be limited (see Chap. 23, Table 23-10), some salted foods are required when sodium is moderately restricted. Salted butter also increases the acceptability of the wheat starch breads. If the sodium is severely restricted, salted fats are not used.

TABLE 24-1. PROTEIN, SODIUM, AND POTASSIUM CONTENT OF FOOD EXCHANGES

FOOD EXCHANGES	HOUSEHOLD MEASURE	GRAMS	PROTEIN (Gm.)	SODIUM (mg.)	POTASSIUM† (mg.)
Milk	½ cup	120	4	60	170
Meat					
Group A	1 ounce	30	7	60	70
Group B	1 ounce	30	7	25	120
Vegetables					
Group A	½ cup	100	1	9	150
Group B	½ cup	100	2	9	240
Fruit					
Group A	varies	varies	1	2	100
Group B	varies	varies	1	2	145
Bread, unsalted					
Group A	varies	varies	2	5	25
Group B	varies	varies	3	5	50
Group C*	1 slice	23	0.2	15	11
Fat, salted	1 teaspoon	5	0	50	0

* Values for Dietetic Paygel-P.
† Handbook No. 8, U.S.D.A., 1963.

TABLE 24-2. PROTEIN, SODIUM AND POTASSIUM EXCHANGE LISTS

MILK EXCHANGES

1 serving contains 4 Gm. of protein, 60 mg. of sodium, 170 mg. of potassium

Milk, whole	½ cup
Milk, skim	½ cup
Light cream 18%	½ cup
Heavy cream 40%	¾ cup
Half and half	½ cup
Ice cream, regular	½ cup
Sherbet, regular	1 cup

MEAT EXCHANGES: GROUP A

1 serving contains 7 Gm. of protein, 60 mg. sodium, 70 mg. potassium

Oysters, raw	4 in number
Lobster, shrimp fresh or canned in water without salt	1 ounce
Tuna, canned in water	¼ cup

MEAT EXCHANGES: GROUP B

1 serving contains 7 Gm. of protein, 25 mg. sodium, 120 mg. of potassium

Beef, lamb, pork, rabbit	1 ounce
Chicken, turkey	1 ounce
Haddock	1 ounce
Egg*	1

* 70 mg. of sodium

VEGETABLE EXCHANGES: GROUP A

1 serving contains 1 Gm. of protein, 9 mg. sodium, 150 mg. potassium

Beans, green or wax	½ cup
Beets*	½ cup
Cabbage	½ cup
Corn, whole kernel	½ cup
Eggplant	½ cup
Summer squash	½ cup
Zucchini	½ cup

All vegetables *cooked* or *canned* without salt and *well-drained.*

* Reduce to ⅓ cup if sodium restricted to less than 500 mg.

VEGETABLE EXCHANGES: GROUP B

1 serving contains 2 Gm. of protein, 9 mg. sodium, 240 mg. potassium

Asparagus	½ cup
Broccoli	½ cup
Brussel sprouts	½ cup
Carrots*	½ cup
Potatoes†	½ cup

VEGETABLE EXCHANGES (*Continued*)

Pumpkin	½ cup
Winter squash	½ cup
Tomatoes	½ cup
Tomato juice, low-sodium dietetic	½ cup
Turnips	⅓ cup

All vegetables *cooked* or *canned* without salt and *well-drained.*

* Reduce to ⅓ cup if sodium restricted to less than 500 mg.

† Pare, soak in water ½ hour, discard water, cook in fresh water.

FRUIT EXCHANGES: GROUP A

1 serving contains 1 Gm. of protein, 2 mg. of sodium, 100 mg. of potassium

Apple, raw	1 small
Apple juice	½ cup
Applesauce	½ cup
Blueberries	⅝ cup
Peach nectar	½ cup
Pears, canned	⅓ cup
Pear nectar	½ cup
Pineapple, canned	1 slice

FRUIT EXCHANGES: GROUP B

1 serving contains 1 Gm. of protein, 2 mg. of sodium, 145 mg. of potassium

Blackberries, fresh or frozen	½ cup
Fruit cocktail	⅓ cup
Grapejuice, canned	½ cup
Grapefruit, raw	½ medium
Grapefruit, juice	⅓ cup
Grapefruit sections	½ cup
Pear, raw	½ medium
Pineapple juice	⅓ cup
Plums, purple, canned	3 medium
Raspberries, red, fresh, frozen	½ cup
Strawberries, fresh, frozen	½ cup
Tangerine	1 medium
Watermelon, raw, cubed	¾ cup

BREAD EXCHANGES: GROUP A

1 serving contains 2 Gm. of protein, 5 mg. of sodium, and 25 mg. of potassium

Low-sodium bread	1 slice
Unsalted cooked cereal	
Rice	½ cup
Farina	¾ cup
Corn grits	¾ cup

Use regular only. Do not use instant or quick-cooking varieties.

TABLE 24-2 (*Continued*)

BREAD EXCHANGES (*Continued*)

Dry cereal

    Puffed rice .... 1 cup
    Unsalted cornflakes .... 1 cup

BREAD EXCHANGES: GROUP B

1 serving contains 3 Gm. of protein, 5 mg. of sodium, 50 mg. of potassium

Dry cereal

    Puffed wheat .... ½ cup

Unsalted cooked

    Macaroni .... ½ cup
    Noodles .... ½ cup
    Spaghetti .... ½ cup

BREAD EXCHANGES: GROUP C

1 serving contains 0.2 Gm. of protein, 15 mg. of sodium, and 11 mg. of potassium

Bread* .... 1 slice

    * Dietetic Paygel-P.

FAT EXCHANGES

1 serving contains 0 protein, 50 mg. of sodium, 0 potassium

Butter, salted .... 1 teaspoon
Margarine, salted .... 1 teaspoon
Mayonnaise, salted .... 1 teaspoon

Unsalted butter and margarine, and vegetable oil may be used as desired.

BEVERAGES

May be used according to fluid allowance.

Pepsi-Cola
Royal Crown Cola
Sodium and potassium may vary according to local water supply.
Juices, milk, ice cream and sherbet must be counted as part of total fluid allowance.

MISCELLANEOUS

These items may be used as desired.

Spices and flavorings

Allspice	Nutmeg
Caraway	Paprika
Cinnamon	Pepper
Curry powder	Peppermint extract
Garlic	Sage
Garlic powder	Thyme
(not salt)	Turmeric
Ginger	Vanilla extract
Mace	Vinegar (limit to
Mustard, dry	1 tablespoon)

Sugars and candies

Hard candies	Lollipops
Honey	Syrup, corn
Jams	Sugar, white
Jellies	

Small amounts of the following may be used in food preparation.

Celery	Mint leaves
Green pepper	Mushrooms
Horseradish, fresh	Onions

Calculating a Diet Pattern for 40 Grams of Protein, 1000 Milligrams of Sodium and 1500 Milligrams of Potassium

Table 24-3 demonstrates how the exchanges in Table 24-1 may be used to calculate a diet pattern. The six Group C bread exchanges (6 slices of wheat starch bread) and the nine fat exchanges provide approximately 1000 calories. (100 calories per 20 Gm. slice of bread and 45 calories per 5 Gm. of butter). The meat, vegetable, fruit canned with sugar and the other cereal exchanges in this diet pattern will provide approximately 500 calories. Other products made with wheat starch such as cookies or pies using the fruit calculated in the diet pattern can provide an additional 200 to 400 calories for a total of approximately 1700 to 1900 calories per day.

Average servings of the additional wheat starch products contain some sodium and potassium and a 4- to 6-ounce serving of coffee or tea contains potassium. These additions correct the discrepancy between the diet as ordered and the totals in Table 24-3 for sodium (1000 mg. vs. 719 mg.) and the potassium (1500 mg. vs. 1281 mg.).

TABLE 24-3. CALCULATIONS OF DIET PATTERN FOR 40 GRAMS PROTEIN, 1000 MILLIGRAMS SODIUM AND 1500 MILLIGRAMS POTASSIUM

FOOD	EXCHANGES	PROTEIN Gm.	SODIUM mg.	POTASSIUM mg.
Breakfast				
Fruit, Group A	1	1	2	100
Bread, Group A	1	2	5	25
Group C	2	0.4	30	22
Fat, salted	3	—	150	—
Milk	1	4	60	170
Noon Meal				
Meat, Group A	1	7	60	70
Bread, Group C	2	0.4	30	22
Fat, salted	3	—	150	—
Vegetables, Group A	1	1	9	150
Fruit, Group B	1	1	2	145
Evening Meal				
Meat, Group B	2	14	25	120
Vegetables, Group B	1	2	9	240
Bread, Group B	1	3	5	50
Group C	2	0.4	30	22
Fat, salted	3	—	150	—
Fruit, Group A	1	1	2	145
Total		37.2	719*	1281*

* Does not include other foods made with wheat starch such as pies, cookies, and puddings which will increase sodium and potassium to the desired levels.

Table 24-4 illustrates a menu using the calculations in Table 24-3.

Diet and the Post-Transplant Patient

After kidney transplant the patient is maintained on steroid therapy, usually prednisone. Therefore, many clinicians order a mildly sodium-restricted diet (see Chap. 23). This diet is also usually bland because individuals on long-term steroid therapy are apt to develop gastrointestinal bleeding (see Chap. 25).

Counseling the Patient

The exchange system for calculating the protein-sodium-potassium-restricted diet given in Tables 24-1 and 24-2, or ones similar to it developed in various institutions, are designed to help the chronic renal failure patient cope with his diet after discharge from the hospital or the uremic patient who is on home dialysis or being prepared as an outpatient for kidney transplant. Because of the multiplicity of restrictions the diet is difficult to manage in the home. In many homes major changes in food preparation are required. Convenience foods and a variety of other processed foods cannot be used. Baking with wheat starch products takes skill and time. Eating in

TABLE 24-4. MENU* FOR 40 GRAMS PROTEIN, 1000 MILLIGRAMS SODIUM, AND 1500 MILLIGRAMS POTASSIUM

BREAKFAST

½ cup apple juice
1 cup puffed rice
½ cup of half and half
2 slices wheat starch bread
3 teaspoons salted butter
½ cup of coffee (4 ounces)

NOON MEAL

½ cup tuna canned in water
2 slices wheat starch bread
1 leaf lettuce
1 teaspoon salted butter
2 teaspoons salted mayonnaise
½ cup unsalted canned green beans (well-drained)
½ cup grapefruit sections (well-drained)
3 wheat starch cookies

EVENING MEAL

2 ounces roast beef
½ cup noodles, seasoned with 1 teaspoon salted butter
½ cup tomatoes
2 slices of wheat starch bread
2 teaspoons salted butter
1 small apple as apple pie made with starch crust

* Provides 360 ml. of fluid of day's total.

restaurants is impossible because salt and other sodium compounds are often added to foods during preparation.

Imagination, patience, understanding and empathy are needed by those who are counseling these patients to live within their dietary limitations and to help them extend their lives for months and even years. The nurse and dietitian, assisted by the physician, will need to work closely with the patient to help him accept this diet and understand why he requires it. Thus, nurse, dietitian and physician need to understand the protein, sodium and potassium composition of foods. (See Introduction to Diet Therapy, pp. 175 to 176.)

KIDNEY STONES

Kidney stones or renal calculi are formed because the concentration of a particular substance in the urine exceeds its solubility. About 95 percent of all kidney stones contain calcium combined with phosphate or another substance and therefore, physicians may order a calcium-restricted diet as part of a patient's therapy.

Table 24-5, Moderately Reduced Calcium and Phosphorus Diet, contains 500 to 700 mg. of calcium and 1,000 to 1,200 mg. of phosphorus. If a more restricted diet is required, it can be achieved by omitting, in addition to those foods listed under foods to be avoided, all milk and

TABLE 24-5. MODERATELY REDUCED CALCIUM AND PHOSPHORUS DIET
(This diet will contain from 500 to 700 mg. of calcium and from 1,000 to 1,200 mg. of phosphorus*)

FOODS USED

Milk
Limited to 1 cup (½ pint) a day. Cream may be substituted for part of the milk.

Cheese
Pot or cottage cheese only. Limited to 2 ozs.

Fats
As desired

Eggs
Limited to 1 a day; egg whites as desired.

Meat, fish, fowl
Limited to 4 ozs. daily of beef, lamb, pork, veal, chicken, turkey, fish. See those to be Avoided.

Soups and broths
All. Cream soups made with milk allowance only.

Vegetables
At least 3 servings besides potato. One or 2 servings of deep green or deep yellow vegetables to be included daily. See list of those to be Avoided.

Fruits
All except rhubarb. Include citrus fruit daily.

Breads, cereals, Italian pastes
White, enriched bread, rolls and crackers except those made from self-rising white flour. Farina (not enriched), cornflakes, corn meal, hominy grits, rice, Rice Krispies, Puffed Rice. Macaroni, spaghetti, noodles.

Desserts
Fruit pies, fruit cobblers, fruit ices, gelatin. Puddings made with allowed milk and egg. Angel food cake. (Do not use packaged mixes.)

Beverages
Coffee, Postum, Sanka, tea, ginger ale

Condiments
Sugar, jellies, honey, salt, pepper, spices

FOODS TO BE AVOIDED

Cheese
All except pot or cottage cheese.

Meat, fish, fowl
Brains, heart, liver, kidney, sweetbreads. Game (pheasant, rabbit, deer, grouse). Sardines, fish roe.

Vegetables
Beet greens, chard, collards, mustard greens, spinach, turnip greens. Dried beans, peas, lentils, soybeans.

Fruits
Rhubarb

Breads, cereals, Italian pastes
Whole-grain breads, cereals and crackers. Rye bread. All breads made with self-rising flour. Oatmeal, brown and wild rice. Bran, Bran Flakes, wheat germ. All dry cereals except those allowed.

Desserts
All except those allowed.

Beverages
Carbonated "soft" drinks; cocoa.

Miscellaneous
Nuts, peanut butter, chocolate, cocoa. Condiments having a calcium or a phosphate base. (Read labels.)

* Adapted from Shorr, E.: Aluminum hydroxide gels in the management of renal stone. J. Urol., 53:507, 1945.

cheese, all breads made with milk or dry skim milk, and deep green leafy vegetables.

STUDY QUESTIONS AND ACTIVITIES

1. Plan a menu, fluid or soft, for a day for a 10-year-old boy who has acute glomerulonephritis. Food must be unsalted, he is allowed 30 Gm. of protein, and fluid is restricted to 800 ml.

2. Why are fluids restricted in kidney failure? On what basis is the amount of fluid allowed calculated?

3. Using the Protein-, Sodium- and Potassium-Restricted Diet Exchange Lists, make out a Pattern Dietary for a 16-year-old boy who is receiving hemodialysis. His physician has ordered a diet containing 60 Gm. of protein, 750 mg. of sodium, 2,000 mg. of potassium, and fluids restricted to 1000 ml. The boy is in school, continually hungry, and rather anxious.

4. Make out a menu for a day for a patient critically ill with uremia. His physician has ordered: 30 Gm. of protein, 500 mg. of sodium, 1500 mg. of potassium, fluids restricted to 800 ml. The patient is anorexic and has some nausea. The diet should be bland and semisoft.

5. Look at Table 4 in Part Four, Sodium and Potassium Content of Foods. What foods are high in sodium? In potassium? Take average servings of foods into account.

6. Make out a menu for a day for a patient who has a calcium phosphate kidney stone, and who has been placed on a moderately low calcium and phosphorus diet. He is young and somewhat of a gourmet.

SUPPLEMENTARY READING ON RENAL DISEASE AND KIDNEY STONES

Berlyne, G. M.: Nutrition in renal failure. Nutr. Rev., 27:219, 1969.

Blagg, C. R., *et al.*: Home hemodialysis: Six years' experience. New Eng. J. Med., 283:1126, 1970.

de St. Joer, S. T., *et al.*: Planning low-protein diets for use in chronic renal failure. J. Am. Dietet. A., 54:34, 1969.

Jordan, W. L., *et al.*: Basic pattern for controlled protein, sodium and potassium diet. J. Am. Dietet. A., 50:137, 1967.

Kossoris, P.: Family therapy: an adjunct to hemodialysis and transplantation. Am. J. Nursing, 70:1730, 1970.

Krane, S. M.: Renal lithiasis. New Eng. J. Med., 267-875, 977, 1962.

Louis, C. J., and Dolan, E. M.: Removal of potassium in potatoes by leaching. J. Am. Dietet. A. 57:42, 1970.

Schlotter, L.: What do you teach dialysis patients? Am. J. Nursing, 70:82, 1970.

Sorensen, M. K.: A yeast-leavened, low-protein, low-electrolyte bread. J. Am. Dietet. A., 56:521, 1970.

Tsaltas, T. T.: Dietetic management of uremic patients. I. Extraction of potassium from foods for uremic patients. Am. J. Clin. Nutr., 22:490, 1969.

WHEAT STARCH* RECIPES

Low Protein Baking Mix. Cellu-Featherweight, Chicago Dietetic Supply, Inc., La Grange, Illinois 60525.

Paygel-P Wheat Starch Recipes. Dietetic Sales, General Mills, Inc., 4620 West 77th Street, Minneapolis, Minnesota 55435.

For further references see Bibliography in Part Four.

* For product, write directly to the producer.

Diet in Gastrointestinal Disease

INTRODUCTION

Diet in gastrointestinal disease is concerned with problems which may occur in the esophagus and stomach; the small and large bowel; or in the appendages to the tract, the pancreas and the liver. There is good evidence that dietary modifications are effective in the treatment of a number of malabsorption syndromes due to: (1) the lack or inadequate amounts of pancreatic or intestinal enzymes required to digest (hydrolyze) certain components in foods such as lactose; (2) the lack of bile from the liver to emulsify fats in preparation for absorption; (3) a structural defect in the small bowel which occurs in celiac disease; and (4) the inability of the small bowel to transport a nutrient such as long-chain fatty acids. Also there is evidence that caffeine and alcohol stimulate the secretion of hydrochloric acid in the stomach.

Otherwise the significance of diet therapy in the treatment of a variety of gastrointestinal diseases such as peptic ulcer and ulcerative colitis is not clear. Physicians vary in their approaches to the dietary treatment of these diseases. Also peptic ulcer disease and ulcerative colitis carry many emotional overtones as well as presenting clear-cut pathological problems.

Symptoms ascribed to gastric disorders may be due to other pathological conditions. For example, nausea and vomiting can be caused by a brain tumor or by an elevated temperature due to infection outside the gastrointestinal tract, especially in young children. Medications such as salicylates in aspirin or Darvon Compound, used in the treatment of other diseases, can cause gastric distress.

Dietary treatment of peptic ulcer disease, malabsorption problems in the small intestine, diseases of the large bowel, and liver disease, are discussed in this chapter. Problems of chewing and swallowing are discussed in Chapter 28.

DIETARY TREATMENT OF PEPTIC ULCER (GASTRIC OR DUODENAL)

Principles of Diet Therapy. The medical treatment of peptic ulcer is basically aimed at neutralizing the hydrochloric acid in the stomach and thus protecting the ulcerated area from irritation and promoting healing. For many years this has been achieved by the use of food in combination with nonabsorbable antacid medication in an attempt to buffer the elevated gastric acid that occurs in ulcer disease. The dietary programs have varied from the severely restricted milk and cream regimen of Sippy to a bland diet regimen or a liberal regimen of frequent feedings of such foods as the patient tolerates. Numerous clinical research studies have been conducted in an attempt to identify the best therapeutic diet plan for the treatment of peptic ulcer, but, as yet, there is no firm evidence for one specific approach to diet therapy in ulcer disease.

Research has shown that all food and fluids stimulate the flow of gastric juice to some extent. Protein can buffer the gastric acid for short periods of time and for this reason milk has been an important part of the diet plan for patients with ulcers. It has also been shown that alcohol and the caffeine in tea and coffee are powerful stimulants to the flow of gastric juice. Therefore, alcohol, coffee, and tea are either not used or restricted in the diet plans. There is some evidence that meat extractives (broth and gravies) may stimulate the flow of gastric juice.

There has been controversy about the use of spices and seasonings in food preparation and most diet plans recommend the avoidance of spices. One group of investigators[1] showed that the addition of considerable amounts of cinnamon, allspice, thyme, sage, paprika, cloves and other spices produced no increase in gastric juice in patients with gastric ulcer. In 5 out of 50 patients in this study, some difficulty was encountered with chili, black pepper, mustard seed and nutmeg. This suggests that spices may be tolerated although there may be some individual differences.

Raw fruits and vegetables, especially those with skins and seeds, and unrefined cereals and flours have usually been excluded because of their fiber content, commonly referred to as roughage. It is suggested that this roughage might be irritating to the ulcer crater. Also some patients do not tolerate citrus juices even when these are diluted with water or taken at the end of a meal rather than at the beginning.

The nutritional adequacy of any diet plan for the treatment of peptic ulcer must be carefully evaluated. With the exclusion of raw fruits and vegetables and a limited use or exclusion of citrus juices, the diet may be inadequate in ascorbic acid. Also the liberal use of milk or milk and cream could lead to an inadequate iron intake. Because the ulcer patient often feels more comfortable with frequent feedings he can easily become obese.

With our present knowledge of the relationship of the type of dietary fat to the development of atherosclerosis (see Chap. 23) the use of a diet high in milk fat is being questioned. It has been observed that ulcer patients experience a higher mortality from heart disease than the general population.[2] This problem may be met by the use of skim or nonfat milk in place of the whole milk or milk and cream, especially for the overweight patient.

The Bland Diet

Many clinicians will use the bland diet or a progression of bland diets in the treatment of the hospitalized peptic ulcer patient. Table 25-1, Progressive Peptic Ulcer Regimen, gives a general plan used to treat the acutely ill patient on admission and the progression to a six meal feeding plan as his condition improves. It is shown that these hourly feedings may be milk and cream, milk or skim milk. The hourly milk feedings are usually discontinued when the patient can tolerate six small meals or three meals with three between-meal feedings.

Table 25-2, Menu for 6-Feeding Convalescent Peptic Ulcer Diet, shows the types of foods that might be served to a patient. It is shown that the food used in this plan illustrates the principles presented in the previous section. The liberal use of milk, meat, eggs and cheese supply protein; coffee and tea, raw fruits and vegetables and spices are avoided. Compare the information in Tables 25-1 and 25-2 with the diet plans for ulcer patients in the diet manual used in your hospital.

In some hospitals it is the responsibility of nursing service to see that the hourly milk feedings and later the feedings given other than at meal time are delivered to and consumed by the patient. Together with the antacids, these feedings are an important part of a patient's therapy. Close cooperation between dietary and nursing service is required to insure that the patient receives them.

Table 25-3, Bland Diet, gives a diet plan that may be used by some physicians as soon as the acutely ill patient with a peptic ulcer has improved. The convalescent ulcer diet plan in Table 25-1 is omitted. The bland diet plan may also be used after discharge from the hospital. Table 25-4 gives a typical day's menu for a bland diet. Most convalescent ulcer patients are advised to distribute this food into three small meals and three between meal feedings. For example, the canned pears and the bread and butter in the noon meal menu can be eaten at 3:00 p.m.

The bland diet may be ordered for patients other than those with peptic ulcers. These may be patients receiving certain medications such as steroids, for example the post renal transplant patient, or the patient with an hiatus hernia or patients recovering from acute gastritis.

The Severely Restricted Regimen (Sippy Regimen). The Sippy regimen, first proposed in 1915, restricted the acutely ill patient to hourly servings of milk and cream for 21 days. Then limited servings of refined cereals, eggs and custard were added. Later this plan was revised from 21 to 14 days. As the patient improved, other simple

[1] Schneider, M. A., *et al.*: Am. J. Gastroent., 26:722, 1956.

[2] Spiro, H. M.: Clinical Gastroenterology. New York, Macmillan, 1970.

TABLE 25-1. PROGRESSIVE PEPTIC ULCER REGIMEN

IN THE ACUTE STAGE

Milk and cream, half and half, or milk, or skim milk
3 oz. every hour alternating with nonabsorbable antacid on the half hour

Supplements (given in 3 small meals, adding 2 or 3 foods each day as tolerated, in addition to hourly milk feedings):

Eggs
Soft cooked or poached

Cereal
Refined, cooked cereals only

Toast and crackers
White, refined bread and crackers

Cottage and cream cheese
May be substituted for an egg

Strained cream soup
Made of bland, low residue vegetables such as asparagus, corn (cream), peas, spinach, and strained

Baked or soft custard, Jello, junket
Purée fruits and vegetables
Those available as infant foods are suitable

CONVALESCENT ULCER DIET
(Served in 6 small meals or 3 meals with 3 between meal feedings)

Milk
Milk, cream, buttermilk

Cheese
Cottage, cream; other mild, soft cheeses. Cheddar cheese may be added later.

Fats
Butter or margarine

Eggs
Soft or hard cooked, poached, scrambled

Meats
Tender beef, lamb, veal; sliced chicken; liver; fish, poached, broiled or baked; crisp bacon; smooth peanut butter

Soups
Cream soups, using only vegetables listed below

Vegetables
Well-cooked or canned: asparagus, beets, carrots, peas, green or wax beans, spinach; mashed squash or pumpkin; mashed or baked white and sweet potato (no skins)

Fruits
Applesauce, baked apples without skin, ripe or baked bananas, diluted fruit juices, stewed or canned pears, peaches and peeled apricots, purée of all dried fruits except figs
It is advisable to take citrus fruit juices after eating some of the other foods of the meal, or to dilute them half and half with water.

Breads, cereals, macaroni products
Enriched white bread, fine whole wheat or light rye bread; refined cereals; all ready-to-eat cereals except those containing bran; oatmeal; macaroni, spaghetti, noodles

Desserts
Ice cream, plain; custard; simple puddings of rice, cornstarch, tapioca or bread without fruit or nuts; gelatin desserts (with fruit as permitted above); sponge and other plain cakes, sugar cookies

Beverages
Milk, cream, buttermilk. Postum, and decaffeinated coffee if allowed by physician

Condiments
Moderate amounts of sugar, jelly and salt; others if permitted by physician

FOODS TO BE AVOIDED

Fats
All fried foods

Meats and fish
Smoked and preserved meats and fish; pork; meat gravies

Soups
All meat soups; all canned soups

Vegetables
All raw vegetables; all gas-forming vegetables, including cabbage, cauliflower, brussels sprouts, broccoli, cucumbers, onions, turnips, radishes

Fruits
All raw fruits except orange juice and ripe banana

Breads and cereal
Coarse breads and cereals; hot breads

Desserts
Pastries, nuts, raisins, currants and candies

Beverages
Coffee, tea, alcoholic and carbonated beverages

Condiments
All condiments except salt, unless permitted by physician

TABLE 25-2. MENU FOR 6-FEEDING CONVALESCENT PEPTIC ULCER DIET

BREAKFAST	DINNER	SUPPER
Orange juice	Chicken, sliced	Cream of spinach soup
Eggs, scrambled	Baked potato (no skin)	Cottage cheese
White toast	String beans purée	White-bread toast
Butter or margarine	White bread	Butter or margarine
Jelly	Butter or margarine	Milk
Milk	Milk	
10 A.M.	**3 P.M.**	**9 P.M.**
Cornflakes with milk	Canned peaches	Baked custard
Milk	Plain cookies	Milk
	Milk	

TABLE 25-3. BLAND DIET

PRINCIPLES

1. Low in fiber and connective tissue
2. Little or no condiments or spices, except salt in small amounts
3. No highly acid foods
4. Foods simply prepared

FOODS USED

Milk

Milk, cream, buttermilk, yoghurt

Cheese

Cream, cottage and other soft, mild cheeses

Fats

Butter and margarine

Eggs

Boiled, poached, scrambled in teflon pan or top of double boiler

Meat, fish, fowl

Roast beef and lamb; broiled steak, lamb or veal chops; stewed, broiled or roast chicken; fresh tongue; liver; sweetbreads; baked, poached or broiled fish

Soups

With milk or cream-sauce foundation

Vegetables

Potatoes, peas, squash, asparagus tips, carrots, tender string beans, beets, spinach. (In severe cases these vegetables are puréed.)

Fruits

Orange juice, ripe bananas, avocados, baked apple (without skin), applesauce, canned peaches, pears, apricots, white cherries, stewed prunes

Bread, cereals, macaroni products

White bread and rolls, crackers, all refined cereals; macaroni, spaghetti, noodles

Desserts

Custard, junket, ice cream, tapioca, rice, bread or cornstarch pudding, gelatin desserts, junket, sponge cake, plain cookies, prune, apricot or peach whip

Beverages

Milk, buttermilk, cocoa, malted milk, fruit juices (if tolerated), coffee or tea (if allowed)

FOODS TO BE AVOIDED

Fats

Fried or fatty foods

Meat, fish

Smoked and preserved meat and fish; pork

Vegetables

All raw; all cooked except those listed above

Fruits

All except those listed above

Desserts, sweets

Pastries, preserves, candies

Beverages

Alcoholic beverages; carbonated drinks unless prescribed by the doctor

Condiments

Pepper, other spices, vinegar, ketchup, horseradish, relishes, gravies, mustard, pickles

TABLE 25-4. TYPICAL MENU FOR BLAND DIET

BREAKFAST	NOON MEAL	EVENING MEAL
Banana, ripe	Roast lamb	Cream of potato soup
Farina with milk	Mashed potatoes	Scrambled eggs
1 egg, poached	Peas	Fresh spinach
White-bread toast	White bread	White bread
Butter or margarine	Butter or margarine	Butter or margarine
Coffee or substitute	Canned pears	Applesauce with sugar cookies
Cream	Tea or milk	Milk
	Cream	Small glass orange juice*
	Small glass tomato juice*	

* If tolerated.

foods were added. Table 25-1 is a further modification of the Sippy regimen combining hourly feedings of milk and servings of eggs, refined cereals and other simple foods for the acutely ill patient with progression to the convalescent diet as tolerated.

The Liberal Dietary Regimen. Some clinicians advocate a liberal diet in the treatment of peptic ulcer. The diet plan is usually based on the patient's usual dietary practices provided that his food choices provide an adequate nutrient intake for him. He should be counseled to omit any food that has regularly caused gastric distress. He should be advised to eat frequently—mid-morning, mid-afternoon and before retiring, together with three small meals—and to avoid excessive use of alcoholic beverages, tea and coffee.[3]

The total calories of the diet of the patient of normal weight should be such as to maintain weight. The obese patient should be assisted to lose weight.

Patient Counseling. The physician's diet order determines the approach to dietary counseling whether a bland or a liberal diet is ordered. The personality of the patient may be a factor in the diet the physician chooses. A patient with an ulcer often expects some dietary restrictions. If he is a worrisome, overanxious individual, he may find a carefully controlled regimen such as a bland diet more to his liking than to be told he can eat what he wants. On the other hand, the patient who is able to take his diagnosis in stride, or who finds dietary restrictions irksome may do very well on a liberal dietary regimen.

Patients who are employed may need some suggestions about what to eat at coffee break time and the homemaker responsible for preparing a bland diet may need some assistance in modifying food preparation methods.

Surgical Treatment. Peptic ulcer tends to be recurrent. If the ulcer proves to be resistant to medical treatment, or if it recurs fairly frequently, surgery is usually necessary. (For the dietary regimen following surgery for peptic ulcer see Chap. 26.)

MALABSORPTION PROBLEMS

Patients hospitalized with malabsorption problems may be of normal weight with mild symptoms of their disease, or they may be grossly underweight and dehydrated from severe diarrhea. Successful treatment depends on the diagnosis of each patient's specific problem. The most common problems in adults are: (1) a lack of or an insufficient amount of the enzyme lactase required to hydrolyze lactose (milk sugar); or (2) gluten-induced enteropathy (celiac disease) due to a structural defect[4] in the mucosa of the duodenum and jejunum that interferes with the digestion of gliadin, a fraction of the cereal protein gluten found in wheat and rye. Cystic fibrosis, a common malabsorption problem in infants and children due to interference with the flow of pancreatic enzymes into the small intestine, is discussed in Chapter 29.

LACTOSE INTOLERANCE

Principles of Diet Therapy. Lactose intolerance is due to a deficiency of the enzyme, lactase. In infants, primary lactase deficiency appears to be genetic; in adults, it may appear as a natural process of aging. In the United States, it seems to occur more frequently in people whose heritage derives from countries in Asia and Africa where

---

[3] Spiro: op. cit.

[4] Spiro: op. cit.

milk, and therefore, lactose, is not consumed post-weaning. Secondary lactase deficiency may occur following subtotal gastrectomy, severe infection in the small bowel or severe malnutrition.

The individual who is lactose intolerant experiences abdominal pain and diarrhea after consuming lactose. His symptoms may be mild or severe. Severe diarrhea can lead to fluid and electrolyte imbalance and the loss of nutrients from the gastrointestinal tract.

Diet in Lactose Intolerance. Lactose is the disaccharide that occurs in mammalian milk—human, cow's, goat and others. Therefore, human, cow's, or goat milk is excluded from the diets of these individuals. The infant formulas, Probana,* Meat-base† and soy formulas currently on the United States market, are free of lactose and can be used to feed the lactose-intolerant infant. Some baby foods have dried milk solids added. Therefore, the mother of a lactose-intolerant infant must be counseled to read labels critically to avoid the lactose in these products. At the same time as the lactose is excluded, the diet of the infant and young child must be adequate in calories and nutrients to support normal growth and development. As the child grows older the limitations discussed in the following paragraphs for the severely lactose-intolerant adult must be observed.

The mildly lactose-intolerant adult may be required to exclude only the major sources of lactose from his diet. This includes milk as a beverage and products made from milk such as cheese, ice cream, iced milk, milk chocolate, puddings, cream-filled pies, soups made with milk, and milk gravies and sauces. Care must also be taken to avoid medications containing lactose.

On the other hand, the severely lactose intolerant adult may need to avoid all sources of milk and milk solids. This includes, in addition to the items listed above, many convenience foods to which milk solids have been added; white bread which is made with 2 to 4 percent dry milk solids; and many other bakery products. French bread and Italian bread is usually made without milk or dry milk solids and can be used by the lactose intolerant individual.

The diet of the lactose-intolerant individual may be inadequate in calcium. The physician may order calcium pills to make up this inadequacy.

Other Disaccharide Intolerances. Sucrase and maltase-isomaltase deficiencies occur but are rare

* Mead Johnson Laboratories, Evansville, Ind.
† Gerber Products, Fremont, Mich.

compared with lactase deficiency. In sucrase deficiency, sucrose (table sugar) is excluded from the diet and in maltase-isomaltase deficiency starch, which yields maltose and isomaltose on digestion by pancreatic enzymes, is reduced.

GLUTEN-INDUCED ENTEROPATHY (CELIAC DISEASE)

Principles of Diet Therapy. Although the term celiac disease was originally applied only to children who exhibited this malabsorption syndrome, it is generally accepted today that what formerly was called nontropical sprue is in reality adult celiac disease and may be referred to as celiac-sprue. It has been observed that a number of patients who developed celiac disease in adult life have a history of the disease in childhood. Today the term gluten-induced enteropathy is generally used and is more useful because it identifies the component in food that is excluded from the diet.

Gluten-induced enteropathy is characterized by diarrhea, with the passing of at least 2 to 3 stools a day. These are described as bulky, foamy, light colored and foul smelling. They contain a high percentage of fat, fatty acids and calcium soaps, resulting from incomplete digestion and absorption in the intestinal tract. The term *steatorrhea* (fatty diarrhea) is applied to this finding.

Due to the loss of fat and other nutrients in the stool, a whole complex of symptoms result. There is often marked weight loss, muscle wasting, anorexia and debilitation; in infants, and sometimes in adults there is a typical "pot belly"; there is anemia due to poor absorption of iron and folic acid; there may be tetany, bone pain and fractures resulting from the poor absorption of calcium and vitamin D; and hypoprothrombinemia and roughening of the skin may be present because fat-soluble vitamins K and A are not absorbed. Occasionally patients have glossitis and peripheral neuritis, possibly due to an inadequate intake of the B vitamins. More recent findings suggest that there may be a deficiency of vitamin E due to faulty fat absorption, and of vitamin B_6.

A biopsy of jejunal tissue of a patient with gluten enteropathy viewed under the electron microscope, reveals marked changes in the jejunal mucosa. Instead of the finger-like projections of the villi with their brush border, the mucosa is flat and thickened and appears to have varying degrees of epithelial cell atrophy, now recognized as characteristic of celiac disease.

In 1953, three Dutch investigators, Dicke, Weijers and van de Kamer[5] reported that wheat, rye and oat cereals were responsible for the steatorrhea and other symptoms of celiac disease in children. When they excluded these cereals from the diets of their patients there was prompt and marked improvement. Further research has shown that gliadin, part of the cereal protein gluten, is the offending substance. Because it is impossible to exclude only the gliadin fraction of cereal protein, the cereal grains—wheat, rye, barley and oats—that contain the most significant amount of gluten are excluded. The cereal grains rice and corn, which are practically free of gluten, are used.

The Gluten-Free Diet. Table 25-5 lists the foods used and the foods avoided in a gluten-free diet. In the patient with severe diarrhea, the diet may be restricted in residue until the diarrhea is controlled.

The exclusion of all cereal grains except corn and rice from the diet may seem to be an easier matter than it actually is. Wheat-flour and wheat-bread products are used in such a variety of ways in food preparation that their elimination poses many problems. Not only must all wheat bread and rolls be omitted, both white and whole wheat, but all breaded products, bread stuffing, gravies and cream sauces thickened with wheat flour, macaroni, spaghetti, noodles, biscuits, crackers, cakes and cookies made from wheat flour must be eliminated from the diet. Oatmeal and rye grain, with the exception of rye breads, pretzels and Ry-Krisp, is less commonly used and, therefore, is omitted more easily. For adults, beer and ale must be omitted, because they may contain cereal grain residues.[6]

In place of the cereals that must be excluded, bread, biscuits and cookies made from rice, corn and soy flour and wheat starch are used. Wheat starch is discussed in Chapter 24, Diet In Renal Disease. A gluten-free bread mix is available from Chicago dietetic Supply House, Le Grange, Illinois. Cornflakes, corn meal, hominy, rice, Rice Krispies, Puffed Rice and precooked rice cereals may be used. Cornstarch and potato flour may be used to thicken gravies and cream sauces.

Because wheat flour is in such common usage, it is well to check the labels on commercially prepared foods for content before using them on this diet to be sure that no wheat flour has been used in their preparation. Postum, malted milk and Ovaltine are examples of commercial products made from or containing cereal grains. Where such content is not included in the label, the food had better be omitted if there is a question.

When the individual has a concurrent lactase deficiency, milk in all forms must also be excluded from the diet.

The physician may augment the diet with mineral and vitamin supplements to correct deficiencies and hasten recovery. Although fat excretion persists to some extent, fat is well tolerated and there is no need to limit it in the diet.

Patient Counseling. Individuals with gluten-induced enteropathy need help in identifying gluten in foods. A very useful booklet for the patient on the gluten-free diet is listed at the end of this chapter.

PROBLEMS OF THE LARGE BOWEL— THE RESIDUE-RESTRICTED DIET

Patients with problems in the terminal ileum and large bowel may require a low residue diet. These patients may have regional ileitis, ulcerative colitis, malignant or nonmalignant lesions of the colon or rectum; or hemorrhoids. Regional ileitis and ulcerative colitis are generally treated medically. Progression of the disease may lead to surgery: ileostomy in regional ileitis, and colostomy or ileostomy in ulcerative colitis. In all situations the low residue diet is generally used as part of medical treatment or in preparation for surgical treatment of the patient.

Principles of Diet Therapy. The foods used in the residue-restricted diets are not only low in fiber but also decrease total fecal output by mechanisms other than fiber such as connective tissue in meats. Fiber is that portion of food (cellulose, hemicellulose and lignin) that is not enzymatically digested in the digestive tract. Fruits, vegetables, nuts and whole grains are the major contributors of fiber. The term "roughage" is also used to refer to fiber.

It is generally agreed that meats free of connective tissue, fats such as butter and margarine, and highly refined carbohydrates such as flour, spaghetti, macaroni, noodles, rice, and sugar add minimal residue to the fecal contents of the large bowel. Bananas and potatoes, which are low in residue, are exceptions in classifying fruits and vegetables as high in residue.

Limited evidence exists which indicates that

[5] Dicke, W. K., *et al.*: Acta Paediat., 42:34, 1953.

[6] Sleisenger, M. H., Rynbergen, H. J., *et al.*: J. Am. Dietet. A. 33:1137, 1957.

TABLE 25-5. GLUTEN-FREE DIET

CHARACTERISTICS

1. All forms of wheat, rye, oatmeal, buckwheat and barley are omitted, except gluten-free wheat starch.

2. All other foods are permitted freely, including fats and starches.

3. The diet should be high in protein and calories. Mineral and vitamin supplements may be needed if malnutrition is present. After that, the diet should be sufficient to maintain normal growth and development in children, and normal weight in adults.

FOODS USED

Milk

2 glasses or more. Flavored if desired. More for children

Cheese

As desired. Cottage and pot cheese only for very young children
Butter and other fats as desired. (Note restrictions under "Foods To Be Avoided.")

Eggs

1 to 2 a day

Meat, fish, fowl

1 or 2 servings daily (not breaded, creamed or served with thickened gravy; no bread dressings). Otherwise prepared as desired

Soups

All clear and vegetable soups; cream soups thickened with cream, cornstarch or potato flour only

Vegetables

As desired, except creamed. Include 2 servings of green or yellow vegetables and at least 1 raw vegetable daily. (The last may be omitted for very young children.) Rice may be substituted occasionally for potato.

Fruits

As desired; 2 or 3 servings daily. Include citrus fruit once a day.

Bread and cereals

Bread made from rice, corn or soybean flour and gluten-free wheat starch only
Cornflakes, corn meal, hominy, rice, Rice Krispies, Puffed Rice, precooked rice cereals

Desserts

Any of the following: jello, fruit jello, ice or sherbet, homemade ice cream, custard, junket, rice pudding, or cornstarch pudding (homemade)

Beverages

Milk, fruit juices, ginger ale, cocoa. (Read label to see that no wheat flour has been added to cocoa or cocoa syrup.) Coffee (made from ground coffee), tea, carbonated beverages

Condiments and sweets

Salt; sugar, white or brown; molasses; jellies and jams; honey; corn syrup

FOODS TO BE AVOIDED

Fats

Cream sauces made with wheat flour; commercial salad dressings except pure mayonnaise. (Read labels.)

Meat, fish, fowl

Meat patties or meat, fish or chicken loaf and pies made with bread or bread crumbs; croquettes; breaded meat, fish or chicken. Chili con carne and other canned meat dishes. Cold cuts unless guaranteed pure meat. Bread stuffings
All gravies or cream sauces thickened with wheat flour

Soups

All canned soups except clear broth. All cream soups unless thickened with cream, cornstarch or potato flour

Vegetables

Any prepared with cream sauce or breaded

Bread, cereals, macaroni products

All bread, rolls, crackers, cake and cookies made from wheat or rye; Ry-Krisp; muffins, biscuits, waffles, pancake flour and other prepared mixes; rusks, Zwieback, pretzels; any product containing oatmeal, barley or buckwheat
Breaded foods, bread crumbs
All wheat and rye cereals; wheat germ, barley, oatmeal, buckwheat, kasha
Macaroni, spaghetti, noodles, dumplings

Desserts

Cakes, cookies, pastry; commercial ice cream and ice-cream cones; prepared mixes, puddings. All homemade puddings thickened with wheat flour

Beverages

Postum, malted milk, Ovaltine. For adults: beer, ale

Sweets

Commercial candies containing cereal products. (Read labels.)

WARNING: *Read labels on all packaged and prepared foods.*

milk may add residue to the fecal contents. As a result there is controversy about the use of milk in residue-restricted diet plans. It has been observed that some adult ulcerative colitis patients have insufficient amounts of lactase and respond favorably to a moderate lactose restriction.[7] (See discussion of lactose intolerance earlier in this chapter.)

Tea, coffee, meat extractives, condiments, spices and carbonated beverages are usually not excluded

from the residue-restricted diet. Fruit and vegetable juices may be excluded in some situations not because of residue, but because the organic acids in these beverages may stimulate peristaltic action.

The Residue-Restricted Diets. Residue-restricted diets may be ordered at various levels of restriction. The nurse is urged to check the residue-restricted regimens in the diet manual used in her hospital. Table 25-6, Diets Varying in Residue, presents one example of levels of residue-restricted diets.

---

[7] Spiro: op. cit.

TABLE 25-6. DIETS VARYING IN RESIDUE

FOODS	RESIDUE-RESTRICTED DIET	MODERATE RESIDUE DIET	MINIMAL RESIDUE DIET
Milk*	Milk, buttermilk, yoghurt, cream	Same	Same
Cheese	Cottage, cream*, Cheddar	Same	Cottage, cream only*
Fat	Butter, margarine	Same	Same
Eggs	Cooked, poached, scrambled in double boiler	Same	Same
Meat, fish, fowl	Tender chicken, fish, sweetbreads, ground beef and lamb	Same	Ground, tender meat; minced chicken and fish
Soups and Broths	Broth, strained meat-base soups	Same	Broth only
Vegetables	Cooked vegetables: asparagus, peas, string beans, spinach, carrots, beets, squash; potatoes—boiled, mashed, baked	Vegetable juice; vegetable purée, cooked asparagus tips, carrots, potatoes—boiled, mashed, baked	Unseasoned vegetable juices in limited amounts*
Fruits	Fruit juices, cooked and canned fruits (without skins, seeds or fiber), bananas	Fruit juice, fruit purée, ripe bananas, cooked, peeled apples, apricots, peaches, pears, plums	Fruit juices, preferably citrus in limited amounts*
Bread, cereals	Refined, enriched bread and cereals; macaroni, spaghetti, noodles, rice, crackers	Refined, enriched bread and cereals only, macaroni, spaghetti, noodles, rice, white crackers	As in moderately low residue
Desserts	Ices, ice cream*, junket*, cereal puddings*, custard*, gelatin, plain cake and cookies; all without fruit and nuts	Same	Same
Beverages	Tea, coffee, carbonated beverages	Same	Tea, coffee as permitted
Condiments	Salt, moderate amounts of pepper, other mild spices, sugar	Salt and sugar	Salt and sugar

---

* If tolerated

The Minimal Residue Diet in Table 25-6 may be used to prepare a patient for bowel surgery or immediately after surgery. It is shown that the foods used in this diet are limited and that this diet can be inadequate in calcium and vitamins A and C. If used for any period of time it should be supplemented with mineral and vitamin preparations.

The Moderate Residue Diet in Table 25-6 may be used to progress a patient after bowel surgery, in the early medical treatment of regional ileitis or ulcerative colitis, or for the symptomatic control of diarrhea. The Residue-Restricted Diet in Table 25-6 is usually the one used over a period of time by individuals with regional ileitis or ulcerative colitis.

The Ulcerative Colitis Patient. The etiology of ulcerative colitis is unknown. No organism has been isolated as a cause. It has been ascribed to allergy, especially to milk proteins. In addition, there are indications that colitis may occur on an emotional basis, since these patients are often very painstaking and meticulous, and seem to be unable to express strong emotions.[8] As a result there are various approaches, including diet therapy, to the treatment of ulcerative colitis.

Depending on the patient's condition some clinicians order a Moderate Residue or Residue-Restricted Diet. Because of the emotional components of the disease some clinicians order a self-selected diet and encourage the patient to try any food that appeals to him.

Whatever the plan of treatment ordered by the physician, the nurse and the dietitian must be supportive and accepting of these patients. Only when both the nurse and the dietitian understand that the patient with ulcerative colitis can be a "difficult" patient can they work together to help him. The hospitalized ulcerative colitis patient is usually underweight and nutritionally debilitated and needs an adequate calorie and nutrient intake.

DIET IN LIVER DISEASE

Although the primary effect of liver disease is on intermediary metabolism, it is classified with gastrointestinal diseases because it also affects the function of the gastrointestinal tract. Dietary modification plays an important role in the therapy of fatty infiltration of the liver, early and late or advanced cirrhosis (generalized fibrosis of liver tissue) or acute liver failure. In some instances liver disease may interfere with the flow of bile into the duodenum which results in the malabsorption of fats.

The ingestion of alcohol is one of the most common causes of liver disease in the United States. It is estimated that one out of 12 chronic alcoholics develops cirrhosis.[9] The effect of alcohol intake on the cells of the liver is under intensive study today. Some investigators indicate that alcohol damages the cells of the liver. Others suggest that alcohol promotes the accumulation of fat in the liver. Liver disease may also be caused by viral hepatitis and toxic chemicals such as carbon tetrachloride; or it may be secondary to systemic disease.

Principles of Diet Therapy. Protein is the key nutrient in the treatment of liver disease. The protein in the diet is normal or increased in fatty infiltration or early cirrhosis of the liver. It is restricted in advanced cirrhosis or may be entirely excluded in acute liver failure (hepatic coma) because the liver is unable to metabolize the nitrogen in protein, resulting in the accumulation of toxic ammonia in the blood.

The work of Patek[10] in 1941 showed that an adequate intake of calories, protein and other nutrients by the nutritionally debilitated, cirrhotic patient resulted in marked improvement. Patek's dietary regimen contained 3000 calories, 2 Gm. of protein per kilogram of body weight, moderate amounts of fat and liberal amounts of minerals and vitamins, especially the B vitamins. Subsequent research has demonstrated that adequate calories, 1½ Gm. protein per kilogram of high biological value and liberal amounts of minerals, especially iron, and vitamins is effective in the treatment of early cirrhosis. When ascites accompanies other symptoms the diet may also be sodium-restricted (see Chap. 23).

In late or advanced cirrhosis, especially for those patients who can easily go into hepatic coma, the protein of the diet is restricted. The individual's tolerance for protein determines the level of restriction. This may vary from 20 to 60 Gm. of protein per day. In the acute phase of hepatic coma protein may be totally excluded from the diet with calories provided by carbohydrate or carbohydrate and fat. Sodium and in some situations fluids are also restricted in advanced cirrhosis.

---

8 Spiro: op. cit.

9 Spiro: op. cit.
10 Patek, A. J. and Post, J.: J. Clin. Invest., 20:481, 1941.

Planning the Protein Modified Diet. Table 25-7, Diet Pattern for 100 Grams of Protein and 2500 Calories, using the Exchange System (see Chap. 20), illustrates the kinds and amounts of food required to provide adequate calories and protein for the patient with early cirrhosis. The quart of milk (4 exchanges), the two 3-ounce servings of meat (6 meat exchanges) and the 10 servings of bread, cereals and potato (10 bread exchanges), are the primary sources of protein in this diet pattern. If a patient does not want to drink one quart of milk the milk in this pattern can be reduced and the amount of meat increased to provide 100 Gm. of protein per day.

The calorie composition of this pattern is 2290 not 2500. Fruits canned with sugar, and sugar, jams, jellies and simple desserts can supply the 210 calories to make 2500 calories, or more if the patient requires more than 2500. Some patients prefer three meals with three between meal feedings, especially if they have had nausea and vomiting prior to admission.

The most important medication order for these patients is mineral and vitamin supplements.

Table 25-8, Diet Pattern for 40 Grams of Protein and 2000 Calories, illustrates a level of protein restriction for a patient with advanced cirrhosis. It is shown that canned fruits and additional sugars and sweets are required to achieve a 2000 calorie intake. Care must be taken that simple desserts do not add significant amounts of protein—for example: apple pie, not custard pie. The restricted-protein diet for the patient with cirrhosis will also be restricted in sodium—to as low as 500 mg. for some patients. These patients usually have ascites and are more comfortable if served six small meals a day. They also should

be cautioned not to "borrow" food from other patient's trays, especially meat, eggs and milk.

Special Problems. Food is the major component in the treatment plan of any patient with liver disease. Patients with hepatitis, including the drug addict, and patients with cirrhosis are usually anorexic and frequently have nausea, vomiting and diarrhea. These patients require help in accepting fluids and foods. Careful daily observation at meal times is essential to insure that, as their appetites improve, they are consuming adequate amounts of foods. Numerous adjustments of diet plans may be needed before an acceptable one is achieved.

To prevent irritation and bleeding, it may be necessary to avoid roughage in the diet of a patient with esophageal varices (enlarged blood vessels in the esophagus), a complication of advanced cirrhosis. The diet plans in Tables 25-7 and 25-8 can also be restricted in residue (see Residue-Restricted Diets in Table 25-6). If the varices hemorrhage, the dietitian receives an order for a protein and sodium restricted tube-feeding because the majority of patients whose varices hemorrhage have advanced cirrhosis and readily go into hepatic coma.

OTHER GASTROINTESTINAL PROBLEMS

Gallbladder Disease. Disease of the gallbladder may be due to infection (cholecystitis) or the presence of gallstones (cholelithiasis). In either case there is a great deal of pain in the region of the gallbladder. It has been thought that the pain is caused by the ingestion of large amounts of dietary fat. A survey of hospitalized patients by

TABLE 25-7. DIET PATTERN FOR 100 GRAMS OF PROTEIN AND 2500 CALORIES

Food	Exchanges	Calories	Protein Gm.	Fat Gm.
Milk	4	680	32	40
Meat	6	450	42	30
Bread	10	700	20	..
Vegetable B	2	70	4	..
Fruit	3	120*	..	..
Fat	6	270	..	30
Totals		2290†	98	100

* Fruit canned with sugar provides more calories.
† Additional calories from sugar, jams, jellies, candy, cookies, cake to provide 2500.

TABLE 25-8. DIET PATTERN FOR 40 GRAMS OF PROTEIN AND 2000 CALORIES

Food	Exchanges	Calories	Protein Gm.	Fat Gm.
Milk	1	170	8	10
Meat	2	150	14	10
Bread	6	420	12	..
Vegetable B	1	35	2	..
Fruit	3	120*	..	..
Fat	6	270	..	..
Totals		1165†	36	50

* Fruit canned with sugar provides more calories.
† Additional calories from sugar, jams, jellies, candies, cookies and fats, if tolerated, to provide 2000 calories.

Koch and Donaldson[11] indicates that some patients with gallbladder disease have pain when they eat fat while others do not.

A fat-restricted diet may be ordered for patients with gallbladder disease. Table 25-9 shows the foods containing significant amounts of fat that must be used in limited quantities and foods high in fat that are omitted. Table 25-10 gives a very low fat, bland diet menu. If the individual is obese, which is relatively typical, the low fat diet may need to be further restricted in total calories to achieve weight loss by decreasing the amount of carbohydrate (see Chap. 21).

---

[11] Koch, J. P. and Donaldson, R. M., Jr.: New Eng. J. Med., 271:657, 1964.

TABLE 25-9. RESTRICTIONS AND OMISSIONS ON A LOW FAT DIET

FOODS LIMITED

Milk to 1 pint daily
Eggs to 1 daily
Butter or margarine to ½ tablespoon daily
Lean meat, fish or fowl to 1 serving daily
    (If skim milk is used, meat may be increased to 2 servings without altering the fat limitation.)

FOODS OMITTED

Cream; cheese other than pot or cottage cheese
All fried foods
Salad oils; salad dressings; gravies
All meat high in fat, such as pork, bacon, ham, goose, duck, fatty fish
Pastry; cake; cookies; ice cream
Nuts, olives, avocados

Pancreatitis. Pancreatitis, acute or chronic, frequently occurs in alcoholism or it may be of unknown origin. On admission to the hospital the patient with acute pancreatitis is usually treated with intravenous fluids. As the patient improves he may be offered small meals consisting of easily digested carbohydrate and protein. The patient with chronic pancreatitis may tolerate a 6-meal bland diet, restricted in fat. He may also be given pancreatic enzymes with each meal.

STUDY QUESTIONS AND ACTIVITIES

1. Explain the principles underlying the dietary treatment of peptic ulcer. What is the purpose of the antacid medication?

2. A patient with a peptic ulcer works in a factory from 7:00 a.m. to 3:30 p.m. and buys his lunch from the vending machines at the plant. What suggestions can you make to enable him to follow his 6-meal bland diet on workdays? How can you help him to have an adequate diet?

3. Using the information in Chapter 11 and the readings in Chapter 18 write a 6-meal bland diet pattern for a Jewish patient who carries his lunch to work; for a Puerto Rican cab driver who works from 4 p.m. to midnight.

4. Calculate a 1500-calorie, 6-meal bland diet for a business executive who has a peptic ulcer and is overweight. The doctors have discovered that he has mild coronary heart disease.

5. Obtain a week's menus from the school lunch program in your community and help a school boy who is lactose intolerant choose the foods in these menus that he can eat.

6. Plan a picnic menu for the mother of a 5-year-old girl who has gluten-induced enteropathy. The rest of the family—mother, father, and

TABLE 25-10. VERY LOW FAT, BLAND DIET MENU IN 6 MEALS*

BREAKFAST	LUNCH	DINNER
Stewed prunes	Cottage cheese	Sliced chicken
Cream of Wheat	Toast, slightly buttered, 2 slices	Baked potato
Milk, whole, ½ cup	Jelly or honey	Soft-cooked string beans
Postum	Applesauce	Canned apricots
Sugar	Tea, sugar	Tea, sugar
10 A.M.	**3 P.M.**	**8 P.M.**
Toast, slightly buttered, 2 slices	Junket made with skim milk	Crackers
Jelly or honey	Crackers	Jelly or honey
Skim milk, 1 glass	Jelly or honey	Skim milk, 1 glass

* This diet will contain approximately 70 Gm. of protein, 25 Gm. of fat, 325 Gm. of carbohydrate and 1,750 calories.

two older brothers—are going on the picnic too. Can you plan a menu that is gluten-free that satisfies the whole family?

7. With the help of nursing and dietary personnel keep a record for 3 days of all the food and beverages consumed by a patient with regional ileitis or ulcerative colitis (or any patient requiring nutritional rehabilitation). Estimate the daily total calorie and protein intake of the individual. Was this intake adequate? Was the intake of other nutrients adequate? If not, how can you help this patient improve?

8. You observe Mr. A., who has advanced cirrhosis and whose diet is restricted to 40 Gm. of protein and 500 mg. of sodium, "borrow" and drink an 8-ounce carton of milk from the patient in the next bed. How would you handle this situation?

9. Using the Exchange Lists in Chapters 20 and 23 plan a diet pattern for a patient with advanced cirrhosis containing 30 Gm. of protein, 500 mg. of sodium, 2000 calories and 1000 ml. of fluid a day.

10. Using the Exchange Lists in Chapter 20 plan a 1200-calorie bland diet for Mrs. A. who is an obese homemaker and has gallstones. The doctors have advised her to lose 50 pounds before surgery.

SUPPLEMENTARY READING ON DIET IN GASTROINTESTINAL DISEASE

Peptic Ulcer

Given, B., and Simons, S.: Care of patient with gastric ulcer. Am. J. Nursing, 70:1472, 1970.
Koch, J. P., and Donaldson, R. M., Jr.: A survey of food intolerances in hospitalized patients. New Eng. J. Med., 271:657, 1964.
Kramer, P., and Caso, E. K.: Is the rationale for gastrointestinal diet therapy sound? J. Am. Dietet. A., 42:505, 1963.
Manier, J. W.: Diet in gastrointestinal disease. Med. Clin. N. Am., 54:1357, 1970.
Piper, D. W.: Milk in treatment of gastric disease. Am. J. Clin. Nutr., 21:191, 1969.

Malabsorption

De Risi, L. L.: Starving in the midst of plenty: adult celiac disease. Am. J. Nursing, 70:1048, 1970.
Nutrition reviews: primary intestinal lactase deficiency. Nutr. Rev., 25:265, 1967.
Rubin, W.: Celiac disease. Am. J. Clin. Nutr., 24:91, 1971.
Sleisenger, M. H.: Malabsorption syndrome. New Eng. J. Med., 281:1111, 1969.
Sleisenger, M. H., Rynbergen, H. J., et al.: A wheat, rye and oat-free diet in the treatment of non-tropical sprue. J. Am. Dietet. A., 33:1137, 1957.
Simoons, F. J.: Primary adult lactose intolerance and the milking habits: a problem in biological and cultural interrelations. II. A cultural historical hypothesis. Am. J. Dig. Dis., 15:695, 1970.

Liver Disease

Crews, R. H., and Faloon, W. W.: The fallacy of a low fat diet in liver disease. JAMA, 181:754, 1962.
Gabuzda, G. J.: Nutrition and liver disease. Med. Clin. N. Am., 54:1455, 1970.
Lieber, C. S., and Rubin, E.: Alcoholic fatty liver. New Eng. J. Med., 280:705, 1969.
Popper, H., et al.: Social impact of liver disease. New Eng. J. Med., 281:1455, 1969.

Other Problems

Hinkle, C. L., and Moller, G. A.: Correlation of symptoms, age, sex and habits with cholecystographic findings in 1,000 consecutive examinations. Gastroenterology, 32:807, 1957.
Small, D. M.: Current concepts: gallstones. New Eng. J. Med., 279:588, 1968.

PATIENT RESOURCES

Celiac Disease Recipes. Hospital for Sick Children, 555 University, Toronto 5, Ontario, Canada.
Low Gluten Diet with Tested Recipes. 3rd rev. Gastrointestinal Section, Univ. of Michigan Medical Center, Ann Arbor, Michigan, 1964.
Sheedy, C. B., and Keifetz, N.: Cooking for Your Celiac Child. New York, The Dial Press, 1969.

For further references see Bibliography in Part Four.

Nutritional Care—
Surgical and
Burn Therapy

26

Principles of Nutritional Care · Postoperative Oral Feeding Routines · Tube Feedings
Diet Therapy after Gastrointestinal Surgery · Nutrition Following Burns

INTRODUCTION

Good nutritional status is an asset for the patient who is to undergo surgery. This is possible for patients undergoing elective surgery for problems that do not interfere with eating an adequate diet. These may be patients who require gynecological or orthopedic surgery or surgery for uncomplicated cholelithiasis, hernias, thyroid diseases and tonsillitis. Patients who are to undergo cardiac surgery or kidney transplant need the appropriate dietary treatment prior to surgery to reduce operative risks (Chaps. 23 and 24).

The obese patient is a special operative risk especially for the anesthesiologist. When possible the obese patient should be counseled to lose weight prior to surgery (Chap. 21).

Patients with cancer of the oral cavity, esophagus, larynx, stomach or colon may come to surgery in a nutritionally debilitated state. The nutritional rehabilitation of these and certain other patients cannot be done until after surgery because these problems may interfere with chewing and swallowing, or digestion, absorption and excretion.

Principles of postoperative nutritional care, postoperative oral feeding routines, tube feedings, and diet therapy used after surgery of the gastrointestinal tract are discussed in this chapter. Also, the nutritional care of the severely burned patient is discussed in the last section.

PRINCIPLES OF NUTRITIONAL CARE

The key factors of postoperative nutritional care arc: (1) maintenance of fluid and electrolyte balance; (2) adequate calorie-protein intake; and (3) adequate total nutrient intake to promote wound healing and resumption of normal activities.

For the majority of patients, in the immediate postoperative period, fluid and electrolyte balance is maintained by the intravenous route. Intravenous solutions of physiologic saline and other electrolytes, if necessary, combined with 5 percent glucose are used. Later oral fluids and foods can be used to maintain fluid and electrolyte balance.

Maintaining adequate calorie-protein intake in the immediate postoperative period is difficult, especially if the patient cannot be returned to food by mouth within a day or two after surgery. A negative nitrogen balance is promoted by the stress reaction that occurs as a result of surgery, or trauma and surgery that frequently happens after an accident. Under stress the amino acids of the body are catabolized to meet the increased energy needs caused by the stress reaction and the nitrogen of the amino acids that is not used for energy is excreted in the urine. As the patient recovers from the stress of surgery this strongly catabolic phase of metabolism changes to a strongly anabolic one with positive nitrogen balance (Chaps. 4 and 9).

The calories provided by the 5 percent glucose in the intravenous solution help to minimize the loss of nitrogen. The return to oral feedings, adequate in calories and protein and all other nutrients, is required as soon as possible to support a positive nitrogen balance and therefore, wound healing.

Total parenteral nutrition is provided for those patients who cannot take food by mouth for long periods of time after surgery. This feeding may be a solution containing 20 percent glucose and 3.5 percent protein as amino acids, providing approximately 0.94 calories per milliliter.[1] It is fed

---

[1] Morgan, A., *et al.*: Med. Clin. N. Am., 54:1363, 1970.

to the patient through a central venous catheter that is inserted at surgery. This solution can meet the calorie-protein needs of such patients. Minerals and vitamins are added to this solution.

In addition to adequate calorie and protein intake, early ambulation also helps promote the change from negative to positive nitrogen balance. Therefore, the nurse who is successful in promoting early ambulation in the postoperative period is giving expert nutritional as well as expert nursing care. Passive exercise during personal care for the postoperative patient who cannot ambulate also helps to reverse the negative nitrogen balance.

An adequate intake of minerals and vitamins, especially vitamins B_6 and C, are also required by the postoperative patient. Vitamin C plays a special role in wound healing (Chap. 8). The B vitamins and vitamin C are often added to the intravenous solutions and vitamin C supplements are often ordered when the patient can take medications by mouth.

Before discharge it should be observed that the postoperative patient is selecting and consuming a diet totally adequate for him to promote his full recovery; and he should be counseled to continue these practices at home without gaining excessive weight.

Because many patients become fatigued easily for a period after surgery, special care should be taken to identify the mother with a large family or the individual who lives alone. They may need assistance after discharge with food buying and preparation at home. Otherwise their recovery may be delayed. If relatives or friends are not available to assist them, a home-health aid (Chap. 1) can be requested to help them two or three times a week, or daily if required. For the patient over 65 this service is provided by Medicare. Some of these individuals may need to transfer to an extended care facility before returning to their own homes. The social worker can assist the nurse and the dietitian in these situations.

POSTOPERATIVE ORAL FEEDING ROUTINES

Anesthesia decreases peristaltic action. Therefore, food and fluids are not given by mouth after surgery until peristalsis returns. For the first oral feeding the patient is offered a clear liquid diet. If this is well tolerated he may progress to a full liquid diet and then to a soft and finally a regular diet. (See Chap. 19 for a description of these diets.) For some patients the progression is directly from clear liquid to regular.

In any event the nurse is frequently responsible for diet progression postoperatively. The physician's order reads "clear liquid diet and progress." It must be remembered that the clear liquid diet is nutritionally inadequate in calories, protein and other nutrients, and therefore, such patients should be observed carefully so that they may progress to an adequate diet as soon as it is tolerated. Because of their cultural expectations of food for illness, an older patient who could be offered a regular diet after clear liquids, may accept a soft diet more readily before progressing to a regular diet.

Patients with a concurrent disease such as diabetes mellitus or heart disease should be returned to their appropriate therapeutic diet. Serious postoperative complications can occur if the appropriate diet is not offered.

TUBE FEEDINGS

Feeding by nasogastric, gastric or jejunal tube is used when it is not possible to take food otherwise. This may occur: when there is an obstruction in

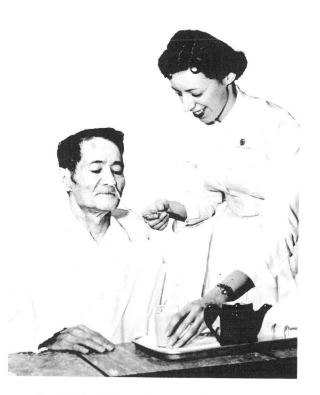

FIG. 26-1. If the patient must be fed by tube, the feeding should be served in an attractive and appetizing manner, so that it reflects that this is food and not a medication. (Paul Parker)

the esophagus or after surgery for oral or esophageal cancer; when the esophagus and, in some cases, the stomach has been injured by strong alkali solutions; after gastrectomy for cancer; or when the patient is unconscious due to trauma to the head or a cerebral vascular accident (stroke). The tube feeding must be liquid, yet contain reasonable proportions of all the nutrients essential for adequate nutrition, especially if it is used permanently or over a considerable period of time.

There are two general types of tube feedings: (1) primarily a milk-base solution; and (2) a milk-base solution with suspended solids from strained or blenderized foods. Commercial preparations of the first type are generally available and used by hospitals.

Nutrient Composition of Tube Feedings

Calories. Standard tube feedings, prepared in the hospital or obtained from commercial sources, contain approximately 1 calorie per milliliter. Therefore, 1,500 ml. of standard tube feeding contain 1,500 calories, and 2,000 ml. contain 2,000 calories. Tube feedings can be prepared which contain ½ calorie per milliliter or 1½ calories per milliliter. The more dilute feeding (½ calorie per milliliter) is generally used as the first feeding to test tolerance. The more concentrated feeding (1½ calorie per milliliter) is used to rehabilitate the nutritionally debilitated patient.

Protein, Fat and Carbohydrate. Tube feedings should contain reasonable proportions of protein, fat and carbohydrate. Whole milk, which contains approximately ⅔ of a calorie per milliliter, evaporated milk, nonfat dry milk solids, pasteurized powdered egg, liquified meats (baby foods) and various carbohydrates are used to provide the protein, fat and carbohydrate in standard nasogastric and gastric tube feedings.

Table 26-1 gives the ingredients and nutrient analyses of 1,000 ml. of an inexpensive, standard tube feeding containing one calorie per ml. or 1,000 calories per 1,000 ml. (1 quart). This feeding contains 42 Gm. of protein, 55 Gm. of fat and 94 Gm. of carbohydrate. Two thousand ml. of this feeding contains 2,000 calories, 84 Gm. of protein, 110 Gm. of fat and 188 Gm. of carbohydrate.

Table 26-2 gives the ingredients and nutrient analysis of a blenderized tube feeding containing 1 calorie per ml. or 1,000 calories per 1,000 ml. (1 quart). This feeding contains 50 Gm. of protein, 46 Gm. of fat and 106 Gm. of carbohydrate. Two thousand ml. of this feeding contains 2,000

calories, 100 Gm. of protein, 92 Gm. of fat and 212 Gm. of carbohydrate. It has been observed that blenderized tube feedings are better tolerated than the standard one.

Minerals and Vitamins. Both the standard and the blenderized tube feedings require supplementation with thiamine. The standard formula requires supplementation with vitamin C and iron if a liquified meat other than liver is used. In some hospitals the vitamins are added during the preparation of the tube feeding; in others, the vitamins are ordered and given to the patient by the nurse. Check the policy in your hospital.

The commercial tube feedings presently available are fortified with vitamins and iron and do not require further supplementation.

Special Considerations

The First Feedings. To avoid adverse reactions to tube feeding such as gastric distention and diarrhea, the first feeding should be dilute—½ to ⅔ calorie per milliliter—*warmed* at least to room temperature, and given *slowly*. The standard tube feeding can be diluted with water, or whole or skim milk can be used for the first feeding.

The volume of the first feeding should not exceed 100 ml. If the patient has had no oral feeding for 3 or more days it is wise to limit this first feeding to 50 ml. If the first feeding is well tolerated, the next feedings can be increased by 50 to 100 ml. increments up to the volume per feeding as ordered—usually 300 to 400 ml. per feeding.

The dilute feeding should be continued for approximately 24 hours. If the patient tolerates these first feedings without gastric distress or diarrhea then the amount of the standard or blenderized tube feeding as ordered, *warmed* to room temperature can be given *slowly*. For the comfort of the patient and to avoid, if possible, adverse reactions all feedings by tube should be *warmed* and given *slowly*.

Recording Intake. After giving the feeding, the amount and type should be recorded separately from the water used to test the patency of the tube or to give medications. Only when this is done can the physician and dietitian appraise the adequacy of the calorie and nutrient intake of a patient with any degree of accuracy.

The Hazards of Tube Feedings. Care must be taken to avoid contaminating the supply of tube feeding and therefore, giving the patient a gastrointestinal infection. The tube feeding made by the dietary department should be prepared *daily*

TABLE 26-1. STANDARD TUBE FEEDING (1 calorie per milliliter)

FOOD	WEIGHT IN GM.	HOUSE-HOLD MEASURE	CALORIES	PROTEIN Gm.	FAT Gm.	CARBO-HYDRATE Gm.	CALCIUM Gm.	IRON mg.	VITAMIN A I.U.	THIAMINE mg.	RIBO-FLAVIN mg.	NIACIN mg.	VITAMIN C mg.
Evaporated milk	400	1 can	548	28.0	31.6	38.6	1.000	0.4	1,280	0.16	1.36	0.8	4.0
Corn syrup	70	¼ c.	200	..	..	52.5	.030	2.7	..	..	..	..	..
Puréed liver*†	100	1 jar	94	14.0	3.1	2.4	.006	6.8	25,655	0.057	2.25	9.4	27.4
Corn oil	20	1½ T	177	..	20.0	..	..	..	..	..	..	..	..
Water—add to make 1,000 ml.													
Totals			1,019	42.0	54.7	93.5	1.036	9.9	26,935	0.217	3.61	10.2	31.4

* Strained baby food.
† Other baby meats can be used, but there is a decrease in mineral and vitamin content.

DIRECTIONS: Place all ingredients in a mechanical blender and mix 10 minutes. Place in sterile containers, label and refrigerate immediately. Shake well before pouring.

TABLE 26-2. BLENDERIZED TUBE FEEDING

FOOD	WEIGHT IN GM.	HOUSE-HOLD MEASURE	CALO-RIES	PROTEIN Gm.	FAT Gm.	CARBO-HYDRATE Gm.	CALCIUM Gm.	IRON mg.	VITAMIN A I.U.	THIA-MINE mg.	RIBO-FLAVIN mg.	NIACIN mg.	VITAMIN C mg.
Milk, whole	244	1c.	160	8.5	8.5	12	.288	0.2	350	.08	.42	0.2	2
Dry skim milk (instant)	16	2 T	58	6.0	..	8	.206	0.2	..	.06	.62	0.2	2
Cream, 20%	100	½ c.	211	3.0	21.0	4	.102	..	840	.03	.15	0.1	1
Egg, pasteurized powder*	30	4 T	163	13.0	12.0	1	.054	2.3	1,180	.11	.30	0.1	..
Corn syrup	70	½ c.	200	..	..	52.5	.030	2.7	..	..	..	..	..
Strained pears†	70	½ jar	48	0.2	..	11.5	.007	0.2	26	.09	.10	0.3	..
Strained peas†	70	½ jar	38	2.8	..	6.3	.007	0.8	350	.05	.06	0.7	7
Strained beef†	100	6 T	99	15.0	4.0	..	.008	2.0	..	.01	.16	3.5	..
Orange juice	100	½ c.	45	1.0	..	11.0	.009	0.1	200	.09	.01	0.3	45
Water, add to make 1,000 ml.													
Totals			1,022	49.5‡	45.5	106.3	.711	8.5	2,946	.52	1.82	5.4	57

* Pasteurized powdered egg is used to avoid salmonella. Fifteen Gm. is equivalent to one egg.
† Strained baby foods. These can be changed daily. This alters nutrient composition somewhat.
‡ Can be increased, if necessary, by addition of protein supplement.

DIRECTIONS: Place all ingredients in a mechanical blender and mix 10 minutes. Strain, place in sterile containers, label and refrigerate immediately. Shake well before pouring.

under clean conditions and delivered to the refrigerator in the nursing unit in *sterile* containers. When opening commercial tube feedings that are packaged in cans, a *sterile opener* should be used. After the nurse has poured out the appropriate amount for a feeding the supply of feeding should be *immediately* refrigerated. With the exception of an unopened can of a commercial product, all tube feedings that have been in the nursing unit refrigerator for *24 hours* are *discarded.*

If watery diarrhea occurs in a patient receiving a tube feeding that has been administered correctly, it may be due to the carbohydrate content. Excessive amounts of milk and therefore, lactose may cause diarrhea in some patients. The dietitian needs to design a tube feeding with a reduced amount or no lactose.

Excessive protein without adequate total fluid intake, especially in the older patient, can lead to dehydration and an elevated blood sodium level.[2] Therefore, when a tube feeding for an older patient provides more than 2 Gm. of protein per kilogram of body weight per day, the fluid intake and output should be carefully measured and recorded daily.

DIET THERAPY AFTER GASTROINTESTINAL SURGERY

Diet After Gastric and Duodenal Surgery. The patient whose gastric or duodenal ulcer does not respond to medical treatment is the most common candidate for gastric surgery. He may have a vagotomy and pyloroplasty or partial gastrectomy and vagotomy.

Principles of Postoperative Diet Therapy. There are various approaches to the feeding of patients after gastric surgery. Two principles appear to apply to all routines: (1) the restriction of the total volume of any feeding during the immediate postoperative period, with gradual increase as tolerated; and (2) the restriction of concentrated carbohydrate, particularly excessive amounts of sucrose, and in some situations, lactose.

After peristalsis has returned and the patient has tolerated clear fluids by mouth—beginning with 30 ml. per feeding on the first day and increasing to 60 ml. on the second day—the patient is offered 6 to 8 small feedings of soft or solid foods, neither very hot or very cold.[3] A small feeding in this situation may be limited to 3 or 4 ounces increasing gradually to 8 to 10 ounces. For example, 1 poached egg and 1 slice of buttered toast is approximately 3 ounces of food.

Fluids including milk may or may not be included in the small frequent feedings. After gastric surgery the contents of the stomach may pass into the small intestine before it is properly prepared and cause distention of the jejunum. When this happens the patient complains of nausea, cramps, diarrhea, light headedness and extreme weakness. This occurs 15 to 30 minutes after meals and is known as early dumping syndrome. It has been observed that this occurs less frequently if the patient avoids too much fluid with his meals.[4]

It has also been observed that excessive amounts of carbohydrate, especially sucrose and in some patients lactose, cause the early dumping syndrome. Therefore, sucrose is usually restricted in the diet of the patient immediately after gastric surgery. Candies, jams, jellies, frosted cakes and beverages sweetened with sucrose are not used. After recovery from gastric surgery many patients tolerate moderate amounts of sugar.

Some but not all individuals, after gastric surgery, develop lactose intolerance; therefore, some clinicians exclude milk after surgery.[5] However, other clinicians exclude milk only after the patient has experienced distention and diarrhea that is relieved by the exclusion of milk.

Nutritional Care of the Patient after Gastric Surgery

Table 26-3 lists the foods used after gastric surgery. These foods can be used in six to eight small meals. If any of the foods listed were not well tolerated by the patient before surgery, it is advisable to avoid them in the postoperative period.

Both the nurse and dietitian should observe these patients closely to check their food acceptance so that the volume of food in a meal can be increased as tolerated. Most patients after recovery from gastric surgery eventually eat normal amounts of food at a meal but they should be advised to increase the amount of food at each meal slowly after discharge.

One dietitian[6] who works closely with patients

[2] Gault, M. H., *et al.*: Ann. Intern. Med., 68:788, 1968.

[3] Malt, R. A.: Nutrition Today, 6:30, (June/July) 1971.

[4] Spiro, H. M.: Clinical Gastroenterology, New York, Macmillan, 1970.

[5] Malt: op. cit.

[6] Personal communication. The Ohio State University Hospital Dietary Department.

TABLE 26-3. FOODS USED AFTER
GASTRIC SURGERY

*Milk**

Eggs and Cheese
    Eggs—boiled, poached, scrambled or omelets

Meat, Fish, Poultry
    Any type—baked, broiled, boiled or in simple mixed dishes

Potato, Rice, Macaroni, Spaghetti, Noodles
    Plain or in simple mixed dishes

Bread, Crackers
    Enriched white bread and rolls toasted or plain in sandwiches
    Saltines and other plain crackers

Vegetables†
    Soft cooked vegetables

Fruits
    Cooked or well-drained canned fruit

Fat
    Butter, margarine, mayonnaise, bacon and cream cheese

Desserts
    Cooked or well-drained canned fruit
    Baked custard or plain vanilla pudding*

---

* If tolerated.
† Avoid gas-forming vegetables. These are cabbage, cauliflower, brussels sprouts, broccoli, cucumbers, onions, turnips, and radishes.

after gastric surgery tests each one's tolerance for concentrated carbohydrate before discharge. She serves a sweet such as cake, ice cream, or jelly with toast at one meal and observes the patient's tolerance carefully.

Late Dumping Syndrome or Postgastrectomy Hypoglycemia

A few patients develop severe dumping syndrome after gastric surgery. After taking sugar by mouth they have an elevated blood glucose level (hyperglycemia). This is followed by a precipitous drop in blood sugar to below normal levels (hypoglycemia) at which time the patient is dizzy, feels faint, and is nauseated. These patients usually have diarrhea, and lose weight. They find it difficult to maintain a normal weight status.

A high-protein, high-fat, low-carbohydrate diet is usually well tolerated by these patients. One diet plan[7] that has been used successfully contains

---

[7] Spiro: op. cit.

20 meat exchanges, 20 fat exchanges, 4 bread exchanges, 3 fruit exchanges and 2 vegetable exchanges (see Chap. 20). This food is served in six meals without fluids. One cup of coffee or tea with 40 percent cream is served 1 hour before breakfast, lunch and dinner. If possible, medications requiring water should also be given 1 hour before meals.

The dietitian plans the diet with these patients daily and the nurse should report to her any symptoms of the dumping syndrome the patient may have.

After the severe symptoms of the syndrome are controlled, individual patients may tolerate an increase in complex carbohydrate such as bread, potatoes and other starches but may need to avoid using sugar in any form. These individuals may also be lactose-intolerant and need to exclude all milk from their diets.

Bowel Surgery

Postoperative Nutritional Care. Many patients require surgery in other sections of the gastrointestinal tract. This may be surgery in the esophagus, small or large bowel resections, hemorrhoidectomy, or an ileostomy or colostomy may be required.

Postoperatively these patients usually are given a residue-restricted diet. They progress from a minimal to a moderate residue diet. (See the residue-restricted diet plans in Table 25-6 in Chap. 25.)

Most patients with colostomies are able before long to return to their regular food practices, provided that these are adequate for their nutritional needs. They should omit foods that were not well tolerated before surgery, but no food is contraindicated once the patient has recovered from the operation.

The ileostomy patient may present a special problem. If a significant portion of the terminal ileum has been removed there is a decrease in vitamin B_{12} absorption because it is absorbed in the terminal ileum. In this case vitamin B_{12} may need to be given parenterally. After recovery from surgery, the ileostomy patient is able to tolerate a regular diet although he may be advised to avoid excessive roughage which has in some patients obstructed the stoma.

Short Bowel Syndrome. In some situations a large portion of the ileum may be removed at surgery. Because of a decrease in the amount of absorptive surface these individuals often have difficulty maintaining a reasonable nutritional status. Some of these patients respond to a diet of small frequent feedings high in protein and carbohydrate and relatively low (less than 100 Gm.) in fat. Medium-chain triglycerides[8] (fatty acids of 12 or less carbons) have been used in these diets to supply calories but in general the results have not been satisfactory.

Recently a "space diet" or an elemental diet has been used in severe cases. This is a mixture of protein hydrolysates and other partially digested nutrients[9] supplemented with minerals and vitamins to provide a complete diet. The nutrients, primarily protein and carbohydrate, are partially digested and therefore, more readily absorbed in the terminal duodenum and jejunum. The product comes in powdered form and six servings dissolved in water provide 1,800 calories and adequate protein and carbohydrate.

NUTRITION FOLLOWING BURNS

Patients with extensive burns present nutritional problems much more far-reaching even than those who have undergone major surgery. As a result of the stress reaction there is massive loss of fluids and electrolytes, and serum proteins are lost by exudation from the burned areas. There is extensive tissue breakdown, lasting for periods of weeks as evidenced by tremendous losses of nitrogen and potassium in the urine. Such nitrogen losses continue for the first 30 days, then gradually diminish as healing takes place. There is also severe heat loss from the burn area, as shown by the rate of oxygen consumption. The energy losses may be as crucial to the ultimate survival of the patient as the loss of protein.

The first need is for fluid and electrolyte replacement, followed as quickly as possible by a diet markedly increased in protein and calories, with supplemental vitamins, particularly ascorbic acid to aid in wound healing and the B complex vitamins to meet the tremendously increased metabolic demands.

If flames or fumes have been inhaled, injuring the respiratory and the gastrointestinal tracts, or if there are burns about the mouth and the face, the oral route of feeding may at first be impossible. Oral or tube feeding may be further contraindicated, as badly burned patients frequently have gastrointestinal atony the first few days after injury.

The early part of treatment consists of the intravenous administration of plasma and whole blood, glucose and electrolyte solutions and solutions of protein hydrolysates. When the patient can take oral feeding he is given a high-calorie, high-protein diet or tube feeding. From 50 to 70 calories per kilogram and 2 to 4 Gm. of protein per kilogram of body weight meet the needs of the severely burned adult patient. Depending on the severity and extent of the burn and on the age, a child may require 70 to 100 calories per kilogram and 3 to 5 Gm. of protein per kilogram of body weight. Greatly increased amounts of ascorbic acid and the B vitamins and two times the allowance of the fat-soluble vitamins should be given as medication.

If tube feeding is used as the first oral feeding, excessive protein without adequate water intake, especially in children, should be avoided. (See Hazards of Tube Feedings in this chapter, page 270.) When food can be eaten in adequate quantities, between-meal feedings of high-calorie, high-protein beverages are used. Because the burn patient may develop gastric hemorrhage it is advisable to give tube feedings spread evenly over the 24-hour period or serve frequent small meals and between-meal beverages.

There is a tremendous need for supportive care of the severely burned patient by nurses, doctors, dietitians and all others with whom he comes in contact. The importance of the greatly increased need for food must be carefully explained to the patient. The diet particularly must be individualized to meet his needs and desires, and close cooperation by all who care for him is essential to meet the nutritional and emotional needs of the burned patient.

STUDY QUESTIONS AND ACTIVITIES

1. List the beverages used on a clear liquid diet. What beverages are used on a full liquid diet?

2. With the help of other members of the nursing team keep a record of the kinds and amounts of clear liquids consumed in a 24-hour period by a postoperative patient. Using Table 1 in Part Four estimate this patient's 24-hour calorie and nutrient intake. Was it nutritionally adequate for him?

3. Using Table 26-3 plan eight small meals for a patient who has had gastric surgery. Describe the size of serving of each food item.

4. What food may be poorly tolerated after gastric surgery? Why?

---

[8] Portagen and MCT Oil, Mead Johnson & Co., Evansville, Indiana.

[9] Vivonex, Vivonex Corporation, Mountain View, California.

5. What are some possible causes of diarrhea in the tube-fed patient? How may it be prevented?

6. What is the nurse's responsibility to the tube-fed patient? How is this accomplished in your hospital?

7. Obtain from the dietitian the kinds and nutrient composition of the high-calorie, high-protein beverages served to burn patients or any other patient receiving a similar beverage. Estimate how much these beverages cost per serving.

8. Which foods are generally gas-forming?

SUPPLEMENTARY READING ON SURGICAL NUTRITION; BURNS

Anderson, E. L.: Eating patterns before and after dentures. J. Am. Dietet. A., 58:421, (May) 1971.

Fason, M. F.: Controlling bacterial growth in tube feedings. Am. J. Nursing, 67:1246, 1967.

Gault, M. H., *et al.*: Hypernatremia, azotemia, and dehydration due to high protein tube feeding. Ann. Intern. Med., 68:788, 1968.

Gormican, A.: Prepackaged tube feedings. Hospitals, 44:58, (Sept. 1) 1970.

Grant, J. A. N., *et al.*: Parenteral hyperalimentation. Am. J. Nursing, 69:2393, 1969.

Malt, R. A.: Keep it simple. Nutrition Today, 6:30, (May/June) 1971.

Morgan, A., Filler, R. M., and Moore, F. D.: Surgical nutrition. Med. Clin. of N. Am., 54:1363, 1970.

Secor, S. M.: Colostomy rehabilitation. Am. J. Nursing, 70:2400, 1970.

Shatz, B., *et al.*: Medical and surgical aspects of hiatus hernia. JAMA, 214:125, 1970.

Tarsitano, J. J., *et al.*: Nursing care after oral surgery. Am. J. Nursing, 69:1493, 1969.

For further references see Bibliography in Part Four.

Special Problems

Allergy · Anemia · Arthritis and Gout · Constipation
Diet-Medication Interrelationships · Hyperthyroidism · Hypoglycemia

ALLERGY

Allergic reactions to foods occur in both children and adults. The protein component of a food is considered to be the causative factor in food allergy, even though foods that cause an allergic reaction may vary widely in protein content. Sensitivity to a food such as honey is explained as due to the associated protein in the pollen grains mixed in the honey, for it has been shown that very minute amounts of a given protein may cause an allergic reaction.

Among the common allergy-producing foods, particularly in children, are oranges, milk, eggs and sometimes wheat. Other common food allergens are fish and shellfish, chocolate, tomatoes, and strawberries. It has been found that members of the same botanic family may have a similar allergic effect. Lemons and grapefruit are likely to cause a reaction if oranges are allergenic. Likewise, if cabbage gives rise to an allergic reaction, so may broccoli, brussels sprouts and cauliflower.

Food allergy is much more common in infants and young children than in adults and is often more severe. In some instances, providing an adequate intake of calories and nutrients to support normal growth is a complex problem for the mother and the child. This is especially true when an infant or child is allergic to milk, wheat, or eggs, or a combination of two or all three of these.

Milk Allergy. The young infant may tolerate boiled or evaporated cow's milk because the heating has changed the protein. A variety of milk-free commercial infant formulas are available with either soybean or meat base.[1] Nutramigen made from partially hydrolyzed casein[2] is also given to the young infant with severe allergy. These preparations are equal in calorie and nutrient value with other commercial infant formulas and when used as directed are well tolerated and support adequate growth.

When solid foods are added to the infant's diet, care must be taken to avoid foods that have milk or nonfat dry milk added during processing. The mother must be advised to read labels carefully so that she can avoid these products. The companies that market baby foods make available to dietitians, nurses and physicians, lists of ingredients in their products.

If the child does not accept the special milks when he is older, it is necessary to supplement his diet with calcium pills and also with riboflavin. It has been observed that as these children get older they may tolerate small amounts of milk such as the bread made with 2 to 4 percent dry milk solids, and small amounts of milk used in food preparation such as cakes, cookies and puddings. But usually, they will not tolerate enough milk to meet their calcium needs. It may also be advisable for the adult who is allergic to milk to use calcium supplements daily.

Wheat Allergy. Because wheat bread and other products made with wheat cereal or flour are basic items in the American diet, the individual who is allergic to wheat finds he cannot eat many common foods. He must learn that baker's rye bread contains some wheat flour; that practically all hot breads, griddle cakes, pastries and crackers are made chiefly or partly from wheat products; that

---

[1] Meat Base, Gerber's, Fremont, Michigan.

[2] Nutramigen, Mead Johnson, Evansville, Indiana.

bran and gluten are wheat derivatives. Thickened gravies, cream soups and sauces are to be avoided unless thickened with corn or rice starch. Even meat dishes, such as meat loaf, hamburger, bologna and sausage may contain wheat flour or bread. All malted beverages must be avoided by the wheat-sensitive individual.

For a complete description of the omissions necessary in wheat sensitivity, see Chapter 25 under Gluten-Free Diet. For the patient allergic to wheat only, the restrictions on rye flour and oatmeal do not apply, but the remaining material proves helpful in insuring that all wheat products are eliminated from the diet.

Egg Allergy. The patient who is allergic to egg must investigate carefully all commercial products before partaking of them. He must remember that even the baking powder used in baked goods may contain dried egg white; that egg white may be used in the clearing of coffee and in the preparation of foaming beverages; and that most desserts, especially cakes, cookies, pastries, puddings and ice cream, contain eggs. These patients may also be allergic to chicken, which must then be omitted from the diet.

Allergy to Citrus Fruit. The major problem for these individuals is an adequate daily intake of vitamin C. Potatoes, other vegetables and fruit can provide an adequate intake although some individuals may take 50 mg. of ascorbic acid as medication each day to insure an adequate intake.

Resources for Patients. At the end of this chapter is a list of sources of recipes for allergy patients. These recipes may help them discover new dishes because allergy diets can become monotonous and uninteresting.

Elimination Test Diets. A series of diets, designed by A. H. Rowe, have been used to identify food allergies. A full description of these diets can be found in the 15th editon of Cooper's Nutrition in Health and Disease.[3]

ANEMIAS

Nutritional Anemia. Anemia in the hospitalized patient may be due to a previous inadequate nutrient intake especially of protein, iron, the B vitamins and vitamin C (see Chap. 6). The anemia in these patients responds to an adequate diet supplemented with vitamin and iron medications. Because iron medication may cause gastric irritation in some patients, it should be given after

meals. Before discharge these patients, usually adolescent girls and young mothers, should have diet counseling in order to avoid a recurrence of their problem.

Acute and Chronic Blood Loss. More frequently anemia in the hospitalized patient is due to acute or chronic blood loss. After treatment of the basic problem, these individuals should be observed carefully to insure that they consume adequate amounts of food to support blood cell production. Vitamin and mineral preparations are also required.

A special problem is the patient who has had numerous blood transfusions due to massive hemorrhage, or at surgery. Adult patients should consume at least 1½ to 2 Gm. protein per kilogram a day, adequate calories and all other nutrients to insure red cell production. The young child may need 2 to 3 Gm. protein per kilogram per day.

Pernicious Anemia. Pernicious anemia, which is due to the lack of a gastric factor required for the absorption of vitamin B_{12}, cannot be treated by diet alone. However, together with injections of B_{12}, a totally adequate nutrient intake is required for the production of normal red cells. These patients, many of whom are in the older age group, often require diet counseling to achieve an adequate nutrient intake (see Chap. 8).

ARTHRITIS AND GOUT

Arthritis. At present there is no known specific diet therapy for the prevention or treatment of arthritis. Many arthritics, however, become the victims of food faddists, self-appointed "arthritis experts" or quacks who advocate quick and miraculous cures with bizarre diet plans. The arthritic patient often brings these diet plans to the hospital and needs expert counseling to understand why the plans are not effective in the treatment of his disease.

Each patient with arthritis should be assisted to consume an adequate diet without excessive calories, especially if his activity is limited. Patients with severely crippled hands may need special equipment to feed themselves (see Chap. 28). The overweight patient benefits from a calorie-restricted diet. With weight loss he may experience some relief from his discomfort and pain and achieve an increase in activity.

Aspirin and steroids that are commonly used in the treatment of arthritis may, with long continued use, lead to gastric hemorrhage. Frequently the patient using either of these medications is advised to use a bland diet and antacids (see Chap. 25).

Gout. Gout, an abnormality of purine metabolism resulting in an elevated blood uric acid level,

[3] Mitchell, H. S., Rynbergen, H. J., Anderson, L., and Dibble, M.: Cooper's Nutrition in Health and Disease. ed. 15. Philadelphia, J. B. Lippincott, 1968.

TABLE 27-1. PURINE CONTENT OF FOODS
PER 100 GRAMS*

GROUP I (0-15 mg.)	GROUP II (50-150 mg.)	GROUP III (150-800 mg.)
Vegetables	Meats, poultry	Sweetbreads
Fruits	Fish	Anchovies
Milk	Sea food	Sardines
Cheese	Beans, dry	Liver
Eggs	Peas, dry	Kidney
Cereals, bread	Lentils	Meat extracts
Sugars, fats	Spinach	Brains

* Adapted from Turner, D.: Handbook of Diet Therapy, ed. 5, Chicago, University of Chicago Press, 1971.

may produce a condition resembling arthritis. Purines are obtained from ingested food and from the catabolism of body protein. In the past a purine-restricted diet was used as part of the treatment of gout but it is seldom used routinely today. In the purine-restricted diet, all foods in Group III in Table 27-1, Purine Content of Foods, were excluded and only limited amounts of those in Group II were used.

Today, some physicians restrict foods that are very high in purine content such as liver, kidney, brains and sweet breads. Patients with gout should be cautioned about fasting, whether it is to lose weight or when on an alcoholic spree, because it has been observed that fasting, even for 1 or 2 days, leads to an increase in blood uric acid.

CONSTIPATION

Constipation is a common disturbance of the digestive tract. In the hospitalized patient it may be a symptom of dehydration or especially of disease in the large bowel, or it may be due to dietary practices. Care must be taken to identify the cause before therapy is undertaken because the diet therapy for uncomplicated constipation—an increased intake of roughage—is contraindicated if there is disease in the large bowel.

There is considerable confusion as to what is meant by the term, constipation. Although a daily bowel movement has been stressed as desirable, there are many people for whom an evacuation every other day or even every third day is normal. Moreover, evacuation may occur regularly until an emotional upset occurs, in which case there may either be an increased number of bowel movements, almost a diarrhea, or retention of the feces for a day or two, resembling constipation. The matter usually straightens itself out when the strain is relieved. However, if the person becomes anxious when no daily bowel movement occurs

and begins to resort to cathartics or enemas, a vicious pattern is set up, and it may be difficult to effect a return to normal habits.

Chronic constipation may be due to the individual's dietary and living habits. Insufficient rest, hurried, irregular meals, a food intake that does not meet the nutritional needs of the body, and too sedentary a life all may contribute to poor bowel function. The problem here is to help the patient to accept a more regular mode of living, including a diet that meets all his nutritive requirements and a reasonable amount of exercise.

Elderly patients may suffer from constipation because muscle tone is relaxed, the dietary intake is inadequate for nutritional needs, and activity is diminished.

Dietary Treatment. In most cases of so-called constipation, a normal diet (see Chap. 10) containing roughage in the form of fresh and cooked fruit and vegetables and including whole-grain bread and cereals provides sufficient bulk to maintain regular bowel evacuation. Where such regularity needs to be reestablished—for instance, following an illness in which the mobility of the patient has been greatly limited—the addition of stewed fruit and of fruit juices to the ordinary diet is found helpful. Prune juice, particularly, taken at bedtime or the first thing in the morning, is usually effective.

Elderly patients should not use foods with a high bran content for fear of impaction. Cooked fruits and vegetables are often better tolerated by the older patient than raw ones, except for bananas.

Immobilized patients, either in a cast or for other reasons, may need help in maintaining regular bowel habits. For such patients the generous inclusion of stewed fruit and stewed fruit juices, especially prune juice, in a well-balanced diet may be all that is necessary to prevent constipation and straining. The patient receiving stool softeners also requires a well-balanced diet with generous amounts of fruit and fruit juice.

DIET-MEDICATION INTERRELATIONSHIPS

A variety of commonly used medications can have an effect on the nutritional status of patients. Some medications cause gastric distress, nausea, vomiting and diarrhea that can lead to a decrease in food intake or a decrease in nutrient absorption. Others may interfere with nutrient absorption from the gastrointestinal tract or with nutrient utilization at the cellular level.

TABLE 27-2. How Various Types of
Medications Affect Nutritional Status*

MEDICATION	NUTRITIONAL EFFECT
Barbiturates and anticonvulsants	Antivitamin action on folic acid
Cancer chemotherapy	Antivitamin action on folic acid
Corticosteroids	Decrease glucose tolerance Decrease in muscle protein Increase in liver fat
Diuretics	Potassium loss
Salicylates and steroids	Possible gastric hemorrhage

* Adapted from Christakis, G., and Miridjanian: J. Am.
Dietet. A., 52:21, 1968.

Salicylates—common aspirin—and the corticosteroids can cause gastric hemorrhage. Corticosteroids also have an effect on electrolyte balance and promote negative nitrogen balance and a decreased glucose tolerance.

The long term use of diuretics in the treatment of cardiac disease can lead to potassium deficiency, especially the thiazide (Diuril) and furosemide (Lasix) ones. Patients using these diuretics may be given potassium medication and be advised to

TABLE 27-3. Mechanisms by Which
Antibiotics Affect Nutritional Status*

Direct action on GI tract	Glossitis, stomatitis, nausea, diarrhea . . . decrease in appetite
Metabolic link with certain nutrients	
Tetracycline	Combines with folic acid
Isoniazid	Combines with B_6
Chloramphenicol	Decreases protein synthesis
Malabsorption syndrome	
Neomycin	Decreases carotene, B_{12}, glucose, cholesterol, fat absorption
Effect on stool	Increase in volume, undigested food, frequency, fibrous material

* Adapted from Christakis, G., and Miridjanian: J. Am.
Dietet. A., 52:21, 1968.

drink fruit juices high in potassium. Other diuretics do not promote potassium deficiency and, therefore, potassium supplements are not given.

Certain medications act as vitamin antagonists. Barbiturates, anticonvulsants and chemotherapeutic agents used in the treatment of cancer are antagonists of folic acid, a B vitamin (see Table 27-2). Every effort should be made to assist patients receiving these medications to consume an adequate diet. In some situations vitamin preparations are given with the medication.

Antibiotics have various effects on nutritional status (Table 27-3). They may cause nausea, vomiting, malabsorption or act as a vitamin antagonist. Tetracycline is an antagonist of folic acid and isoniazid, used in the treatment of tuberculosis, is an antagonist of pyridoxine (vitamin B_6). Pyridoxine is given to patients on isoniazid therapy.

Mono-amine oxidase inhibitors (Parnate) used in the treatment of depressed patients is a special case of food-medication interrelationship. It has been observed that if patients receiving mono-amine oxidase inhibitors consume foods rich in tyramine (a form of phenylalanine), headache, diarrhea, high blood pressure, and even death can occur. Foods rich in tyramine, which are excluded from the diets of these patients, are listed in Table 27-4. Although yeast is high in tyramine, bread

TABLE 27-4. Foods Rich in Tyramine*

Dairy Products	*Meats*
Yogurt	Liver
Aged Cheeses	Game
Cheddar	Dried fish
Gruyere	Herring
Stilton	Cod
Emmentaler	Caplin
Brie	Pickled Herring
Camembert	*Vegetables*
Gouda	Italian Broad Beans with
Mozzarella	Pods (fava beans)
Parmesan	
Provolone	*Others*
Romano	Vanilla
Roquefort	Chocolate
Alcoholic Beverages	Yeast and Yeast Extracts
Beer and Ale	Soya Sauce
Wine	
Chianti	
Sherry	
Riesling	
Sauterne	

* Adapted from Sen, J. P.: J. Food Science, 34:22, 1969.

made with yeast is not excluded from the diet unless symptoms occur.

HYPERTHYROIDISM

The patient with untreated hyperthyroidism, a condition characterized by excessive secretion of the hormone thyroxine that regulates metabolism, experiences hunger and weight loss. Medical or surgical treatment reduces the hypermetabolic state. However, before treatment can effect this change, these patients may require 4,000 to 5,000 calories a day (adequate in all nutrients) to meet their metabolic needs and prevent further weight loss. Supplementary vitamins and minerals may be prescribed, and all stimulants such as tea, coffee, alcohol and tobacco are limited or omitted.

In addition to regular meal service sizable snacks of sandwiches and other items should be available to the hospitalized patients at their request to avoid hunger. In the event they require food at 2:00 or 3:00 a.m., and if no food is available in the nursing unit, sandwiches and candy from the vending machines for employees can be used.

HYPOGLYCEMIA

Functional hypoglycemia without demonstrable organic disease may occur in adults. The symptoms of an attack are almost identical with those produced by an overdose of insulin and are due to a low blood sugar. There is weakness, trembling, sweating and extreme hunger. In severe cases there may be convulsions, hysterical symptoms and, eventually, unconsciousness. The attacks do not occur in the fasting state. They are caused by overstimulation of the pancreas resulting in the production of excess insulin following a meal, particularly one high in quickly digested and absorbed carbohydrate. Abdominal discomfort, which is also characteristic, is sometimes ascribed to peptic ulcer because the symptoms are similar.

Dietary Treatment. The objective of dietary treatment is to prevent a marked rise in the blood sugar that stimulates the pancreas to overproduce insulin. For this reason the individual must avoid the quickly digested sugars and limit other carbohydrate foods. The more slowly digested proteins and fats may be ingested freely.

The diet should contain from 120 to 150 Gm. of protein, from 75 to 100 Gm. of carbohydrate, and sufficient fat to meet caloric requirements. No candy, sugar, jellies, jams, desserts and soft drinks containing sugar should be eaten. Saccharin may be substituted for sugar. The low carbohydrate vegetables and fruits (see Chap. 20), and limited quantities of bread, cereal and potatoes should provide the carbohydrate of the diet. A generous serving of meat, fish, fowl, eggs or cheese must be included at each meal. Because milk contains the sugar lactose, it must be limited to a pint a day in the adult. Butter or margarine, cream, bacon, mayonnnaise and other oil dressing and meat fats supply the fat needed for calories. It is best to divide the food intake into five to eight meals a day. The patient may find it useful to carry crackers and a cube of cheese with him to control attacks if they are frequent.

STUDY QUESTIONS AND ACTIVITIES

1. What are some common allergenic foods?
2. Using the producers' literature, make a list of popular baby foods that cannot be fed to an infant who is allergic to cow's milk.
3. Plan an inexpensive dinner menu for a family of four—two adults and two children—with one child who is allergic to wheat.
4. At time of discharge from the obstetrical unit, Mrs. A is advised to be sure to eat high iron foods. She dislikes liver in any form. What foods would you suggest she eat to supply an adequate daily intake of iron? (See Chap. 6.)
5. Why may a patient who needs large doses of aspirin also be taking an antacid medication?
6. What would you suggest to an elderly patient who complains of constipation and has been found to be free of disease of the bowel?

SUPPLEMENTARY READING ON SPECIAL PROBLEMS

Christakis, G., and Miridjanian, A.: Diets, drugs, and their interrelationships. J. Am. Dietet. A., 52:21, 1968.

Ellis, R. S.: Allergic rhinitis—seasonal and nonseasonal. Geriatrics, 25:113, 1970.

Frier, S., *et al.*: Intolerance to milk protein. J. Pediat., 75:623, 1969.

Headache, tyramine, serotonin and migrane. Nutr. Rev., 26:40, 1968.

Pearson, H. A., *et al.*: Anemia related to age: study of a community of young black Americans. JAMA, 215:1982, 1971.

Sen, N. P.: Analysis and significance of tyramine in foods. J. Food Science, 34:29, 1969.

Traut, E. F., and Thrift, C. B.: Obesity in athritis: related factors: dietary therapy. J. Am. Geriat. Soc., 17:710, 1969.

Waxman, S., *et al.*: Drugs, toxins and dietary amino acids affecting vitamin B_{12} or folic acid absorption or utilization. Am. J. Med., 48:599, 1970.

White, H. S.: Iron deficiency in young women. Am. J. Public Health, 60:659, 1970.

SOURCES OF RECIPES: ALLERGY DIETS

Allergy Recipes ($1.00). American Dietetic Association, 620 N. Michigan Avenue, Chicago, Illinois 60611.

Allergy Recipes from the Blue Flame Kitchen ($.50). Metropolitan Utilities District, 1723 Harney Street, Omaha, Nebraska 68102.

Baking for People with Food Allergies ($.10). Superintendent of Documents, U.S. Government Printing Office, Washington, D.C. 20402.

Celiac Disease Recipes ($1.25). Hospital for Sick Children, 555 University, Toronto 5, Ontario, Canada.

Cooking with Imagination for Special Diets. Grocery Store Products Company, West Chester, Pennsylvania.

Easy, Appealing Milk-Free Recipes. Mead-Johnson and Company, Evansville, Indiana 47221.

Great Recipes for Allergy Diets ($.50), and Helps for Allergics ($.10). Good Housekeeping Institute, 959 Eighth Avenue, New York, New York 10019.

Good Recipes to Brighten the Allergy Diet. Best Foods, Division of Corn Products Company, 10 E. 56th Street, New York, New York 10022.

Low Gluten Diet with Tested Recipes ($1.00). Arthur B. French, M.D., Clinical Research Unit, W 4644 University Hospital, Ann Arbor, Michigan 48104.

Recipes for the Allergic Individual. Kannengiesser and Company, 76 Ninth Avenue, New York, New York 10011.

Recipes for Using Soya Bean Powder. Fearn Soya Foods, 1206 N. 31st Avenue, Melrose Park, Illinois 60160.

For further references see Bibliography in Part Four.

Feeding the Handicapped

28

Skills Necessary for Self-Feeding • Motor Performance Problems
Special Nutritional Care Problems • Special Programs

INTRODUCTION

Patients with physical handicaps may have difficulty achieving an adequate nutrient intake because they may be unable to feed themselves; or they may be limited in their ability or unable to suck, bite, chew, or swallow fluids and/or foods. Severe arthritis may affect the joints of the fingers, the elbow and the shoulder to such an extent that the adult patient cannot feed himself; or affect the jaw so that he may even have difficulty biting and chewing. Some patients after a cerebral vascular accident (stroke) may be unable to swallow clear liquids but may be able to swallow semisolids such as "soupy" mashed potatoes or soft ice cream.

Infants and children with neuromuscular defects such as cerebral palsy may present numerous problems that require carefully planned and consistently implemented feeding training programs in order to achieve their potential for self-feeding. Until a cleft palate with or without a cleft lip is repaired surgically an infant with this congenital anomaly has special feeding problems.

It is necessary to assess the individual needs of each handicapped patient when determining the method of feeding and/or feeding training to be used to assist him in achieving his potential. There are two major aspects of this assessment: (1) the individual's nutritional needs; and (2) his physi-

cal capacity. In assessing his nutritional needs the patient's age, height, weight, activity level and any disease requiring diet modification must be identified. His physical capacity must be evaluated to set reasonable goals for his self-feeding or feeding training program. In certain situations special attention must be given to the consistency of food required to overcome the difficulty.

The skills necessary for self-feeding: coping with problems of positioning, sucking, biting, chewing and swallowing; adaptive equipment; selected nutritional care problems; and special programs for the handicapped are discussed in the following sections of this chapter. The nutritional needs of infants, children and adults are presented in other chapters and are not repeated here.

SKILLS NECESSARY FOR SELF-FEEDING

Table 28-1 lists the progressive levels of motor performance necessary for self-feeding. Although it is not necessary that all skills at each level be completely mastered before progressing to the next one, some evidence of skill or readiness is necessary at all levels if self-feeding is to be achieved. These are the developmental tasks the normal infant and young child goes through in achieving the ability to feed himself, and the skills the normal individual uses throughout life.

The neurologically handicapped infant may present problems in progressing to one or more levels in sequence, while the recently handicapped adult may lose his ability to perform at one or more levels. Suggestions for coping with the prob-

This chapter was written in cooperation with Nancy D. Herrick, M.S., M.P.H., Chief of Nutrition, and Marian F. Chase, M.S., L.P.T., Chief of Physical Therapy, Nisonger Center, The Ohio State University Affiliated Center for Mental Retardation and Developmental Defects.

TABLE 28-1. PROGRESSIVE LEVELS OF MOTOR
SKILLS NECESSARY FOR SELF-FEEDING

Sucking

Sitting and head balance

Upper extremity control sufficient to bring hand
  to mouth

Cup and utensil grasp

Ability to sip and take liquids from cup

Ability to take food from spoon with lips

Ability to bite, chew and swallow with a minimum
  of drooling

lems of positioning, sucking, biting, chewing, and
swallowing are presented in the next section.

MOTOR PERFORMANCE PROBLEMS
Positioning

The normal feeding position for humans is upright and requires the ability to sit up and control
the balance of the head. Proper positioning of
the handicapped patient should be based on the
assessment of his ability to hold himself upright.
Aspiration of fluids or food into the bronchi can
be hazardous to the individual who cannot maintain head balance.

Patients with limited ability to support the
trunk may be helped to sit at the table by stabilizing the trunk with a binder or strap secured at the
pelvis. The patient is also more stable if his feet
are firmly positioned flat on the floor or on a foot
stool. Figure 28-1 illustrates this method. If the
patient is in a wheelchair, the foot rest is used.
This method permits the patient to concentrate
on his food rather than worrying about falling off
his chair. It also eliminates constricting the chest
or "hanging" which happens frequently when a
binder is placed under the arms.

If the patient is seated in an armchair, pillows
at each side and a head rest may be used for
stabilization. A lap board, or over-bed table
adjusted to the appropriate height, is useful to
the patient in a wheelchair or armchair. When a
lap board is used it is advisable to have it equipped

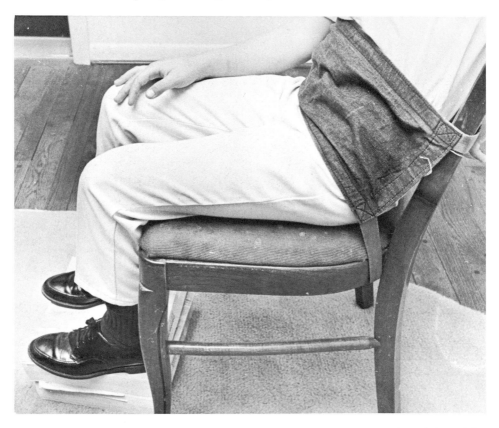

FIG. 28-1. A child with poor trunk control stabilized by a binder at the pelvis and feet
supported. (Note use of telephone directories as a foot stool.)

with a raised edge so that the patient with poor motor skills is not frustrated by having dishes and other equipment slide off the board onto the floor. For the small child, a high chair is often appropriate because of the protection it offers on all four sides. For the larger child it is helpful to use a cutout table with a strap placed across the back of the chair to hold him close to the table.

Sucking—Straw Drinking

The problems encountered in the neurologically handicapped infant may include limitation in the ability to suck. Initially the mother is taught to stroke the infant's cheek and stimulate the oral area to elicit the sucking reflex. However, the infant may need to be tube fed during the first months to insure adequate fluid, electrolyte and nutrient intake. Stimulation and some oral feed-ing may be done even though tube feeding is necessary.

Straw drinking, a form of sucking, may be used with the neurologically handicapped child or the handicapped adult. It aids in the development of the facial and oral musculature, and with breath control—an important aspect of speech develop-ment. Also, many severely involved patients are helped to obtain an adequate fluid intake through straw drinking.

Initially a short straw with a small diameter should be used. The patient should be instructed to take one sip at a time until he is able to suck continuously. If he has difficulty holding his lips closed around the straw, light pressure may be applied with the fingers. Figure 28-2 illustrates this method in the feeding training program for a child. Flex straws (Fig. 28-2) may be helpful

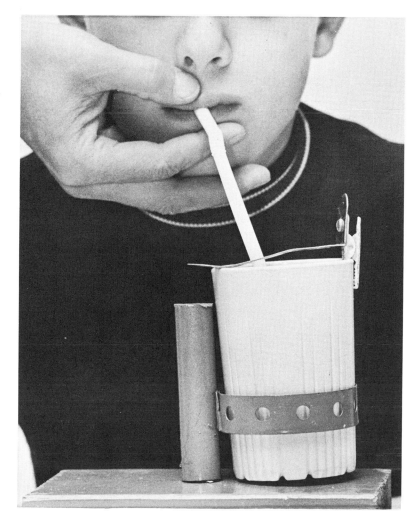

FIG. 28-2. Applying light pressure to lips to help patient develop ability to drink through straw. Note adap-tive cup holder and straw holder.

in some situations. For the severely involved patient a plastic straw with an inch or two of rubber tubing attached to the mouth end is often helpful because it prevents crushing the straw (see Fig. 28-3). As the patient progresses in his ability to suck through the straw the length and diameter may be increased. This allows him to take thicker fluids that usually contain more calories and nutrients than thinner fluids.

Biting, Chewing and Swallowing

The patient who has the ability to bite and chew, or who can reestablish this ability, can be offered food of various texture and, therefore, a more acceptable diet. Patients with neurological diseases who have difficulty biting and chewing and, at the same time, can take food without choking, should be encouraged to bite off small amounts of soft or semisolid foods; for example: a small bite of mashed potato or a well-cooked carrot strip. The food should be directed to alternate sides of the mouth and the patient encouraged to use his tongue to move the food in his mouth. The patient should chew and swallow each bite before he takes more food. Food may become lodged between the teeth and inside of the cheeks in patients with facial paralysis or a very high palate and it may become necessary to use a finger to dislodge it.

It is obvious that any patient who is unable to

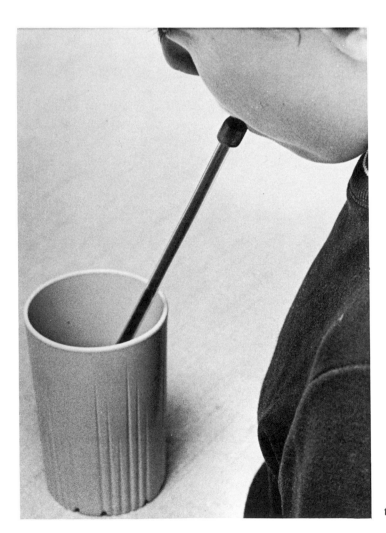

FIG. 28-3. Plastic straw with rubber tip to prevent crushing end of straw.

swallow cannot be offered fluids or foods by mouth and must be tube fed (see Chap. 26). On the other hand, these patients need to be evaluated continuously so that if there is any indication that the ability to swallow is developing or has been reestablished he is offered fluids and food by mouth. One indication of this would be his ability to swallow his saliva.

Adaptive Equipment

Adaptive equipment may be used in the beginning of any feeding training program. However, the objective is to move from adaptive equipment to independent skill as soon as possible if the situation permits. For the quadraplegic adult or the neurologically handicapped child, adaptive equipment may be a part of his life if he is to achieve and maintain some degree of self-feeding skills. Figure 28-4 shows the device a neurologically handicapped child might need to help him feed himself.

There are many adaptive devices on the market today to help those who need them. However, many devices can be constructed easily in the hospital or home to fit the needs of the individual. The basic areas in which adaptive devices are most often required are: difficulty in sucking which has been discussed previously, poor grasp, poor upper extremity strength, and poor coordination of hand-to-mouth movements.

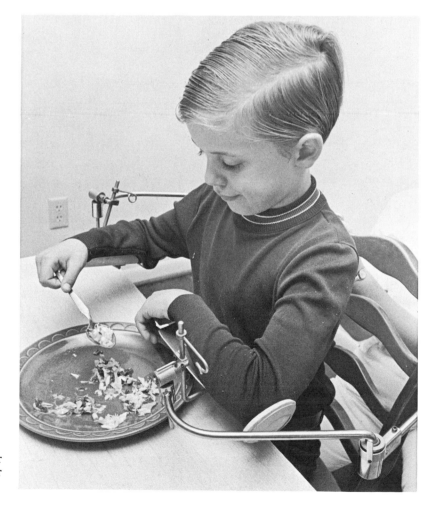

Fig. 28-4. Swivel feeder for patient with very weak upper extremities.

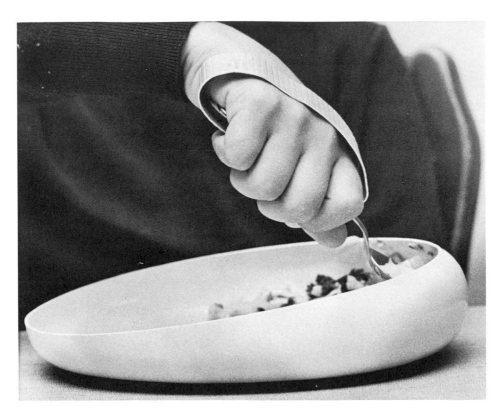

FIG. 28-5. Spoon with loop handle and scoop guard plate.

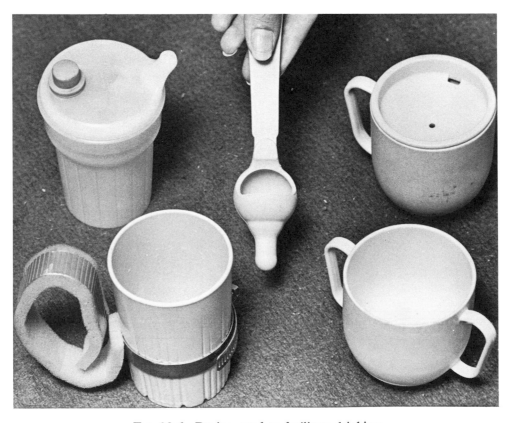

FIG. 28-6. Devices used to facilitate drinking.

Poor grasp may be aided by the use of a "loop handle" on a spoon or fork (see Fig. 28-5). The use of the fork is encouraged, especially if hand-to-mouth coordination is good, because it is often easier to "spear" bits of food than get them on a spoon. Handles that are built up with tape, sponge or foam rubber, wood or other materials to fit the patients' needs are effective and relatively inexpensive to replace when they become soiled. Cups with handles on both sides (bouillon cups) or small, lightweight cups can be more easily grasped with both hands (see Fig. 28-6).

A patient with poor upper extremity strength may be helped by raising the height of the table. Swivel feeders as shown in Figure 28-4 may be used with patients who have very weak upper extremities.

The scoop plate (see Fig. 28-5) or the plate with a guard attached to one side, can be used with the patient with poor coordination in the upper extremities. A piece of wet foam rubber under the plate, or a hole in a lap board cut to fit a plate, keeps the dish from sliding. Plates with suction cups attached to the underside are also available. As illustrated in Figure 28-2 cup holders and straw holders stabilize these items.

Table 28-2 lists the most common handicapping conditions and the feeding disability most frequently encountered by these patients.

TABLE 28-2. HANDICAPPING CONDITIONS AND FEEDING DISABILITIES

HANDICAPPING CONDITIONS	FEEDING DISABILITIES				
	INABILITY TO SUCK, CLOSE LIPS	INABILITY TO BITE, CHEW, SWALLOW	POOR GRASP	POOR HAND-MOUTH COORDINATION	POOR TRUNK AND UPPER EXTREMITIES CONTROL
Cardio-Vascular Accident					
with facial paralysis	+	+		+	
with hemiplegia on dominant side	+	+	+	+	+
Cerebral Palsy					
athetoid type	+	+	+	+	+
ataxic type			+ −	+	+
spastic type				+ −	+
Traumatic Spinal Cord Injury					
paraplegia					
quadraplegia			+	+	+
Muscular Dystrophy					
Duchenne's			+	+	+
fascio-scapular-humeral	+ +	+	+	+	+
Multiple Sclerosis	+	+	+	+	+
Parkinson's Disease	+	+	+	+	+
Myasthenia Gravis			+	+	+
Rheumatoid Arthritis			+	+	+ −
Severe and Profound Mental Retardation	+	+	+	+	+

+ Moderate
++ Severe
+− Varies

SPECIAL NUTRITIONAL CARE PROBLEMS

Fluid Intake

The handicapped patient, especially those who can take only sips of fluids slowly by mouth, present a special problem. Care must be taken that he does not become dehydrated or become overhydrated if he is also receiving intravenous fluids. Accurate records of his fluid intake and output are a very important part of his nursing care plan. If the patient cannot help himself he must be offered fluids frequently. If he can manage himself care must be taken that his glass, cup or an adapted drinking device is conveniently placed within his reach. Adequate fluid intake is important in the prevention of urinary tract infection and, for some patients, the prevention of kidney stones.

Consistency of Food

Two concerns should be kept in mind regarding the consistency of food offered the handicapped patient: (1) its nutritional value and (2) the progression from semiliquid to more solid foods as the patient progresses.

Generally, it is difficult to keep a reasonable proportion of protein, fat and carbohydrate in semiliquid diets (see tube feeding in Chap. 26). Also if milk is used extensively as a beverage, with mashed potatoes and cereals, and in other foods, the daily calcium intake may be excessive while the iron intake may be inadequate. At this time the relationship of calcium intake to the formation of kidney stones in the relatively immobile patient is not well understood but, it is probably advisable that daily calcium intake not exceed the NRC's Recommended Dietary Allowance (see Chap. 10).

Continuous evaluation of a patient's progress is necessary if he is to be helped to progress from semisolid to solid foods when ready. It has been observed that individuals may not progress because they are not encouraged and assisted to try more solid foods.

Weight Control

Weight control is a very important aspect of the nutritional care of the handicapped patient. Persons with paralysis or other motor dysfunctions that permanently limit physical activity require fewer calories to meet their energy needs. In these situations the diet pattern must be carefully planned so that adequate nutrients, without excessive calories, are consumed each day. The patient who is obese when he acquires his handicapping condition should be helped to lose weight for his own benefit and for the benefit of those who give him physical care.

Constipation

Persons with paralysis or hypotonia often become constipated due to immobility and a diet low in roughage. Regular bowel movements may be encouraged through promoting as much physical movement as possible and a diet with adequate roughage (see Chap. 27).

SPECIAL PROGRAMS

Feeding Training of the Neurologically Handicapped Infant

In a number of centers in the United States, intensive study of the training of the neurologically handicapped infant and child is in progress to assist these children in developing their fullest potential for participation in the activities of daily living. The feeding training aspect of this program is concerned not only with the nutritional needs of these children but also with the development of self-feeding skills, so they may eat with their families at home and with others when away from home.

Careful study of each stage in the self-feeding process is being done. For example, the elements of feeding oneself with a spoon are: grasping the spoon; getting food onto it; lifting the spoon to the mouth; placing the spoon in the mouth; taking the food from the spoon with the lips; removing the spoon from the mouth; returning it to the plate; and chewing and swallowing the food.

It has been observed that using the fingers is the best way to begin the program. Peanut butter, pudding or mashed potatoes on the fingers often encourages hand-to-mouth action. When spoon feeding is introduced foods which stick to the spoon are used such as cooked cereal, mashed potatoes or mashed carrots, and thick puddings.

The staffs of these centers recognize that the key to success in the feeding training programs are repeating the activity, giving gentle yet consistent encouragement, giving only the required amount of help, and knowing when the child does not need assistance.

When the neurologically handicapped child who has been carefully trained to achieve his potential for self-feeding is admitted to a pediatric unit for an acute illness, nurses should seek the help of the mother so that he can maintain the skills he has acquired and not regress.

The Handicapped Homemaker

The homemaker who is handicapped can often perform her usual activities of meal preparation by using specialized equipment and methods. These activities can be programmed by an occupational therapist or through use of manuals such as the *Mealtime Manual for the Aged and Handicapped* by Klinger, *et al.*[1] or *Homemaking for the Handicapped* by May, *et al.*[2]

STUDY QUESTIONS

1. If you have not done so in a class in the fundamentals of nursing, have a classmate or friend feed you liquids and solids while you are lying on your back without your head raised. What difficulties do you encounter with sipping, chewing, and swallowing?

2. Feed or assist with the feeding of a patient recovering from a stroke. How long did it take?

---

[1] Klinger, J. L., *et al.*: Mealtime Manual for the Aged and Handicapped. New York, Simon & Schuster, 1970.

[2] May, E. E., *et al.*: Homemaking for the Handicapped. New York, Dodd, Mead & Co., 1966.

Did the patient consume a reasonable calorie and nutrient intake at this meal ($\frac{1}{4}$ to $\frac{1}{2}$ of his daily needs)?

3. Why is it more valuable to the other members of the health care team for you to record what the patient in question No. 2 ate than what he did not eat?

SUPPLEMENTARY READING

Committee on Children with Handicaps: The Pediatrician and the Child with Mental Retardation. Evanston, Ill., American Academy of Pediatrics, 1971.

Holser-Buehler, Patricia: The Blanchard method of feeding the cerebral palsied. Am. J. Occup. Ther., 20:1, 31, 1966.

Jernigan, A. K.: Diet for the stroke patient. Hospitals, 44:66, (June 16) 1970.

Klinger, J. L., *et al.*: Mealtime Manual for the Aged and Handicapped. New York, Simon & Schuster, 1970.

Zickefoose, M.: Feeding the child with a cleft palate. J. Am. Dietet. A., 36:129, 1960.

Zickefoose, M., and Frey, P. W.: Helping the disabled person to help himself to good nutrition. Hospitals, 37:91, 1963.

Nutrition in Diseases of Infancy and Childhood

29

The Acutely Ill Infant and Young Child · **Underfed and Overfed Children**
Epilepsy · **Malabsorption Syndromes** · **Inborn Errors of Metabolism**

INTRODUCTION

The infant or child admitted to a pediatric hospital or the pediatric unit of a general hospital may be acutely ill or have a birth defect or long-term illness. The majority of infants and children requiring hospitalization need a normal diet for age. This applies even to the acutely ill child after the treatment of the critical problem, such as the establishment of fluid and electrolyte balance, or to the child who has undergone surgery. Some of the children with a birth defect or long-term illness may need modifications in consistency or feeding methods such as the child with a cleft palate or the child with cerebral palsy. Other children may need modifications in nutrient intake such as a sodium-restricted diet for the child with a congenital anomaly of the heart or the restriction of phenylalanine, an essential amino acid, in phenylketonuria (PKU).

Normal diet for age is presented in Chapters 15 and 16 and is not reviewed in this chapter. The nurse is advised to study these chapters because the information also applies to the majority of hospitalized children in her care. The following topics are discussed in this chapter: the nutritional needs of the acutely ill infant or child; meals for the sick child in the home or hospital; the problems of the underfed or overfed child; and special problems of the nutritional care of the infant or child with a birth defect or long-term illness including inborn errors of metabolism such as PKU. The problems of the child with a neuromuscular impairment are discussed in Chapter 28, Feeding the Handicapped.

THE ACUTELY ILL INFANT OR YOUNG CHILD

Many infants and young children are admitted to the hospital today with an acute infection complicated by vomiting and diarrhea. The first need of these patients is fluids, glucose and electrolytes since moderate to severe dehydration in the infant or young child is life-threatening. Also, in the very young infant, severe dehydration and an elevated temperature may damage the developing nervous system. After reestablishing the fluid and electrolyte balance, the nutrient and calorie needs of each patient must be met to make up for his losses during the acute phase of his illness and to support his normal progress in growth and development.

The Infant 0 to 1 Year. The same principles that apply to tube feedings for the adult patient apply to formula feeding of the infant being treated for diarrhea and dehydration (see Chap. 26). These principles may also be applied to the infant recovering from major surgery. After reestablishing fluid and electrolyte balance with intravenous fluids, if necessary, the infant should be offered a glucose solution and then a dilute formula.

The dilute formula may be a commercial one containing 13 calories per ounce compared with the standard formulas that contain 20 calories per ounce (see Chap. 15). Or the infant may be offered skim milk containing 10 calories per ounce. If these dilute feedings are tolerated, the infant then progresses to a standard formula with 20 calories per ounce or, if needed, one with 24 calories per ounce.

In the past, boiled skim milk was offered to infants with diarrhea. This is no longer recommended because the boiling reduces the total water content of the milk, which results in an increase in the total amount of sodium and potassium per ounce. In the very young infant care must be taken to see that he gets only the amount of sodium and potassium his kidneys can handle— not too much or too little.

After severe diarrhea, some infants may not tolerate the lactose in milk for a short period. Therefore, a lactose free formula is offered these infants. Two lactose free formulas commonly used are Nutramigen* and Cho-Free†. Glucose or fructose is added to Cho-Free to provide 20 calories per ounce. The protein in both of these products is partially hydrolyzed (digested) and therefore, more readily absorbed by the gastrointestinal tract. Also, these formulas do not contain excessive amounts of sodium or potassium.

In addition to recording the total amount of fluid *taken* and *retained* at each feeding, it is strongly recommended that the calories per ounce in the feeding be recorded in the nursing notes. With the use of commercial formulas, this is not a difficult task since the calories per ounce are stated on each bottle. This information recorded in the nursing notes helps the physician make a quick estimate of the total calorie intake in a 24-hour period without referring back to the order sheet. He can then more readily correlate an infant's total calorie intake with daily weights and other information in evaluating progress. This system should also protect against giving an infant a dilute formula longer than necessary.

When an infant is also taking baby foods, the *kind* and *amount* should be recorded as precisely as possible. If dry infant cereals are used, the kind and amount of cereal and the kind and amount of fluid added to the cereal should be recorded separately. If there is any suspicion that an infant has an allergy to a food, it can be identified more easily if the kinds of food he is fed are recorded.

The guidelines for calorie and nutrient needs for the first year of life given in Chapter 15 can be used to assess the adequacy of an infant's feeding program during recovery from an acute illness. One hundred fifty ml. of fluid and 120 to 100 calories per kilogram per day can be used as a rough guide to the adequacy of the daily intake.

---

* Mead Johnson Laboratories, Evansville, Ind.
† Borden Co., Columbus, Ohio.

To make up for previous losses he may need more than the recommended calories and nutrients for his age. A critical evaluation of the daily weight gains and intake identifies these infants.

Frequently infants with mild infection and diarrhea are seen in the outpatient clinic or pediatrician's office. The infant is not admitted to the hospital and the mother is advised to offer her child Karo water with or without a specific amount of salt (NaCl) added. When the infant's diarrhea improves, she is advised to offer him skim milk. These mothers need precise directions and follow-up. Infants have been seen still on skim milk formula 2 weeks after recovery because the mother did not understand that she should resume the normal feeding program. Also, if the salt is not measured carefully and too much is given, the infant can become critically ill.

The Young Child 1 to 4 Years. Acute infection with diarrhea and dehydration is critical in this age group although not as devastating as in the infant unless accompanied by encephalitis or meningitis. Children 1 to 2 years of age who have previously been weaned to a cup may prefer to take fluids from a nursing bottle. Older children with elevated temperatures may more readily accept fluids other than milk.

In addition to water and milk, fruit juices, fruit drinks fortified with vitamin C, and carbonated beverages are commonly used to meet fluid needs. Some clinicians use cola syrups to supply glucose and potassium. Carbonated beverages are usually more acceptable to the yearling if the beverage is poured in advance of offering to the child to reduce the fizziness.

Before offering carbonated beverages to a child, it is well to check with the parents. They may not serve these beverages to the child at home and may not want them used in the hospital. Because there are various other fluids the child is familiar with and usually accepts, there is no reason why the parents' wishes cannot be met.

As these children recover they usually tolerate a soft or simple regular diet adequate to support the nutritional needs of their age group (see Chap. 15). Fluid and food intake, both in kind and amount, should be recorded after each feeding.

FEEDING THE HOSPITALIZED CHILD

It is recognized that when children are ill, they tend to regress to an earlier developmental level.

This is extensively covered in pediatric nursing textbooks and is not discussed in this book. Rather, some specifics about food and feeding are presented.

The sick child often finds it difficult to cope with new food experiences. Therefore, it is helpful if on admission or as soon as possible after admission the nurse or dietitian obtains from the mother of the young child or directly from the older child a list of the foods he likes. From experience with the children who enter a pediatric unit, the food served by the dietary department usually reflects these likes. This does not solve the problem because the methods of food preparation vary and the taste of a food prepared in the hospital may differ from the same dish prepared at home. Also, today the child may not be comparing the food served in the hospital with that served at home but with his past experiences eating away from home —at McDonald's or other fast-food service chains.

The size of a serving offered the child is also important. "Appetite poor" recorded in the nursing notes may mean that a child was served too much food. A serving of 4 ounces (120 ml.)

of soup and ½ a sandwich is adequate for many 2- to 3-year-olds while a 12-year-old boy may need a "man size" serving. Table 29-1, using the Exchange System, illustrates the amount of food needed in a day to meet the calorie needs of children 2 to 6 years old. It is shown that when this food is distributed in three meals and two or three between meal feedings the servings are small by adult standards.

Five or six 3- to 4-year-olds eating together is helpful for both the child and the staff. Children often eat better around a table with other children of the same age; also, it takes the time of only one staff member to help these children in a group compared with the number of staff required if the children are served in their rooms or at the bedside in a ward.

Finally, parents have rights. The mother who spends the day with her hospitalized child usually wants to contribute to his care. Choosing the food and feeding the child may be the only contribution she can make. This is especially true if the child has a terminal illness. These mothers may be demanding: they have a right to be demanding and their demands should be met if possible.

TABLE 29-1. DAILY AMOUNTS OF FOODS TO MEET CALORIE NEEDS OF
2- TO 6-YEAR-OLD CHILDREN

FOOD EXCHANGES	2 TO 3 YEARS		3 TO 4 YEARS		4 TO 6 YEARS	
	AMT.	CALORIES*	AMT.	CALORIES	AMT.	CALORIES
Milk	3 c.	510	3 c.	510	4 c.	680
Meat	1 oz.	75	2 oz.	150	2 oz.	150
Egg	1	75	1	75	1	75
Bread	4	280	4	280	5	350
Fruit	2 servings	80	2 servings	80	2 servings	80
Vegetables B	1 serving	35	1 serving	35	1 serving	35
Fat	2 tsp.	90	3 tsp.	135	3 tsp.	135
Dessert†	⅔ serving	100	1 serving	150	1 serving	150
Totals		1,245		1,415		1,655
NRC–RDA	1,250 Cals.		1,400 Cals.		1,600 Cals.	

* Exchange System. Chapter 20.
† Chocolate Pudding. Table 1, Part Four.

Fig. 29-1. Meals taste better when they are eaten in company with other children in the hospital. (Arkansas Children's Hospital, Little Rock, Arkansas)

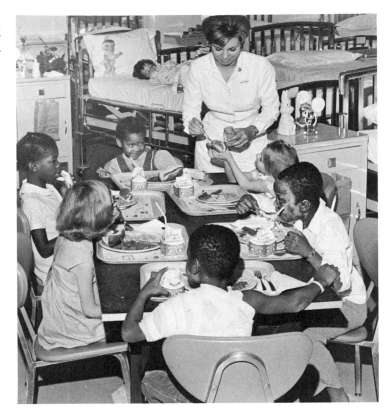

UNDERFED AND OVERFED CHILDREN

Growth Failure Due to Underfeeding. When the physician records an infant's or child's "failure-to-thrive" he is dealing with an unknown or unrecognized factor or factors. Many of these are being identified, such as inborn errors of metabolism discussed later in the chapter.

Other factors besides disease may be responsible for a child's failure-to-thrive. The problem of the severely growth-retarded infant, usually under 18 months of age, who has no disease or birth defect, has been called emotional, environmental or maternal deprivation. When these infants are admitted to the hospital they may be severely dehydrated due to infection and obviously malnourished. Some may even be marasmic. They may also be retarded in motor development and most of them take very little interest in their environment.

Bowlby[1] and others have shown that if the in-fant is to achieve the developmental milestones of the first year of life, there must be social interaction between the mother and infant as well as routine physical care. This applies to the infant's own mother or other caretaking persons. It has been observed that the infant with growth failure without disease has not experienced adequate mother-child interaction; and that the mothers of these infants are overburdened with their own personal problems and are unable to meet the physical or psycho-social needs of their infants. Whitten[2] and co-workers have shown that the physical growth failure of these infants is due to underfeeding and that the mothers are not aware that they are underfeeding them.

On admission to the hospital these infants require the same care as any acutely ill infant (see previous section on acutely ill infant). In addition, it is advisable that these infants be fed and played with by one caretaking person as frequently as possible within the staffing schedules of the nurs-

---

[1] Bowlby, J.: Attachment and Loss. Vol. I. New York, Basic Books, 1969.

[2] Whitten, F., *et al.*: JAMA, 209:1675, 1969.

ing unit. A volunteer, or a nursing student, with a particular interest in this problem may be willing to commit herself for 8 or 9 consecutive days to give intensive care to one of these infants and to help them achieve their developmental milestones.

The future of these children depends on two factors: (1) the age at which the underfeeding occurs; and (2) the help the mother and the family receive to solve their problems. Chase and co-workers[3] indicate that when the nutritional deprivation occurs early in infancy, the infant may not achieve his growth potential. At the same time as the infant is being rehabilitated in the hospital the family should be receiving intensive counseling. This counseling needs to be continued if the child is to be protected from future episodes of nutritional deprivation.

Overfeeding. With the realization that much adult obesity has its origins in infancy, childhood and adolescence, the prevention of obesity begins with infant feeding. Many mothers are not aware that they may be overfeeding their infants. In any contact with the mother of infants—in an outpatient clinic or the pediatrician's office—it is strongly recommended that the *amounts* and *kinds* of foods and fluids being consumed by the infants be appraised for at least their calorie value. If the young infant is receiving more than 120 calories per kilogram (50 calories per pound) or if the older infant is receiving more than 100 calories per kilogram (40 calories per pound) per day this information together with other data such as height and weight plotted on a growth chart should be evaluated. The infant may be overfed or he may be growing at a greater rate than others of his age. If the problem is overfeeding, the mother should be given assistance (see Chap. 15). Care must be taken to assure that the diet is adequate in nutrients, particularly iron and vitamins. Obesity in childhood and adolescence is discussed in Chapters 13, 15 and 16.

LONG-TERM ILLNESSES

Allergy, cardiac disease, renal disease and diabetes occur in children as in adults and are discussed in detail in previous chapters—allergy in Chapter 27; cardiac disease in Chapter 23; renal disease in Chapter 24; and diabetes in Chapter 22.

Only the ketogenic diet for epilepsy is presented in this section.

Epilepsy—the Ketogenic Diet

For those young patients with petit mal epilepsy who do not respond to drug therapy, the ketogenic diet, abandoned for many years, is again being used.[4] The diet was successful in controlling attacks, and had a favorable effect on the restlessness, hypermobility and irritability found in children with convulsive disorders. Some children previously considered dull or mentally retarded, became alert, bright and sociable when the seizures were controlled by the diet.

There are many drawbacks, however, to the use of the diet. It demands the use of gram scales for the weighing of all food, careful menu planning and rigid control. Parents must be able to cope with the restrictions and be carefully instructed in the details of the diet if the treatment is to be successful.

Principles of Diet Therapy. The goal of the ketogenic diet is to *produce* mild ketosis: the reverse of the goal in the therapy of diabetes— to *prevent* ketosis. On page 219 in Chapter 22 it is pointed out that 58 percent of protein and 10 percent of fat in the diet forms glucose in intermediary metabolism, and 100 percent of the carbohydrate in the diet forms glucose. This actual and potential glucose is antiketogenic. Ninety percent of the fat and the remainder of the protein in the diet are ketogenic; that is, they have the potential to form ketone bodies. When the ratio of fatty acids to available glucose exceeds 2:1, ketosis occurs. However, to be effective the ketogenic-antiketogenic (K-AK) ratio must be at least 3:1 at the beginning of treatment and maintained at a ratio of 4:1.

Diet Prescription. The method for calculating the diet prescription for a child using Mike's[5] method in given in Table 29-2. It is shown that for a 4-year-old child weighing 18 Kg. the diet order for a 4:1 K-AK ratio is 1,300 calories, 18 Gm. of protein, 130 Gm. of fat and 14.5 Gm. of carbohydrate. A 1,300 calorie diet for a normal 4-year-old weighing 18 Kg. would contain approximately 30 Gm. of protein, 60 Gm. of fat and 160 Gm. of carbohydrate. It is readily apparent that the food served on the ketogenic diet is very different from that served to the average child.

---

[3] Chase, H. P., and Martin, H. P.: New Eng. J. Med., 282:933, 1970.

[4] Edit.: JAMA, 197:580, 1966.
[5] Mike, E. M.: Am. J. Clin. Nutr., 17:399, 1965.

TABLE 29-2. METHOD FOR CALCULATING A KETOGENIC DIET*

Calorie requirements, rounded to the nearest 100

AGE (years)	CAL./KG. BODY WEIGHT
2-3	100-80
3-5	80-60
5-10	75-55

Protein requirement

1 Gm./Kg. body weight for young children
1.5 Gm./Kg. body weight for older children

To calculate for a 3:1 ratio	*To calculate for a 4:1 ratio*
1 Gm. fat = 9 Cal. × 3 = 27 Cal.	1 Gm. fat = 9 Cal. × 4 = 36 Cal.
1 Gm. P + C = 4 Cal. × 1 = 4 Cal.	1 Gm. P + C = 4 Cal. × 1 = 4 Cal.
31 Cal.	40 Cal.
per unit	per unit

Example: 4-year-old child, weighing 18 Kg. × 70 Cal's = 1,260 or 1,300 Calories

For a 3:1 K-AK ratio (31 Cal./unit)	For a 4:1 K-AK ratio (40 Cal./unit)
1,300 Cal.: 31 Cal. = 42 units	1,300 Cal.: 40 Cal. = 32.5 units
Fat 42 × 3 = 126 Gm.	Fat 32.5 × 4 = 130 Gm.
P + C 42 × 1 = 42 Gm.	P + C 32.5 × 1 = 32.5 Gm.
P (1 Gm./Kg.) 18 Gm.	P (1 Gm./Kg.) = 18 Gm.
C (by difference) 24 Gm.	C (by difference) = 14.5 Gm.
The diet prescription with a 3:1 K-AK ratio will therefore contain 18 Gm. of protein, 126 Gm. of fat and 24 Gm. of carbohydrate	The diet prescription for a 4:1 K-AK ratio will contain 18 Gm. of protein, 130 Gm. of fat and 14.5 Gm. of carbohydrate See menu in Table 29-3.

* From Mike, E. M.: Practical Guide and Dietary Management of Children with Seizures Using the Ketogenic Diet. Am. J. Clin. Nutr., 17:399, 1965.

To establish ketosis nothing is given by mouth except 500 to 1,000 ml. of water for 24 to 72 hours. Hunger disappears as ketosis develops. When a high degree of ketosis has been achieved, the diet is begun with a 3:1 K-AK ratio, then changed to the 4:1 K-AK ratio for the duration of treatment. There may be nausea or vomiting at first, but this disappears. A strongly positive ketonuria should be maintained at all times.

The diet is continued for 1 to 3 years, then a gradual return to a normal diet is made by slowly reducing the fat and increasing the protein and carbohydrate as directed by the physician.

Planning the Ketogenic Diet. Mike's article includes tables of food values and many suggestions for using the fat to make the diet as palatable as possible. The dietitian is responsible for planning the ketogenic diet. Table 29-3 gives a menu for a diet with a 4:1 K-AK ratio to show the kinds of meals served.

All food should be eaten at each meal. The diet is supplemented with an aqueous solution of multiple vitamins, with calcium gluconate or calcium lactate (not as a syrup that contains carbohydrate), and with an iron medication to provide the amount of iron needed by the child.

Nursing Responsibilities. The child on a ketogenic diet needs constant supervision to see that he does not receive any fluid except water or any food other than that provided by the dietitian. A piece of candy, a glass of fruit juice or a carton of milk would upset the K-AK ratio. Counseling sessions with the dietitian should be arranged for the mother early in her child's hospitalization so that she has adequate time to learn how to manage the diet at home.

TABLE 29-3. MENU FOR A KETOGENIC DIET WITH A 4:1 K-AK RATIO, CONTAINING 18 GM. OF PROTEIN, 130 GM. OF FAT AND 14.5 GM. OF CARBOHYDRATE*

FOOD	WEIGHT (Gm.)	PROTEIN	FAT	CARBOHYDRATE
Breakfast				
Orange	30	0.3	0.1	3.0
Heavy cream (diluted with water for drinking)	75	1.6	28.1	2.3
Egg, cooked in	25	3.2	2.9	—
Butter	15	—	12.0	—
		5.1	43.1	5.3
Dinner				
Meat, medium fat, cooked in	20	5.6	3.2	—
Butter	15	—	12.0	—
Asparagus	30	.6	—	1.5
Lettuce	20	.4	—	1.0
Mayonnaise	20	.2	16.0	—
Oil (added to mayonnaise)	10	—	10.0	—
Cantaloupe	20	.2	—	2.0
		7.0	41.2	4.5
Supper				
Egg, hard cooked	25	3.2	2.9	—
Spinach, cooked in	30	.6	—	1.5
Butter	10	—	8.1	—
Lettuce	20	.4	—	1.0
Mayonnaise	20	.2	16.0	—
Heavy cream, whipped with	50	1.1	18.8	1.5
Apple sauce	10	.1	—	.5
		5.6	45.8	4.5
Totals for the day		17.7	130.1	14.3

* All figures obtained from Mike, E. M.: Practical Guide and Dietary Management of Children with Seizures Using the Ketogenic Diet. Am. J. Clin. Nutr., 17:399, 1965.

MALABSORPTION SYNDROMES

Cystic Fibrosis

Cystic fibrosis is one of the most common long-term illnesses of infants and children. It is an inherited disease affecting the mucous and the sweat glands of the body. The mucous glands excrete an abnormally thick mucous and the sweat glands produce salty sweat, high in sodium chloride. The disease may first manifest itself in the lungs where the thick mucous obstructs the air passages; or there may be diarrhea with fatty stools and growth failure, due to mucous plugs in the fine pancreatic ducts, blocking the release of pancreatic digestive enzymes.

Until recently, cystic fibrosis was thought of

primarily as a disease of young children, usually fatal. With the use of techniques to clear the lungs of mucous, of antibiotics to control infections, of pancreatic enzymes and a nutritionally adequate diet, moderately restricted in fat, patients are now growing into young adulthood.

Dietary Treatment. Protein foods are the foods most readily digested by the patient with cystic fibrosis, and fat is digested least well. A high protein low fat formula such as Probana* is fed to the young infant. With the addition of solids to supply adequate calories, skim milk may be used in later infancy. In the older child, the diet is increased in protein, normal in carbohydrate, and restricted in excessively fatty foods such as butter and margarine, peanut butter, cream, fatty meats, vegetable oils, fried food and pastry rich in shortening. If tolerated, homogenized whole milk may be used.

A preparation of pancreatic enzymes is given with meals and all between meal snacks. Both water-soluble and fat-soluble vitamins, including vitamin E, are prescribed. During the summer months, when there is danger of heat prostration from excessive loss of sodium chloride in the sweat, extra salt must be added to the diet.

The child with cystic fibrosis, who has no concurrent infection, has a large appetite, eats well and is able to maintain good nutritional status. The child with cystic fibrosis hospitalized for the treatment of an acute infection presents numerous problems. A major one is the scheduling of postural drainage and meals. To prevent regurgitation when the child is clearing mucous from his lungs, postural drainage should not be done too soon after a meal. Also food and beverages should be available to these children whenever they request them. The older child with cystic fibrosis may have diabetes secondary to the destruction of the insulin-secreting cells of the pancreas.

Celiac Disease—Gluten-Induced Enteropathy

Celiac disease is not observed in infants until cereal with a significant quantity of gluten is added to their diets. Infants who have celiac disease are fed rice cereal and other baby foods free of gluten, together with formula or homogenized milk. The older child is treated with the gluten-free diet described in Chapter 25 (see p. 261 to 262). If a child has had severe diarrhea before his problem has been diagnosed, some physicians prefer to use a low-roughage, gluten-free diet until the child has recovered. Then the restriction of roughage is discontinued.

Care must be taken to see that other children in a pediatric unit do not share their bread, crackers or snacks containing gluten with the toddler or young child who has celiac disease. Mothers of these children face this same problem in the home and the neighborhood and when the child goes to school.

Lactose Intolerance

Lactose intolerance is discussed in Chapter 25 in detail and is not repeated here.

Glucose-Galactose Malabsorption

In this rare disorder, the mechanism for the active transport of glucose and galactose in the intestinal mucosa is not functioning. The digestion of sucrose and starch each yield glucose, and the end products of lactose digestion are glucose and galactose. Infants with this disorder cannot be kept free from symptoms unless all sources of carbohydrate are omitted with the exception of fructose. Cho-Free* formula with fructose added can be used to feed these infants. Lindquist[6] gives details of a formula and the subsequent diet for children with this disorder.

INBORN ERRORS OF METABOLISM

In the last 30 years, as our knowledge of the control of metabolic processes by enzymes has increased, a growing number of diseases due to an inborn error of metabolism (lack of an enzyme) are being identified. This includes diseases of carbohydrate metabolism such as the glycogen storage diseases and galactosemia. An ever-increasing list of amino acid disorders are grouped under the name aminoacidurias. Recently a defect in the metabolism of short-chain fatty acids C:4 and C:6 has been reported.[7] Inborn errors of the metabolism of minerals and vitamins are also known. Many of the defects are of genetic origin as shown by family histories.

The effects of disease due to a metabolic defect

---

* Mead Johnson and Co., Evansville, Ind.

* Cho-Free, Borden Co., Columbus, Ohio.
[6] Lindquist, B., and Meeuwisse, G.: J. Am. Dietet. A., 48:307, 1966.
[7] Sidbury, J. B., *et al.*: J. Pediatrics, 70:8, 1967.

may be extremely serious, especially if it occurs in newborn infants and young children. Death intervenes in some, because, even when the disease is recognized, there is no known therapy for it. In several diseases of inborn metabolic errors, mental retardation occurs unless the disease is treated promptly. In others, the child may live on for a few years but die eventually. And in a few, such as alkaptonuria, an amino acid defect in which the urine becomes dark on standing, the condition is harmless, at least in infancy and childhood, although some pathologic effects become evident by the third decade of life. In the following pages only phenylketonuria and galactosemia, for which dietary treatment has been used successfully for some years, is discussed in detail. Several other diseases due to inborn metabolic errors are mentioned briefly. For full discussion the student is referred to the survey articles included in the Supplementary Reading at the end of the chapter, and to the Bibliography in Part Four.

Phenylketonuria (PKU)

Phenylketonuria is a familial disease inherited through a simple autosomal recessive gene and is characterized by the presence of phenylpyruvic acid in the urine. Affected individuals lack the liver enzyme phenylalanine hydroxylase that converts the amino acid phenylalanine to tyrosine under normal circumstances (see Fig. 29-2). As soon as a newborn infant with phenylketonuria begins to take milk, his serum phenylalanine and

phenylpyruvic acid levels rise. Later these substances are excreted in the urine.

If the disease goes untreated, about 90 percent of individuals develop severe mental retardation. It is estimated that from ½ to 1 percent of all patients in institutions for the mentally retarded are phenylketonurics. The continued high level of phenylalanine and its metabolites in the blood is believed in some way to be responsible for the cerebral damage.

Phenylketonurics also usually show neurological disturbances such as irritability, hyperactivity and convulsive seizures. Because tyrosine is involved in the formation of melanine pigments in the body (see Fig. 29-2), these patients are often blond, fair skinned and blue eyed, even when other family members are of darker coloration.

Treatment of the disease was delayed for many years because there was no known method for limiting phenylalanine in the diet. All foods except oils and sugars contain protein. Because all proteins are estimated to contain from 4 to 6 percent of phenylalanine, the diet is an extremely restricted one. With the development of a satisfactory phenylalanine-restricted diet described later in the section, it has been possible for these children to achieve their growth potential both mentally and physically if the diet is started in the first few months of life. Therefore dietary treatment is recommended for all phenylketonurics early in infancy. When the disease is discovered later, dietary treatment is not effective in preventing mental retarda-

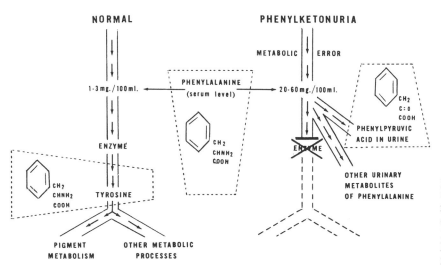

Fig. 29-2. The pathway of phenylalanine metabolism, normally and in phenylketonuria. (Phenylketonuria. Children's Bureau Publ. No. 388, 1965. U.S. Department of Health, Education and Welfare)

tion, although the behavior of the child appears to improve with such treatment.

Principles of Diet Therapy. Phenylalanine is an essential amino acid that the body needs for growth and maintenance. For the phenylketonuric child the diet is planned to provide adequate calories, protein and all other nutrients while the phenylalanine content of the diet is restricted to the amount required by the individual for growth and maintenance and, at the same time, maintain the blood levels of phenylalanine between 5 to 10 mg. per 100 ml. To maintain the blood level, the phenylketonuric infant at one month of age requires 70 to 90 mg. of phenylalanine per kilogram of body weight. With the decreasing rate of growth throughout the first year of life, the requirement decreases to 25 to 35 mg. of phenylalanine per kilogram of body weight by 2 years of age. Children 2 to 10 years of age require on the average 30 mg. of phenylalanine per kilogram.[8]

The Diet Prescription. The diet prescription gives the calories, grams of protein and milligrams of phenylalanine required by the child. For example, the diet order for a 2-month-old infant weighing 4.5 Kg. should be: 540 calories (120 calories × 4.5 Kg.); 10 Gm. of protein (2.2 Gm. × 4.5 Kg.) and 315 mg. of phenylalanine (70 mg. × 4.5 Kg.).

Food for the Phenylalanine-Restricted Diet. A substitute for milk, Lofenalac*, is available for feeding the infant and child who has PKU. This product is made from partially digested protein, adequate in amino acid composition with the exception of phenylalanine. Fat, carbohydrate and certain minerals and vitamins are added to the protein to make a complete formula. The product is marketed in powdered form and one measure (1 tablespoon, 9.5 Gm.) of Lofenalac contains 1.4 Gm. protein and 7.5 mg. of phenylalanine. This amount added to 60 ml. of water contains 20 calories per ounce. It has almost the same appearance and consistency as milk, but a markedly different flavor. Most infants and young children accept it without difficulty. It is the main source of protein in the diet throughout the years of treatment.

When formula is the only source of nutrients for the infant, limited quantities of cow's milk are

TABLE 29-4. AVERAGE NUTRIENT CONTENT OF SERVING LISTS*

LIST	PHENYL-ALANINE mg.	PROTEIN Gm.	CALORIES
Vegetables	15	0.5	10
Fruits			
Strained and Junior	15	0.6	150
Table and Juices	15	0.6	70
Breads and Cereals	30	0.6	30
Fats	5	0.1	60
Desserts†	30	varies	varies

* From The Phenylalanine Restricted Diet—for Professional Use, 1966. The Bureau of Public Health Nutrition of the California State Department of Public Health.

† Average of dessert recipes in Phenylalanine-Restricted Diet Recipe Book, The Bureau of Public Health Nutrition of the California State Department of Health.

added to the Lofenalac to provide adequate amounts of phenylalanine and calories and protein. Generally 1 to 2 ounces of cow's milk are required.

When the infant is ready for baby foods, fruits and vegetables containing no more than 1 percent of protein are added. The physician decides this on the basis of the infant's blood phenylalanine level and his calorie and protein requirements for expected increases in length and weight.

As the child grows older, other foods of known phenylalanine content are added to the diet. Table 29-4 gives the average content of phenylalanine, protein and calories for the food groups used in the phenylalanine diet—actually a modification of the exchange system. Table 29-5 gives the specific food list for each group.

The Bread and Cereal List in Table 29-5 gives only cereal and crackers. Regular bread is not included. One slice of bread made with 1 to 2 percent nonfat dry milk solids contains 99 mg. of phenylalanine. Some mothers of young children find the special bread for renal patients (see Chap. 24) an acceptable substitute for regular bread. With butter and jelly this bread can provide calories with very limited amounts of phenylalanine.

---

[8] Hunt, M. H., *et al.*: Am. J. Dis. Child., 122:1, 1971.
* Mead Johnson Laboratories: op. cit.

TABLE 29-5. SERVING LISTS FOR PHENYLALANINE RESTRICTED DIET*

FOOD	AMOUNT	PHENYLALANINE mg.	PROTEIN Gm.	CALORIES

VEGETABLES
Each serving as listed contains 15 milligrams of phenylalanine

Baby and Junior

FOOD	AMOUNT	PHENYLALANINE mg.	PROTEIN Gm.	CALORIES
Beets	7 tbsp.	15	1.1	35
Carrots	7 tbsp.	15	0.7	28
Creamed Spinach	1 tbsp.	16	0.4	6
Green Beans	2 tbsp.	15	0.3	7
Squash	4 tbsp.	14	0.4	14

Table Vegetables

FOOD	AMOUNT	PHENYLALANINE mg.	PROTEIN Gm.	CALORIES
Asparagus, cooked	1 stalk	12	0.6	4
Beans, green, cooked	4 tbsp. (¼ cup)	14	0.6	9
Beans, yellow, wax, cooked	4 tbsp. (¼ cup)	15	0.6	9
Bean sprouts, mung, cooked	2 tbsp.	18	0.6	5
Beets, cooked	8 tbsp. (½ cup)	14	0.8	34
Beet greens, cooked	1 tbsp.	14	0.2	3
Broccoli, cooked	1 tbsp.	11	0.3	3
Brussels sprouts, cooked	1 medium	16	0.6	5
Cabbage, raw, shredded	8 tbsp. (½ cup)	15	0.7	12
Cabbage, cooked	5 tbsp. (⅓ cup)	16	0.8	12
Carrots, raw	1/6 large (¼ cup)	16	0.5	16
Carrots, cooked	8 tbsp. (½ cup)	17	0.5	23
Cauliflower, cooked	3 tbsp.	18	0.6	6
Celery, cooked, diced†	4 tbsp. (¼ cup)	15	0.4	6
Celery, raw†	1—8 inch stalk	16	0.5	7
Chard leaves, cooked	2 tbsp.	19	0.6	6
Collards, cooked	1 tbsp.	16	0.5	5
Cucumber slices, raw	8 slices, ⅛″ thick	16	0.7	12
Eggplant, diced raw	3 tbsp.	18	0.4	9
Kale, cooked	2 tbsp.	20	0.5	5
Lettuce†	3 small leaves	13	0.4	5
Mushrooms, cooked†	2 tbsp.	14	0.4	35
Mushrooms, fresh†	2 small	16	0.5	3
Mustard greens, cooked	2 tbsp.	18	0.6	6
Okra, cooked†	2—3″ pods	13	0.4	7
Onion, raw, chopped	5 tbsp. (⅓ cup)	14	0.5	20
Onion, cooked	4 tbsp. (¼ cup)	14	0.5	19
Onion, young scallion	5—5″ long	14	0.5	23
Parsley, raw, chopped†	3 tbsp.	13	0.4	5
Parsnips, cooked, diced†	3 tbsp.	13	0.3	18
Peppers, raw, chopped†	4 tbsp.	13	0.4	12
Pickles, Dill	8 slices—⅛″ thick	16	0.7	12
Pumpkin, cooked	4 tbsp. (¼ cup)	14	0.5	16
Radishes, red, small†	4	13	0.4	8
Rutabagas, cooked	2 tbsp.	16	0.3	10

Soups

FOOD	AMOUNT	PHENYLALANINE mg.	PROTEIN Gm.	CALORIES
Beef broth (Campbell's condensed)	1 tbsp.	14	0.5	3
Celery (Campbell's condensed)	2 tbsp.	18	0.4	19
Minestrone (Campbell's condensed)	1 tbsp.	17	1.5	25

* From The Phenylalanine-Restricted Diet—for Professional Use, 1966. The Bureau of Public Health Nutrition of the California State Department of Public Health.
† Phenylalanine calculated as 3.3 percent of total protein.

TABLE 29-5. SERVING LISTS FOR PHENYLALANINE RESTRICTED DIET* (*Continued*)

FOOD	AMOUNT	PHENYLALANINE mg.	PROTEIN Gm.	CALORIES
VEGETABLES (*Continued*)				
Mushroom (Campbell's condensed)	1 tbsp.	11	0.2	17
Onion (Campbell's condensed)	1 tbsp.	14	0.6	8
Tomato (Campbell's condensed)	1 tbsp.	11	0.2	11
Vegetarian Veg. Soup (Campbell's condensed)	1½ tbsp.	17	0.4	14
Spinach, cooked	1 tbsp.	15	0.4	3
Squash, summer, cooked	8 tbsp. (½ cup)	16	0.6	16
Squash, winter, cooked	3 tbsp.	16	0.6	14
Tomato, raw	½ small	14	0.5	10
Tomato, cooked	4 tbsp. (¼ cup)	15	0.6	10
Tomato juice	4 tbsp. (¼ cup)	17	0.6	12
Tomato catsup	2 tbsp.	17	0.6	34
Turnip greens, cooked	1 tbsp.	18	0.4	4
Turnips, diced, cooked	5 tbsp. (⅓ cup)	16	0.4	12
FRUITS				
Each serving as listed contains 15 milligrams of phenylalanine				
Baby and Junior				
Applesauce and apricots	16 tbsp. (1 cup)	15	0.6	205
Applesauce and pineapple	16 tbsp. (1 cup)	11	0.5	176
Apricots with tapioca	16 tbsp. (1 cup)	16	0.6	187
Bananas	8 tsbp. (½ cup)	14	0.6	97
Bananas and pineapple	16 tbsp. (1 cup)	18	0.6	187
Peaches	10 tbsp.	15	0.7	124
Pears	12 tbsp. (¾ cup)	16	0.5	106
Pears and pineapple	16 tbsp. (1 cup)	17	1.0	166
Plums with tapioca	12 tbsp. (¾ cup)	16	0.5	163
Prunes with tapioca	12 tbsp. (¾ cup)	16	0.5	152
Fruit Juices				
Apricot nectar	6 oz. (¾ cup)	14	0.6	102
Cranberry juice	12 oz. (1½ cup)	15	0.6	39
Grape juice	4 oz. (½ cup)	14	0.5	80
Grapefruit juice	8 oz. (1 cup)	16	1.2	104
Orange juice	6 oz. (¾ cup)	16	1.2	84
Peach nectar	5 oz. (⅔ cup)	15	0.5	75
Pineapple juice	6 oz. (¾ cup)	16	0.6	90
Prune juice	4 oz. (½ cup)	16	0.5	84
Table Fruits				
Apple, raw	4 small 2½″ diam.	16	0.8	176
Applesauce	16 tbsp. (1 cup)	12	0.6	192
Apricots, raw	1 medium	12	0.5	25
Apricots, canned	2 medium 2 tbsp. syrup	14	0.6	80
Avocado, cubed or mashed†	5 tbsp. (⅓ cup)	16	0.6	80
Banana, raw, sliced	4 tbsp. (¼ cup)	15	0.4	32
Blackberries, raw†	5 tbsp. (⅓ cup)	14	0.6	25
Blackberries, canned, in syrup†	5 tbsp. (⅓ cup)	13	0.5	55
Blueberries, raw or frozen†	12 tbsp. (¾ cup)	16	0.6	60
Blueberries, canned, in syrup†	10 tbsp.	16	0.6	140
Boysenberries, frozen, sweetened†	8 tbsp. (½ cup)	16	0.6	72
Cantaloupe	5 tbsp. (⅓ cup)	16	0.4	15

† Phenylalanine calculated as 2.6 percent of total protein.

TABLE 29-5. SERVING LISTS FOR PHENYLALANINE RESTRICTED DIET* (*Continued*)

FOOD	AMOUNT	PHENYLALANINE mg.	PROTEIN Gm.	CALORIES
FRUITS (*Continued*)				
Cherries, sweet, canned, in syrup†	8 tbsp. (½ cup)	16	0.6	104
Dates, pitted, chopped	3 tbsp.	18	0.7	96
Figs, raw†	1 large	18	0.7	40
Figs, canned, in syrup†	2 figs 4 tsp. syrup	16	0.6	90
Figs, dried†	1 small	16	0.6	40
Fruit cocktail†	12 tbsp. (¾ cup)	16	0.6	120
Grapes, American type	8 grapes	14	0.5	24
Grapes, American slipskin	5 tbsp. (⅓ cup)	16	0.6	25
Grapes, Thompson seedless	8 tbsp. (½ cup)	13	0.8	64
Guava, raw†	½ medium	13	0.5	35
Honeydew melon†	¼ small 5″ melon	13	0.5	32
Mango, raw†	1 small	18	0.7	66
Nectarines, raw	1—2″ high, 2″ diam.	15	0.4	45
Oranges, raw	1 medium 3″ diam. or ⅔ cup sections	15	1.1	60
Papayas, raw†	¼ med. or ½ cup	14	0.6	36
Peaches, raw	1 medium	15	0.5	46
Peaches, canned, in syrup	2 medium halves	18	0.6	88
Pears, raw	1—3″ × 2½″	14	1.3	100
Pears, canned, in syrup	2 med. halves 2 tbsp. syrup	14	1.3	78
Pineapple, raw†	16 tbsp. (1 cup)	16	0.6	80
Pineapple, canned, in syrup†	2 small slices	13	0.5	93
Plums, raw	½—2″ plum	12	0.3	15
Plums, canned, in syrup	3—2 tbsp. syrup	16	0.5	91
Prunes, dried	2 large	14	0.4	54
Raisins, dried seedless	2 tbsp.	14	0.5	54
Raspberries, raw†	5 tbsp. (⅓ cup)	13	0.5	25
Raspberries, canned, in syrup†	6 tbsp.	14	0.5	78
Strawberries, raw†	8 large	16	0.6	32
Strawberries, frozen†	6 tbsp.	14	0.5	108
Tangerines	1½ large	15	1.2	66
Watermelon†	½ cup cubes	13	0.5	28

BREADS AND CEREALS
Each serving as listed contains 30 milligrams of phenylalanine

Baby and Junior

Cereals, ready to serve				
Barley	3 tbsp.	32	0.8	24
Oatmeal	2 tbsp.	34	0.8	16
Rice	5 tbsp. (⅓ cup)	30	0.6	40
Wheat	2 tbsp.	30	0.6	17
Creamed corn	3 tbsp.	30	0.5	27
Sweet Potatoes (Gerber's)	3 tbsp.	32	0.5	31
Table Foods				
Cereals, cooked				
Cornmeal	4 tbsp. (¼ cup)	29	0.6	29
Cream of rice	4 tbsp. (¼ cup)	35	0.7	34
Cream of wheat	2 tbsp.	27	0.6	16
Farina	2 tbsp.	25	0.5	18

† Phenylalanine calculated as 2.6 percent of total protein.

TABLE 29-5. SERVING LISTS FOR PHENYLALANINE RESTRICTED DIET* (*Continued*)

FOOD	AMOUNT	PHENYLALANINE mg.	PROTEIN Gm.	CALORIES
BREADS AND CEREALS (*Continued*)				
Malt-o-meal	2 tbsp.	27	0.5	17
Oatmeal	2 tbsp.	32	0.7	18
Pettijohns	2 tbsp.	24	0.5	19
Ralstons	2 tbsp.	34	0.7	18
Rice, brown or white	4 tbsp. (¼ cup)	35	0.7	34
Wheatena	2 tbsp.	27	0.5	19
Cereals, ready to serve				
Alpha bits	4 tbsp. (¼ cup)	32	0.6	28
Cheerios	3 tbsp.	32	0.6	20
Corn Chex	4 tbsp. (¼ cup)	29	0.6	32
Cornfetti	5 tbsp. (⅓ cup)	31	0.6	46
Cornflakes	5 tbsp. (⅓ cup)	29	0.6	30
Crispy Critters	4 tbsp. (¼ cup)	30	0.6	28
Kix	5 tbsp. (⅓ cup)	31	0.6	31
Krumbles	3 tbsp.	32	0.7	26
Rice Chex	6 tbsp.	32	0.7	49
Rice flakes	5 tbsp. (⅓ cup)	33	0.6	32
Rice Krispies	6 tbsp.	30	0.6	40
Rice, puffed	12 tbsp. (¾ cup)	30	0.6	38
Sugar Crisp puffed wheat	4 tbsp. (¼ cup)	30	0.6	46
Sugar sparkled flakes	5 tbsp. (⅓ cup)	29	0.6	55
Wheat Chex	10 biscuits	30	0.6	22
Wheaties	3 tbsp.	26	0.5	20
Wheat, puffed	6 tbsp.	30	0.6	16
Crackers				
Barnum Animal	5	30	0.6	45
Graham (65/lb.)	1	26	0.5	30
Ritz (no cheese)	2	24	0.5	34
Saltines (140/lb.)	2	29	0.6	28
Soda (63/lb.)	1	36	0.7	30
Wheat thins (248/lb.)	5	30	0.6	45
Corn, cooked	2 tbsp.	32	0.7	17
Hominy	2 tbsp.	32	0.7	17
Macaroni, cooked	1½ tbsp.	31	0.7	20
Noodles, cooked	3 tbsp.	32	0.7	20
Popcorn, popped	5 tbsp. (⅓ cup)	31	0.6	17
Potato chips	4—2″ diam.	30	0.6	44
Potato, Irish, cooked	3 tbsp.	33	0.8	31
Spaghetti, cooked	1 tbsp.	24	0.5	14
Sweet potato, cooked	2 tbsp.	25	0.4	31
Tortilla, corn	1½—6″ diam.	30	0.8	31
FATS				
Each serving as listed contains 5 milligrams of phenylalanine				
Butter	1 tbsp.	5	0.1	100
French dressing, commercial	1 tbsp.	5	0.1	59
Mayonnaise, commercial	1 tbsp.	5	0.1	100
Margarine	½ tbsp.	5	0.1	30
Olives, green or ripe	1 medium	5	0.1	12

TABLE 29-5. SERVING LISTS FOR PHENYLALANINE RESTRICTED DIET* (*Continued*)

FOOD	AMOUNT	PHENYLALANINE mg.	PROTEIN Gm.	CALORIES

DESSERTS
Each serving as listed contains 30 milligrams of phenylalanine

Cake†	1/12 of cake
Cookies—Rice flour†	2
Corn starch†	2
Cookies, Arrowroot	1½
Ice Cream—Chocolate†	⅔ cup
Pineapple†	⅔ cup
Strawberry†	⅔ cup
Jello	⅓ cup
Puddings†	½ cup
Sauce, Hershey	2 tbsp.
Wafers, sugar, Nabisco	5

FREE FOODS
Contain little or no phenylalanine. May be used as desired.

Apple juice	Cherries, Maraschino	Popsicles, with artificial fruit
Beverages, carbonated	Fruit ices (if no more than ½	flavor
Gingerbread‡	cup used daily)	Rich's Topping
Guava Butter	Cornstarch	Salt
Candy	Jell-quik	Shortening, vegetable
Butterscotch	Jellies	Soy sauce
Cream Mints	Kool-ade	Sugar, brown, white, or
Fondant	Lemonade	confectioner's
Gum drops	Molasses	Syrups, corn or maple
Hard	Oil	Tang
Jelly beans	Pepper, black, ground	Tapioca
Lollipops		

† Low phenylalanine recipes—in Phenylalanine-Restricted Diet Recipe Book.

‡ Special recipe must be used—in Phenylalanine-Restricted Diet Recipe Book.

Diet Planning and Parent Education. The dietitian has the responsibility for planning the diet and instructing the mother of an infant or child with PKU. She works with the mother of a newly diagnosed infant daily during hospitalization and then weekly or every other week on an outpatient basis until the infant is 5 to 6 months of age. She continues to work with the mother as long as the child is on a phenylalanine-restricted diet. The continuous contact with the dietitian in cooperation with the physician is required to monitor and maintain the blood level of phenylalanine between 5 to 10 mg. per 100 ml. and, at the same time, provide adequate calories and nutrients to support growth and development. Educational materials that are used by the dietitian and others are listed at the end of the chapter.

It becomes evident that cooperation and understanding of the parents, and indeed of the whole family, is essential if this difficult regimen is to be successful. It is strongly recommended that the phenylketonuric child be followed at a center that can provide the services of physician, nutritionist, social worker and public health nurse, supported by competent laboratory facilities. The frequent monitoring of blood serum phenylalanine levels and urinary excretion of phenylpyruvic acid, and the necessary adjustment of the diet can thus be accomplished quickly and with least danger to the child.

Nursing Responsibilities. Special care must be taken to assure that the newly diagnosed hospitalized infant with PKU is offered the correct feeding. Formula made from Lofenalac powder must be correctly reconstituted under sterile conditions either in the infant formula laboratory or in the sterile supply room. All feeding bottles must be clearly labeled with the infant's name to avoid errors. The number of ounces taken and retained at each feeding must be accurately recorded in the nurse's notes and made readily available to the dietitian so that she can estimate daily the infant's calorie, protein and phenylalanine intake.

For the older hospitalized infant who is taking solids, only the kinds and amounts of baby foods provided by the dietitian can be fed. The amount of baby food accepted at each feeding must also be recorded accurately.

An older child with PKU who is admitted for surgery or because he has an infection that results in an elevated phenylalanine blood level needs careful observation at mealtime to see that the correct meal is served and that he accepts the food. At snack time the child with PKU can be served only the food or fluid planned by the dietitian. Care must also be taken that other children or parents of other children do not offer food to the child with PKU.

Duration of Treatment. At present there is no agreement on the length of time the diet must be continued. Dietary control varies as the infant becomes mobile and maintaining the diet becomes more difficult. Because the critical period for the development of the nervous system is 0 to 4 years of age, some physicians offer a less restricted diet to the child with PKU after age 4 or 5. The increase in the phenylalanine content of the diet is made slowly. This appears to have no ill effects on physical and mental development although this is presently being investigated at a number of PKU centers.

Galactosemia

Galactosemia is an inherited disorder of carbohydrate metabolism. It is characterized by an inability to convert galactose to glucose in the liver, due to the absence of an enzyme. In this disorder an intermediary product of galactose metabolism, galactose-1-phosphate, accumulates in the blood and is thought to be responsible for the symptoms. In the majority of patients symptoms develop in early infancy. These include jaundice, enlargement of the liver, digestive disturbances and failure to grow and thrive. If the infant survives, cataracts may develop and mental and physical growth is retarded.

Dietary Treatment. Treatment is directed toward rigid exclusion of galactose from the diet.

Because galactose is a component of lactose, the sugar found in milk, milk and all foods containing milk must be omitted.

In place of a cow's milk formula, Nutramigen*, an infant formula free of lactose, Meat Base† formula or soy formulas are used. Some physicians do not use soy formulas because soy beans contain a complex carbohydrate, stachyose, that contains galactose. It is not known if this is released during digestion and absorbed.

The lactose-free diet discussed in Chapter 25 is galactose-free and applies to the dietary treatment of the child with galactosemia as well as to the child with lactose intolerance.

Leucine-Induced Hypoglycemia

Hypoglycemic reactions in infants induced by the amino acid leucine is another inborn error of metabolism of familial origin. It may be manifested from birth, or it may appear later in the first year of life. The symptoms are precipitated by a high-protein meal or a fasting state. In the early stages there are irritability and twitching movements of the extremities, and, if the disease is not treated, hypoglycemic convulsions, with blood sugar levels as low as 20 mg. percent. Eventually failure-to-thrive and mental and psychomotor retardation occur. Control of the hypoglycemia as early as possible is therefore imperative.

A dietary regimen consisting of leucine restriction and postprandial carbohydrate feedings has been devised by Roth and Segal.[9] Leucine restriction is achieved by limitation of dietary protein, including only sufficient amounts to meet the minimal requirements for growth. Enfamil‡ and Similac§ are two infant formulas relatively low in leucine. Roth and Segal give lists of foods to be omitted and those allowed, and a series of menus calculated for leucine content are included. The menus and the times for the administration of sugar must be followed exactly if the diet is to be effective. The diet has been used by these investigators and by others,[10] with good results. Hypoglycemia and the attendant symptoms were controlled, and the children have developed normally. Fortunately, the disease appears to be self-limiting,

---

* Mead Johnson Laboratories: op. cit.
† Gerber Products Co., Fremont, Mich.
‡ Mead Johnson Laboratories: op. cit.
§ Ross Laboratories, Columbus, Ohio.
[9] Roth, H., and Segal, H.: Pediatrics, 34:831, 1964.
[10] Snyder, R. D., and Robinson, A.: Am. J. Dis. Child., 113:566, 1967.

and by the time the child is 5 to 6 years old he is able to tolerate a normal diet.

Maple Syrup Urine Disease

This disease, an inborn error of metabolism, is so called because of the odor of maple syrup of the urine. Infants with this disease cannot metabolize the three-branched chain amino acids—leucine, isoleucine and valine. The symptoms develop a few days after birth, and babies die with severe neurologic symptoms and high levels of unmetabolized amino acids in the body fluids. Several children with this disease are being treated with some success with a mixture of amino acids, omitting those that are not tolerated, plus small additions of natural foods.[11]

STUDY QUESTIONS AND ACTIVITIES

1. Using the information in Table 29-1 plan a day's menu for a 2½-year-old hospitalized child. Do your food selections meet this child's Recommended Dietary Allowance of protein? (See Table 10-1, Chapter 10 for NRC-RDA.)

2. Using the recordings in the nursing notes of formula and food intake estimate the 24-hour calorie intake of an infant to whom you are giving care. Record the infant's length, daily weight and head circumference on a growth chart. Is the infant progressing normally?

3. What effect may an emotionally disturbed mother have on the nutritional status of her infant?

4. Why would you report immediately to your nursing instructor if you found an epileptic child, on a ketogenic diet, drinking a glass of homogenized milk?

5. Why should obesity in the young child be treated promptly? Which foods must be included in a calorie-restricted diet to maintain an adequate nutrient intake?

6. Make out a menu for a day for a 2-year-old child with gluten induced enteropathy. Does this menu meet the child's nutrient needs?

7. Why is it important to treat the infant with PKU as early as possible?

8. List some of the problems that a family may encounter daily in maintaining a 3-year-old child with PKU on a phenylalanine-restricted diet.

9. Why must medications be closely scrutinized when an infant or child is on a lactose- or galactose-free diet?

---

[11] Snyderman, S. E.: Am. J. Dis. Child., 113:68, 1967.

SUPPLEMENTARY READING IN DISEASES OF CHILDREN

General

Bellam, G.: The first year of life. Am. J. Nursing, 69:1244, 1969.

Jernigan, A. K.: Suggestions for feeding hospitalized children. Hospitals, 44:86, (May 16) 1970.

Ziegler, E. E., and Fomon, S. J.: Fluid intake, renal solute load, and water balance. J. Pediat., 78:561, 1971.

Allergy

Feeney, M. C.: Nutritional and dietary management of food allergy in children. Am. J. Clin. Nutr., 22:103, 1969.

Failure to Thrive

Chase, H. P., and Martin, H. P.: Undernutrition and child development. New Eng. J. Med., 282:933, 1970.

Fischoff, J., Whitten, C. F., and Pettit, M. G.: A psychiatric study of mothers of infants with growth failure secondary to maternal deprivation. J. Pediat., 79:209, 1971.

Leonard, M. F., and Solnit, A. J.: Growth failure, maternal deprivation and undereating. JAMA, 212:822, 1970.

Pavenstedt, E.: To help infants weather disorganized family life. Am. J. Nursing, 69:1668, 1969.

Whitten, C. F.: Evidence that growth failure from maternal deprivation is secondary to undereating. JAMA, 209:1675, 1969.

Epilepsy

Mike, E. M.: Practical guide and dietary management of children with seizures using the ketogenic diet. Am. J. Clin. Nutr., 17:399, 1965.

Malabsorption

Handwerger, J., et al.: Glucose intolerance in cystic fibrosis. New Eng. J. Med., 281:451, 1969.

Shwachman, H., et al.: Studies in cystic fibrosis: report of 130 patients diagnosed under 3 months of age over a 20 year period. Pediatrics, 46:335, 1970.

Inborn Errors—General

Craig, J. W.: Present knowledge of nutrition in inborn errors of metabolism. Nutrition Rev., 26:161, 1968.

Phenylketonuria

Composition of Lofenalac. J. Am. Dietet. A., 52:48, 1968.

Frisch, R. O., et al.: Responses of children with phenylketonuria to dietary treatment. J. Am. Dietet. A., 58:32, 1971.

Hunt, M. H., et al.: Nutrition management of phenylketonuria. Am. J. Dis. Child., 122:1, 1971.

Rinic, M. M., and Rogers, P. J.: A low-protein, low-phenylalanine vegetable casserole. J. Am. Dietet. A., 55:353, 1969.

Smith, B. A., and Waisman, H. A.: Adequate phenylalanine intake for optimum growth and development in the treatment of phenylketonuria. Am. J. Clin. Nutr., 24:423, 1971.

Sutherland, B. S., *et al.*: Growth and nutrition in treated phenylketonuric patients. JAMA, 211:270, 1970.

Galactosemia

Hansen, R. G.: Hereditary galactosemia. JAMA, 208:2077, 1969.

Maple Syrup Urine Disease

Goodman, S. I., *et al.*: The treatment of maple syrup urine disease. J. Pediat., 75:485, 1969.

Snyderman, S. E., *et al.*: Maple syrup urine disease with particular reference to dietotherapy. Pediatrics, 34:454, 1964.

RESOURCES FOR PARENTS OF CHILDREN WITH PKU

PKU—A Diet Guide, 1970. Available from P. B. Acosta Dr. P. H., Chief Nutritionist, Division of Child Development, Children's Hospital at Los Angeles. 4650 Sunset Boulevard, Los Angeles, California 90054.

The Low Phenylalanine Diet ($1.00 per copy). Available from Bureau of Public Health Nutrition, Michigan Department of Public Health, Lansing, Michigan.

A Diet Guide for Parents of Children with Phenylketonuria, 1966. Available to residents of the State of California only from Bureau of Public Health Nutrition, California Department of Public Health, 2151 Berkeley Way, Berkeley, California 94704.

Other treatment centers and state departments of public health have materials for parents of children with PKU. Check the nearest resource.

For further references see Bibliography in Part Four.

PART FOUR

Tabular Material
and Bibliography

Tables

EXPLANATION OF TABLES

Table 1. Composition of Foods—Edible Portion

This table of food values gives proximate composition and mineral and vitamin content of most foods in common use in the United States. It includes processed and prepared foods where such foods would not be consumed in the natural state. The foods have been arranged alphabetically for convenience. The values for 100-Gm. portions are given for all natural foods, but for some processed foods the common unit of package or can is given where a 100-Gm. portion would seldom be used.

Most of the values are taken from the second edition of Handbook No. 8[6] and a few values from other sources.[1,2,3,4,5]

RELIABILITY OF DATA

Research in food values has demonstrated repeatedly that the composition of foods is variable, due to differences in variety, soil and climate in which grown, the method of handling, and the sampling and the analyzing. The values given are usually averages of several determinations on a variety of samples and frequently include a wide range of values; therefore, it seems unnecessary to retain decimals where they are of questionable significance. Thus the values for calories and for grams of protein, fat, carbohydrate and water are given in whole numbers, and fiber is carried to one decimal place only.

Minerals and vitamins are all measured in milligrams (mg.), except for vitamin A, which is still usually given in International Units (I.U.). In order to be consistent in the use of mg., it is necessary to use decimals for measuring the B complex vitamins because they are present in such small amounts.

The common measures for 100-Gm. or other quantities commonly used are only approximate. For instance, 100 Gm. of most liquids would measure about ⅜ of a cup. Since this is not a convenient fraction for measuring, the designation ½ *cup scant* has been used. This would mean about 1½ tbsp. less than ½ cup.

The individual nutrients in foods have been determined by many different laboratories and the data assembled by the Department of Agriculture or other agencies.

FOOD ENERGY

Calorie values have been calculated by using specific factors for individual foods, taking into consideration the digestibility and the physiologic value of nutrients. It is still possible to estimate caloric value of a food by applying the factors 4, 9 and 4 calories per gram of protein, fat and carbohydrate, respectively, but the values will be slightly different from those calculated by the more accurate method mentioned.

NIACIN VALUES

The values for niacin are for the preformed niacin present in the food. Since niacin may be formed in the body from tryptophan in food protein, the total niacin equivalent will be larger than the figure given in most cases. "The average diet in the United States, which contains a generous amount of protein, provides enough tryptophan to increase the niacin value by about a third."[5]

Table 2. Selected Fatty Acids and Cholesterol in Common Foods

This tables gives the total fat; the total saturated fat; the unsaturated fatty acids, oleic (monounsaturated) and linoleic (polyunsaturated); and the cholesterol content of common foods. Values are taken from Handbook No. 8[6] and from Hardinge and Crooks.[3]

Table 3. Amino Acid Content of Foods per 100 Grams—Edible Portion

The essential amino acid content of selected foods is listed in an order convenient for nurses and dietitians dealing with inborn errors of metabolism. The values are given in micrograms rather than milligrams to avoid the use of decimals.

Table 4. Sodium, Potassium and Magnesium Content of Foods

Table 4 gives sodium, potassium and magnesium content of foods. Copper values are omitted because the values given in the literature are conflicting and incomplete. References to pertinent articles are given at the end of Table 4.

Table 5. Alcoholic and Carbonated Beverages

The calorie, carbohydrate and alcohol content of common alcoholic and carbonated beverages are listed in this table to assist the nurse in planning and assessing dietary intake.

Table 6. Equivalent Weights and Measures

This table which lists weight, volume and linear equivalents; comparative temperatures for centigrade and Fahrenheit scales; and approximate weights for common measures, should serve as a ready reference for nurses.

Table 7. Height and Weight for Age— Percentile Standards—Boys and Girls

Heights and weights for boys and girls for each year from 2 to 18 years are listed according to their percentile standards. This table permits the nurse to compare and evaluate height and weight in terms of percentile when assessing growth.

Table 8. Desirable Weights for Men and Women Aged 25 and Over

This table gives the desirable adult weight for height according to the size of the individual's frame—small, medium or large. It is based on the concept that there is no need for an increase in weight once adult height is achieved.

Signs and Symbols Used

An asterisk in the table indicates an item for which the composition has been calculated from a recipe.

Dots (. .) show that no basis could be found for imputing a value, although there was some reason to believe that a measurable amount of the constituent might be present.

The designation Tr. (trace) is used to indicate values that would round to zero when calculated to the number of decimal places used in each column.

REFERENCES USED IN COMPILING FOOD TABLES

1. Burger, M., *et al.*: Vitamin, mineral and proximate composition of frozen fruits, juices and vegetables. J. Agr. & Food Chem., 4:417, 1956.
2. Church, C. E., and Church, H. N.: Food Values of Portions Commonly Used. ed. 11. Philadelphia, J. B. Lippincott, 1970.
3. Hardinge, M. G., and Crooks, H.: J. Am. Dietet. A., 34:1065, 1958.
4. Orr, M. L., and Watt, B. K.: Home Econ. Res. Report No. 4. U.S.D.A., Washington, D.C., 1957.
5. Nutrition Value of Foods. Home and Garden Bulletin No. 72. Agricultural Research Service, U.S.D.A., Washington, D.C., 1960.
6. Watt, B. K., and Merrill, A. L.: Composition of Foods—Raw, Processed, Prepared. Agr. Handbook No. 8. ed. 2. U.S.D.A., Washington, D.C., 1963.

For additional references on food values see Bibliography in Part Four.

TABLE 1. Composition of Foods—Edible Portion

Food and Description	Wt. Gm.	Approximate Measure	Food Energy Cal.	Protein Gm.	Fat Gm.	Carbohydrate Total Gm.	Carbohydrate Fiber Gm.	Water Gm.	Minerals Ca Mg.	Minerals P Mg.	Minerals Fe Mg.	Vitamins Vitamin A I.U.	Vitamins Thiamine Mg.	Vitamins Riboflavin Mg.	Vitamins Niacin Mg.	Vitamins Ascorbic Acid Mg.
Acerola (West Indian cherry) raw	100	1 c.	28	Tr.	Tr.	7	0.4	92	12	11	0.2	..	0.02	0.06	0.4	1,300†
Almonds, dried	100	⅔ c.	598	19	54	20	2.6	5	234	504	4.7	0	0.24	0.92	3.5	Tr.
salted	15	12-15	94	3	9	3	0.4	1	35	75	0.7	0	0.04	0.14	0.5	Tr.
Apples:																
Raw, pared	100	medium	54	Tr.	Tr.	14	0.6	85	6	10	0.3	40	0.03	0.02	0.1	2
Frozen, sliced, sweetened	100	⅔ c.	93	Tr.	Tr.	24	0.7	75	5	6	0.5	20	0.01	0.03	0.2	7
Apple Betty*	100	½ c. scant	151	2	4	30	0.5	64	18	22	0.6	100	0.06	0.04	0.4	1
Apple juice, bottled or canned	100	½ c. scant	47	Tr.	0	12	0.1	88	6	9	0.6	..	0.01	0.02	0.1	1
	250	1 c.	120	Tr.	0	30	..	220	15	22	1.5	..	0.03	0.05	0.3	3
Apple sauce, canned:																
Unsweetened	100	½ c. scant	41	Tr.	Tr.	11	0.6	88	4	5	0.5	40	0.02	0.01	Tr.	1
Sweetened	100	½ c. scant	91	Tr.	Tr.	24	0.5	76	4	5	0.5	40	0.02	0.01	Tr.	1
Apricots:																
Raw	100	3 medium	51	1	Tr.	13	0.6	85	17	23	0.5	2,700	0.03	0.04	0.6	10
Canned: Solids and liquid water pack	100	½ c. scant	38	1	Tr.	10	0.4	89	12	16	0.3	1,830	0.02	0.02	0.4	4
Syrup pack (heavy syrup)	100	½ c. scant	86	1	Tr.	22	0.4	77	11	15	0.3	1,740	0.02	0.02	0.4	4
Dried, sulfured uncooked	100	20 large or 30 small halves	260	5	Tr.	67	3.0	25	67	108	5.5	10,900	0.01	0.16	3.3	12
Cooked, sweetened fruit and liquid*	100	⅓ c.	122	1	Tr.	31	0.9	66	19	31	1.6	2,600	Tr.	0.04	0.9	2
Frozen, sweetened	100	½ c.	98	1	Tr.	25	0.6	73	10	19	0.9	1,680	0.02	0.04	0.8	28‡

Tr. (trace) is used to indicate values that would round to zero with the number of decimal places carried in this table. Thus Tr. means 0.4 Gm. or less of protein, fat, carbohydrate or water.

* Values are calculated from a recipe.
† Value for fully ripe fruit. Av. for firm ripe is 1,900; Av. for partially ripe is 2,500.
‡ Varying amounts of ascorbic acid are added in processing.

TABLE 1. COMPOSITION OF FOODS—EDIBLE PORTION (Continued)

FOOD AND DESCRIPTION	WT. Gm.	APPROXIMATE MEASURE	FOOD ENERGY Cal.	PROTEIN Gm.	FAT Gm.	CARBOHYDRATE Total Gm.	CARBOHYDRATE Fiber Gm.	WATER Gm.	MINERALS Ca Mg.	MINERALS P Mg.	MINERALS Fe Mg.	VITAMINS Vitamin A I.U.	VITAMINS Thiamine Mg.	VITAMINS Riboflavin Mg.	VITAMINS Niacin Mg.	VITAMINS Ascorbic Acid Mg.
Asparagus:																
Fresh, cooked	100	6-7 spears	20	2	Tr.	4	0.7	94	21	50	0.6	900	0.16	0.18	1.4	26
Frozen, cooked	100	6-7 spears	22	3	Tr.	4	0.8	92	22	67	1.1	780	0.16	0.14	1.1	26
Canned:																
Green, drained, solids	100	½ c. cut or 6-7 spears	21	2	Tr.	3	0.8	93	19	53	1.9	800	0.06	0.10	0.8	15
Avocados, raw commercial																
varieties	100	½ peeled	167	2	16	6	1.6	74	10	42	0.6	290	0.11	0.20	1.6	14
Baby Foods:																
Cereals, pre-cooked:																
Mixed, dry, with added nutrients	100	3½ ozs.	368	15	3	71	1.1	7	820	741	56.4	..	3.15	1.35	22.3	0
Dessert:																
Custard pudding	100	3½ ozs.	100	2	2	19	0.2	77	64	62	0.3	100	0.02	0.12	0.1	1
Fruits:																
Apple sauce	100	3½ ozs.	72	Tr.	Tr.	19	0.5	81	4	7	0.4	40	0.01	0.02	0.1	Tr.
Apple sauce and apricot	100	3½ ozs.	86	Tr.	Tr.	23	0.5	77	4	14	0.3	600	0.01	0.02	0.1	2
Apricot, pineapple, and/ or orange with tapioca	100	3½ ozs.	84	Tr.	Tr.	22	0.2	78	15	9	0.4	450	0.02	0.01	0.2	4
Peaches	100	3½ ozs.	81	1	Tr.	21	0.5	78	6	14	0.3	500	0.01	0.02	0.7	3
Pears	100	3½ ozs.	66	Tr.	Tr.	17	1.0	82	7	8	0.2	30	0.02	0.02	0.2	2
Prunes with tapioca	100	3½ ozs.	86	Tr.	Tr.	22	0.3	77	7	21	0.9	400	0.02	0.06	0.4	4
Meats, Poultry and Eggs:																
Beef, strained	100	3½ ozs.	99	15	4	0	0	80	8	127	2.0	..	0.01	0.16	3.5	0
junior	100	3½ ozs.	118	19	4	0	0	76	8	163	2.5	..	0.02	0.20	4.3	0
Beef heart	100	3½ ozs.	93	14	4	Tr.	0	81	5	155	3.7	..	0.06	0.62	3.6	0
Chicken	100	3½ ozs.	127	14	8	0	0	77	..	129	1.9	..	0.02	0.16	3.5	0
Egg yolk, strained	100	3½ ozs.	210	10	18	Tr.	0	70	81	256	3.0	1,900	0.12	0.22	Tr.	Tr.
Lamb, strained	100	3½ ozs.	107	15	5	0	0	79	9	124	2.1	..	0.02	0.17	3.3	..
junior	100	3½ ozs.	121	18	5	0	0	76	13	156	2.7	..	0.02	0.21	4.1	..
Liver, strained	100	3½ ozs.	97	14	3	2	0	80	6	182	5.6	24,000	0.05	2.00	7.6	10
Pork, strained	100	3½ ozs.	118	15	6	0	0	78	8	130	1.5	..	0.19	0.20	2.7	..
junior	100	3½ ozs.	107	19	3	0	0	74	8	144	1.2	..	0.23	0.23	2.8	..
Veal, strained	100	3½ ozs.	91	16	3	0	0	81	10	145	1.7	..	0.03	0.20	4.3	..
junior	100	3½ ozs.	134	19	6	0	0	77	8	157	1.6	..	0.03	0.22	6.0	..

Vegetables:

Beans, green	100	3½ ozs.	22	1	Tr.	5	0.8	93	33	25	1.1	400	0.02	0.06	0.3	3
Beets	100	3½ ozs.	37	1	Tr.	8	0.6	89	18	27	0.7	20	0.02	0.03	0.1	3
Carrots	100	3½ ozs.	29	1	Tr.	7	0.6	92	23	21	0.5	13,000	0.02	0.03	0.1	3
Mixed vegetables	100	3½ ozs.	37	2	Tr.	9	0.5	89	22	36	0.9	4,700	0.05	0.04	0.6	2
Peas	100	3½ ozs.	54	4	Tr.	9	0.8	86	11	63	1.2	500	0.08	0.09	1.2	10
Spinach, creamed	100	3½ ozs.	43	2	1	8	0.4	88	64	63	0.6	5,000	0.02	0.13	0.3	6
Squash	100	3½ ozs.	25	1	Tr.	6	0.8	92	24	17	0.4	2,400	0.02	0.04	0.3	8
Sweet potatoes	100	3½ ozs.	67	1	Tr.	16	0.5	82	16	34	0.4	4,900	0.04	0.03	0.4	8
Tomato soup	100	3½ ozs.	54	2	Tr.	14	0.2	83	24	52	0.4	1,000	0.05	0.12	0.7	3
Bacon, broiled or fried	100	12 strips	611	30	52	3	0	8	14	224	3.3	0	0.51	0.34	5.2	0
	16	2 strips	100	5	8	1	0	1	2	37	0.5	0	0.08	0.06	0.8	0
Bacon, Canadian, broiled or fried	100	3½ ozs.	277	28	18	Tr.	0	50	19	218	4.1	0	0.92	0.17	5.0	0
Bananas, raw	100	1 small	85	1	Tr.	22	0.5	76	8	26	0.7	190	0.05	0.06	0.7	10
Barley, pearled, light uncooked	100	½ c.	349	8	1	79	0.5	11	16	189	2.0	0	0.12	0.05	3.1	0
Beans, common or kidney:																
Red kidney, canned or cooked, solids and liquids	100	½ c. scant	90	6	Tr.	16	0.9	76	29	109	1.8	0	0.05	0.04	0.6	..
Canned, baked:																
Pork and molasses	100	½ c. scant	150	6	5	21	1.7	66	63	114	2.3	..	0.06	0.04	0.5	..
Pork and tomato sauce ..	100	½ c. scant	122	6	3	19	1.4	71	54	92	1.8	130	0.08	0.03	0.6	2
Beans, Lima:																
Fresh, cooked	100	⅔ c.	111	8	Tr.	20	1.8	71	47	121	2.5	280	0.18	0.10	1.3	17
Frozen, cooked	100	⅔ c.	99	6	Tr.	19	1.6	74	20	90	1.7	230	0.07	0.05	1.0	17
Canned, drained solids ...	100	½ c. scant	96	5	Tr.	18	1.8	75	28	70	2.4	190	0.03	0.05	0.5	6
Beans:																
Snap green:																
Cooked, fresh or frozen	100	¾ c.	25	2	Tr.	5	1.0	92	50	37	0.6	540	0.07	0.09	0.5	12
Canned, drained solids..	100	¾ c.	24	1	Tr.	5	1.0	92	45	25	1.5	470	0.03	0.05	0.3	4
Wax or yellow:																
Canned, drained solids..	100	½ c.	22	1	Tr.	5	1.0	93	50	37	0.6	230	0.07	0.09	0.5	13
Bean Sprouts, mung, raw ...	100	1 c.	35	4	Tr.	7	0.7	89	19	64	1.3	20	0.13	0.13	0.8	19
Beef, trimmed to retail basis, cooked:																
Cuts, braised, simmered or pot-roasted:																
Lean and fat	100	3½ ozs.	289	27	19	0	0	53	12	134	3.4	30	0.05	0.21	4.2	0

TABLE 1. COMPOSITION OF FOODS—EDIBLE PORTION (*Continued*)

FOOD AND DESCRIPTION	WT. Gm.	APPROXIMATE MEASURE	FOOD ENERGY Cal.	PROTEIN Gm.	FAT Gm.	CARBOHYDRATE		WATER Gm.	MINERALS			VITAMINS				
						TOTAL Gm.	FIBER Gm.		CA Mg.	P Mg.	FE Mg.	VITA-MIN A I.U.	THIA-MINE Mg.	RIBO-FLAVIN Mg.	NIA-CIN Mg.	ASCORBIC ACID Mg.
Beef: (*Continued*)																
Lean only (from above serving)	85	3 ozs.	165	26	6	0	0	52	12	128	3.2	10	0.05	0.19	3.2	0
Hamburger, broiled:																
Market ground	100	3½ ozs.	286	25	20	0	0	54	11	194	3.2	40	0.09	0.21	5.4	0
Ground lean	100	or 2 patties	219	27	11	0	0	60	12	230	3.5	20	0.09	0.23	6.0	0
	50	1 patty	109	14	6	0	0	30	6	115	1.8	10	0.05	0.12	3.0	0
Roast, oven-cooked no water added Relatively fat such as rib:																
Lean and fat	100	3½ ozs.	417	21	36	0	0	42	9	175	2.7	70	0.06	0.16	3.8	0
Lean only (from above serving)	63	2.2 ozs.	135	18	6	0	0	38	7	153	2.3	12	0.04	0.14	3.3	0
Relatively lean such as round:																
Lean and fat	100	3½ ozs.	317	25	23	0	0	51	11	207	3.1	40	0.06	0.19	4.5	0
Lean only (from above serving)	76	2.8 ozs.	145	23	5	0	0	47	10	186	2.8	7	0.06	0.17	4.0	0
Steak, broiled Relatively fat such as sirloin:																
Lean and fat	100	3½ ozs.	387	23	32	0	0	44	10	191	2.9	50	0.06	0.18	4.7	0
Lean only (from above serving)	66	2.3 ozs.	136	21	5	0	0	39	8	173	2.6	7	0.06	0.17	4.2	0
Relatively lean such as round:																
Lean and fat	100	3½ ozs.	261	29	15	0	0	55	12	250	3.5	30	0.08	0.22	5.6	0
Lean only (from above serving)	81	2.9 ozs.	152	25	5	0	0	50	11	218	3.0	8	0.07	0.19	4.9	0
Beef, canned:																
Corned beef	100	3½ ozs.	185	26	8	0	0	62	21	110	4.5	..	0.02	0.25	3.5	0
Corned beef hash	100	3½ ozs.	181	9	11	11	1	67	13	67	2.0	..	0.01	0.09	2.1	..
Beef, dried or chipped	100	3½ ozs.	203	34	6	0	0	48	20	404	5.1	0	0.07	0.32	3.8	0
cooked, creamed	100	3½ ozs.	154	8	10	7	0	72	105	140	0.8	360	0.06	0.19	2.6	Tr.
Beef and vegetable stew canned	100	½ c.	79	6	3	7	0.3	83	12	45	0.9	970	0.03	0.05	1.0	3

Food	Grams	Measure	Calories	Protein (g)	Fat (g)	Carbohydrate (g)	Fiber (g)	Water (%)	Calcium (mg)	Phosphorus (mg)	Iron (mg)	Vit. A (I.U.)	Thiamine (mg)	Riboflavin (mg)	Niacin (mg)	Ascorbic Acid (mg)
Beets, cooked, drained	100	½ c.	32	1	Tr.	7	0.8	91	14	23	0.5	20	0.03	0.04	0.3	6
canned, solids	100	½ c.	37	1	Tr.	9	0.8	90	19	18	0.7	20	0.01	0.03	0.1	3
Beet greens, cooked	100	⅔ c.	18	2	Tr.	3	1.1	94	99†	25	1.9	5,100	0.07	0.15	0.3	15
Beverages, carbonated:																
Ginger ale	100	3½ ozs.	31	..	..	8	..	92	..	..	..	..	..	..	..	..
Other, including cola type	100	3½ ozs.	40	..	..	10	..	90	..	..	..	..	..	..	..	..
Biscuits, baking powder, made with enriched flour*	100	3 biscuits 2-in. diam.	369	7	17	46	0.2	27	121	175	1.6	Tr.	0.21	0.21	1.8	Tr.
Blackberries: including dewberries, boysenberries																
Raw	100	⅔ c.	58	1	1	13	4.2	85	32	19	0.9	200	0.03	0.04	0.4	21
Canned, solids and liquids:																
Water pack	100	½ c. scant	40	1	1	9	2.8	89	22	13	0.6	140	0.02	0.02	0.2	7
Syrup pack	100	½ c. scant	91	1	1	22	2.6	76	21	12	0.6	130	0.01	0.02	0.2	7
Blueberries:																
Raw	100	⅔ c.	62	1	1	15	1.5	83	15	13	1.0	100	0.03	0.06	0.5	14
Frozen without sugar	100	⅔ c.	55	1	Tr.	14	1.5	85	10	13	0.8	70	0.03	0.06	0.5	7
Canned, solids and liquids:																
Water pack	100	½ c. scant	39	Tr.	Tr.	10	1.0	89	10	9	0.7	40	0.01	0.01	0.2	7
Syrup pack	100	½ c. scant	101	Tr.	Tr.	26	1.0	73	9	8	0.6	40	0.01	0.01	0.2	6
Bouillon cubes	100	25 cubes	120	20	5	4	0	..	..	..	..	..	..	..	..	..
	4	1 cube	2	Tr.	Tr.	Tr.	0	Tr.	..	..	..	..	..	..	..	..
Brains, all kinds, raw	100	3½ ozs.	125	10	9	1	0	79	10	312	2.4	0	0.23	0.26	4.4	18
Bran (breakfast cereal, almost wholly bran)	28	1 oz.	95	3	1	21	2.0	1	24	350	2.9	0	0.11	0.09	5.0	0
Bran flakes (40 percent bran) with added thiamine	100	2½ c.	303	10	2	81	3.6	3	71	495	4.4	0	0.40	0.17	6.2	0
	28	¾ c. 1 oz.	85	3	1	23	1.0	1	20	138	1.2	0	0.11	0.05	1.7	0
Bran flakes with raisins added thiamine	100	2 c.	287	8	1	79	3.0	7	56	396	4.0	..	0.32	0.13	5.3	0
Brazil nuts, shelled	100	⅔ c.	654	14	67	11	3.1	5	186	693	3.4	Tr.	0.96	0.12	1.6	0

* Values are calculated from a recipe.

† Calcium may not be available because of the presence of oxalic acid.

TABLE 1. COMPOSITION OF FOODS—EDIBLE PORTION (*Continued*)

Food and Description	Wt. Gm.	Approximate Measure	Food Energy Cal.	Protein Gm.	Fat Gm.	Carbohydrate Total Gm.	Carbohydrate Fiber Gm.	Water Gm.	Ca Mg.	P Mg.	Fe Mg.	Vitamin A I.U.	Thiamine Mg.	Riboflavin Mg.	Niacin Mg.	Ascorbic Acid Mg.
Breads: *																
Boston brown bread made with degermed corn meal, enriched	100	2 sl. 3 x ¾ in.	211	6	1	46	0.7	45	90	160	1.9	..	0.11	0.06	1.2	0
Cracked wheat bread made with enriched flour	100	4 sl.	263	9	2	52	0.5	35	88	128	1.1	0	0.12	0.09	1.3	Tr.
	23	1 sl.	60	2	Tr.	12	0.1	8	20	29	0.3	0	0.03	0.02	0.3	Tr.
French or Vienna breads: unenriched	100	3½ ozs.	290	9	3	55	0.2	31	43	85	0.7	0	0.08	0.08	0.8	Tr.
enriched	100	3½ ozs.	290	9	3	55	0.2	31	43	85	2.2	0	0.28	0.22	2.5	Tr.
Italian bread: unenriched	100	3½ ozs.	276	9	1	56	0.2	32	17	77	0.7	0	0.09	0.06	0.8	0
enriched	100	3½ ozs.	276	9	1	56	0.2	32	17	77	2.2	0	0.29	0.20	2.6	0
Raisin bread	100	4 sl.	262	7	3	54	0.2	35	71	87	1.3	Tr.	0.05	0.09	0.7	Tr.
	23	1 sl.	60	2	1	13	Tr.	7	16	20	0.3	Tr.	0.01	0.02	0.2	0
Rye bread, American (⅓ rye, ⅔ wheat flour)..	100	4 sl.	243	9	1	52	0.4	36	75	147	1.6	0	0.18	0.07	1.4	0
	23	1 sl.	56	2	Tr.	12	0.1	9	17	34	0.4	0	0.04	0.02	0.3	0
White bread, unenriched: 4 percent nonfat dry milk	100	4 sl.	270	9	3	51	0.2	36	84	97	0.7	Tr.	0.07	0.09	1.1	Tr.
	23	1 sl.	62	2	1	12	Tr.	8	19	22	0.2	Tr.	0.02	0.02	0.3	Tr.
White bread, enriched: 1-2 percent nonfat dry milk	100	4 sl.	269	9	3	50	0.2	36	70	87	2.4	Tr.	0.25	0.17	2.3	Tr.
	23	1 sl.	62	2	1	12	0.1	9	16	20	0.6	Tr.	0.06	0.04	0.5	Tr.
3-4 percent nonfat dry milk†	100	4 sl.	270	9	3	50	0.2	36	84	97	2.5	Tr.	0.25	0.21	2.4	Tr.
	23	1 sl.	62	2	1	12	0.1	9	19	22	0.6	Tr.	0.06	0.05	0.6	Tr.
5-6 percent nonfat dry milk	100	4 sl.	275	9	4	50	0.2	35	96	102	2.5	Tr.	0.27	0.20	2.4	Tr.
	23	1 sl.	63	2	1	12	0.1	9	22	24	0.6	Tr.	0.06	0.05	0.6	Tr.
Whole wheat, graham, entire wheat bread, 2 percent dry milk	100	4 sl.	243	10	3	48	1.6	37	99	228	2.3	Tr.	0.26	0.12	2.8	Tr.
	23	1 sl.	56	2	1	11	0.4	9	23	53	0.6	Tr.	0.06	0.03	0.6	Tr.
Bread crumbs, dry	100	1 c.	392	13	5	73	0.3	7	122	141	3.6	Tr.	0.22	0.30	3.5	Tr.

Breakfast foods. See individual grain, as corn, oatmeal, etc.

Food	g	Measure														
Broccoli, flower stalks, fresh or frozen	100	⅔ c.	32	4	Tr.	6	1.5	89	103	78	1.1	2,500	0.10	0.23	0.9	113
cooked	100	⅔ c.	26	3	Tr.	5	1.5	91	88	62	0.8	2,500	0.09	0.20	0.8	90
Brussels sprouts, fresh or frozen, cooked	100	¾ c.	36	4	Tr.	6	1.6	88	32	72	1.1	520	0.08	0.14	0.8	87
Buckwheat flour, light	100	1 c. sifted	347	6	1	80	0.5	12	11	88	1.0	0	0.08	0.04	0.4	0
Bun, hamburger. See Rolls.																
Butter	100	½ c. scant	716	1	81	Tr.	0	16	20	16	0	3,300‡	..	..	..	0
	14	1 tbsp.	100	Tr.	11	Tr.	0	2	3	2	0	460‡	..	..	..	0
Buttermilk, cultured (made from skim milk)	100	½ c. scant	36	4	Tr.	5	0	91	121	95	Tr.	Tr.	0.04	0.18	0.1	1
Cabbage: Raw	100	wedge 3½ x 4½ in.	24	1	Tr.	5	0.8	92	49	29	0.4	130	0.05	0.05	0.3	47§
Cooked (short time)	100	1⅔ c.	20	1	Tr.	4	0.8	94	44	20	0.3	130	0.04	0.04	0.3	33
Cabbage, celery or Chinese, raw	100	1 c., 1-in. pieces	14	1	Tr.	3	0.6	95	43	40	0.6	150	0.05	0.04	0.6	25
Cakes: home recipes: Chocolate (devil's food with icing)	100	1 piece	369	4	16	56	0.3	22	70	131	1.0	160	0.02	0.10	0.2	Tr.
Fruit cake, dark type	100	3 pieces 2 x 2 x ½ in.	379	5	15	60	0.6	18	72	113	2.6	120	0.13	0.14	0.8	Tr.
Plain or cup cake, no icing	100	2 cupcakes	364	5	14	56	0.1	25	64	102	0.4	170	0.02	0.09	0.2	Tr.
Sponge cake	100	2 pieces	297	8	6	54	0	32	30	112	1.2	450	0.05	0.14	0.2	Tr.
Cakes: made from mixes: Angel food	100	2 pieces	259	6	Tr.	59	Tr.	34	95	119	0.3	0	Tr.	0.11	0.1	0
Coffee cake	100	2 pieces	322	6	10	52	0.1	30	61	174	1.6	160	0.18	0.16	1.4	Tr.
Yellow cake, chocolate icing	100	3-in. piece	337	4	11	58	0.2	26	91	182	0.6	140	0.02	0.08	0.2	Tr.
Cake icing, mix: Chocolate fudge	100	3½ ozs.	378	2	14	67	0.5	15	16	66	1.0	270	0.01	0.04	0.2	0

* Values are calculated from a recipe.
† When the amount of nonfat milk solids in commercial bread is unknown, use bread with 3 to 4 percent nonfat milk solids.
‡ Year-round average.
§ Freshly harvested av. 51 Mg.; stored av. 42 Mg.

TABLE 1. Composition of Foods—Edible Portion (Continued)

FOOD AND DESCRIPTION	WT. Gm.	APPROXIMATE MEASURE	FOOD ENERGY Cal.	PROTEIN Gm.	FAT Gm.	CARBOHYDRATE TOTAL Gm.	CARBOHYDRATE FIBER Gm.	WATER Gm.	MINERALS CA Mg.	MINERALS P Mg.	MINERALS FE Mg.	VITAMINS VITAMIN A I.U.	VITAMINS THIAMINE Mg.	VITAMINS RIBOFLAVIN Mg.	VITAMINS NIACIN Mg.	VITAMINS ASCORBIC ACID Mg.
Candy:																
Candied or glacé peel—lemon, orange or grape-fruit peel	100	3½ ozs.	316	Tr.	Tr.	81	..	17	..	..	..	..	..	..	..	..
Butterscotch	28	1 oz.	111	..	1	26	0	..	5	2	0.4	40	0	0	0	..
Caramels, plain	28	1 oz.	109	1	3	27	0.1	..	42	34	0.4	3	0.01	0.05	0.1	Tr.
Chocolate, plain, milk	28	1 oz.	146	2	9	16	0.1	Tr.	64	65	0.3	75	0.02	0.10	0.1	Tr.
Chocolate, milk with almonds	28	1 oz.	150	3	10	14	0.2	Tr.	64	76	0.4	64	0.02	0.11	0.2	Tr.
Chocolate covered peanuts	28	1 oz.	157	4	12	11	0.3	Tr.	32	84	0.4	Tr.	0.10	0.05	2.4	Tr.
Fudge, plain chocolate	28	1 oz.	112	1	3	21	Tr.	2	22	24	0.3	Tr.	0.01	0.03	0.1	Tr.
Hard candy	28	1 oz.	108	0	Tr.	27	0	Tr.	7	2	0.7	0	0	0	0	0
Marshmallows	28	1 oz.	85	1	Tr.	22	0	5	5	2	0.4	0	0	0	0	0
Peanut bar	28	1 oz.	144	5	9	13	0.3	Tr.	12	74	0.5	0	0.12	0.02	2.6	0
Peanut brittle	28	1 oz.	118	2	3	22	0.1	Tr.	10	28	0.6	0	0.04	0.01	0.9	0
Cantaloupe, raw netted type	100	⅙ melon, 5 in. diam.	30	1	Tr.	8	0.3	91	14	16	0.4	3,400	0.04	0.03	0.6	33
Carrots:																
Raw	100	2 carrots, 5½ x 1 in. or 1 c. grated	42	1	Tr.	10	1.0	88	37	36	0.7	11,000	0.06	0.05	0.6	8
Cooked, drained	100	⅔ c.	31	1	Tr.	7	1.0	92	33	31	0.6	10,500	0.05	0.05	0.5	6
Canned: Drained solids	100	⅔ c.	30	1	Tr.	7	0.8	92	30	22	0.7	15,000	0.02	0.03	0.4	2
Cashew nuts, roasted or cooked	100	3½ ozs.	561	17	46	29	1.4	5	38	373	3.8	100	0.43	0.25	1.8	0
	28	1 oz.	168	5	14	9	0.4	1	11	112	1.1	30	0.13	0.08	0.5	0
Cauliflower:																
Raw	100	1 c. flower buds	27	3	Tr.	5	0.9	91	25	56	1.1	60	0.11	0.10	0.7	78
Cooked, drained	100	1 c. scant	22	2	Tr.	4	0.9	93	21	42	0.7	60	0.09	0.08	0.6	55
Frozen, raw	100	1 c. scant	22	2	Tr.	4	0.8	93	19	42	0.6	30	0.06	0.06	0.5	56
Celery, bleached:																
Raw	100	2 large stalks or 1 c. diced	17	1	Tr.	4	0.6	94	39	28	0.3	240	0.03	0.03	0.3	9
Cooked	100	¾ c. diced	14	1	Tr.	3	0.6	95	31	22	0.2	230	0.02	0.03	0.3	6

Chard, leaves and stalks, cooked

Food	g	Measure													
Chard, leaves and stalks, cooked	100	⅔ c.	18	2	Tr.	3	0.7	94	73†	24	1.8	5,400	0.04	0.11	0.4	16
Cheeses:																
Blue mold, or Roquefort	100	3½ ozs.	368	22	31	2	0	40	315	339	0.5	1,240	0.03	0.61	1.2	0
	28	1 oz.	110	6	9	1	0	11	88	95	0.1	343	0.01	0.18	0.4	0
Camembert	100	3½ ozs.	299	18	25	2	0	52	105	184	0.5	1,010	0.04	0.75	0.8	0
	28	1 oz.	84	5	7	1	0	15	29	52	0.2	282	0.01	0.22	0.2	0
Cheddar, American, regular	100	3½ ozs.	398	25	32	2	0	37	750	478	1.0	2,310	0.03	0.46	0.1	0
	28	1 oz.	120	7	9	1	0	10	210	134	0.3	650	0.01	0.14	Tr.	0
Cheddar, American, processed	100	3½ ozs.	370	23	30	2	0	40	697	771	0.9	1,220	0.02	0.41	Tr.	0
	28	1 oz.	107	6	8	1	0	11	195	218	0.3	340	0.01	0.11	Tr.	0
Cottage, from skim milk creamed	100	3½ ozs.	106	14	4	3	0	78	94	152	0.3	170	0.03	0.25	0.1	0
	28	1 oz.	30	4	1	1	0	23	28	43	0.1	48	0.01	0.07	Tr.	0
Cream cheese	100	3½ ozs.	374	8	38	2	0	51	62	95	0.2	1,540	0.02	0.24	0.1	0
	28	1 oz.	113	2	10	1	0	14	17	27	0.1	430	0.01	0.07	Tr.	0
Parmesan	100	3½ ozs.	393	36	26	3	0	30	1,140	781	0.4	1,060	0.02	0.73	0.2	0
	28	1 oz.	110	11	8	1	0	9	312	218	0.1	296	0.01	0.20	0.1	0
Pimiento, American, processed	100	3½ ozs.	371	23	30	2	Tr.	40	..	..	..	..	..	..	..	..
	28	1 oz.	103	6	8	1	Tr.	11	..	..	..	..	..	..	..	0
Swiss, processed	100	3½ ozs.	355	26	27	2	0	40	887	867	0.9	1,100	0.01	0.40	0.1	0
	28	1 oz.	109	7	8	1	0	11	245	240	0.3	310	Tr.	0.11	Tr.	0
Cherries:																
Sour, red, raw	100	1 c. whole or pitted	58	1	Tr.	14	0.2	84	22	19	0.4	1,000	0.05	0.06	0.4	10
Sweet, raw	100	⅔ c.	70	1	Tr.	17	0.4	80	22	19	0.4	110	0.05	0.06	0.4	10
Red, sour, canned, heavy syrup	100	½ c. scant	89	1	Tr.	23	0.1	76	14	12	0.3	650	0.03	0.02	0.2	5
Maraschino	100	½ c. scant	116	Tr.	Tr.	29	0.3	70	..	..	..	..	..	..	..	..
Chicken, cooked																
Light meat	100	3½ ozs.	166	32	3	0	0	64	11	265	1.3	60	0.04	0.10	11.6	0
no skin, roasted, fried	100	3½ ozs.	197	32	6	1	0	60	12	280	1.3	50	0.05	0.25	12.9	0
Dark meat	100	3½ ozs.	176	28	6	0	0	64	13	229	1.7	150	0.07	0.23	5.6	0
no skin, roasted, fried	100	3½ ozs.	220	30	9	2	0	58	14	225	1.8	130	0.07	0.45	6.8	0
Canned, boneless	100	3½ ozs.	198	22	12	0	0	65	21	247	1.5	230	0.04	0.12	4.4	4
Chickpeas or garbanzos, dry, whole seed, raw	100	½ c.	360	21	5	61	5.3	11	150	331	6.9	50	0.31	0.15	2.0	..
Chili sauce	100	½ c. scant	104	3	Tr.	25	0.7	68	20	52	0.8	1,400	0.09	0.07	1.6	..
	17	1 tbsp.	18	1	Tr.	4	0.1	11	3	9	0.1	238	0.02	0.01	0.3	..

† Calcium may not be available because of the presence of oxalic acid.

TABLE 1. COMPOSITION OF FOODS—EDIBLE PORTION (*Continued*)

FOOD AND DESCRIPTION	WT. Gm.	APPROXIMATE MEASURE	FOOD ENERGY Cal.	PROTEIN Gm.	FAT Gm.	CARBOHYDRATE TOTAL Gm.	FIBER Gm.	WATER Gm.	MINERALS Ca Mg.	P Mg.	FE Mg.	VITAMINS VITAMIN A I.U.	THIAMINE Mg.	RIBOFLAVIN Mg.	NIACIN Mg.	ASCORBIC ACID Mg.
Chocolate:																
Bitter or unsweetened	100	3½ ozs.	505	11	53	29	2.5	2	78‖	384	6.7	60	0.05	0.24	1.5	0
	28	1 oz. square	142	3	15	8	0.8	1	23‖	116	2.0	18	0.01	0.07	0.5	0
Bittersweet	100	3½ ozs.	477	8	40	47	1.8	2	58‖	284	5.0	40	0.03	0.17	1.0	0
	28	1 oz.	143	2	12	14	0.5	1	17‖	85	1.5	12	0.01	0.05	0.3	0
Chocolate syrup, thin type ...	100	⅓ c.	245	2	2	63	0.6	32	17‖	92	1.6	Tr.	0.02	0.07	0.4	0
	20	1 tbsp.	49	Tr.	Tr.	13	0.1	6	3‖	18	0.3	Tr.	Tr.	0.01	0.1	0
Clams, long and round:																
Raw, meat only	100	3½ ozs.	76	13	2	2	..	82	69	162	6.1	100	0.10	0.18	1.3	10
Canned, solids and liquid ..	100	3½ ozs.	52	8	1	3	..	86	55	137	4.1	..	0.01	0.10	1.1	..
Cocoa beverage, made with all milk*	100	½ c. scant	95	4	5	11	0.1	79	119	114	0.4	160	0.04	0.19	0.2	1
	250	1 c.	236	10	12	27	0.3	198	298	285	1.0	400	0.10	0.46	0.5	3
Coconut:																
Fresh, meat	100	1 c. shredded	346	4	35	9	4.0	51	13	95	1.7	0	0.05	0.02	0.5	3
Dried, shredded (sweetened)	100	3½ ozs.	548	4	39	53	4.1	3	16	112	2.0	0	0.04	0.03	0.4	0
Coleslaw, French dressing ...	100	¾ c.	95	1	7	8	0.7	84	42	26	0.4	110	0.04	0.04	0.3	29
Collards: leaves only Cooked (boiled in small amount of water)	100	½ c.	33	4	1	5	1.0	90	188	52	0.8	7,800	0.11	0.20	1.2	76
Cookies:*																
Assorted, commercial	25	1 cookie	120	1	5	18	Tr.	1	9	41	0.2	20	0.01	0.01	0.1	Tr.
Brownie with nuts	50	1 bar	242	3	16	25	0.5	5	20	74	1.0	100	0.10	0.06	0.4	Tr.
Chocolate chip	25	3 small	129	1	8	15	0.1	1	8	25	0.5	28	0.03	0.03	0.2	Tr.
Macaroons, coconut	20	1 cookie	95	1	5	13	0.4	1	5	17	0.2	0	0.01	0.03	0.1	0
Oatmeal with raisins	20	1 cookie	90	1	3	15	0.1	1	4	20	0.6	10	0.02	0.02	0.1	Tr.
Sandwich type, commercial	20	1 cookie	99	1	5	14	Tr.	Tr.	5	48	0.1	0	0.01	0.01	0.1	0
Corn, sweet:																
Cooked, fresh on cob	100	1 small ear	91	3	1	21	0.7	74	3	89	0.6	400†	0.11	0.10	1.4	9
Canned:																
Cream style	100	½ c. scant	82	2	1	20	1.0	76	3	56	0.6	330†	0.03	0.05	1.0	5
Whole kernel	100	½ c. scant	66	2	1	16	0.8	81	4	50	0.4	270†	0.03	0.05	0.9	5

Corn bread or muffins*
made with:

Food	g	Measure													
Whole ground corn meal	100	2 muffins, 2¾ in. diam.	215	7	6	35	0.6	49	141	216	1.7	130‡	0.15	0.18	0.8	0
Enriched, degermed corn meal	100	2 muffins, 2¾ in. diam.	219	7	5	37	0.2	49	139	155	1.9	130§	0.17	0.23	1.3	0

Corn Cereals:

Food	g	Measure													
Cornflakes (added thiamine, niacin and iron)	100	4 c.	386	8	Tr.	86	0.6	4	17	45	1.4	0	0.42	0.07	2.1	0
	28	1 c., 1 oz. pkg.	108	2	Tr.	24	0.2	1	5	13	0.4	0	0.12	0.02	0.6	0
Corn, puffed, sweetened	100	4 c.	379	4	Tr.	90	0.3	5	11	28	1.8	0	0.42	0.17	2.1	0
	28	1 oz. package	106	1	Tr.	25	0.1	1	3	8	0.5	0	0.11	0.05	0.6	0
Corn shredded (added thiamine and niacin)	100	2½ c.	389	7	Tr.	87	0.6	3	5	39	2.4	0	0.42	0.18	2.1	0
	28	¾ c., 1 oz. pkg.	109	2	Tr.	25	0.2	1	1	11	0.7	0	0.12	0.05	0.6	0

Corn grits, degermed, white:

Food	g	Measure													
Unenriched, cooked*	100	½ c. scant	51	1	Tr.	11	0.1	87	1	10	0.1	Tr.	0.02	0.01	0.2	0
Enriched, cooked*	100	½ c. scant	51	1	Tr.	11	0.1	87	1	10	0.3	Tr.	0.04	0.03	0.4	0

Corn meal, white or yellow:

Food	g	Measure													
Degermed, unenriched, cooked*	100	½ c. scant	50	1	Tr.	11	0.1	88	1	14	0.2	60†	0.02	0.01	0.1	0
Degermed, enriched, cooked*	100	½ c. scant	50	1	Tr.	11	0.1	88	1	14	0.4	60†	0.06	0.04	0.5	0

Food	g	Measure													
Cowpeas, immature seeds, cooked	100	⅔ c.	108	8	1	18	1.8	72	24	146	2.1	350	0.30	0.11	1.4	17

Crabs, Atlantic and Pacific,

Food	g	Measure													
hard shell, steamed	100	3½ ozs.	93	17	2	1	..	79	43	175	0.8	2,170	0.16	0.08	2.8	2
Canned, meat only	100	3½ ozs.	101	17	3	1	..	77	45	182	0.8	..	0.08	0.08	1.9	..

Crackers:

Food	g	Measure													
Graham	14	2 medium	55	1	1	10	0.1	1	3	28	0.3	0	0.04	0.02	0.2	0
Saltines	8	2 crackers	34	1	1	6	Tr.	1	2	7	0.1	0	Tr.	Tr.	0.1	0
Soda, plain or oyster crackers	14	2 crackers	60	1	1	5	..	..	..	..	..	..	..	..	..	..
Ritz type	7	1 cracker	34	1	2	4	..	..	..	..	..	..	..	..	..	..

* Values are calculated from a recipe.
† Vitamin A based on yellow corn: white corn contains only a trace.
‡ Based on recipe using white corn meal: if yellow, the vitamin A value is 330 I.U.
§ Based on recipe using white corn meal: if yellow, the vitamin A value is 250 I.U.
‖ Calcium may not be available because of the presence of oxalic acid.

TABLE 1. COMPOSITION OF FOODS—EDIBLE PORTION (Continued)

FOOD AND DESCRIPTION	WT. Gm.	APPROXIMATE MEASURE	FOOD ENERGY Cal.	PRO-TEIN Gm.	FAT Gm.	CARBO-HYDRATE Total Gm.	CARBO-HYDRATE Fiber Gm.	WATER Gm.	MINERALS CA Mg.	MINERALS P Mg.	MINERALS FE Mg.	VITAMINS VITA-MIN A I.U.	VITAMINS THIA-MINE Mg.	VITAMINS RIBO-FLAVIN Mg.	VITAMINS NIA-CIN Mg.	VITAMINS ASCORBIC ACID Mg.
Cranberries:																
Raw	100	1 c.	46	Tr.	1	11	1.4	88	14	11	0.5	40	0.03	0.02	0.1	11
Juice, cocktail	100	½ c. scant	65	Tr.	Tr.	17	Tr.	83	5	3	0.3	Tr.	0.01	0.01	Tr.	40†
Sauce, sweetened, canned strained	100	½ c. scant	146	Tr.	Tr.	38	0.2	62	6	4	0.2	20	0.01	0.01	Tr.	2
Cream:																
Light, table or coffee	100	½ c. scant	211	3	21	4	0	72	102	80	Tr.	840	0.03	0.15	0.1	1
	15	1 tbsp.	31	Tr.	3	1	0	11	15	12	0	125	Tr.	0.02	Tr.	Tr.
Heavy or whipping	15	1 tbsp.	53	Tr.	6	1	0	8	12	9	0	230	Tr.	0.02	Tr.	Tr.
Cucumbers, raw pared	100	⅓ of 7-8 in. cucumber	14	1	Tr.	3	0.3	96	17	18	0.3	Tr.	0.03	0.04	0.2	11
Currants, red & white, raw	100	1 c.	50	1	Tr.	12	3.4	86	32	23	1.0	120	0.04	0.05	0.1	41
Custard, baked*	100	½ c. scant	115	5	6	11	0	77	112	117	0.4	350	0.04	0.19	0.1	Tr.
Dandelion greens, raw	100	1 c.	45	3	1	9	1.6	86	187	66	3.1	14,000	0.19	0.26	..	35
cooked	100	½ c.	33	2	1	6	1.3	90	140	42	1.8	11,700	0.13	0.16	..	18
Dates, "fresh" and dried	100	½ c. pitted	274	2	1	73	2.4	23	59	63	3.0	50	0.09	0.10	2.2	0
Doughnuts, cake type made with enriched flour*	100	2 or 3 doughnuts	391	5	19	51	0.1	24	40	190	1.4	80	0.16	0.16	1.2	Tr.
Duck, domestic raw, flesh only	100	3½ ozs.	165	21	8	0	0	69	12	203	1.3	..	0.10	0.12	7.7	..
Eels, raw, American	100	3½ ozs.	233	16	18	0	0	66	18	202	0.7	1,610	0.22	0.36	1.4	..
Eggplant, boiled, drained	100	3½ ozs.	19	1	Tr.	4	0.9	94	11	21	0.6	10	0.05	0.04	0.5	3
Eggs, fresh, stored or frozen: Raw or cooked:																
Whole	100	2 medium	163	13	12	1	0	74	54	205	2.3	1,180	0.10	0.29	0.1	0
	50	1 medium	81	7	6	Tr.	0	38	27	102	1.2	590	0.05	0.15	Tr.	0
White	100	3 medium	51	11	0	1	0	89	9	15	0.1	0	0	0.27	0.1	0
	31	1 medium	16	3	0	Tr.	0	27	3	5	Tr.	0	0	0.08	Tr.	0
Yolk	100	6 medium	348	16	31	1	0	51	141	569	5.5	3,400	0.27	0.44	0.1	0
	17	1 medium	58	3	5	Tr.	0	9	24	96	0.9	580	0.05	0.07	Tr.	0

Food	Amount (g)	Measure	Calories	Protein (g)	Fat (g)	Carbohydrate (g)	Fiber (g)	Water (g)	Calcium (mg)	Phosphorus (mg)	Iron (mg)	Vitamin A (I.U.)	Thiamine (mg)	Riboflavin (mg)	Niacin (mg)	Ascorbic Acid (mg)
Cooked, omelet or scrambled*	100	made with 2 small eggs	173	11	13	2	0	73	80	189	1.7	1,080	0.08	0.28	0.1	0
Dried, whole	100	1 c.	592	47	41	4	0	5	187	800	8.7	4,290	0.33	1.20	0.2	0
Endive or escarole, raw	100	3½ ozs.	20	2	Tr.	4	0.9	93	81	54	1.7	3,300	0.07	0.14	0.5	10
Evaporated milk. See milk.																
Farina: quick cooking Unenriched, cooked*	100	½ c. scant	43	1	Tr.	9	0	89	4	13	0.2	0	0.01	0.01	0.1	0
Enriched, cooked	100	½ c. scant	43	1	Tr.	9	0	89	60	13	5.0	0	0.05	0.03	0.4	0
Fats, cooking (vegetable fat or oil)	100	½ c.	884	0	100	0	0	0	0	0	0	0	0	0	0	0
	12.5	1 tbsp.	110	0	13	0	0	0	0	0	0	0	0	0	0	0
Figs: Raw	100	3 small	80	1	Tr.	20	1.2	78	35	22	0.6	80	0.06	0.05	0.4	2
Canned, heavy syrup, solids and liquid	100	3 figs and 2 tbsp. syrup	84	1	Tr.	22	0.7	77	13	13	0.4	30	0.03	0.03	0.2	1
Dried	100	5 figs	274	4	1	69	5.6	23	126	77	3.0	80	0.10	0.10	0.7	0
Filberts or hazelnuts	100		634	13	62	17	3.0	6	209	337	3.4	..	0.46	..	0.9	Tr.
Fig Bars	100	4 large	350	4	5	76	1.7	14	69	69	1.3	0	0.02	0.06	0.9	0
	25	1 large	88	1	1	19	0.4	3	17	17	0.3	0	0.01	0.01	0.2	0
Fish: Bluefish: Baked or broiled	100	3½ ozs.	159	26	5	0	0	68	29	287	0.7	50	0.11	0.10	1.9	..
Fried	100	3½ ozs.	205	23	10	5	0	61	35	257	0.9	..	0.11	0.11	1.8	..
Cod: Broiled	100	3½ ozs.	170	29	5	0	0	65	31	274	1.0	180	0.08	0.11	3.0	..
Dried	100	3½ ozs.	375	82	3	0	0	12	..	891	3.6	0	0.08	0.45	10.9	0
Flounder, baked	100	3½ ozs.	202	30	8	0	0	58	23	344	1.4	..	0.07	0.08	2.5	..
Haddock, fried	100	3½ ozs.	165	20	6	6	0	67	40	247	1.2	..	0.04	0.07	3.2	..
Halibut, broiled	100	3½ ozs.	171	25	7	0	0	67	16	248	0.8	680	0.05	0.07	8.3	2
Herring: Atlantic, raw	100	3½ ozs.	176	17	11	0	0	69	..	256	1.1	110	0.02	0.15	3.6	..
Pacific, raw	100	3½ ozs.	98	18	3	0	0	79	..	225	1.3	100	0.02	0.16	3.5	..
Canned in tomato sauce	100	3½ ozs.	176	16	11	4	0	67	..	243	..	..	..	0.11	3.5	..
Smoked, kippered	100	3½ ozs.	211	22	13	0	0	61	66	254	1.4	30	..	0.28	3.3	..

* Values are calculated from a recipe.

† Ascorbic acid added in processing.

TABLE 1. COMPOSITION OF FOODS—EDIBLE PORTION (*Continued*)

FOOD AND DESCRIPTION	WT. Gm.	APPROXIMATE MEASURE	FOOD ENERGY Cal.	PROTEIN Gm.	FAT Gm.	CARBOHYDRATE Total Gm.	Fiber Gm.	WATER Gm.	MINERALS CA Mg.	P Mg.	FE Mg.	VITAMINS VITAMIN A I.U.	THIAMINE Mg.	RIBOFLAVIN Mg.	NIACIN Mg.	ASCORBIC ACID Mg.
Fish: (*Continued*)																
Mackerel:																
Atlantic, broiled	100	3½ ozs.	236	22	16	0	0	62	6	280	1.2	530	0.15	0.27	7.6	..
Pacific, canned, solids and liquid	100	3½ ozs.	180	21	10	0	0	66	260	288	2.2	30	0.03	0.33	8.8	..
Salmon:																
Cooked, broiled or baked	100	3½ ozs.	182	27	7	0	0	63	..	414	1.2	160	0.16	0.06	9.8	..
Canned: solid & liquid																
Chinook or King	100	3½ ozs.	210	20	14	0	0	65	154	289	0.9	230	0.03	0.14	7.3	..
Pink or humpback ...	100	3½ ozs.	141	21	6	0	0	70	196	286	0.8	70	0.03	0.18	8.0	..
Sockeye or red	100	3½ ozs.	171	20	9	0	0	67	259	344	1.2	230	0.04	0.16	7.3	..
Smoked	100	3½ ozs.	176	22	9	0	0	59	14	245	..	..	..	..	..	..
Sardines:																
Atlantic type, canned in oil, drained solids	100	3½ ozs.	203	24	11	0	Tr.	62	437‡	499‡	2.9	220	0.03	0.20	5.4	..
Pacific type,																
In brine or mustard ..	100	3½ ozs.	196	19	12	2	..	64	303	354	5.2	30	0.01	0.30	7.4	..
In tomato sauce	100	3½ ozs.	197	19	12	2	..	64	449	478‡	4.1	30	0.01	0.27	5.3	..
Shad, baked	100	3½ ozs.	201	23	11	0	0	64	24	313	0.6	30	0.13	0.26	8.6	..
Swordfish, broiled	100	3½ ozs.	174	28	7	0	0	65	27	275	1.3	2,050	0.04	0.05	10.9	..
Tuna fish, canned in oil drained solids	100	3½ ozs.	197	29	8	0	0	61	8	234	1.9	80	0.05	0.12	11.9	0
Canned in water solids and liquid	100	3½ ozs.	127	28	1	0	0	70	16	190	1.6	..	..	0.10	13.3	..
White fish, cooked baked, stuffed	100	3½ ozs.	215	15	14	6	..	63	..	246	0.5	2,000	0.11	0.11	2.3	Tr.
Frog legs, raw	100	3½ ozs.	73	16	Tr.	0	0	82	18	147	1.5	0	0.14	0.25	1.2	..
Fruit cocktail, canned, light syrup solids and liquids	100	½ c. scant	60	Tr.	Tr.	16	0.4	84	9	12	0.4	140	0.02	0.01	0.5	2
Gelatin, dry:																
Plain	100	⅔ c.	335	86	Tr.	0	0	13	0	0	0	0	0	0	0	0
	10	1 tbsp.	34	9	0	0	0	1	0	0	0	0	0	0	0	0

Food, measure, and weight (per 100 Gm.)	Gm.	Measure	Food energy (cal.)	Protein (g)	Fat (g)	Carbohydrate (g)	Water (%)	Calcium (mg)	Phosphorus (mg)	Iron (mg)	Vitamin A (I.U.)	Thiamine (mg)	Riboflavin (mg)	Niacin (mg)	Ascorbic acid (mg)
Gelatin dessert, ready to serve:															
Plain	100	½ c. heaping	59	2	0	14	84	0	0	0	0	0	0	0	0
With fruit added	100	½ c. heaping	67	1	Tr.	16	82	6	11	0.3	110	0.03	0.02	0.2	3
Gingerbread from a mix	100	2 pieces, 2 x 2 x 2 in.	276	3	7	51	37	90	100	1.6	Tr.	0.03	0.09	0.8	Tr.
Grapefruit: white															
Raw, pulp only	100	½ small	41	1	Tr.	11	88	16	16	0.4	80	0.04	0.02	0.2	38
Canned in syrup, solids and liquid	100	½ c. scant	70	1	Tr.	18	81	13	14	0.3	10	0.03	0.02	0.2	30
Grapefruit juice:															
Fresh or frozen reconstituted	100	½ c. scant	41	1	Tr.	10	90	10	17	0.1	10	0.04	0.02	0.2	38
Canned:															
Unsweetened	100	½ c. scant	41	1	Tr.	10	89	8	14	0.4	10	0.03	0.02	0.2	34
Sweetened	100	½ c. scant	53	1	Tr.	13	86	8	14	0.4	10	0.03	0.02	0.2	31
Grapefruit-orange juice blend, canned or frozen reconstituted:															
Unsweetened	100	½ c. scant	43	1	Tr.	10	89	10	15	0.3	100	0.05	0.02	0.2	34
Sweetened	100	½ c. scant	50	1	Tr.	12	87	9	15	0.3	100	0.05	0.02	0.2	34
Grapes, raw:															
American type (slip skin) as Concord, Delaware, Niagara and Scuppernong	100	1 bunch 3½ x 3 in.	69	1	1	16	82	16	12	0.4	100	0.05	0.03	0.3	4
European type (adherent skin) as Malaga, muscat, sultana, Thompson seedless and Tokay	100	⅔ c.	67	1	Tr.	17	82	12	20	0.4	100	0.05	0.03	0.3	4
Grape juice, bottled, commercial	100	3½ ozs.	66	Tr.	0	17	83	11	12	0.3	..	0.04	0.03	0.2	Tr.
Guavas, common, raw	100	1 large	62	1	0.6	15	83	23	42	0.9	280	0.05	0.05	1.2	242†
Heart:															
Beef, lean, braised	100	3½ ozs.	188	31	6	1	61	6	181	5.9	30	0.25	1.22	7.6	1
Chicken, cooked	100	3½ ozs.	173	25	7	Tr.	67	4	107	3.6	30	0.06	0.92	5.3	4
Pork, cooked	100	3½ ozs.	195	31	7	Tr.	61	4	121	4.9	40	0.20	1.72	6.7	1

‡ Includes skin and bones; if discarded, Ca 54 mg;; P319 per 100 Gm.

† Range for varieties grown in U.S.—23 to 1,160 mg.

TABLE 1. COMPOSITION OF FOODS—EDIBLE PORTION (*Continued*)

Food and Description	Wt. Gm.	Approximate Measure	Food Energy Cal.	Protein Gm.	Fat Gm.	Carbohydrate Total Gm.	Carbohydrate Fiber Gm.	Water Gm.	Ca Mg.	P Mg.	Fe Mg.	Vitamin A I.U.	Thiamine Mg.	Riboflavin Mg.	Niacin Mg.	Ascorbic Acid Mg.
Honey, strained or extracted	21	1 tbsp.	64	Tr.	0	17	..	4	1	1	0.1	0	Tr.	0.01	Tr.	Tr.
Honeydew melon, raw	100	wedge 1½ x 7 in.	33	1	Tr.	8	0.6	91	14	16	0.4	40	0.05	0.03	0.6	23
Ice cream, plain, 12 percent fat	100	¾ c.	207	4	13	21	0	62	123	99	0.1	520	0.04	0.19	0.1	1
	62	1 container	129	3	8	13	0	37	76	61	0.1	320	0.03	0.12	0.1	1
Ice milk	100	⅔ c.	152	5	5	22	0	67	156	124	0.1	210	0.05	0.22	0.1	1
Infant Foods See Baby Foods.																
Jams, marmalades, preserves	20	1 tbsp.	55	Tr.	Tr.	14	0.2	6	4	2	0.2	Tr.	Tr.	Tr.	Tr.	2†
Jellies	20	1 tbsp.	50	0	0	14	0	7	4	2	0.3	Tr.	Tr.	Tr.	Tr.	1†
Kale: leaves only																
Cooked, fresh	100	1 c.	39	5	1	6	..	87	187	58	1.6	8,300	0.10	0.18	1.6	93
Frozen, boiled, drained	100	1 c.	31	3	1	5	0.9	90	121	48	1.0	8,200	0.06	0.15	0.7	38
Kidneys, raw:																
Beef	100	3½ ozs.	130	15	7	1	0	76	11	219	7.4	690	0.36	2.55	6.4	15
Lamb	100	3½ ozs.	105	17	3	1	0	78	13	218	7.6	690	0.51	2.42	7.4	15
Pork	100	3½ ozs.	106	16	4	1	0	78	11	218	6.7	130	0.58	1.73	9.8	12
Kohlrabi:																
Raw	100	¾ c. diced	29	2	Tr.	7	1.1	90	41	51	0.5	20	0.06	0.05	0.2	66
Cooked	100	⅔ c.	24	2	Tr.	7	1.1	92	33	41	0.3	20	0.06	0.03	0.2	43
Lamb, trimmed to retail basis, cooked: Chop, thick, broiled																
Lean and fat	100	3½ ozs.	359	22	29	0	0	47	9	172	1.3	..	0.12	0.23	5.0	..
Lean only (from above serving)	66	2.4 ozs.	125	19	5	0	0	41	8	145	1.3	..	0.10	0.18	4.1	..
Leg, roasted																
Lean and fat	100	3½ ozs.	266	26	17	0	0	55	11	212	1.8	..	0.15	0.27	5.6	..
Lean only (from above serving)	85	3 ozs.	121	19	4	0	0	41	8	157	1.5	..	0.11	0.20	4.1	..

Food	g	Measure														
Shoulder, roasted																
Lean and fat	100	3½ oz.	338	22	27	0	0	50	10	172	1.2	..	0.13	0.23	4.7	..
Lean only (from above serving)	74	2.7 ozs.	150	20	7	0	0	46	9	162	1.4	..	0.11	0.21	4.3	..
Lard	100	½ c.	902	0	100	0	0	0	0	0	0	0	0	0	0	0
	14	1 tbsp.	126	0	14	0	0	0	0	0	0	0	0	0	0	0
Lemons, peeled fruit	100	1 medium, 2¾ x 2 in.	27	1	Tr.	8	0.4	90	26	16	0.6	20	0.04	0.02	0.1	53
Lemon juice, fresh and canned, unsweetened	100	½ c. scant	24	Tr.	Tr.	8	0	91	7	10	0.2	20	0.03	0.01	0.1	42
Lentils, mature, cooked	100	3½ ozs.	106	8	Tr.	19	1.2	72	25	119	2.1	20	0.07	0.06	0.6	0
Lettuce, crisp, headed	100	¼ head	13	1	Tr.	3	0.6	96	20	22	0.5	330	0.06	0.06	0.3	6
leafy types, Boston, Bibb ..	100	4 large leaves	14	1	Tr.	3	0.5	95	35	26	2.0	970	0.06	0.06	0.3	8
Limes, peeled fruit	100	2 medium	28	1	Tr.	10	0.5	89	33	18	0.6	10	0.03	0.02	0.2	37
Lime juice, fresh	100	½ c. scant	26	Tr.	0	9	0	90	9	11	0.2	10	0.02	0.01	0.1	32
Liver:																
Beef:																
Raw	100	3½ ozs.	140	20	4	5	0	70	8	352	6.5	43,900	0.25	3.26	13.6	31
Fried	100	3½ ozs.	229	26	11	5	0	56	11	476	8.8	53,400	0.26	4.19	15.6	27
Calf, fried	100	3½ ozs.	261	30	13	4	0	51	13	537	14.2	32,700	0.24	4.17	16.5	37
Chicken, simmered	100	3½ ozs.	165	27	4	3	0	65	11	159	8.5	12,300	0.17	2.69	11.7	16
Lamb, broiled	100	3½ ozs.	261	32	12	3	0	50	16	572	17.9	74,500	0.49	5.11	24.9	36
Pork, fried	100	3½ ozs.	241	30	12	3	0	54	15	539	29.1	14,900	0.34	4.36	22.3	22
Lobster:																
Raw	100	3½ ozs. meat	91	17	2	1	0	79	29	183	0.6	..	0.40	0.05	1.5	..
Canned or cooked	100	3½ ozs.	95	19	2	Tr.	0	77	65	192	0.8	..	0.10	0.07	..	..
Loganberries, raw	100	⅔ c.	62	1	1	15	3.0	83	35	17	1.2	200	0.03	0.04	0.4	24
Luncheon meat: Canned, ham or pork	100	3½ oz. slice	294	15	25	1	0	55	9	108	2.2	0	0.31	0.21	3.0	..
Macaroni: Unenriched: Cooked,* firm	100	⅔ c. elbow type	148	5	1	30	0.1	64	11	65	0.5	0	0.02	0.02	0.4	0
Enriched: Cooked,* firm	100	⅔ c. elbow type	148	5	1	30	0.1	64	11	65	1.1	0	0.18	0.10	1.4	0

† Variable according to fruit used.
* Values are calculated from a recipe.

TABLE 1. Composition of Foods—Edible Portion (Continued)

Food and Description	Wt. Gm.	Approximate Measure	Food Energy Cal.	Protein Gm.	Fat Gm.	Carbohydrate Total Gm.	Fiber Gm.	Water Gm.	Ca Mg.	P Mg.	Fe Mg.	Vitamin A I.U.	Thiamine Mg.	Riboflavin Mg.	Niacin Mg.	Ascorbic Acid Mg.
Macaroni and cheese, baked* made with enriched macaroni	100	½ c.	215	8	11	20	0.1	58	181	161	0.9	430	0.10	0.20	0.9	Tr.
Mangos, raw	100	½ medium	66	1	Tr.	17	0.9	81	10	13	0.4	4,800	0.05	0.05	1.1	35
Margarine, fortified	100	½ c. scant	720	1	81	Tr.	0	16	20	16	0	3,300	..	..	..	0
	14	1 tbsp.	101	Tr.	11	Tr.	0	2	3	2	0	460	..	..	..	0
Marmalades. See Jams, citrus	100	½ c. scant	257	1	Tr.	70	0.4	29	35	9	0.6	..	0.02	0.02	0.1	6
	14	1 tbsp.	36	Tr.	Tr.	10	0.1	4	5	1	0.1	..	Tr.	Tr.	Tr.	1
Mayonnaise. See Salad dressings.																
Meat. See Beef, Lamb, Pork, Veal.																
Milk, cow: Fluid (pasteurized and raw): Whole	100	½ c. scant	65	3.5	3.5	5	0	87	118	93	Tr.	140	0.03	0.17	0.1	1
	244	1 c.	160	8.5	8.5	12	0	212	288	226	0.2	350	0.08	0.42	0.2	2
Nonfat (skim)	100	½ c. scant	36	3.6	Tr.	5	0	91	121	95	Tr.	Tr.	0.04	0.18	0.1	1
	246	1 c.	88	8.8	Tr.	13	0	224	297	234	0.2	Tr.	0.10	0.44	0.2	2
Canned: Evaporated (unsweetened)	100	½ c. scant	137	7	8	10	0	74	252	205	0.1	320	0.04	0.34	0.2	1
Condensed (sweetened)	100	⅓ c.	321	8	9	54	0	27	262	206	0.1	360	0.08	0.38	0.2	1
Dried: Whole	100	1 c. scant	502	26	28	38	0	2	909	708	0.5	1,130	0.29	1.46	0.7	6
	8	1 tbsp.	40	2	2	3	0	Tr.	72	56	0.1	90	0.02	0.12	0.1	1
Skim, instant	100	1¼ c.	359	36	1	52	0	4	1,293	1,005	0.6	30	0.35	1.78	0.9	7
	8	1 tbsp.	29	3	Tr.	4	0	Tr.	103	80	0.1	2	0.03	0.31	0.1	1
Malted†: Dry powder	30	1 oz.	115	4	2	20	0	Tr.	81	107	0.6	285	0.09	0.15	..	0
Beverage with whole milk powder	270	1 c.	281	12	12	32	0	210	364	328	0.8	670	0.17	0.56	..	2

Food	(g)	Measure														
Chocolate flavored*	100	½ c. scant	76	3	2	11	0	83	108	91	0.2	80	0.04	0.16	0.1	1
made with skim milk	250	1 c.	190	7	6	27	0	207	272	228	0.5	200	0.10	0.40	0.2	2
Milk, goat, fluid	100	½ c. scant	67	3	3	5	0	87	129	106	0.1	160	0.04	0.11	0.3	1
	244	1 c.	164	7	7	12	0	212	315	259	0.2	390	0.10	0.26	0.7	2
Molasses, cane:																
First extraction or light	100	⅓ c.	252	..	..	65	..	24	165	45	4.3	..	0.07	0.06	0.2	..
Second extraction or medium	100	⅓ c.	232	..	..	60	..	24	290	69	6.0	..	..	0.12	1.2	..
Third extraction or blackstrap	100	⅓ c.	213	..	..	55	..	24	579	85	11.3	..	0.12	0.18	2.0	..
Muffins, made with enriched wheat flour*	100	2 muffins, 3¾-in. diam.	294	8	10	42	0.1	38	104	151	1.6	100	0.17	0.23	1.4	Tr.
Corn, enriched, ungerminated meal	100		314	7	10	48	0.2	33	105	169	1.7	300	0.20	0.23	1.6	Tr.
Mushrooms, cultivated, raw	100	½ c.	28	3	Tr.	4	0.8	90	6	116	0.8	Tr.	0.10	0.46	4.2	3
canned, solids and liquid	100	½ c.	17	2	Tr.	2	0.6	93	6	68	0.5	Tr.	0.02	0.25	2.0	2
Muskmelons See Cantaloupe.																
Mustard greens: Cooked	100	⅔ c.	23	2	Tr.	4	0.9	92	138	32	1.8	5,800	0.08	0.14	0.6	48
Frozen, cooked	100	⅔ c.	20	2	Tr.	3	0.9	93	104	43	1.5	6,000	0.03	0.10	0.4	20
Nectarines, raw	100	1 small	64	1	Tr.	17	0.4	82	4	24	0.5	1,650	..	..	..	3
Noodles (containing egg), enriched, cooked*	100	⅔ c.	125	4	2	23	0.1	70	10	59	0.9	70	0.14	0.08	1.2	0
Oat cereal, ready-to-eat (added vitamins and minerals)	100	4 c.	397	12	6	75	1.1	3	177	408	4.7	0	0.98	0.18	1.9	0
	25	1 c.	100	3	2	19	0.3	1	44	102	1.2	0	0.25	0.04	0.5	0
Oatmeal or rolled oats: Cooked*	100	⅔ c.	55	2	1	10	0.2	87	9	57	0.6	0	0.08	0.02	0.1	0
Oils, salad or cooking	100	½ c.	884	0	100	0	0	0	0	0	0	0	0	0	0	0
	14	1 tbsp.	124	0	14	0	0	0	0	0	0	0	0	0	0	0
Okra, cooked	100	9 pods	29	2	Tr.	6	1.0	90	92	41	0.5	490	0.13	0.18	0.9	20

* Values are calculated from a recipe.　　† Based on unfortified products.

TABLE 1. COMPOSITION OF FOODS—EDIBLE PORTION (Continued)

FOOD AND DESCRIPTION	WT. Gm.	APPROXIMATE MEASURE	FOOD ENERGY Cal.	PROTEIN Gm.	FAT Gm.	CARBOHYDRATE TOTAL Gm.	CARBOHYDRATE FIBER Gm.	WATER Gm.	CA Mg.	P Mg.	FE Mg.	VITAMIN A I.U.	THIAMINE Mg.	RIBOFLAVIN Mg.	NIACIN Mg.	ASCORBIC ACID Mg.
Olives, pickled:																
Green	100	16 olives	116	1	13	1	1.3	78	61	17	1.6	300	..	..	..	..
Ripe, Mission	100	10 olives	184	1	20	3	1.5	73	106	17	1.7	70	Tr.	Tr.	..	..
	20	2 olives	37	Tr.	2	Tr.	0.3	15	21	3	0.3	14	..	..	..	..
Onions:																
Mature:																
Raw	100	1 onion, 2½-in. diam.	38	2	Tr.	9	0.6	89	27	36	0.5	40	0.03	0.04	0.2	10
Cooked, drained	100	½ c.	29	1	Tr.	7	0.6	92	24	29	0.4	40	0.03	0.03	0.2	7
Young, green, raw bulb and white top	100	12 small, without tops	45	1	Tr.	11	1.8	88	40	39	0.6	Tr.	0.05	0.04	0.4	25
Oranges, all varieties peeled fruit	100	1 small	49	1	Tr.	12	0.6	86	41	20	0.4	200	0.10	0.04	0.4	50‡
Orange juice:																
Fresh	100	½ c. scant	45	1	Tr.	11	0.1	88	11	17	0.2	200	0.09	0.03	0.4	50‡
Canned, unsweetened	100	½ c. scant	48	1	Tr.	11	0.1	88	10	18	0.4	200	0.07	0.02	0.3	40
Orange juice, concentrate,																
Frozen:																
Undiluted	100	3½ ozs.	158	2	Tr.	38	0.2	58	33	55	0.4	710	0.30	0.05	1.2	158
Reconstituted, 3 parts water	100	3½ ozs.	45	1	Tr.	11	Tr.	88	9	16	0.1	200	0.09	0.01	0.3	45
Oysters, meat only, raw Av. Eastern	100	5-8 medium	66	8	2	3	..	85	94	143	5.5	310	0.14	0.18	2.5	..
Oyster stew:																
1 part oysters to 3 parts milk by volume	100	½ c. scant	86	5	5	5	..	84	117	109	1.4	280	0.06	0.18	0.7	..
Pancakes (griddlecakes).*																
Wheat (home recipe), with enriched flour	100	4 cakes, 4 in. diam.	231	7	7	34	0.1	50	101	139	1.3	120	0.17	0.22	1.3	Tr.
Buckwheat, with milk and egg pancake mix	100	4 cakes	200	7	9	24	0.4	58	220	337	1.3	230	0.12	0.16	0.7	Tr.

Food	Gm	Measure	Water %	Food energy	Protein	Fat	Carbohydrate	Calcium	Phosphorus	Iron	Vit. A	Thiamine	Riboflavin	Niacin	Ascorbic acid
Papayas, raw	100	½ c., ½ in. cubes	89	39	1	Tr.	10	20	16	0.3	1,750	0.04	0.04	0.3	56
Parsley, common, raw	3½	1 tbsp. chopped	3	1	Tr.	0	Tr.	7†	2	0.2	300	Tr.	0.01	0.1	7
Parsnips, cooked	100	⅔ c.	82	66	2	1	15	45	62	0.6	30	0.07	0.08	0.1	10
Peaches: Raw	100	1 peach, 2½ x 2 in. diam.	89	38	1	Tr.	10	8	19	0.5	1,330§	0.02	0.05	1.0	7
Canned, solids and liquid:															
Water pack	100	½ c. scant	91	31	Tr.	Tr.	8	4	13	0.3	450	0.01	0.03	0.6	3
Syrup pack, heavy	100	½ c. scant	79	79	Tr.	Tr.	20	4	12	0.3	430	0.01	0.02	0.6	3
Frozen, sliced	100	3½ ozs.	77	88	Tr.	Tr.	23	4	13	0.5	650	0.01	0.03	0.7	40‖
Dried, sulfured:															
Uncooked	100	⅔ c.	25	262	3	1	68	48	117	6.0	3,900	0.01	0.19	5.3	18
Cooked, sugar added*	100	4-5 halves / 2 tbsp. fluid	67	119	1	Tr.	31	13	32	1.6	1,070	Tr.	0.05	1.4	2
Peanuts: roasted and salted	100	⅔ c.	2	585	26	50	19	74	401	2.1	0	0.32	0.13	17.2	0
	9	1 tbsp. chopped	Tr.	52	2	5	2	7	36	0.2	0	0.03	0.01	1.6	0
Peanut butter, made with small am't added fat	100		2	581	28	49	17	63	407	2.0	0	0.13	0.13	15.7	0
	15	1 tbsp.	Tr.	87	4	7	3	10	61	0.3	0	0.02	0.02	2.3	0
Pears: Raw, including skin	100	1 med. pear, 2½ x 2 in.	83	61	1	Tr.	15	8	11	0.3	20	0.02	0.04	0.1	4
Canned, solids and liquid:															
Water pack	100	½ c. scant	91	32	Tr.	Tr.	8	5	7	0.2	Tr.	0.01	0.02	0.1	1
Syrup pack, light	100	2 med. halves	84	61	Tr.	Tr.	16	5	7	0.2	Tr.	0.01	0.02	0.1	1
Peas, green: Immature: Cooked fresh or frozen	100	⅔ c. drained	82	72	5	Tr.	12	22	93	1.9	610	0.27	0.10	2.0	16
Canned: Solids and liquid	100	½ c. scant	83	66	4	Tr.	13	20	66	1.7	450	0.09	0.05	0.9	9
Drained solids	100	⅔ c.	77	88	5	1	17	26	76	1.9	690	0.09	0.06	0.8	8
Mature dry seeds, split	100	½ c.	9	348	24	1	62	33	268	5.1	120	0.74	0.28	3.0	..
Pecans, shelled	100	1 c. halves	3	687	9	71	15	73	289	2.4	130	0.86	0.13	0.9	2
	7½	1 tbsp. chopped	Tr.	51	1	5	1	5	22	0.2	10	0.06	0.01	0.1	Tr.

* Values are calculated from a recipe.
‡ Year-round average.
† Calcium may not be available because of the presence of oxalic acid.
‖ Ascorbic acid added in processing.
§ Based on yellow varieties; White types 50 I.U. 100 Gm.

Table 1. Composition of Foods—Edible Portion (Continued)

Food and Description	Wt. Gm.	Approximate Measure	Food Energy Cal.	Protein Gm.	Fat Gm.	Carbohydrate Total Gm.	Carbohydrate Fiber Gm.	Water Gm.	Minerals Ca Mg.	P Mg.	Fe Mg.	Vitamins Vitamin A I.U.	Thiamine Mg.	Riboflavin Mg.	Niacin Mg.	Ascorbic Acid Mg.
Peppers, green:																
Raw	100	1 large	22	1	Tr.	5	1.4	93	9	22	0.7	420	0.08	0.08	0.5	128
Cooked, boiled and drained	100	1 large or 2 small	18	1	Tr.	4	1.4	95	9	16	0.5	420	0.06	0.07	0.5	96
Persimmons, Japanese, raw	100	1 medium	77	1	Tr.	20	1.6	79	6	26	0.3	2,710	0.03	0.02	Tr.	11
Pickles:																
Dill, cucumber	100	1 large	11	1	Tr.	2	0.5	93	26	21	1.0	100	Tr.	0.02	Tr.	6
Fresh, cucumber (as bread and butter pickles)	100	½ c.	73	1	Tr.	18	0.5	79	32	27	1.8	140	Tr.	0.03	Tr.	9
Sour, cucumber or mixed	100	½ c.	10	1	Tr.	2	0.5	95	17	15	3.2	100	Tr.	0.02	Tr.	7
Sweet, cucumber or mixed	100	½ c.	146	1	Tr.	37	..	61	12	16	1.2	90	Tr.	0.02	Tr.	6
Pies:*		⅙ of 9-in. pie														
Apple	160		410	3	18	61	0.6	76	1	35	0.5	48	0.03	0.03	0.6	2
Blueberry	160		387	4	17	56	1.1	82	18	37	1.0	48	0.03	0.03	0.5	5
Cherry	160		418	4	18	62	0.2	74	22	40	0.5	705	0.03	0.03	0.8	Tr.
Chocolate chiffon	160		525	11	25	70	0.3	53	38	155	1.9	496	0.05	0.16	0.3	0
Custard	150		327	9	17	35	Tr.	87	144	170	0.9	345	0.08	0.24	0.4	0
Mince	160		434	4	18	66	0.6	69	45	61	1.6	Tr.	0.11	0.06	0.6	2
Pecan	160		668	8	37	82	0.8	31	75	165	4.5	256	0.25	0.11	0.5	Tr.
Pumpkin	150		317	6	17	37	0.8	94	76	104	0.8	3,700	0.04	0.15	0.8	Tr.
Pimientos, canned solid and liquid	38	1 medium	10	Tr.	Tr.	2	0.2	35	3	6	0.6	875	0.01	0.02	0.1	36
Pizza:																
Cheese topping	100	⅙ of 14-in. pie	236	12	8	28	0.3	48	221	195	1.0	630	0.06	0.20	1.0	8
Sausage topping	100		234	8	9	30	0.3	51	17	92	1.2	560	0.09	0.12	1.5	9
Pineapple:																
Raw	100	¾ c. diced or 1 med. slice	52	Tr.	Tr.	14	0.4	85	17	8	0.5	70	0.09	0.03	0.2	17
Canned, solids and liquid																
in juice	100	1 med. slice	58	Tr.	Tr.	15	0.3	84	16	8	0.4	60	0.10	0.03	0.3	10
in heavy syrup	100	1 med. slice	74	Tr.	Tr.	19	0.3	80	11	5	0.3	50	0.08	0.02	0.2	7
Frozen, chunks	100	3½ ozs.	86	Tr.	Tr.	22	0.3	77	9	4	0.4	30	0.10	0.03	0.3	8

Food	Measure	g														
Pineapple juice, canned																
unsweetened	½ c. scant	100	55	Tr.	Tr.	14	0.1	86	15	9	0.3	50	0.05	0.02	0.2	9
Frozen, reconstituted	½ c. scant	100	52	Tr.	Tr.	13	0.1	87	11	8	0.3	10	0.07	0.02	0.2	12
Pine nuts:																
Pignolias	3½ ozs.	100	552	31	47	12	0.9	6	..	..	..	..	0.62	..	..	..
Piñon	3½ ozs.	100	635	13	61	21	1.1	3	12	604	5.2	30	1.28	0.23	4.5	Tr.
Pistachio nuts	3½ ozs.	100	594	19	54	19	1.9	5	131	500	7.3	230	0.67	..	1.4	0
Plantain, raw, baking banana	1 small	100	119	1	Tr.	31	0.4	66	7	30	0.7	..	0.06	0.04	0.6	14
Plums:																
All, excluding prunes, raw	2 medium	100	48	1	Tr.	12	0.6	87	12	18	0.5	250	0.03	0.03	0.5	6
Italian prunes, canned, syrup pack, solids and liquid	½ c. scant or 3 med. prunes	100	83	Tr.	Tr.	22	0.3	77	9	10	0.9	1,210	0.02	0.02	0.4	2
Popcorn, popped	1 c.	14	54	2	1	10	0.3	1	2	39	0.4	0	..	0.02	0.3	0
Pork, fresh, trimmed to retail basis, cooked:																
Chop, thick:																
Lean and fat	1 large chop	100	391	25	32	0	0	42	12	268	3.4	0	0.96	0.28	5.6	..
Lean only from 1 chop	3½ ozs.	72	195	22	11	0	0	38	9	248	2.7	0	0.82	0.24	4.9	..
Roast, loin or shoulder	3½ ozs.	100	373	23	31	0	0	45	10	232	2.9	0	0.50	0.23	4.9	..
Lean only from above serving	2.9 ozs.	77	182	22	10	0	0	44	9	226	2.8	0	0.46	0.22	4.2	..
Picnic cut simmered																
Lean and fat	3½ ozs.	100	374	23	31	0	0	46	10	139	3.0	0	0.54	0.25	4.8	..
Lean only from above serving	2.6 ozs.	74	157	21	7	0	0	45	9	130	2.7	0	0.49	0.22	4.4	..
Pork, smoked ham																
Ham, cooked																
Lean and fat	3½ ozs.	100	289	21	22	0	0	54	9	172	2.6	0	0.47	0.18	3.6	..
Lean only from above serving	3 ozs.	84	157	21	7	0	0	52	9	170	2.7	0	0.49	0.19	3.8	..
Ham, canned	3½ ozs.	100	193	18	12	1	0	65	11	156	2.7	0	0.53	0.19	3.8	..
Pork, fat, salted raw	3½ ozs.	100	783	4	85	0	0	8	Tr.	Tr.	0.6	0	0.18	0.04	0.9	..

* Values are calculated from a recipe.

TABLE 1. COMPOSITION OF FOODS—EDIBLE PORTION (Continued)

Food and Description	Wt. Gm.	Approximate Measure	Food Energy Cal.	Protein Gm.	Fat Gm.	Carbohydrate Total Gm.	Carbohydrate Fiber Gm.	Water Gm.	Minerals Ca Mg.	Minerals P Mg.	Minerals Fe Mg.	Vitamins Vitamin A I.U.	Vitamins Thiamine Mg.	Vitamins Riboflavin Mg.	Vitamins Niacin Mg.	Vitamins Ascorbic Acid Mg.
Potatoes:																
Baked in skin	100	1 med.	93	3	Tr.	21	0.6	75	9	65	0.7	Tr.	0.10	0.04	1.7	20‡
Boiled, pared before cooking	100	1 med.	65	2	Tr.	15	0.5	83	6	48	0.5	Tr.	0.09	0.03	1.2	16
French fried	100	20 pieces 2 x ½ x ½ in.	274	4	13	36	1.0	45	15	111	1.3	Tr.	0.13	0.08	3.1	21
Fried from raw	100	⅔ c.	268	4	14	33	1.0	47	15	101	1.1	Tr.	0.12	0.07	2.8	19
Hash brown after holding overnight	100	½ c.	229	3	12	29	0.8	54	12	79	0.9	Tr.	0.08	0.05	2.1	9
Mashed, milk and table fat added	100	½ c.	94	2	4	12	0.4	80	24	53	0.4	170	0.08	0.05	1.0	9
Dehydrated Flakes, prep. with water, milk and butter added	100	3½ ozs.	93	2	3	15	0.3	79	31	47	0.3	130	0.04	0.04	0.9	5
Potato chips	20	10 med. or 7 large	114	1	8	10	0.1	1	8	28	0.4	Tr.	0.04	0.02	1.0	3
Potato flour	100	1 c. sifted	351	8	1	80	1.6	8	33	178	17.2	Tr.	0.42	0.14	3.4	19
Pretzels	5	5 small sticks	19	Tr.	Tr.	4	Tr.	Tr.	1	6	Tr.	0	Tr.	Tr.	Tr.	0
Prunes:																
Dried, softenized uncooked	100	⅔ c. medium	255	2	1	67	1.6	28	51	79	3.9	1,600	0.09	0.17	1.6	3
Cooked, no sugar added	100	6 prunes, 2 tbsp. juice	119	1	Tr.	31	0.8	66	24	37	1.8	750	0.03	0.07	0.7	1
Cooked, sugar added	100	6 prunes, 2 tbsp. juice	172	1	Tr.	45	0.6	53	19	30	1.5	600	0.03	0.06	0.6	1
Prune juice, canned	100	½ c. scant	77	Tr.	0	19	..	80	14	20	4.1	..	0.01	0.01	0.4	2
Prune whip*	100	¾ c.	148	3	Tr.	37	0.7	59	26	42	1.8	460	0.04	0.11	0.7	2
Pudding, chocolate*	100	½ c.	148	3	5	26	0.2	66	96	98	0.5	150	0.02	0.14	0.1	Tr.
Pumpkin, canned	100	⅞ c.	33	1	Tr.	8	1.2	90	25	26	0.4	6,400	0.03	0.05	0.6	5
Radishes, raw	40	4 small	7	Tr.	Tr.	1	0.1	37	12	12	0.4	Tr.	0.01	0.01	0.1	10

Food	Wt. (gm.)	Measure	Water	Cal.	Pro.	Fat	Carb.	Fiber	Ca.	P.	Fe.	Vit. A	Thia.	Ribo.	Niac.	Asc.
Raisins, natural dried, seedless (unbleached)	100	⅔ c.	18	289	3	Tr.	77	0.9	62	101	3.5	20	0.11	0.08	0.5	1
	10	1 tbsp.	2	29	Tr.	Tr.	8	0.1	6	10	0.3	Tr.	0.01	0.01	Tr.	Tr.
Raspberries:																
Black, raw	100	¾ c.	81	73	2	1	16	5.1	30	22	0.9	0	0.03	0.09	0.9	18
Red:																
Raw	100	¾ c.	84	57	1	1	14	3.0	22	22	0.9	130	0.03	0.09	0.9	25
Frozen, sweetened	100	3½ ozs.	74	98	1	Tr.	25	2.2	13	17	0.6	70	0.02	0.06	0.6	21
Rhubarb, stems only:																
Raw	100	¾ c. diced	95	16	1	Tr.	4	0.7	96‡	18	0.8	100	0.03	0.07	0.3	9
Cooked, sugar added or canned in syrup*	100	⅓ c.	63	141	Tr.	Tr.	36	0.6	78‡	15	0.6	80	0.02	0.05	0.3	6
Rice:																
Brown, cooked	100	⅔ c.	70	119	3	1	26	0.3	12	73	0.5	0	0.09	0.02	1.4	0
White, milled enriched, cooked	100	⅔ c.	73	109	2	Tr.	24	0.1	10	28	0.9§	0	0.11§	0.01	1.0§	0
Parboiled, converted, cooked	100	⅔ c.	73	106	2	Tr.	23	0.1	19	57	0.8	0	0.11	0.03	1.2	0
Precooked, instant, cooked	100	⅔ c.	73	109	2	Tr.	24	0.1	3	19	0.8	0	0.13§	0.01	1.0§	0
Rice products (added thiamine and niacin):																
Flakes	30	1 c.	1	118	2	Tr.	26	0.2	9	40	0.5	0	0.11	0.02	1.6	0
Krispies	30	1 c.	Tr.	107	2	Tr.	25	0.1	7	33	0.5	0	0.11	0.01	2.0	0
Puffed, presweetened	14	1 c.	Tr.	55	1	Tr.	12	Tr.	6	10	0.3	0	0.05	..	0.6	0
Rice pudding with raisins	100	⅔ c.	66	146	4	3	27	0.1	98	94	0.4	110	0.03	0.14	0.2	Tr.
Rolls:*		one roll														
Hard, enriched	35	average	9	109	3	1	21	0.1	16	32	0.8§	Tr.	0.09§	0.08§	0.9§	Tr.
Plain, enriched (pan roll) ..	38	average	12	113	3	2	20	0.1	28	32	0.7§	Tr.	0.11§	0.07§	0.8§	Tr.
Hamburger bun	30	1 large	10	89	3	2	16	0.1	22	26	0.6§	Tr.	0.08§	0.05§	0.7§	Tr.
Sweet roll, enriched	55	average	16	178	5	4	30	0.3	35	57	0.3	0	0.03	0.07	0.6	0
Danish pastry	35	1 small	8	148	3	8	16	Tr.	17	38	0.3	108	0.02	0.05	0.3	Tr.
Rutabagas, boiled, drained ..	100	⅔ c. diced	91	35	1	Tr.	8	1.4	59	31	0.3	550	0.06	0.06	0.8	26
Rye wafers or "Swedish health bread" or Rye Krisp	13	2 wafers 1⅞ x 3½ in.	1	43	2	Tr.	10	0.3	6	52	0.6	0	0.04	0.03	0.6	0

* Values are calculated from a recipe.

† Year-round average. Recently dug potatoes contain about 24 mg. of ascorbic acid per 100 Gm. The value is only half as high after 3 months of storage and about one third as high when potatoes have been stored as long as 6 months.

‡ Calcium may not be available because of the presence of oxalic acid.

§ Based on minimum levels of enrichment specified in standard of identity. F.D.A., for iron, thiamine, riboflavin and niacin.

TABLE 1. COMPOSITION OF FOODS—EDIBLE PORTION (Continued)

Food and Description	Wt. Gm.	Approximate Measure	Food Energy Cal.	Protein Gm.	Fat Gm.	Carbohydrate Total Gm.	Carbohydrate Fiber Gm.	Water Gm.	Ca Mg.	P Mg.	Fe Mg.	Vitamin A I.U.	Thiamine Mg.	Riboflavin Mg.	Niacin Mg.	Ascorbic Acid Mg.
Salad dressings:																
French, commercial	100	½ c.	410	1	39	18	0.3	39	11	14	0.4	..	..	..	..	..
	15	1 tbsp.	61	Tr.	6	3	Tr.	6	2	2	0.1	..	..	..	..	..
Italian	15	1 tbsp.	83	Tr.	9	1	Tr.	4	2	1	Tr.	..	..	..	..	..
Mayonnaise, commercial	100	½ c.	718	.1	80	2	Tr.	15	18	28	0.5	280	0.02	0.04	Tr.	..
	13	1 tbsp.	93	Tr.	10	Tr.	Tr.	2	2	4	0.1	36	Tr.	0.01	Tr.	..
Salad dressing,																
Mayonnaise type	100	½ c.	435	1	42	14	..	41	14	26	0.2	220	0.01	0.03	Tr.	..
	15	1 tbsp.	65	Tr.	6	2	..	6	2	4	Tr.	33	Tr.	Tr.	Tr.	..
Homemade, cooked	100	½ c. scant	164	4	10	15	0	68	89	93	0.6	490	0.05	0.16	0.2	Tr.
	17	1 tbsp.	28	1	2	3	0	12	15	16	0.1	83	0.01	0.03	Tr.	Tr.
Thousand Island	100	½ c.	502	1	50	15	0.3	32	11	17	0.6	320	0.02	0.03	0.2	3
	15	1 tbsp.	75	Tr.	8	2	Tr.	5	2	3	0.1	48	Tr.	Tr.	Tr.	Tr.
Sauerkraut, canned, drained solids	100	⅔ c.	18	1	Tr.	4	0.7	93	36	18	0.5	50	0.03	0.04	0.2	14
Sausage:																
Bologna	100	3½ ozs.	304	12	28	1	0	56	7	128	1.8	..	0.16	0.22	2.6	..
Frankfurter, cooked	100	2 medium	309	13	28	2	0	56	7	133	1.9	..	0.16	0.20	2.7	..
Liver, liverwurst	100	3½ ozs.	307	16	26	2	0	54	9	238	5.4	6,350	0.20	1.30	5.7	..
Pork, links or bulk, cooked	100	3½ ozs.	476	18	44	0	0	35	7	162	2.4	0	0.79	0.34	3.7	..
Pork, bulk, canned	100	3½ ozs.	381	18	33	0	0	43	11	210	2.8	0	0.20	0.24	3.0	..
Vienna sausage, canned	100	3½ ozs.	240	14	20	0	0	63	8	153	2.1	0	0.08	0.13	2.6	..
Scallops, cooked, steamed	100	3½ ozs.	112	23	1	..	..	73	115	338	3.0	..	..	..	..	..
Sherbet, * orange	100	½ c.	134	1	1	31	0	67	16	13	0	60	0.01	0.03	Tr.	2
Shortbread *	16	2 squares, 1¾ x 1¾ in.	81	1	4	10	Tr.	1	2	9	0.1	0	0.01	Tr.	0.1	0
Shrimp, French fried	100	3½ ozs.	225	20	11	10	..	57	72	191	2.0	..	0.04	0.08	2.7	0
Canned, dry pack or drained	100	3½ ozs.	116	24	1	1	..	70	115	263	3.1	60	0.01	0.03	1.8	0
Soups, canned:†‡ prepared to serve																
Bean with pork	100	2/5 c.§	67	3	2	9	0.6	84	25	51	0.9	260	0.05	0.03	0.4	1
Beef bouillon	100	2/5 c.	13	2	0	1	Tr.	96	Tr.	13	0.2	Tr.	Tr.	0.01	0.5	..

Food	gm	Measure§†‡														
Celery, cream of	100	2/5 c.	69	3	4	6	0.2	86	81	63	0.3	160	0.02	0.11	0.3	1
Chicken, cream of	100	2/5 c.	73	3	4	6	0.1	85	70	62	0.2	250	0.02	0.11	0.3	Tr.
Chicken noodle	100	2/5 c.	26	1	1	3	0.1	93	4	15	0.2	20	0.01	0.01	0.3	Tr.
Clam chowder, Manhattan with tomato, no milk ...	100	2/5 c.	33	1	1	5	0.2	92	14	19	0.4	360	0.01	0.01	0.4	..
Minestrone	100	2/5 c.	43	2	1	6	0.3	90	15	24	0.4	960	0.03	0.02	0.4	..
Mushroom, cream of	100	2/5 c.	88	3	6	7	0.1	83	78	69	0.2	100	0.02	0.14	0.3	Tr.
Onion	100	2/5 c.	27	2	1	2	0.2	93	12	11	0.2	Tr.	Tr.	0.01	Tr.	..
Pea (green), made with water	100	2/5 c.	53	2	1	9	0.4	86	18	46	0.4	140	0.02	0.02	0.4	3
Tomato, with water	100	2/5 c.	36	1	1	6	0.2	91	6	14	0.3	410	0.02	0.02	0.5	5
Made with milk	100	2/5 c.	69	3	3	9	0.2	84	67	62	0.3	480	0.04	0.10	0.5	6
Vegetable beef	100	2/5 c.	32	2	1	4	0.2	92	5	20	0.3	1,100	0.02	0.02	0.4	..
Soups, frozen: prepared																
Clam chowder, N.E. style with milk	100	2/5 c.	86	4	5	7	0.1	83	98	82	0.4	100	0.03	0.12	0.2	Tr.
Shrimp, cream of	100	2/5 c.	99	4	7	6	0.2	82	77	68	0.2	120	0.03	0.11	0.2	Tr.
Soybeans, canned,																
immature, boiled	100	3½ ozs.	103	9	5	7	1.4	77	67	114	2.8	340	0.06	..	..	2
Soybean flour or grits:																
High fat	100	1 c.	380	41	12	33**	2.2	8	240	650	9.0	..	0.89	0.36	2.3	0
Low fat	100	1 c.	356	43	7	37**	2.5	8	263	634	9.1	80	0.83	0.36	2.6	0
Defatted	100	1 c.	326	47	1	38**	2.3	8	265	655	11.1	40	1.09	0.34	2.6	0
Soybean Products:																
Soybean milk, fluid	100	½ c. scant	33	3	2	2	0	92	21	48	0.8	40	0.08	0.03	0.2	0
Soybean curd (Tofu)	100	3½ ozs.	72	8	4	2	0.1	85	128	126	1.9	0	0.06	0.03	0.1	0
Fermented (Natto)	100	3½ ozs.	167	17	7	12	3.2	63	103	182	3.7	0	0.07	0.05	..	0
Soy sauce	15	1 tbsp.	10	1	Tr.	1	0	10	12	16	0.7	0	Tr.	0.04	0.1	0
Soybean sprouts, cooked																
boiled, drained	100	1 c.	38	5	1	4	0.8	89	43	50	0.7	80	0.16	0.15	0.7	4
Spaghetti: Enriched:																
Cooked* plain	100	⅔ c.	149	5	1	30	0.2	61	9	65	1.1	0	0.18	0.10	1.4	0
With tomato and cheese sauce*	100	⅔ c.	104	4	4	15	0.2	77	32	54	0.9	430	0.10	0.07	0.9	5

* Values are calculated from a recipe.

† All ready-to-serve soups are calculated from equal weights of the condensed soup and water, except cream soup, which is based on equal weights of the condensed soups and milk.

‡ Dehydrated soups have about the same nutritive values as canned soups when each is prepared as directed on can or package.

§ Usual serving of soups is 1 cup, 2½ times amount given here.

** Approximately 40 percent of this total amount of carbohydrate calculated by difference is sugar, starch and dextrin. The remaining portion is made up of materials thought to be utilized only poorly, if at all, by the body.

TABLE 1. Composition of Foods—Edible Portion (Continued)

Food and Description	Wt. Gm.	Approximate Measure	Food Energy Cal.	Protein Gm.	Fat Gm.	Carbohydrate Total Gm.	Carbohydrate Fiber Gm.	Water Gm.	Ca Mg.	P Mg.	Fe Mg.	Vitamin A I.U.	Thiamine Mg.	Riboflavin Mg.	Niacin Mg.	Ascorbic Acid Mg.
Spaghetti: *(Continued)*																
With meat balls in tomato sauce, canned	100	⅔ c.	103	5	4	11	0.1	78	21	45	1.3	400	0.06	0.07	0.9	2
Spinach:																
Raw	100	3½ ozs.	26	3	Tr.	4	0.6	91	93‖	51	3.1	8,100	0.10	0.20	0.6	51
Cooked	100	½ c. packed	23	3	Tr.	4	0.6	91	93‖	38	2.2	8,100	0.07	0.14	0.5	28
Canned:																
Drained solids	100	½ c. packed	24	3	1	4	1.0	91	118‖	26	2.6	8,000	0.02	0.12	0.3	14
Frozen, cooked drained	100	3½ ozs.	23	3	Tr.	4	0.8	92	113‖	44	2.1	7,900	0.07	0.15	0.4	19
Squash:																
Summer:																
Cooked, diced, fresh or frozen	100	½ c.	15	1	Tr.	3	0.6	95	25	25	0.4	440	0.05	0.08	0.8	11
Winter:																
Baked	100	3½ ozs.	63	2	Tr.	15	1.8	86	28	48	0.8	4,200	0.05	0.13	0.7	13
Boiled, mashed	100	½ c.	38	2	Tr.	9	1.4	89	19	32	0.5	3,500	0.04	0.10	0.4	8
Starch, pure (including arrowroot, corn, etc.)	100	¾ c.	362	Tr.	Tr.	87	0.1	12	0	0	0	0	0	0	0	0
	8	1 tbsp.	29	0	0	7	Tr.	1	0	0	0	0	0	0	0	0
Strawberries:																
Raw	100	⅔ c.	37	1	1	8	1.4	90	21	21	1.0	60	0.03	0.07	0.6	59
Frozen, sugar added	100	3½ ozs.	109	1	Tr.	28	0.8	71	14	17	0.7	30	0.02	0.06	0.5	53
Sugars:																
Granulated, cane or beet	100	½ c.	385	0	0	100	0	1	..	..	..	0	0	0	0	0
	12	1 tbsp.	46	0	0	12	0	..	..	..	..	0	0	0	0	0
Powdered	100	¾ c.	385	0	0	100	0	1	..	..	3.4	0	0	0	0	0
Brown	100	½ c.	373	0	0	96	0	3	88	19	2.6	0	0.01	0.03	0.2	0
Maple	100	3½ ozs.	348	..	..	90	0	8	143	11	1.4	..	..	..	..	..
Sweet potatoes:																
Baked in skin	100	1 small	141	2	1	33	0.9	64	40	58	0.9	8,100	0.09	0.07	0.7	22
Boiled in skin	100	½ medium	114	2	Tr.	26	0.7	71	32	47	0.7	7,900	0.09	0.06	0.6	17
Candied	100	½ medium	168	1	3	34	0.6	60	37	43	0.9	6,300	0.06	0.04	0.4	10

Food		Measure															
Canned, vacuum or solid pack	100	½ c.	108	2	Tr.	25	1.0	72	25	41	0.8	7,800	0.05	0.04	0.5	14
Syrup, table blends (chiefly corn syrup)	100	⅓ c.	290	0	0	75	..	24	46	16	4.1	0	0	0	0	0
	20	1 tbsp.	58	0	0	15	..	5	9	3	0.8	0	0	..	..	0
Tangerines (including other Mandarin type oranges)	100	1 medium	46	1	Tr.	11	0.5	87	40	18	0.4	420	0.06	0.02	0.1	31
Tangerine juice, unsweetened: Fresh or frozen reconstituted	100	½ c. scant	43	1	Tr.	10	..	89	18	14	0.2	420	0.06	0.02	0.1	31
Canned, unsweetened	100	½ c. scant	43	1	Tr.	10	..	89	18	14	0.2	420	0.06	0.02	0.1	22
Tapioca, cream pudding	100	½ c.	134	5	5	17	0	72	105	109	0.4	290	0.04	0.18	0.1	1
Tomatoes: Raw	100	1 small	22	1	Tr.	5	0.5	94	13	27	0.5	900	0.06	0.04	0.7	23
Canned or cooked	100	½ c.	23	1	Tr.	5	0.4*	94	6	19	0.5	900	0.05	0.03	0.7	20
Tomato juice, canned	100	½ c. scant	19	1	Tr.	4	0.2	94	7	18	0.9	800	0.05	0.03	0.8	16
Tomato ketchup	17	1 tbsp.	18	Tr.	Tr.	4	0.1*	12	4	5	0.1	340	0.02	0.01	0.3	3
Tomato purée, canned	100	½ c. scant	39	2	Tr.	9	0.4	87	13	34	1.7	1,000	0.09	0.05	1.4	33
Tongue beef, canned	100	3½ ozs.	267	19	20	Tr.	0	57	10	180	2.5	0	0.05	0.22	2.5	0
Tortillas	30	1 tortilla	63	2	Tr.	13	0.3	8	35	57	0.3	0	0.03	0.07	0.6	..
Tuna fish. See Fish.																
Turkey, total edible roasted	100	3½ ozs.	263	27	16	0	0	55	..	..	..	Tr.	0.09	0.14	8.0	0
Flesh only, roasted	100	3½ ozs.	190	32	6	0	0	61	8	251	1.8	..	0.05	0.18	7.7	0
Turnips: Raw	100	¾ c. diced	30	1	Tr.	7	0.9	92	39	30	0.5	Tr.	0.04	0.07	0.6	36
Cooked, boiled, drained	100	⅔ c. diced	23	1	Tr.	5	0.9	94	35	24	0.4	Tr.	0.04	0.05	0.3	22
Turnip greens, boiled in small amount of water, short time	100	⅔ c.	20	2	Tr.	4	0.7	93	184	37	1.1	6,300	0.15	0.24	0.6	69

|| Calcium may not be available because of presence of oxalic acid.

TABLE 1. COMPOSITION OF FOODS—EDIBLE PORTION (Continued)

FOOD AND DESCRIPTION	WT. Gm.	APPROXIMATE MEASURE	FOOD ENERGY Cal.	PRO-TEIN Gm.	FAT Gm.	CARBO-HYDRATE TOTAL Gm.	FIBER Gm.	WATER Gm.	MINERALS CA Mg.	P Mg.	FE Mg.	VITAMINS VITA-MIN A I.U.	THIA-MINE Mg.	RIBO-FLAVIN Mg.	NIA-CIN Mg.	ASCORBIC ACID Mg.
Veal, cooked:																
Cutlet, broiled	100	3½ ozs.	234	26	13	0	0	59	11	225	3.2	..	0.07	0.25	5.4	..
Roast, medium fat, rib 82 percent lean	100	3½ ozs.	269	27	17	0	0	55	12	248	3.4	..	0.13	0.31	7.8	..
Stew meat without bone medium fat, cooked	100	3½ ozs.	303	26	21	0	0	52	12	138	3.3	..	0.05	0.24	4.6	..
Vinegar, distilled	100	½ c. scant	12	0	..	5	0	95	..	..	..	..	..	..	..	..
Waffles, made with enriched flour*, egg and milk	100	2 small waffles, 4½ x 5½ x ½ in.	279	9	10	38	0.1	41	113	173	1.7	330	0.17	0.25	1.3	Tr.
Walnuts, Persian or English	100	1 c. of halves	651	15	64	16	2.1	4	99	380	3.1	30	0.33	0.13	0.9	2
	8	1 tbsp. chopped	52	1	5	1	0.2	Tr.	8	31	0.2	Tr.	0.03	0.01	0.1	Tr.
Watermelons	100	3½ oz. portion	26	1	Tr.	6	0.3	92	7	10	0.5	590	0.03	0.03	0.2	7
Wheat flours:																
Whole (from hard wheat)	100	1 c. scant	333	13	0	71	2.3	12	41	372	3.3	0	0.55	0.12	4.3	0
Self-rising, enriched	100	1 c. scant	352	9	1	74	0.4	12	265	466	2.9†	0	0.44	0.26	3.5	0
Patent:																
All purpose or family flour:																
Unenriched	100	1 c. scant	364	11	1	76	0.3	12	16	87	0.8	0	0.06	0.05	0.9	0
Enriched	100	1 c. scant	364	11	1	76	0.3	12	16	87	2.9†	0	0.44	0.26	3.5	0
Bread flour:																
Unenriched	100	1 c. scant	365	12	1	75	0.3	12	16	95	0.9	0	0.08	0.06	1.0	0
Enriched	100	1 c. scant	365	12	1	75	0.3	12	16	95	2.9†	0	0.44	0.26	3.5	0
Cake or pastry flour	100	1 c. level	364	8	1	79	0.2	12	17	73	0.5	0	0.03	0.03	0.7	0
Wheat products:																
Flakes (added iron, thiamine and niacin)	100	4 c.	354	10	2	81	1.6	4	41	309	4.4	0	0.64	0.14	4.9	0
	35	1 c.	125	4	1	28	0.6	1	..	107	1.5	0	0.22	0.05	1.7	0
Germ, commercially milled	100	3½ ozs., 1 c.	363	27	11	47	2.5	12	72	1,118	9.4	0	2.01	0.68	4.2	0
Germ cereal with added nutrients	28	1 oz.	110	8	3	14	0.5	1	13	310	2.5	0	0.55	0.27	1.5	0

	grams	measure													
Puffed (added iron, thiamine and niacin)	100	8 c.	363	15	2	79	2.0	3	28	322	4.2	0	0.55	0.23	7.8	0
	12	1 c.	43	2	Tr.	10	0.2	Tr.	3	39	0.5	0	0.07	0.03	0.9	0
Rolled, cooked*	100	½ c. scant	75	2	Tr.	17	0.5	80	8	76	0.7	0	0.07	0.03	0.9	0
Shredded, plain	30	1 large biscuit, 4 x 2¼ in.	107	3	1	24	0.7	2	13	117	1.0	0	0.07	0.03	1.3	0
Wheat, whole meal cooked*	100	⅓ c. scant	45	2	Tr.	9	0.3	88	7	52	0.5	0	0.06	0.02	0.6	0
Wheat and malted barley cereal quick cooking, cooked	100	½ c. scant	65	2	Tr.	13	0.2	84	9	59	0.4	0	0.05	0.01	..	0
White sauce, medium*	100	½ c. scant	162	4	13	9	0	73	115	93	0.2	460	0.04	0.17	0.2	Tr.
Wild rice, parched, raw	100	⅔ c.	353	14	1	75	1.0	9	19	339	..	0	0.45	0.63	6.2	0
Yeast: Dried, brewer's	8	1 tbsp.	22	3	Tr.	3	0.1	1	16	141	1.4	0	1.24	0.35	3.0	0
Yoghurt, from partially skimmed milk	100	⅓ c.	50	3	2	5	0	89	120	94	Tr.	70	0.04	0.18	0.1	1
	246	1 c.	123	8	4	13	0	218	295	230	Tr.	170	0.10	0.43	0.2	2

* Values are calculated from a recipe.

† Based on the minimum level of enrichment specified under the Food, Drug and Cosmetic Act.

TABLE 2. SELECTED FATTY ACIDS AND CHOLESTEROL IN COMMON FOODS

	AMOUNT IN 100 GM. EDIBLE PORTION				
ITEM AND DESCRIPTION	TOTAL FAT	TOTAL SATURATED FAT	UNSATURATED FATTY ACIDS		CHOLESTEROL Mg.
			OLEIC	LINOLEIC	
Almonds, shelled	54.2	4	36	11	..
Avocado, raw	16.4	3	7	2	..
Bacon, broiled or fried	52.0	17	25	5	100
Beef, edible, raw, chuck	31.4	15	14	1	70
Porterhouse steak	36.2	17	16	1	..
Round, entire	12.3	6	5	Tr.	125
Round, separable lean	4.7	2	2	Tr.	..
Rump, total edible	25.3	12	11	1	..
Hamburg, regular	21.2	10	9	Tr.	..
lean	10.0	5	4	Tr.	..
Beef, corned, canned	12.0	6	5	Tr.	..
Brazil nuts, shelled	66.9	13	32	17	..
Bread, white, 3-4% milk solids	3.2	1	2	Tr.	..
Butter	81.0	46	27	2	250
Cake, plain, from mix with milk, egg and vegetable shortening	12.0	3	7	1	45
Candy, made with chocolate, nuts and vegetable shortening Chocolate-coated peanuts	41.3	11	22	7	..
Fudge with walnuts	17.4	6	5	6	..
Cashew nuts	45.7	8	32	3	..
Cheese, cheddar, natural	32.2	18	11	1	100
cottage, creamed	4.2	2	1	Tr.	15
Chicken, raw, edible portion Fryer	7.2	2	2	2	60-90
Roasting	12.6	4	6	2	60-90
Stewing	25.0	6	11	6	60-90

TABLE 2. SELECTED FATTY ACIDS AND CHOLESTEROL IN COMMON FOODS (*Continued*)

	AMOUNT IN 100 GM. EDIBLE PORTION				
ITEM AND DESCRIPTION	TOTAL FAT	TOTAL SATURATED FAT	UNSATURATED FATTY ACIDS		CHOLESTEROL Mg.
			OLEIC	LINOLEIC	
Chocolate, bitter, cooking	53.0	30	20	1	..
Coconut, shredded, sweetened	39.1	34	3	Tr.	..
Cookies, sugar, with v. f.*	16.8	4	10	1	50
Cornbread or muffins, v. f.*	8.4	3	4	1	46
Crackers, Graham, v. f.*	10.0	2	6	1	..
plain soda, v. f.*	10.2	2	6	1	..
Cream, light, coffee	20.6	11	7	1	67
Cream, heavy whipping	37.6	21	12	1	120
Custard, baked, milk and egg	5.5	3	2	Tr.	86
Duck, raw, edible portion	28.6	7	11	7	..
Eggs, whole	11.5	6	5	1	468
yolks only	30.6	10	13	2	1,500
Filberts, shelled	62.4	3	34	10	..
Herring, raw	11.3	2	Tr.	2	..
Ice cream, 12% fat	12.5	7	4	Tr.	45
Ice milk	5.1	3	2	Tr.	..
Lamb, raw, leg, edible portion	16.2	9	6	Tr.	70
shoulder, edible portion	23.9	13	9	1	70
Lard	100	38	46	10	106
Liver, pork, raw	3.7	1	1	Tr.	300
Luncheon meat	24.2	9	10	2	..
Margarine, hydrogenated	81.0	18	47	14	..
Milk, whole, cow's	3.7	2	1	Tr.	11-15
canned, evaporated	7.9	4	3	Tr.	..
dry, whole	27.5	15	9	1	85

* v.f.—vegetable fat.

TABLE 2. SELECTED FATTY ACIDS AND CHOLESTEROL IN COMMON FOODS (*Continued*)

ITEM AND DESCRIPTION	AMOUNT IN 100 GM. EDIBLE PORTION				
	TOTAL FAT	TOTAL SATURATED FAT	UNSATURATED FATTY ACIDS		CHOLESTEROL Mg.
			OLEIC	LINOLEIC	
Noodles, egg, dry form	4.6	1	2	Tr.	..
Oils: corn	100	10	28	53	..
cottonseed	100	25	21	50	..
olive	100	11	76	7	..
peanut	100	18	47	29	..
safflower seed	100	8	15	72	..
soybean	100	15	20	52	..
Olives, ripe, Mission type	20.1	2	15	1	..
Oysters, raw or canned	2.0	..	..	..	200
Peanuts, roasted, shelled	48.7	11	21	14	..
Peanut butter, oil added	50.6	9	25	14	..
Pecans, shelled	71.2	5	45	14	..
Pistachio nuts, shelled	53.7	5	35	10	..
Popcorn, popped, plain	5.0	1	1	3	..
Pork, fresh, raw ham, edible portion	26.6	10	11	2	70-105
Pork, loin, edible portion	24.9	9	10	2	70-105
cured, ham, edible portion	23.0	8	10	2	70-105
canned	12.3	4	5	1	70-105
Potatoes, French-fried	13.2	3	3	7	..
mashed, milk and butter	4.3	2	1	Tr.	..
Potato chips	39.8	10	8	20	..
Salad dressings: made with soybean, cottonseed or corn oil French, commercial	38.9	7	8	20	..
Italian, commercial	60.0	10	13	31	..
Mayonnaise with egg	79.9	14	17	40	..

TABLE 2. SELECTED FATTY ACIDS AND CHOLESTEROL IN COMMON FOODS (*Continued*)

ITEM AND DESCRIPTION	AMOUNT IN 100 GM. EDIBLE PORTION				
	TOTAL FAT	TOTAL SATURATED FAT	UNSATURATED FATTY ACIDS		CHOLESTEROL Mg.
			OLEIC	LINOLEIC	
Russian	50.8	9	11	26	..
Salmon, canned, pink	5.9	2	1	Tr.	..
Salt pork	85.0	32	39	5	..
Sausage, country style	31.1	11	13	3	70-105
pork, link, cooked	44.2	16	19	4	..
Shrimp, raw	.8	..	..	..	125
Tuna fish, canned in oil, drained solids	8.2	3	2	2	..
Turkey, dark meat	9.6	3	4	2	16-26
light meat	4.6	1	2	1	8-15
Veal, total edible, raw Chuck, medium fat	10.0	5	4	Tr.	90
Rib, medium fat	14.0	7	6	Tr.	90
Walnuts, shelled, black	59.3	4	21	28	..
English type	64.0	4	10	40	..
Wheat germ, commercial	11.5	2	3	6	..

Figures in this table are taken from Table 3, Handbook No. 8. Washington, U.S.D.A., 1963, and from Hardinge, M. G., and Crooks, H.: J. Am. Dietet. A., 34:1065, 1958.

TABLE 3. AMINO ACID CONTENT OF FOODS PER 100 GRAMS—EDIBLE PORTION*

Food Item	Nitrogen Conversion Factor	Protein Content Percent	Phenylalanine Mg.	Isoleucine Mg.	Leucine Mg.	Valine Mg.	Sulfur Containing			Tryptophan Mg.	Threonine Mg.	Lysine Mg.	Tyrosine Mg.	Arginine Mg.	Histidine Mg.
							Methionine Mg.	Cystine Mg.	Total Mg.						
Milk, Milk Products															
Fluid, whole	6.38	3.5	170	223	344	240	86	31	117	49	161	272	178	128	92
Canned, evap. unsweetened	6.38	7.0	340	447	688	481	171	63	234	99	323	545	357	256	185
Dried, non-fat	6.38	35.6	1,724	2,271	3,493	2,444	870	318	1,188	502	1,641	2,768	1,814	1,300	937
Cheese, Cheddar, processed	6.38	23.2	1,244	1,563	2,262	1,665	604	131	735	316	862	1,702	1,109	847	756
Cottage	6.38	17.0	917	989	1,826	978	469	147	616	179	794	1,428	917	802	549
Eggs, whole															
fresh or stored	6.25	12.8	739	850	1,126	950	401	299	700	211	637	819	551	840	307
Meat, Poultry, Fish															
Beef, chuck, med. fat	6.25	18.6	765	973	1,524	1,033	461	235	696	217	821	1,625	631	1,199	646
Hamburg, reg.	6.25	16.0	658	837	1,311	888	397	202	599	187	707	1,398	543	1,032	556
Rib roast	6.25	17.4	715	910	1,425	590	432	220	652	203	768	1,520	590	1,122	604
Round	6.25	19.5	802	1,020	1,597	1,083	484	246	730	228	861	1,704	661	1,257	677
Rump	6.25	16.2	666	848	1,327	899	402	205	607	189	715	1,415	550	1,045	562
Lamb, med. fat															
Leg	6.25	18.0	732	933	1,394	887	432	236	668	233	824	1,457	625	1,172	501
Rib	6.25	14.9	606	772	1,154	734	358	195	553	193	682	1,206	517	970	415
Pork, fresh, med. fat															
Ham	6.25	15.2	598	781	1,119	790	379	178	557	197	705	1,248	542	931	525
Loin	6.25	16.4	646	842	1,207	853	409	192	601	213	761	1,346	585	1,005	567
Pork, cured															
Bacon, med. fat	6.25	9.1	434	399	728	434	141	106	247	95	306	587	234	622	246
Ham	6.25	16.9	646	841	1,306	879	411	273	684	162	692	1,420	652	1,068	544
Luncheon meat, canned, spiced	6.25	14.9	570	741	1,151	775	362	241	603	143	610	1,252	879	942	479
Veal, med. fat															
Round	6.25	19.5	792	1,030	1,429	1,008	446	231	677	256	846	1,629	702	1,270	627
Poultry, flesh only															
Chicken, fryer	6.25	20.6	811	1,088	1,490	1,012	537	277	814	250	877	1,810	725	1,302	593
Turkey	6.25	24.0	960	1,260	1,836	1,187	664	330	994	..	1,014	2,173	..	1,513	649
Fish															
Cod, fresh, raw	6.25	16.5	612	837	1,246	879	480	222	702	164	715	1,447	446	929	..
Haddock, raw	6.25	18.2	676	923	1,374	930	530	245	775	181	789	1,596	492	1,025	..

Amino acid content of foods* (amino acid content in milligrams)

Food	Conv. factor	Protein													
Halibut, raw	6.25	18.6	690	943	1,405	991	542	250	792	185	806	1,631	503	1,048	..
Salmon, Pacific, raw	6.25	17.4	646	883	1,314	927	507	234	741	173	754	1,526	470	980	..
Canned, sockeye or red	6.25	20.2	750	1,025	1,526	1,076	588	271	859	200	876	1,771	546	1,138	..
Meat Products	6.25														
Liver, calf	6.25	19.0	958	994	1,754	1,195	447	234	681	286	903	447	711	1,158	505
Bologna sausage	6.25	14.8	540	718	1,061	744	313	185	498	126	606	1,191	481	1,028	398
Frankfurters	6.25	14.2	518	688	1,018	713	300	177	477	120	582	1,143	461	986	382
Liverwurst	6.25	16.7	759	818	1,400	1,037	347	203	550	187	724	1,301	510	1,034	497
Legumes, dry and Nuts															
Bean, red kidney, canned	6.25	5.7	315	324	490	346	57	57	114	53	247	423	220	343	162
Peanuts	5.46	26.9	1,557	1,266	1,872	1,532	271	463	734	340	828	1,099	1,104	3,296	749
Peanut Butter	5.46	26.1	1,510	1,228	1,816	1,487	263	449	712	330	803	1,066	1,071	3,198	727
Pecans	5.30	9.4	564	553	773	525	153	216	369	138	389	435	316	1,185	273
Walnuts	5.30	15.0	767	767	1,228	974	306	320	626	175	589	441	583	2,287	405
Grains and Their Products															
Bread, white, 4% milk solids	5.70	8.5	465	429	668	435	142	200	342	91	282	225	243	340	192
Cereal combinations															
Infant food, precooked mixed cereal & dry milk	6.25	19.4	543	..	1,368	900	310	137	447	118	..	273	447	776	233
Oat-corn-rye, puffed	5.83	14.5	933	841	..	..	388	234	622	172	545	343	622	..	326
Corn Products	6.25														
Corn grits	6.25	8.7	395	402	1,128	444	161	113	274	53	347	251	532	306	180
Corn meal, degermed	6.25	7.9	359	365	1,024	403	147	102	249	48	315	228	483	278	163
Cornflakes	6.25	8.1	354	306	1,047	386	135	152	287	52	275	154	283	231	226
Hominy	6.25	8.7	333	349	810	398	99	..	..	84	316	358	331	444	203
Oatmeal, rolled oats	5.83	14.2	758	733	1,065	845	209	309	518	183	470	521	524	935	261
Rice, white or converted	5.95	7.6	382	356	655	531	137	103	240	82	298	300	347	438	128
Rice, products, flakes or puffed	5.95	5.9	286	..	..	..	44	..	56	46	..	..	124	137	137
Wheat products	5.70														
Farina	5.70	10.9	579	..	891	..	143	184	327	124	356	199	447	424	268
Flakes	5.70	10.8	478	496	..	572	127	191	318	121	356	360	311	559	231
Macaroni or Spaghetti	5.70	12.8	669	642	849	728	193	243	436	150	499	413	422	582	303

* Figures for the amino acid content of foods are taken from Orr, M. L., and Watt, B. K.: Amino Acid Content of Foods. Home Economics Research Report No. 4. Washington, U.S.D.A., 1957. Amino acid content is given in milligrams, using whole numbers, rather than in grams, using decimals. The order of listing the amino acids has been arranged for the convenience of dietitians dealing with inborn errors of metabolism. For further explanation of the nitrogen conversion factors see reference above.

TABLE 3. AMINO ACID CONTENT OF FOODS PER 100 GRAMS—EDIBLE PORTION* (Continued)

| FOOD ITEM | NITROGEN CONVERSION FACTOR | PROTEIN CONTENT PERCENT | PHENYLALANINE Mg. | ISOLEUCINE Mg. | LEUCINE Mg. | VALINE Mg. | SULFUR CONTAINING | | | TRYPTOPHAN Mg. | THREONINE Mg. | LYSINE Mg. | TYROSINE Mg. | ARGININE Mg. | HISTIDINE Mg. |
							METHIONINE Mg.	CYSTINE Mg.	TOTAL Mg.						
Grains and Their Products (Continued)															
Noodles, made with															
egg	5.70	12.6	610	621	834	745	212	245	457	133	533	411	312	621	301
Shredded wheat	5.83	12.8	755	..	..	..	..	246	..	136	..	466	481	742	371
Fruits															
Bananas, ripe	6.25	1.2	..	..	..	..	11	..	..	18	..	55	31	..	..
Grapefruit	6.25	0.5	..	..	..	..	10	..	24	1	..	30	21	42	19
Muskmelon	6.35	0.6	..	..	..	..	2	..	..	1	..	15	..	..	..
Oranges or orange juice	6.25	0.9	..	..	..	..	2	..	..	3	..	22	..	..	..
Pineapple	6.25	0.4	..	..	..	..	1	..	..	5	..	9	..	..	..
Vegetables															
Asparagus, canned	6.25	1.9	60	69	83	92	27	..	24	23	57	89	..	106	31
Beans, snap, canned	6.25	1.0	24	45	58	48	14	10	24	14	38	52	21	42	19
lima, canned	6.25	3.8	197	233	306	246	41	42	83	49	171	240	131	230	125
Beets, canned	6.25	0.9	15	29	31	28	3	..	..	8	19	48	..	16	12
Beet greens	6.25	2.0	116	84	129	101	34	..	..	24	76	108	..	83	26
Broccoli	6.25	3.3	119	126	163	170	50	..	..	37	122	147	..	192	63
Cabbage	6.25	1.4	30	40	57	43	13	28	41	11	39	66	30	105	25
Carrots, raw	6.25	1.2	42	46	65	56	10	29	39	10	43	52	20	41	17
Cauliflower	6.25	2.4	75	104	162	144	47	..	..	33	102	134	34	110	48
Celery	6.25	1.3	..	..	..	..	15	6	21	12	..	..	..	..	..
Corn, sweet, white or yellow, canned	6.25	2.0	112	74	220	125	39	33	72	12	82	74	67	94	52
Cucumber	6.25	0.7	..	..	..	..	8	..	..	14	..	..	..	..	..
Eggplant	6.25	1.1	48	56	68	65	6	..	..	10	38	30	..	37	19
Lettuce	6.25	1.2	..	..	..	..	4	..	..	..	..	70	..	..	..
Onions, mature	6.25	1.4	39	21	37	31	13	..	..	21	22	64	46	180	14
Peas, canned	6.25	3.4	131	156	212	139	27	37	64	28	125	160	83	302	55
Potatoes cooked or canned	6.25	1.7	75	75	85	91	21	16	37	18	67	91	30	84	24
Pumpkin	6.25	1.2	32	44	63	45	11	..	..	16	28	58	16	43	19
Radishes	6.25	1.2	..	..	..	30	2	..	..	5	59	34	..	..	..
Spinach	6.25	2.3	99	107	176	126	39	46	85	37	102	142	73	116	49
Squash, summer	6.25	0.6	16	19	27	22	8	..	..	5	14	23	..	27	9
Tomatoes, all types	6.25	1.0	28	29	41	28	7	..	..	9	33	42	14	29	15
Turnips	6.25	1.1	20	20	..	..	12	..	..	..	..	57	29	..	..

TABLE 4. SODIUM, POTASSIUM AND MAGNESIUM CONTENT OF FOODS

Food	Na	K	Mg	Food	Na	K	Mg
	Mg. per 100 Grams				Mg. per 100 Grams		
Acerola	8	83	..	Rye, regular	557	145	42
Almonds, shelled	4	773	270	unsalted	30	115	42
Apples:				White, enriched	507	105	22
Raw, pared	1	110	5	unsalted	30	180	22
Frozen slices, sweetened	14	68	4	Whole wheat, regular	527	273	78
Apple juice, canned	1	101	4	unsalted	30	230	78
Applesauce, canned,				Raisin	365	233	24
sweetened	2	65	5	Broccoli, frozen	13	244	21
Apricots:				Brussels sprouts, raw	14	390	29
Raw	1	281	12	Butter:			
Canned	1	246	7	Salted	987	23	2
Dried	26	979	62	Unsalted	10	23	2
Frozen	4	229	9	Buttermilk, cultured	130	140	14
Nectar	Tr.	151	..	Cabbage:			
Asparagus:				Common	20	233	13
Fresh, cooked	1	183	20	Chinese	23	253	14
Frozen, cooked	1	238	14	Candy:			
Avocados	4	604	45	Butterscotch	66	2	..
Bacon:				Caramels	226	192	..
Broiled or fried	1,021	236	25	Chocolate, milk	94	384	..
Canadian, broiled or fried	2,555	432	24	Fudge	190	147	..
Baking powders*				Hard candy	32	4	Tr.
Bananas	1	370	33	Peanut brittle	31	151	..
Barley, pearled	3	160	37	Cantaloupe or honeydew	12	251	16
Beans, baked				Carrots, raw	47	341	23
canned, no pork	338	268	37	Cashew nuts	15	464	267
Beans:				Cauliflower, raw	13	295	24
Snap, canned	236	95	14	Celery, raw	126	341	22
Canned, low-sodium	2	95	14	Cereals:			
Frozen, cooked	1	152	21	Corn flakes	1,005	120	16
Lima, cooked, frozen	101	426	48	Corn grits, cooked	..	11	3
Beef:				Cornmeal, yellow or white	1	120	106
Lean, cooked	60	370	29	Farina, cooked	690	188	3
Heart, raw	86	193	18	Oatmeal, cooked	218	61	21
Liver, cooked	184	380	18	Rice, puffed, unsalted	2	100	..
Tongue, raw	73	197	16	Wheat, shredded, unsalted	3	348	133
Beets:				Wheat, puffed, unsalted	4	340	..
Canned, solids	236	167	15	Chard, raw	147	550	65
Cooked, unsalted	46	167	15	Cheese:			
Beet greens, raw	130	570	106	Cheddar	700	82	45
Beverages, carbonated†				Cottage, creamed	229	85	..
Blackberries	1	170	30	Parmesan	734	149	48
Blueberries, raw or frozen	1	81	6	Cherries, sweet or sour	2	191	8-14
Boysenberries, frozen	1	153	18	Chestnuts, fresh	6	454	41
Brazil nuts	1	715	225	Chicken, cooked,			
Breads:				white meat	64	441	19
Boston, brown	251	292	..	dark meat	86	321	..
Cracked, wheat	529	134	35	liver	61	151	16
				Chicory greens, raw	..	420	13

* Baking powders vary greatly in sodium and potassium content. The label on the package tells the type. One tsp. or 5 Gm. of baking powder contains:

	Mg. Na	Mg. K
Alum type	500	8
Phosphate type	450	9
Tartrate type	360	250
Low-sodium type	2	500

† The sodium content of carbonated beverages depends upon the sodium content of the water in the area where they are manufactured. See JAMA, 195:236, 1966.

TABLE 4. SODIUM, POTASSIUM AND MAGNESIUM CONTENT OF FOODS (*Continued*)

Food	Na	K	Mg	Food	Na	K	Mg
	Mg. per 100 Grams				Mg. per 100 Grams		
Chives, raw	..	250	32	Lobster, cooked	210	180	22
Chocolate, bitter	4	830	292	Loganberries, raw	1	170	25
Chocolate syrup	52	282	63	Macaroni, plain, cooked	1	61	18
Clams, meat only	120	181	..	Mangos, raw	7	189	18
Coconut, shredded	..	353	77	Margarine:			
Coffee, instant dry powder	72	3,256	456	Regular	987	23	..
Collards, raw	43	401	57	Unsalted	10 or less	10	..
Corn: sweet, cooked	15	165	..	Marmalade, citrus	14	33	4
frozen, cooked	1	184	22	Milk:			
canned	236	97	19	Whole or skim	50	144	13
Cornbread, from mix	744	127	13	Evap., unsweetened	118	303	25
Crab, cooked meat, canned	1,000	110	34	Molasses, light	15	917	46
Crackers:				Mushrooms:			
Graham	670	384	51	Canned	400	197	8
Soda	1,100	120	29	Fresh	15	414	13
Cranberries:				Mussels	289	315	24
Juice	1	10	2	Mustard greens, cooked	18	220	25
Sauce	1	30	2	Nectarines	6	294	13
Cream, light, coffee	43	122	11	Noodles, cooked	2	44	..
Cress, garden	14	606	..	Okra, fresh or frozen	2	168	47
Cucumbers	6	160	11	Olives:			
Currants, raw, red	2	257	15	Green	2,400	55	22
Dates, natural and dry	1	648	58	Ripe	750	27	..
Eggplant, cooked	1	150	16	Onions, mature, raw	10	157	12
Eggs:				Oranges or orange juice	1	200	11
Whole	122	129	11	Oysters, raw	73	121	32
Whites	146	139	9	Pancakes, from mix	451	156	..
Yolk	52	98	16	Papaya, raw	3	234	..
Endive or Escarole	14	294	10	Parsley	45	727	41
Figs, dried	34	640	71	Parsnips, cooked	8	379	32
Filberts (hazelnuts)	2	704	184	Peaches:			
Fish:				Raw	1	202	10
Cod, broiled	110	407	28	Canned	2	130	6
Haddock, fried	177	348	24	Peanuts, roasted, unsalted	5	701	175
Halibut, broiled	134	525	..	Peanut butter	606	652	173
Salmon, baked, broiled	116	443	30	Pears:			
Sardines, canned in oil	823	590	24	Raw	2	130	7
Tuna, canned, water	41	279	..	Canned	1	84	5
Gooseberries	1	155	9	Peas:			
Grapefruit:				Canned, regular	236	96	20
Pulp	1	135	12	Frozen	115	135	24
Juice	1	162	12	Low sodium, canned	3	96	24
Grapes:				Pecans	Tr.	603	142
American type	3	158	13	Peppers, raw	13	213	18
European type	3	173	6	Persimmons	6	174	8
Grape juice, canned	2	116	12	Pickles:			
Guava, common, raw	4	289	13	Dill	1,428	200	12
Honey, strained	5	51	3	Sweet	527	..	1
Ice cream, regular	63	181	14	Pineapple:			
Ice milk	68	195	..	Raw	1	146	13
Jams, jellies, average	15	81	12	Canned, heavy syrup	1	96	8
Lamb, any cut, broiled or roasted	70	290	19	Juice, unsweetened	1	149	12
Leeks, raw	5	347	23	Pistachio nuts	..	972	158
Lemon juice, fresh or frozen	1	141	7	Plums:			
Lettuce, iceberg	9	175	11	Raw	1	170	9
Lime juice	1	104	..	Purple, canned, in syrup	1	142	5

TABLE 4. SODIUM, POTASSIUM AND MAGNESIUM CONTENT OF FOODS (*Continued*)

Food	Na	K	Mg	Food	Na	K	Mg
	Mg. per 100 Grams				Mg. per 100 Grams		
Pork:				Soybean curd (tofu)	7	42	111
All cuts, fresh cooked	65	390	23	Spinach, cooked	50	324	63
Ham, cured, cooked	930	326	17	Squash:			
Sausage, pork, cooked	958	269	16	Summer, cooked, unsalted ...	1	141	16
Potatoes:				Winter, cooked, unsalted	1	141	17
Peeled, boiled, unsalted	2	285	22	Strawberries, raw	1	164	12
French fried, unsalted	6	853	25	Sweet potato, baked	12	300	31
Mashed, milk added	301	261	12	Tangerine, raw	1	126	..
Potato chips	1,000‡	1,130	..	Tomatoes, raw	3	244	14
Pretzels	1,680	130	..	Tomato juice:			
Prunes:				Canned	200	227	10
Dried, uncooked	8	694	40	Canned, low sodium	3	227	10
Cooked	4	327	20	Tomato catsup:			
Pumpkin, canned, unsalted	2	240	12	Regular	1,338	370	21
Radishes, raw	18	322	15	Low sodium	5-35	370	21
Raisins, uncooked	27	763	35	Turkey, roasted	130	367	28
Raspberries:				Turnips:			
Raw, red	1	168	20	Raw	49	268	20
Black	1	199	30	Cooked, unsalted	34	188	20
Rhubard, cooked	2	203	13	Turnip greens, frozen	17	149	26
Rice:				Veal, all cuts, cooked	80	500	18
Cooked, regular, salted	374	28	8	Walnuts, English	2	450	131
Cooked without salt	2	28	8	Watercress	52	282	20
Rutabagas, cooked, unsalted ...	4	167	15	Watermelon	1	100	8
Salad dressings:				Wheat:			
French	1,370	79	10	Flour	2	95	25
Italian	2,092	15	..	Bran	9	1,121	490
Mayonnaise	597	34	2	Germ	3	827	336
Russian	868	157	..	Yams	..	600	..
Scallops, cooked	265	476	..	Yoghurt	51	143	..
Shrimp, cooked	186	229	51	Zweiback	250	150	..
Syrup, maple	10	176	11				

‡ Potato chips vary in sodium according to amount of salt added.

Sodium, potassium and magnesium figures from Composition of Food, Raw, Processed Prepared. Agr. Handbook No. 8. U.S.D.A., Washington, D.C., 1963; or from Church, C. E., and Church, H. N.: Food Values of Portions Commonly Used, ed. 11. Philadelphia, J. B. Lippincott, 1970.

Values for these minerals in canned and processed foods subject to variation because of methods of processing.

Additional References on Sodium, Potassium and Magnesium Content of Foods
Cancio, M.: Sodium and potassium in Puerto Rican meats and fish. J. Am. Dietet. A., 38:341, 1961.
Cancio, M., and Leon, J. M.: Sodium and potassium in Puerto Rican foods and waters. J. Am. Dietet. A., 35: 1165, 1959.
Chan, S. L., and Kennedy, B. M.: Sodium in Chinese vegetables. J. Am. Dietet. A., 37:573, 1960.
Clifford, P. A.: Sodium content of food. J. Am. Dietet. A., 31:21, 1955.
Dahl, L. K.: Sodium in foods for a 100 Mg. diet. J. Am. Dietet. A., 34:717, 1958.
Davidson, C. S., *et al.*: Sodium-restricted diets. The rationale, complications, and practical aspects of their use. National Academy of Science–National Research Council Publ. No. 325. Washington, D.C., 1954.
Holinger, B. W., *et al.*: Analyzed sodium values in foods ready to serve. J. Am. Dietet. A., 48:501, 1966.

Hopkins, H. T.: Minerals and proximate composition of organ meats. J. Am. Dietet. A., 38:344, 1961.
Hopkins, H. T., and Eisen, J.: Mineral elements in fresh vegetables from different geographical areas. J. Agr. Food Chem., 7:633, 1959.
Nelson, G. Y., and Gram, M. R.: Magnesium content of accessory foods. J. Am. Dietet. A., 38:437, 1961.
Oglesby, L. M., and Bannister, A. C.: Sodium and potassium in salt-water fish. J. Am. Dietet. A., 35:1163, 1959.
Thurston, C. E.: Sodium and potassium content of 34 species of fish. J. Am. Dietet. A., 34:396, 1958.
Thurston, C. E., and Osterhaug, K. L.: Sodium content of fish flesh. J. Am. Dietet. A., 36:212, 1960.

Copper Content of Foods

Tables giving the copper content of certain foods are too conflicting and incomplete to be included in the above table. For persons interested in the copper content of foods in dealing with Wilson's Disease the following references are listed:

Silverberg, M., and Gellis, S. S.: Wilson's Disease. Am. J. Dis. Child., 113:178, 1967 (Lists foods to be avoided).
———: Preventing Wilson's Disease Sequelae. JAMA, 200:41, 1967.
Hook, L., and Brandt, I. K.: Copper content of some low copper foods. J. Am. Dietet. A., 49:202, 1966.
Review: Dietary copper in Wilson's Disease. Nutr. Rev., 23:301, 1965.

TABLE 5. ALCOHOLIC AND CARBONATED BEVERAGES

BEVERAGE	AVERAGE PORTION	WEIGHT Gm.	CALORIES	CARBO-HYDRATE Gm.	ALCOHOL* Gm.
Alcoholic Beverages:					
Ale, mild	8 oz. glass	230	98	8	9
Beer, average	8 oz. glass	240	114	11	9
Benedictine	cordial glass	20	69	7	7
Brandy, California	brandy glass	30	73	..	11
Cider, fermented	6 oz. glass	180	71	2	9
Cordial, anisette	cordial glass	20	74	7	7
Creme de menthe	cordial glass	20	67	6	7
Curaçao	cordial glass	20	54	6	6
Daiquiri	cocktail glass	100	122	5	15
Eggnog, Christmas	4 oz. punch cup	123	335	18	15
Gin Rickey	4 oz. glass	120	150	1	21
Gin, dry	1 jigger, 1½ oz.	43	105	..	15
Highball, average	8 oz. glass	240	166	..	24
Manhattan	cocktail glass, 3½ oz.	100	164	8	19
Old Fashioned	4 oz. glass	100	179	4	24
Planter's punch	3½ oz. glass	100	175	8	22
Rum	1 jigger, 1½ oz.	43	105	..	15
Tom Collins	10 oz. glass	300	180	9	22
Whiskey, rye	1 jigger, 1½ oz.	43	119	..	17
Scotch	1 jigger, 1½ oz.	43	105	..	15
Wines:					
Champagne	4 oz. glass	120	84	3	11
Muscatel or port	3½ oz. glass	100	158	14	15
Sauterne	3½ oz. glass	100	84	4	10
Sherry, domestic	2 oz. glass	60	84	5	9
Table type	3½ oz. glass	100	85	..	10
Vermouth, dry	3½ oz. glass	100	105	1	15
Vermouth, sweet	3½ oz. glass	100	167	12	18
Carbonated Beverages:					
Coca-cola	6 oz. bottle	170	78	20	..
Ginger ale	6 oz. bottle	230	80	21	..
Pepsi-cola	8 oz. bottle	230	106	28	..
Soda, fruit flavor	8 oz. bottle	230	94	24	..
Root beer	8 oz. bottle	230	106	28	..

Values taken from Church, C. F., and Church, H. N.: Food Values of Portions Commonly Used. ed. 11. Philadelphia, J. B. Lippincott, 1970.

* Alcohol yields 7 calories per gram.

TABLE 6. EQUIVALENT WEIGHTS AND MEASURES

Weight Equivalents

	MILLIGRAM	GRAM	KILOGRAM	GRAIN	OUNCE	POUND
1 microgram (mcg.)	0.001	0.000001				
1 milligram (mg.)	1.	0.001		0.0154		
1 gram (Gm.)	1,000.	1.	0.001	15.4	0.035	0.0022
1 kilogram (Kg.)	1,000,000.	1,000.	1.	15,400.	35.2	2.2
1 grain (gr.)	64.8	0.065		1.		
1 ounce (oz.)		28.3		437.5	1.	0.063
1 pound (lb.)		453.6	0.454		16.0	1.

Volume Equivalents

	CUBIC MILLIMETER	CUBIC CENTIMETER	LITER	FLUID OUNCE	PINT	QUART
1 cubic millimeter (cu. mm.)	1.	0.001				
1 cubic centimeter (cc.)	1,000.		0.001			
1 liter (L.)	1,000,000.	1,000.	1.	33.8	2.1	1.05
1 fluid ounce		30.(29.57)	0.03	1.		
1 pint (pt.)		473.	0.473	16.	1.	
1 quart (qt.)		946.	0.946	32.	2.	1.

Linear Equivalents

	MILLIMETER	CENTIMETER	METER	INCH	FOOT	YARD
1 millimeter (mm.)	1.	0.1	0.001	0.039	0.00325	0.0011
1 centimeter (cm.)	10.	1.		0.39	0.0325	0.011
1 meter (M.)	1,000.	100.	1.	39.37	3.25	1.08
1 inch (in.)	25.4	2.54	0.025	1.	0.083	0.028
1 foot (ft.)	304.8	30.48	0.305	1.12	1.	0.33
1 yard (yd.)	914,4	91.44	0.914	36.0	3.	1.

Comparative Values of Weight and Volume of Water

1 liter	=	1 kilo.	=	2.2 lbs.
1 fluid ounce	=	30 Gm.	=	1.04 ozs.
1 pint	=	473 Gm.	=	1.04 lbs.
1 quart	=	.946 kilo.	=	2.1 lbs.

Table of Common Measures and Metric Equivalents

1 tsp.	=	5 cc.
1 tbsp.	=	14 cc. (approx. 15 Gm.)
1 cup	=	225 cc. (approx. 240 Gm.)

Comparative Temperatures

	CENTIGRADE	FAHRENHEIT
Boiling water, sea level	100	212
Body temperature	37	98.6
Tropical temperature	30	89
Room temperature, average	20	70
Freezing	0	32

Table of Measures and Approximate Weights

3 teaspoons	1 tbsp.	*1 tablespoon liquid	½ oz.
16 tablespoons	1 cup	1 tablespoon flour	¼ oz.
½ cup	1 gill	1 tablespoon sugar	⅗ oz.
2 cups	1 pt.	*1 cup liquid	8 ozs.
4 cups	1 qt.	1 cup flour	4½ ozs.
2 pints	1 qt.	1 cup butter	8 ozs.
4 quarts	1 gal.	1 cup sugar	10 ozs.
1 tablespoon butter	½ oz.		

* Water or milk.

TABLE 7. HEIGHT AND WEIGHT FOR AGE—PERCENTILE STANDARDS—BOYS AND GIRLS

AGE YEARS	HEIGHT PERCENTILES					WEIGHT PERCENTILES				
	10	25	50	75	90	10	25	50	75	90
BOYS										
	Ins.	Ins.	Ins.	Ins.	Ins.	Lbs.	Lbs.	Lbs.	Lbs.	Lbs.
2............	32.7	33.2	33.8	34.3	34.6	24.2	25.8	27.3	28.7	30.6
3............	36.0	36.6	37.2	37.6	38.1	28.9	30.4	31.7	33.5	35.5
4............	39.0	39.7	40.2	40.8	41.4	30.0	33.1	34.8	35.9	37.9
5............	41.7	42.4	43.0	43.6	44.3	37.3	38.8	40.6	42.8	45.4
6............	44.1	44.9	45.7	46.3	47.0	41.7	43.2	45.4	48.3	51.6
7............	46.3	47.2	48.1	48.9	49.9	46.1	47.8	50.9	54.7	58.6
8............	48.5	49.4	50.5	51.4	52.6	50.5	52.9	57.4	61.9	66.6
9............	50.6	51.7	52.8	53.8	54.8	55.1	58.6	64.4	70.1	75.2
10............	52.5	53.7	54.9	56.1	57.0	60.4	64.8	71.4	78.0	84.2
11............	54.3	55.4	56.7	58.2	59.1	65.7	71.2	78.9	86.4	93.5
12............	56.0	57.1	58.7	60.3	61.5	71.0	77.8	86.0	94.8	102.7
13............	58.1	59.3	61.2	62.6	64.3	76.9	85.3	95.7	105.8	114.6
14............	60.4	62.1	64.1	65.5	67.2	88.0	98.5	111.1	119.5	128.7
15............	63.0	65.0	66.9	68.3	69.8	101.6	112.2	124.3	134.5	143.3
16............	65.6	67.3	68.9	70.4	71.7	112.4	122.6	133.8	146.4	157.4
17............	66.5	68.2	69.8	71.2	72.4	120.4	130.1	139.8	153.9	169.3
18............	67.1	68.6	70.2	71.5	72.7	127.0	134.3	142.4	158.7	173.3
GIRLS										
2............	31.8	32.7	33.5	34.3	34.9	21.6	23.6	25.8	27.6	29.1
3............	34.9	35.8	37.0	38.0	38.7	25.6	27.3	30.6	32.4	34.4
4............	37.8	38.9	40.4	41.3	42.0	29.3	31.3	35.5	37.5	40.1
5............	40.5	41.6	43.3	44.3	45.0	33.1	35.9	40.3	43.4	45.9
6............	43.1	44.0	45.9	47.2	47.7	37.0	40.6	45.4	49.6	51.6
7............	45.4	46.2	48.5	49.8	50.3	41.4	45.2	51.1	55.8	60.0
8............	47.7	48.4	51.0	52.2	52.8	46.2	50.0	58.0	61.9	70.5
9............	49.8	50.7	53.5	54.6	55.2	51.1	56.0	65.7	70.5	82.5
10............	51.9	53.1	55.6	56.9	58.0	56.0	62.2	74.3	81.8	93.9
11............	53.7	55.7	58.1	59.7	60.9	60.8	69.4	83.8	94.6	104.7
12............	55.5	59.0	61.3	62.6	63.6	70.5	80.9	96.1	106.5	115.1
13............	58.3	61.0	63.9	65.1	65.9	79.4	91.5	108.9	114.9	124.8
14............	60.5	62.2	65.0	66.1	67.2	85.5	98.3	116.6	121.7	133.6
15............	61.8	63.2	65.6	66.5	67.7	89.1	102.7	121.0	127.0	140.7
16............	62.4	63.8	65.9	66.8	68.0	91.5	106.0	123.9	131.0	144.2
17............	62.6	64.1	66.1	67.0	68.3	93.0	108.5	125.7	133.8	145.9
18............	62.7	64.3	66.2	67.6	68.9	93.7	110.0	126.1	135.4	146.8

From Hathaway, M. L.: Heights and Weights of Children and Youth in the United States. Home Economics Res. Bulletin No. 2. U.S.D.A., Washington, D.C., 1957.

TABLE 8. DESIRABLE WEIGHTS FOR MEN AND WOMEN AGED 25 AND OVER*

Weight in Pounds According to Frame (In Indoor Clothing)

HEIGHT		SMALL FRAME	MEDIUM FRAME	LARGE FRAME	HEIGHT		SMALL FRAME	MEDIUM FRAME	LARGE FRAME
MEN					WOMEN†				
Feet	Inches				Feet	Inches			
5	2	112–120	118–129	126–141	4	10	92– 98	96–107	104–119
5	3	115–123	121–133	129–144	4	11	94–101	98–110	106–122
5	4	118–126	124–136	132–148	5	0	96–104	101–113	109–125
5	5	121–129	127–139	135–152	5	1	99–107	104–116	112–128
5	6	124–133	130–143	138–156	5	2	102–110	107–119	115–131
5	7	128–137	134–147	142–161	5	3	105–113	110–122	118–134
5	8	132–141	138–152	147–166	5	4	108–116	113–126	121–138
5	9	136–145	142–156	151–170	5	5	111–119	116–130	125–142
5	10	140–150	146–160	155–174	5	6	114–123	120–135	129–146
5	11	144–154	150–165	159–179	5	7	118–127	124–139	133–150
6	0	148–158	154–170	164–184	5	8	122–131	128–143	137–154
6	1	152–162	158–175	168–189	5	9	126–135	132–147	141–158
6	2	156–167	162–180	173–194	5	10	130–140	136–151	145–163
6	3	160–171	167–185	178–199	5	11	134–144	140–155	149–168
6	4	164–175	172–190	182–204	6	0	138–148	144–159	153–173

* Metropolitan Life Insurance Company.
† For girls between 18 and 25, subtract 1 pound for each year under 25.

Bibliography

PART ONE

PRINCIPLES OF NUTRITION

GENERAL REFERENCES

Books:

Anderson, L., and Browe, J. H.: Nutrition and Family Health Services. Philadelphia, W. B. Saunders, 1960.

Beaton, G. H., and McHenry, E. W.: Nutrition. A Comprehensive Treatise. Vol. III. Nutritional Status, Assessment and Application. New York, Academic Press, 1966.

Bogert, L. J., Briggs, G. M., and Calloway, D. H.: Nutrition and Physical Fitness. ed. 8. Philadelphia, W. B. Saunders, 1966.

Eppright, E., Pattison, M., and Barbour, H.: Teaching Nutrition. Ames, Iowa. Iowa State College Press, 1963.

Fleck, H. C.: Introduction to Nutrition. ed. 2. New York, Macmillan, 1971.

Guthrie, H. A.: Introductory Nutrition. ed. 2. St. Louis, C. V. Mosby, 1971.

Heinz Handbook of Nutrition. ed. 3. New York, McGraw-Hill, 1967.

Krause, M. V.: Food, Nutrition and Diet Therapy. ed. 4. Philadelphia, W. B. Saunders, 1966.

Martin, E. A.: Nutrition In Action. ed. 3. New York, Holt, Rinehart & Winston, 1971.

Mitchell, H. S., Rynbergen, H. J., Anderson, L., and Dibble, M. V.: Cooper's Nutrition in Health and Disease, ed. 15. Philadelphia, J. B. Lippincott, 1968.

Pike, R. L., and Brown, M. L.: Nutrition: An Integrated Approach. New York, John Wiley & Sons, 1967.

Present Knowledge of Nutrition. ed. 3. New York, Nutrition Foundation Inc., 1967.

Robinson, C. H.: Normal and Therapeutic Nutrition. ed. 14. New York, Macmillan, 1972.

Taylor, C. M., and Pye, O. F.: Foundations of Nutrition. ed. 6. New York, Macmillan, 1966.

Wayler, T. J., and Klein, R. S.: Applied Nutrition. New York, Macmillan, 1965.

Williams, S. R.: Nutrition and Diet Therapy. St. Louis, C. V. Mosby, 1969.

Wilson, E. D., Fisher, K. H., and Fuqua, M. E.: Principles of Nutrition. ed. 2. New York, John Wiley & Sons, 1966.

Wohl, M. G., and Goodhart, R. S.: Modern Nutrition in Health and Disease. ed. 4. Philadelphia, Lea & Febiger, 1968.

Journals and Annuals:

American Journal of Nursing
American Journal of Public Health
American Journal of Clinical Nutrition
Borden's Review of Nutrition Research
Journal of the American Dietetic Association
Journal of Home Economics
Journal of Nutrition
Journal of Nutrition Education
Metabolism
Nutrition Abstracts and Reviews
Nutrition Reviews
Nutrition Today
World Review of Nutrition and Dietetics

Journal Articles:

Goldsmith, G. A.: Clinical nutritional problems in the United States today. Nutr. Rev., 23:1, 1965.

Hodges, R. E.: Nutrition and "the Pill." J. Am. Dietet. A., 59:212, 1971.

King, C. G.: Notes on the history of nutrition in America. J. Am. Dietet. A., 56:188, 1970.

Ross, M. L.: The long view. J. Am. Dietet. A., 56:295, 1970.

Sebrell, W. H.: Changing concepts of malnutrition. Am. J. Clin. Nutr., 20:653, 1969.

Todhunter, E. N.: The evolution of nutrition concepts. J. Am. Dietet. A., 46:120, 1965.

TABLES OF FOOD COMPOSITION

Church, C. F., and Church, H. N.: Food Values of Portions Commonly Used. ed. 11. Philadelphia, J. B. Lippincott, 1970.

FAO: Review of Food Composition Tables. Rome, Food Consumption and Planning Branch, FAO, 1965. (Food Composition Tables from around the world.)

————: Amino Acid Content of Foods. Nutr. Studies, No. 24. Rome, 1967.

Hardinge, M. G., and Crooks, H.: Lesser known vitamins in foods. J. Am. Dietet. A., 38:240, 1961.

Orr, M. L., and Watt, B. K.: Amino Acid Content of Foods. U.S.D.A., Washington, D.C., U.S. Gov't. Print. Off., 1957.

U.S.D.A.: Folic Acid Content of Foods. Handbook No. 29. Washington, D.C., U.S. Gov't. Print. Off., 1951.

————: Nutritive Value of Foods. Home and Garden Bull. No. 72. Washington, D.C., U.S. Gov't. Print. Off., 1970.

————: Pantothenic Acid, Vitamin B_6, and Vitamin B_{12} in Food. Home Econ. Res. Report No. 36. Washington, D.C., 1969.

Watt, B. K., and Merrill, A. L.: Composition of Foods —Raw, Processed, Prepared. U.S.D.A. Handbook No. 8. Washington, D.C., U.S. Gov't. Print. Off., 1963.

Widdowson, E. M.: British Food Composition Tables. J. Am. Dietet. A., 50:363, 1967.

RELIABLE SOURCES FROM WHICH TO OBTAIN NUTRITION INFORMATION

American Dietetic Ass., 620 N. Michigan Ave., Chicago, Ill. 60611.

American Home Economics Ass., 1600 Twentieth St., Washington, D.C. 20009.

Council on Foods and Nutrition, or Bureau of Investigation, American Medical Ass., 535 N. Dearborn St., Chicago, Ill. 60610.

Food and Nutrition Board, National Academy of Sciences–National Research Council, 2101 Constitution Ave., Washington, D.C. 20418.

Food and Nutrition Section, American Public Health Ass., 1740 Broadway, New York, N.Y. 10019.

Food and Drug Administration, U.S. Dept. H.E.W., Washington, D.C. 20204.

Federal Trade Commission, Bureau of Investigation, Washington, D.C.

The Nutrition Foundation, Inc., 99 Park Ave., New York, N.Y. 10016.

United States Department of Agriculture, Washington, D.C.

U.S. Department of Health, Education and Welfare, Washington, D.C.

Better Business Bureaus

Cooperative Extension—State and Federal (USDA)

State Health Departments

Food and Nutrition Dept. of State University

FACTORS INFLUENCING FOOD HABITS

Books and Pamphlets:

Lowenberg, M., Todhunter, E. N., and Wilson, E. D.: Food and Man. New York, John Wiley & Sons, 1968.

Mead, M.: Food Habits Research: Problems of the 60's. National Academy of Sciences–National Research Council Publ. No. 1225. Washington, D.C., 1964.

Pyke, M.: Food and Society. London, John Murray, 1968.

Journal Articles:

Adams, R. N.: Nutrition, anthropology, and the study of man. Nutr. Rev., 17:97, 1959.

Babcock, C.: Attitudes and the use of food. J. Am. Dietet. A., 38:546, 1961.

Fathauer, G. H.: Food habits—an anthropologist's view. J. Am. Dietet. A., 37:335, 1960.

Feeding drug addicts. Hospitals, 45: (Part I) 80, (Aug. 1) 1971.

Kallen, D. J.: Nutrition and society. JAMA, 215:94, 1971.

Lowenberg, M. E.: Socio-cultural bases of food habits. Food Technology, 24:27, 1970.

Manning, M. L.: The psychodynamics of dietetics. Nurs. Outlook, 13:57, 1965.

Mead, M.: Changing significance of food. J. Nutr. Educa., 2:17, 1970.

Parrish, J. B.: Implications of changing food habits for nutrition educators. J. Nutr. Educa., 2:140, 1971.

Queen, G. S.: Culture, economics and food habits. J. Am. Dietet. A., 33:1044, 1957.

Simoans, F. J.: The geographic approach to food prejudices. Food Technology, 20:42, 1966.

FOOD PATTERNS AND NUTRITIONAL STATUS U.S.A.

Books and Pamphlets:

Food Intake and Nutritive Value of Diets of Men, Women and Children in the United States, Spring 1965. Agr. Research Service, U.S.D.A., Washington, D.C., 1969.

Household Food Consumption Survey 1965-66 Report No. 6: Dietary Levels of Households in the United States, Spring 1965. Agr. Research Service, U.S.D.A., Washington, D.C., 1969.

Hunger U.S.A. A Report of the Citizen's Board of Inquiry into Hunger and Malnutrition in the U.S. Washington, D.C., New Community Press, 1968.

Nutrition and Human Needs. Hearings before the Select Committee on Nutrition and Human Needs of the U.S. Senate. Parts I et seq. Washington, D.C., U.S. Gov't Print. Off., 1969.

Stewart, M. S.: Hunger in America. Public Affairs Pamphlet 457. New York, Public Affairs Committee, 1970.

White House Conference on Food, Nutrition and Health—Final Report. Washington, D.C., U.S. Gov't Print. Off., 1970.

Journal Articles:

Beloian, A. M.: Seasonal variations in U.S. diets. Family Economics Rev., March 1971.

Council on Foods and Nutrition: Malnutrition and hunger in the United States. JAMA, 213:272, 1970.

Davis, T. R. A., *et al.*: Review of studies of vitamin and mineral nutrition in the United States (1950-1968). J. Nutr. Educa., 1:41 (Supplement), 1969.

Kelsay, J. L.: A compendium of nutritional status studies and dietary evaluation studies conducted in the United States. J. Nutr., 99:123 (Supplement I, Part II), 1969.

Mayer, J.: One year later. J. Am. Dietet. A., 58:300, 1971.

Schaefer, A. E.: The national nutrition survey. J. Am. Dietet. A., 54:371, 1969.

THE ROLE OF THE NURSE, DIETITIAN, NUTRITIONIST AND HEALTH AIDE IN PROMOTING GOOD NUTRITION

Journal Articles:

Callan, L. B.: Supervision, the key to success with aides. Public Health Rep., 85:780, 1970.

Cauffman, J. G., *et al.*: Community health aides: how effective are they? Am. J. Public Health, 60:1904, 1970.

D'Onofrio, C. N.: Aides—pain or panacea. Public Health Rep., 85:788, 1970.

Erlander, D.: Dietetics—a look at the profession. Am. J. Nursing, 70:2402, (Nov.) 1970.

Heath, A. M., and Pelz, D. R.: Perception of functions of health aides by themselves and by others. Public Health Rep., 85:767, 1970.

Hildebrand, G. I.: Guidelines for effective use of non-professionals. Public Health Rep., 85:773, 1970.

Jamann, J. A.: Health as a function of ecology. Am. J. Nursing, 71:970, (May) 1970.

Morris, E.: How does a nurse teach nutrition to patients? Am. J. Nursing, 60:1, 1960.

Sipple, H. L.: Problems and progress in nutrition education. J. Am. Dietet. A., 59:18, 1971.

Spindler, E. B., *et al.*: Action programs to improve nutrition. J. Home Econ., 61:635, 1969.

The American Dietetic Association: Position paper on the nutrition component of health services delivery systems. J. Am. Dietet. A., 58:538, 1971.

CARBOHYDRATES

(*See also* references under Digestion, Absorption and Metabolism and Diabetes)

Journal Articles:

Anderson, J. T.: Dietary carbohydrate and serum triglycerides. Am. J. Clin. Nutr., 20:168, 1967.

Antar, M. A., *et al.*: Changes in retail market food supplies in the U.S. in the last seventy years in relation to the incidence of coronary heart disease, with special reference to dietary carbohydrates and essential fatty acids. Am. J. Clin. Nutr., 14:169, 1964.

Bloom, W. L.: Carbohydrates and water balance. Am. J. Clin. Nutr., 20:157, 1967.

Gryboski, J. D.: Diarrhea from dietetic candies (sorbitol). New Eng. J. Med., 275:718, 1966.

Hardinge, M. G., *et al.*: Carbohydrates in foods. J. Am. Dietet. A., 46:197, 1965.

Hartles, R. L.: Carbohydrate consumption and dental caries. Am. J. Clin. Nutr., 20:152, 1967.

Hodges, R. E.: Present knowledge of carbohydrates. Nutr. Rev., 24:65, 1966.

Hodges, R. E., and Krehl, W. A.: The role of carbohydrates in lipid metabolism. Am. J. Clin. Nutr., 17:334, 1965.

McGandy, R. B., *et al.*: Dietary carbohydrate and serum cholesterol levels in man. Am. J. Clin. Nutr., 18:237, 1966.

Review: Blood lipids and various dietary carbohydrates. Nutr. Rev., 24:35, 1966.

————: Carbohydrate intake and respiratory quotient. Nutr. Rev., 22:104, 1964.

Speirs, R. L.: The systemic influence of carbohydrates on teeth. Proc. Nutr. Soc., 23:129, 1964.

Stevens, H. A., and Ohlson, M. A.: Estimated intake of simple and complex carbohydrates. J. Am. Dietet. A., 48:294, 1966.

Yudkin, J.: Evolutionary and historical changes in dietary carbohydrates. Am. J. Clin. Nutr., 20:108, 1967.

FATS AND LIPIDS

(*See also* references under Digestion, Absorption and Metabolism and Atheroslerosis)

Books and Pamphlets:

Beaton, G. H., and McHenry, E. W.: Nutrition—A Comprehensive Treatise. Vol. I. Macronutrients and Nutrient Elements. Chap. 2. New York, Academic Press, 1964.

Food and Nutrition Board: Dietary Fat and Human Health. National Academy of Science–National Research Council Publ. No. 1147. Washington, D.C., 1966.

Home Economics Research Report, No. 7: Fatty Acids in Food Fats. Agr. Research Service, U.S.D.A., Washington, D.C., 1959.

Journal Articles:

Bernfeld, P., *et al.*: Fatty acid contents of margarines and other table fats. Am. J. Clin. Nutr., 11:554, 1962.

Council of Foods and Nutrition, A.M.A.: Regulation of dietary fat. JAMA, 181:441, 1962.

Eastwood, G., *et al.*: Fatty acids and other lipids in mayonnaise. J. Am. Dietet. A., 42:518, 1963.

Hansen, A. E., *et al.*: Role of linoleic acid in infant nutrition. Pediatrics, 31:171, 1963.

Hegsted, D. M., *et al.*: Quantitative effects of dietary fats on serum cholesterol in man. Am. J. Clin. Nutr., 17:281, 1965.

Horvath, R. A., *et al.*: Variation in the fatty acid distribution of filled milk beverages. Am. J. Clin. Nutr., 24:397, 1971.

Hughes, A. A., *et al.*: Linoleic acid—an essential nutrient: its content in infant formulas and precooked cereals. Clin. Pediat., 2:555, 1963.

Mead, J. F.: Present knowledge of fat. Nutr. Rev., 24:33, 1966.

Miljanich, P., and Ostwald, R.: Fatty acids in newer brands of margarine. J. Am. Dietet. A., 56:29, 1970.

Review: Body fat and adipose tissue. Nutr. Rev., 22:99, 1964.

———: Dietary fat in essential hyperlipemia. Nutr. Rev., 24:103, 1966.

———: Fatty acid composition of fish oils. Nutr. Rev., 23:51, 1963.

Rice, E. E.: Composition of modern margarines. J. Am. Dietet. A., 41:319, 1962.

Scheig, R.: What is Dietary Fat? Am. J. Clin. Nutr., 22:651, 1969.

Symposium: Intravenous fat emulsions. Am. J. Clin. Nutr., 16:1, 1965.

PROTEIN

(*See also* references under Digestion, Absorption and Metabolism)

Books and Pamphlets:

FAO: Protein—At the Heart of the World Food Problem. Rome, FAO, 1967.

———: Amino Acid Content of Foods and Biological Data on Proteins. Nutr. Studies No. 24. Rome, FAO, 1970.

FAO/WHO Joint Expert Group: Protein Requirements. Rome, FAO, 1965.

Food and Nutrition Board: Evaluation of Protein Nutrition. National Academy of Science–National Research Council Publ. No. 711. Washington, D.C., 1959.

———: Evaluation of Protein Quality. National Academy of Science–National Research Council Publ. No. 1100. Washington, D.C., 1963.

———: Progress in Meeting Protein Needs of Infants and Children. National Academy of Science–National Research Council Publ. No. 843. Washington, D.C., 1961.

Orr, M. L., and Watt, B. K.: Amino Acid Content of Food. Home Econ. Res. Report No. 4. U.S.D.A., Washington, D.C., 1957.

Journal Articles:

Bradfield, R. B.: Protein deprivation: comparative response of hair roots, serum protein and urinary nitrogen. Am. J. Clin. Nutr., 24:405, 1971.

Coltman, C. A., *et al.*: The amino acid content of sweat in normal adults. Am. J. Clin. Nutr., 18:373, 1966.

Committee Report: Assessment of protein nutritional status. Am. J. Clin. Nutr., 23:803, 1970.

Fisher, H., *et al.*: Reassessment of amino acid requirements of young women on low nitrogen diets. I. Lysine and tryptophan. Am. J. Clin. Nutr., 22:1190, 1969.

Hardinge, M. G., *et al.*: Nutritional studies of vegetarians. J. Am. Dietet. A., 48:25, 1966.

Hegsted, D. M.: Amino acid fortification and the protein problem. Am. J. Clin. Nutr., 21:688, 1968.

———: Minimum protein requirements of adults. Am. J. Clin. Nutr., 21:352, 1968.

Hegsted, D. M., and Irwin, M. I.: A conspectus of research on protein requirements of man. J. Nutr., 101:385, 1971.

Holt, L. E., and Snyderman, S. E.: Protein and amino acid requirements of infants and children. Nutr. Abstr. & Rev., 35:1, 1965.

Mitchell, H. S.: Protein limitation and human growth. J. Am. Dietet. A., 44:165, 1966.

Review: Evaluation of a peanut-soybean mixture. Nutr. Rev., 23:75, 1965.

———: Histidine requirements in infancy. Nutr. Rev., 22:114, 1964.

———: The concept of protein stores. Nutr. Rev., 21:45, 1963.

Roels, O. A.: Marine proteins. Nutr. Rev., 27:35, 1969.

Rose, W. C.: Amino acid requirements of adult man. Nutr. Abstr. & Rev., 27:631, 1957.

Scrimshaw, N. S.: Nature of protein requirements; ways they can be met in tomorrow's world. J. Am. Dietet. A., 54:94, 1969.

Standal, B. R.: Nutritional value of proteins of oriental soybean foods. J. Nutr., 81:279, 1963.

Watts, J. H.: Evaluation of protein in selected American diets. J. Am. Dietet. A., 46:116, 1965.

Young, V. R., *et al.*: Plasma tryptophan response curve and its relation to tryptophan requirements in young adult men. J. Nutr., 101:45, 1971.

Protein-Calorie Malnutrition

Journal Articles:

Ashworth, A.: Growth rates in children recovering from protein-calorie malnutrition. Brit. J. Nutr., 23:835, 1969.

Bowie, M. D., *et al.*: Diarrhoea in protein-calorie malnutrition. Lancet, 2:550, 1963.

Cabak, V., *et al.*: (Yugoslavia Pediatric Clinic) Effect of undernutrition in early life on physical and mental development. Arch. Dis. Child., 40:532, 1965.

Cravioto, J., and DeLecardie, E. R.: The long-term consequences of protein calorie malnutrition. Nutr. Rev., 29:107, 1971.

Downs, E. F.: Nutritional dwarfing: A syndrome of early protein-calorie malnutrition. Am. J. Clin. Nutr., 15:275, 1965.

György, P.: Protein-rich foods in calorie-protein malnutrition. Problems of evaluation. Am. J. Clin. Nutr., 14:7, 1964.

Jansen, G. R., and Howie, E. E.: World problems in protein nutrition. Am. J. Clin. Nutr., 15:262, 1964.

Jelliffe, D. B.: Incidence of protein-calorie malnutrition in early childhood. Am. J. Public Health, 53:905, 1963.

Pretorius, P. J., and Wehmeyer, A. S.: An assessment of nutritive value of fish flour in the treatment of convalescent kwashiorkor patients. Am. J. Clin. Nutr., 14:147, 1964.

Webb, J. K., *et al.*: Peanut protein and milk protein blends in the treatment of kwashiorkor. Am. J. Clin. Nutr., 14:331, 1964.

ENERGY METABOLISM

Books and Pamphlets:

FAO Committee on Calorie Requirements: Calorie Requirements. FAO Nutrition Studies No. 15. Rome, FAO, 1957.

Richardson, M., and McCracken, E. C.: Energy Expenditures of Women Performing Selected Activities. Home Econ. Res. Report No. 11. Agr. Research Service, Washington, D.C., 1960.

Sargent, D. W.: An Evaluation of Basal Metabolic Data for Children and Youth in the United States. Home Econ. Res. Report No. 14. Agr. Research Service, Washington, D.C., 1961.

———: An Evaluation of Basal Metabolic Data for Infants in the United States. Home Econ. Res. Report No. 18. Agr. Research Service, Washington, D.C., 1962.

Journal Articles:

Ashworth, A.: Malnutrition and metabolic rates. Nutr. Rev., 28:279, 1970.

Buskirk, E. R., *et al.*: Human energy expenditure studies in the National Institute of Arthritis and Metabolic Diseases. I. Interaction of cold environment and special dynamic effect. II. Sleep. Am. J. Clin. Nutr., 8:602, 1960.

Call, D. L.: An examination of calorie availability and consumption in the United States, 1909-1963. Am. J. Clin. Nutr., 16:374, 1965.

Durnin, J. V.: Energy—requirements, intake and balance. Proc. Nutr. Soc., 27:188, 1968.

Hunscher, H. A.: Pertinent factors in interpreting metabolic data. J. Am. Dietet. A., 39:209, 1961.

Johnson, O. C.: Present knowledge of calories. Nutr. Rev., 25:257, 1967.

Konishi, F.: Food energy equivalents of various activities. J. Am. Dietet. A., 46:186, 1965.

Mason, E. D., *et al.*: Racial group differences in basal metabolism and body composition of Indian and European women in Bombay. Human Biol., 36:374, 1964.

Mayer, J.: Why people get hungry. Nutrition Today, 1:2, 1966.

Review: Body fat in adolescent boys. Nutr. Rev., 22:72, 1964.

———: Diet and work metabolism. Nutr. Rev., 21:211, 1963.

———: Eating at various times before exercise. Nutr. Rev., 21:40, 1963.

Sasaki, T.: Relation of basal metabolism to changes in food composition and body composition. Fed. Proc., 25(2):1165, 1966.

Southgate, D. A. T.: Assessing the energy value of the human diet. Nutr. Rev., 29:131, 1971.

Weaver, E. I., and Elliot, D. E.: Factors affecting energy expended in home-making tasks. J. Am. Dietet. A., 39:205, 1961.

Yoshimura, M., *et al.*: Climatic adaptation of basal metabolism. Fed. Proc., 25(2):1169, 1966.

WATER AND MINERALS
General

Books and Pamphlets:

Underwood, E. J.: Trace Elements in Human and Animal Nutrition. New York, Academic Press, 1968.

Journal Articles:

Cadell, J. L.: Mineral deficiency . . . in extremis. Nutrition Today, 2:14, 1967.

McCall, J. T., *et al.*: Implications of trace metals in human diseases. Fed. Proc., 30:1011, 1971.

Review: Loss of nutrients through the skin. Nutr. Rev., 21:266, 1963.

———: Mineral elements in wheat, flour and bread. Nutr. Rev., 22:223, 1964.

Roe, D.: Nutrient toxicity with excessive intake. II. Mineral overload. N.Y. State J. Med., 66:1233, 1966.

Zook, E. G., and Morris, E. R.: Nutrient composition of selected wheats and wheat products. VI. Distribution of manganese, copper, nickel, zinc, magnesium, lead, tin, cadmium, chromium, and selenium as determined by atomic spectroscopy and calorimetry. Cereal Chemistry, 47:720, 1971.

Fluids and Electrolytes
(Water, Sodium and Potassium)

Books and Pamphlets:

Snively, W. D., Jr.: Sea Within: The Story of Our Body Fluid. Philadelphia, J. B. Lippincott, 1960.

Journal Articles:

Baker, E. M., et al.: Water requirements of men as related to salt intake. Am. J. Clin. Nutr., 12:394, 1963.

Consolazio, C. F., et al.: Excretion of sodium, potassium, magnesium and iron in human sweat and the relation of each to balance requirements. J. Nutr., 79:407, 1963.

Cooper, G. R., and Heap, B.: Sodium ion in drinking water. II. Importance, problems, and potential applications of sodium-ion-restricted therapy. J. Am. Dietet. A., 50:37, 1967.

Fielo, S. B.: Teaching fluid and electrolyte balance. Nurs. Outlook, 13:43, 1965.

Gundersen, K., and Shen, G.: Total body water in obesity. Am. J. Clin. Nutr., 19:77, 1966.

Krehl, W. A.: The potassium depletion syndrome. Nutrition Today, 1:20, (June) 1966.

————: Sodium: a most extraordinary dietary essential. Nutrition Today, 1:16, 1966.

Potassium imbalance: programmed instruction. Am. J. Nursing, 67:343, 1967.

Review: Dietary sodium and experimental dental caries. Nutr. Rev., 23:117, 1965.

————: Potassium deficiency and the kidney. Nutr. Rev., 19:242, 1961.

————: Salt supplementation during fasting in the cold. Nutr. Rev., 23:45, 1965.

Robinson, J. B.: Water, the indispensible nutrient. Nutrition Today, 5:16, 1970.

Segar, W. E.: Multiple episodes of potassium deficiency. Am. J. Dis. Child., 109:295, 1965.

White, J. M., et al.: Sodium ion in drinking water. I. Properties, analysis, and occurrence. J. Am. Dietet. A., 50:32, 1967.

Calcium, Phosphorus and Magnesium

Books and Pamphlets:

FAO/WHO Expert Committee on Calcium Requirements: Calcium Requirements. Rome, FAO, 1962.

Hathaway, M. L.: Magnesium in Human Nutrition. Home Econ. Res. Report No. 19. Agr. Research Service, U.S.D.A., Washington, D.C., 1962.

Swanson, P. P.: Calcium in Nutrition. Chicago, National Dairy Council, 1963.

Journal Articles:

Alvarez, W. C.: Osteoporosis, a disease that attacks millions. Geriatrics, 25:77, 1970.

Barzel, U. S.: Symposium Report: Osteoporosis: The state of the art. Am. J. Clin. Nutr., 23:833, 1970.

Birge, S. J., Jr., et al.: Osteoporosis, intestinal lactase deficiency and low dietary calcium intake. New Eng. J. Med., 276:445, 1967.

Briscoe, A., and Ragan, C.: Bile and endogenous calcium in man. Am. J. Clin. Nutr., 16:281, 1965.

————: Effect of magnesium on calcium metabolism in man. Am. J. Clin. Nutr., 19:296, 1966.

Caddell, J. L., and Goddard, D. R.: Studies in protein-calorie malnutrition. I. Chemical evidence for magnesium deficiency. New Eng. J. Med., 276:533, 1967.

Caniggia, A.: Medical problems in senile osteoporosis. Geriatrics, 20:300, 1965.

Copp, D. H.: Endocrine control of calcium metabolism. Physiol. Rev., 32:61, 1970.

Dunn, M. M., and Walser, M.: Magnesium depletion in normal man. Metabolism, 15:884, 1966.

Hankin, J. H., et al.: Contributions of hard water to calcium and magnesium intakes of adults. J. Am. Dietet. A., 56:212, 1970.

Heaney, R. P.: A unified concept of osteoporosis. Am. J. Med., 36:877, 1965.

Hegsted, D. M.: Nutrition, bone and calcified tissue. J. Am. Dietet. A., 50:105, 1967.

————: Present knowledge of calcium, phosphorus and magnesium. Nutr. Rev., 26:65, 1968.

Krehl, W. A.: Magnesium. Nutrition Today, 2:16, (Sept.) 1967.

Lotz, M.: Evidence for a phosphorus-depletion syndrome in man. New Eng. J. Med., 278:409, 1968.

Lutwak, L.: Nutritional aspects of osteoporosis. J. Am. Geriatrics Soc., 17:115, 1969.

————: Osteoporosis—a mineral deficiency disease? J. Am. Dietet. A., 44:173, 1964.

Munson, P. L., and Gray, T. K.: Function of thyrocalcitonin in normal physiology. Fed. Proc., 29:1206, 1970.

Review: Calcium in sweat. Nutr. Rev., 21:13, 1963.

————: Exercise and calcium utilization. Nutr. Rev., 19:42, 1961.

————: Intestinal calcium and bone formation. Nutr. Rev., 23:6, 1965.

————: Human renal calculus formation and magnesium. Nutr. Rev., 24:43, 1966.

————: Phosphate influence on experimental dental caries. Nutr. Rev., 22:311, 1964.

Seelig, M. S.: The requirement of magnesium by the normal adult. Summary and analysis of published data. Am. J. Clin. Nutr., 14:342, 1964.

Sullivan, J. F., et al.: Magnesium metabolism in alcoholism. Am. J. Clin. Nutr., 13:297, 1963.

Wacker, W. E., and Parisi, A. F.: Magnesium metabolism. New Eng. J. Med., 278:658, 712, 772, 1968.

IRON AND COPPER

Books and Pamphlets:

Bothwell, T. H., and Finch, C. A.: Iron Metabolism. Boston, Little, Brown & Co., 1962.

Journal Articles:

Ausman, D. C.: Cobalt-iron therapy for iron-deficiency anemia. J. Am. Geriat. Soc., 13:425, 1965.

Bothwell, T. H.: The control of iron absorption. Brit. J. Haematology, 14:453, 1968.

Bothwell, T. H., *et al.*: Iron overload in Bantu subjects; studies on the availability of iron in Bantu beer. Am. J. Clin. Nutr., 14:47, 1964.

Callender, S. T.: Iron absorption. Proc. Nutr. Soc., 26:59, 1967.

Callender, S. T., and Warner, G. T.: Iron absorption from bread. Am. J. Clin. Nutr., 21:1170, 1968.

Cartwright, G. E., and Wintrobe, M. M.: Copper metabolism in normal subjects. Am. J. Clin. Nutr., 14:224, 1964.

————: The question of copper deficiency in man. Am. J. Clin. Nutr., 15:94, 1964.

Coltman, C., and Rowe, N.: The iron content of sweat in normal adults. Am. J. Clin. Nutr., 18:270, 1966.

Conrad, M. W.: Iron balance and iron deficiency anemia. Borden's Rev. Nutr. Res., 28 (No. 3):49, (July-Sept.) 1967.

Council on Foods and Nutrition: Iron deficiency in the U.S. JAMA, 203:407, 1968.

Crosby, W. H.: Control of iron absorption by intestinal luminal factor. Am. J. Clin. Nutr., 21:1189, 1968.

————: Food pica and iron deficiency. Archives Int. Med., 127:960, 1971.

————: Intestinal response to the body's requirement for iron: Control of iron absorption. JAMA, 208:347, 1969.

Dowdy, R. P.: Copper metabolism. Am. J. Clin. Nutr., 22:887, 1969.

Elwood, P. C., *et al.*: Absorption of iron from bread. Am. J. Clin. Nutr., 21:1162, 1968.

Filer, L. J., Jr.: The United States today: Is it free of public health nutrition problems?—Anemia. Am. J. Public Health, 59:327, 1969.

Finch, C. A.: Iron balance in man. Nutr. Rev., 23:129, 1965.

————: Iron-deficiency anemia. Am. J. Clin. Nutr., 22:512, 1969.

————: Iron metabolism. Nutrition Today, 4:2, (Summer) 1969.

Freiman, H. D., *et al.*: Iron absorption in the healthy aged. Geriatrics, 18:716, 1963.

Heinrich, H. C.: Iron deficiency without anemia. Lancet, 2:460, 1968.

Hook, L., and Brandt, K.: Copper content of some low-copper foods. J. Am. Dietet. A., 49:202, 1966.

Jacobs, A., and Greenman, D. A.: Availability of food iron. Brit. Med. J., 1:673, 1969.

Layrisse, M., *et al.*: Effect of interaction of various foods on iron absorption. Am. J. Clin. Nutr., 21:1175, 1968.

Monsen, E. R.: The need for iron fortification. J. Nutr. Educa., 2:152, 1971.

Pearson, H. A., *et al.*: Anemia related to age. Study of a community of young black Americans. JAMA, 215:1982, 1971.

Peden, J.: Present knowledge of iron and copper. Nutr. Rev., 25:321, 1967.

Prockop, D. J.: Role of iron in the synthesis of collagen in connective tissue. Fed. Proc., 30:984, 1971.

Review: Copper deficiency in malnourished infants. Nutr. Rev., 23:164, 1965.

————: Fortification of bread with iron. Nutr. Rev., 27:138, 1969.

————: Gastric function and structure in iron deficiency. Nutr. Rev., 24:326, 1966.

————: Iron absorption. Nutr. Rev., 24:247, 1967.

————: Symptoms of iron deficiency anemia. Nutr. Rev., 25:86, 1967.

————: The therapeutic effectiveness of various compounds containing iron. Nutr. Rev., 24:232, 1966.

Schaffrin, R. M., *et al.*: The effects of blood donation on serum iron and hemoglobin levels in young women. Canad. Med. A. J., 104:229, 1971.

Schroeder, H. A., *et al.*: Essential trace metals in man. Copper. J. Chron. Dis., 19:1007, 1966.

Scott, D. E., and Pritchard, J. A.: Iron deficiency in healthy young college women. JAMA, 199:897, 1967.

Sturgeon, P., and Shoden, A.: Total liver storage iron in normal populations of the U.S.A. Am. J. Clin. Nutr., 24:469, 1971.

White, H. S.: Iron deficiency in young women. Am. J. Public Health, 60:659, 1970.

White, H. S., and Gynne, T. N.: Utilization of inorganic elements by young women eating iron-fortified foods. J. Am. Dietet. A., 59:27, 1971.

Iodine

Journal Articles:

Harrison, M. T., *et al.*: Nature and availability of iodine in fish. Am. J. Clin. Nutr., 17:73, 1965.

Lowenstein, F. W.: Iodized salt in the prevention of endemic goiter: a world wide survey of present programs. Am. J. Public Health, 57:1815, 1967.

Review: Goiter and iodine deficiency. Nutr. Rev., 22:169, 1964.

Vought, R. L., and London, W. T.: Dietary sources of iodine. Am. J. Clin. Nutr., 14:186, 1964.

Fluorine

Pamphlet:

Adler, P., *et al.*: Fluorides and Human Health. WHO Monograph Series, No. 59. Geneva, Switzerland, 1970.

Journal Articles:

Ast, D. B., *et al.*: Time and cost factors to provide regular periodic dental care for children in a fluoridated and nonfluoridated area. Am. J. Public Health, 57:1635, 1969.

Bernstein, D. S.: Prevalence of osteoporosis in high and low fluoride areas in North Dakota. JAMA, 198:499, 1966.

Bonner, F.: Fluoridation —issue or obsession? Am. J. Clin. Nutr., 22:1346, 1969.

Cohn, S. H., *et al.*: Effects of fluoride on calcium metabolism in osteoporosis. Am. J. Clin. Nutr., 24:20, 1971.

Goggin, J. E., *et al.*: Incidence of femoral fractures in postmenopausal women before and after water fluoridation. Public Health Rep., 80:1005, 1965.

Hodge, H. C.: Metabolism of fluorides. JAMA, 177: 313, 1961.

Morrey, L. W., *et al.*: Fluoridation of water and dental caries. J. Am. Dent. A., 65:587, 1962.

Review: Fluoride bone crystal structure, and calcium balance. Nutr. Rev., 21:165, 1963.

———: Potential toxicity of fluorides. Nutr. Rev., 21:291, 1963.

Waldbott, G. L.: Fluoride in food. Am. J. Clin. Nutr., 12:455, 1963.

Other Minerals

Book:

Prasad, A. S.: Zinc Metabolism. Springfield, Ill., Charles C Thomas, 1966.

Journal Articles:

Glinsman, W. H., *et al.*: Plasma chromium after glucose administration. Science, 152:1243, 1966.

Hopkins, L. L., Jr., and Majaj, A. S.: Normalization of impaired glucose utilization and hypoglycemia by Cr(III) in malnourished infants. Fed. Proc., 25: 303, 1966.

Lanier, V. C., Jr., *et al.*: Zinc and wound healing. Am. J. Clin. Nutr., 23:514, 1970.

Leach, R. M.: Role of manganese in mucopolysaccharide metabolism. Fed. Proc., 30:991, 1971.

Luecke, R. W.: The significance of zinc in nutrition. Borden's Rev. Nutr. Res., 26:45, 1965.

Mayer, J.: Zinc deficiency: a cause of growth retardation. Postgrad. Med., 35:206, 1964.

McBean, L. D., *et al.*: Correlation of zinc concentrations in human plasma and hair. Am. J. Clin. Nutr., 24:509, 1971.

Mills, C. F., *et al.*: Metabolic role of zinc. Am. J. Clin. Nutr., 22:1240, 1969.

O'Dell, B. L.: Effect of dietary components upon zinc availability: A review with original data. Am. J. Clin. Nutr., 22:1315, 1969.

Reinhold, J. G., *et al.*: Zinc and copper concentrations in hair of Iranian villagers. Am. J. Clin. Nutr., 18: 294, 1966.

Review: Relation of zinc metabolism to a syndrome characterized by anemia, dwarfism, and hypogonadism. Nutr. Rev., 21:264, 1963.

———: Manganese balance in children. Nutr. Rev., 23:236, 1965.

———: Trivalent chromium in human nutrition. Nutr. Rev., 25:50, 1967.

Schroeder, H. A.: Renal cadmium and essential hypertension. JAMA, 187:358, 1964.

———: Cadmium as a factor in hypertension. J. Chron. Dis., 18:647, 1965.

Sullivan, J. F., and Lankford, H. G.: Zinc metabolism and chronic alcoholism. Am. J. Clin. Nutr., 17:57, 1965.

Westmoreland, N.: Connective tissue alterations in zinc deficiency. Fed. Proc., 30:1001, 1971.

VITAMINS

General

Books and Pamphlets:

Conserving the Nutritive Values in Foods. Home and Garden Bulletin No. 90. U.S.D.A., Washington, D.C., U.S. Gov't. Print. Off., 1963.

Report of a Joint FAO/WHO Expert Group: Requirements of Ascorbic Acid, Vitamin D, Vitamin B_{12}, Folate, and Iron. Rome, FAO, 1970.

———: Requirements of Vitamin A, Riboflavin and Niacin. Rome, FAO, 1967.

Wagner, A. F., and Folkers, K.: Vitamins and Coenzymes. New York, Interscience Publishers, 1964.

Journal Articles:

Campbell, J. A., and Morrison, A. B.: Some factors affecting the absorption of vitamins. Am. J. Clin. Nutr., 12:162, 1963.

Gershoff, S. N.: Effects of dietary levels of macronutrients on vitamin requirements. Fed. Proc., 23: 1077, 1964.

Levy, G., and Hewitt, R. R.: Evidence in man for different specialized intestinal transport mechanisms for riboflavin and thiamine. Am. J. Clin. Nutr., 24: 401, 1971.

Mayer, J.: Vitamins and mental disorders. Postgrad. Med., 45:268, 1969.

Review: Lipids and fat-soluble vitamins in cellular metabolism. Nutr. Rev., 24:272, 1966.

Roe, D. A.: Nutrient toxicity with excessive intake. I. Vitamins. N.Y. State J. Med., 66:869, 1966.

Symposium: Advances in the detection of nutrition deficiencies in man. Am. J. Clin. Nutr., 20: June, 1967.

Vitamin A

Journal Articles:

Ames, S. R.: Factors affecting absorption, transport and storage of vitamin A. Am. J. Clin. Nutr., 22: 934, 1969.

Council on Foods and Nutrition: Fortification of nonfat milk solids with vitamins A and D. JAMA, 198: 1107, 1966.

DiBenedetto, R. J.: Chronic hypervitaminosis A in an adult. JAMA, 201:130, 1967.

Goodman, D. S.: Biosynthesis of vitamin A from β-carotene. Am. J. Clin. Nutr., 22:963, 1969.

Hughes, J. D., and Wooten, R. L.: The orange people. JAMA, 197:730, 1966.

McLaren, D. S.: Nutritional Disease and the Eye. Borden's Rev. Nutr. Res., 25:1, 1964.

———: Xerophthalmia: a neglected problem. Nutr. Rev., 22:289, 1964.

————: Xerophthalmia in Jordan. Am. J. Clin. Nutr., 17:117, 1965.

Muenter, M. D., *et al.*: Chronic vitamin A intoxication in adults. Am. J. Med., 50:129, 1971.

Olson, J. A.: Metabolism and function of vitamin A. Fed. Proc., 28:1670, 1969.

————: The alpha and the omega of vitamin A metabolism. Am. J. Clin. Nutr., 22:953, 1969.

Reddy, V., and Srikantia, S. G.: Serum vitamin A in kwashiorkor. Am. J. Clin. Nutr., 18:105, 1966.

Review: An active metabolite of retinoic acid. Nutr. Rev., 24:113, 1966.

————: Etiology of follicular hyperkeratosis. Nutr. Rev., 21:106, 1963.

————: The influence of vitamin A on sulfate and hexosamine metabolism. Nutr. Rev., 24:204, 1966.

————: Interrelationships between vitamins A and E. Nutr. Rev., 23:82, 1965.

————: Intestinal absorption of vitamin A. Nutr. Rev., 22:86, 1964.

————: Toxic reactions of vitamin A. Nutr. Rev., 22:109, 1964.

————: Transport of vitamin A in the lymphatic system. Nutr. Rev., 24:16, 1966.

————: Vitamin A intoxication in infancy. Nutr. Rev., 23:263, 1965.

————: Vitamin A transport in man. Nutr. Rev., 25:199, 1967.

————: Vitamin A and vascularization. Nutr. Rev., 23:248, 1965.

Roels, O. A.: Present knowledge of vitamin A. Nutr. Rev., 24:129, 1966.

————: Vitamin A and protein metabolism. N.Y. State J. Med., 64:288, 1964.

————: Vitamin A physiology. JAMA, 214:1097, 1970.

Wolf, G.: International symposium on metabolic function of vitamin A. Am. J. Clin. Nutr., 22:903, 1969.

Vitamin D

Journal Articles:

Broadfoot, B. V. R., *et al.*: Vitamin D intakes of Canadian children. Canad. Med. A. J., 94:332, 1966.

Committee on Nutrition: The prophylactic requirement and toxicity of vitamin D. Pediatrics, 31:512, 1963.

————:Vitamin D intake and the hypercalcemic syndrome. Pediatrics, 35:1022, 1965.

Dale, A. E., and Lowenberg, M. E.: Consumption of vitamin D in fortified and natural foods and in vitamin preparations. J. Pediat., 70:952, 1967.

DeLuca, H. F.: Recent advances in the metabolism and function of vitamin D. Fed. Proc., 28:1678, 1969.

Favus, M. J.: Treatment of vitamin D intoxication. New Eng. J. Med., 283:1468, 1970.

Fomon, S. J., *et al.*: Vitamin D and growth of infants. J. Nutr., 88:345, 1965.

Forbes, G. B.: Present knowledge of vitamin D. Nutr. Rev., 25:225, 1967.

Harrison, H. E.: The disappearance of rickets. Am. J. Public Health, 56:734, 1966.

Hurwitz, S., *et al.*: Role of vitamin D in plasma calcium regulation. Am. J. Physiol., 216:254, 1969.

Nichols, B. L., *et al.*: Nutritional rickets among indigent children in Houston. Texas Med. (formerly Texas State Journal of Medicine), 66:74, 1970.

Review: Effect of vitamin A on vitamin D toxicity. Nutr. Rev., 20:315, 1962.

————: Nutritional rickets and parathyroid function. Nutr. Rev., 21:271, 1963.

————: Safe levels of vitamin D intake for infants. Nutr. Rev., 24:230, 1966.

————: Serum transport of vitamin D. Nutr. Rev., 24:149, 1966.

————: Vitamin D and protein synthesis. Nutr. Rev., 24:18, 1966.

Seelig, M. S.: Vitamin D and cardiovascular renal and brain damage in infancy and childhood. Ann. N.Y. Acad. Sci., 147:537, 1969.

Taylor, A. N., and Wasserman, R. H.: Correlations between vitamin D-induced calcium binding protein and intestinal absorption of calcium. Fed. Proc., 28:1834, 1969.

Vitamin E

Journal Articles:

Bunnell, R. H., *et al.*: Alpha-tocopherol content of foods. Am. J. Clin. Nutr., 17:1, 1965.

Committee on Nutrition: Vitamin E in human nutrition. Pediatrics, 31:324, 1963.

Draper, H. H., and Callany, A. S.: Metabolism and function of vitamin E. Fed. Proc., 28:1690, 1969.

Green, J., and Bunyan, J.: Vitamin E and the biological antioxidant theory. Nutr. Abst. Rev., 39:321, 1969.

Gross, S., and Guilford, M. V.: Vitamin E-lipid relationships in premature infants. J. Nutr., 100:1099, 1970.

Herting, D. C.: Perspective on Vitamin E. Am. J. Clin. Nutr., 19:210, 1966.

Herting, D. C., and Drury, E. E.: Plasma tocopherol levels in man. Am. J. Clin. Nutr., 17:351, 1965.

Horwitt, M. K.: Role of vitamin E, selenium, and polyunsaturated fatty acids in clinical and experimental muscle disease. Fed. Proc., 24:68, 1964.

Kelleher, J., and Losowsky, M. S.: The absorption of α-tocopherol in man. Brit. J. Nutr., 24:1033, 1970.

Leonard, P. J., and Losowsky, M. S.: Effect of alpha-tocopherol administration on red cell survival in vitamin E-deficient human subjects. Am. J. Clin. Nutr., 24:388, 1971.

Review: Antioxidant replacements for vitamin E. Nutr. Rev., 19:217, 1961.

————: Erythrocyte hemolysis, lipid peroxidation, and vitamin E. Nutr. Rev., 20:60, 1962.

————: Interrelationships between vitamins A and E. Nutr. Rev., 23:82, 1965.

————: Metabolic role of vitamin E. Nutr. Rev., 23:90, 1965.

————: Vitamin E and amino acid transport. Nutr. Rev., 24:203, 1966.

————: Vitamin E status of adults on a vegetable oil diet. Nutr. Rev., 24:41, 1966.

Roels, O. A.: Present knowledge of vitamin E. Nutr. Rev., 25:33, 1967.

Tappel, A. L.: Will antioxidant nutrients slow aging processes? Geriatrics, 23:97, 1968.

Vitamin K

Journal Articles:

Aballi, A. J.: The action of vitamin K in the neonatal period. Southern Med. J., 58:1, 48, 1965.

Committee on Nutrition: Vitamin K compounds and the water soluble analogues. Pediatrics, 28:501, 1961.

Goldman, H. I., and Amades, P.: Vitamin K deficiency after the newborn period. Pediatrics, 44:745, 1969.

Johnson, B. C.: Dietary factors and vitamin K. Nutr. Rev., 22:225, 1964.

Nammacher, M. A., et al.: Vitamin K deficiency in infants beyond the neonatal period. J. Pediat., 76:549, 1970.

Shoshkes, M., et al.: Vitamin K_1 in neonatal hypoprothrombinemia. J. Am. Dietet. A., 38:380, 1961.

Suttie, J. W.: Control of clotting factor biosynthesis by vitamin K. Fed. Proc., 28:1696, 1969.

Wefring, K. W.: Hemorrhage in the newborn and vitamin K prophylaxis. J. Pediat., 63:663, 1963.

Thiamine

Journal Articles:

Noble, L. I.: Thiamine and riboflavin retention in braised meat. J. Am. Dietet. A., 47:205, 1965.

Review: Carbohydrates and thiamine synthesis. Nutr. Rev., 20:216, 1962.

Rogers, E. F.: Thiamine antagonists. Ann. N.Y. Acad. Sci., 98:412, 1962.

Sebrell, W. H.: A clinical evaluation of thiamine deficiency. Ann. N.Y. Acad. Sci., 98:563, 1962.

Wurst, H. M.: The history of thiamine. Ann. N.Y. Acad. Sci., 98:385, 1962.

Ziporin, Z. Z., et al.: Excretion of thiamine and its metabolites in the urine of young adult males receiving restricted intakes of the vitamins. J. Nutr., 85:287, 1965.

————: Thiamine requirement in the adult human as measured by urinary excretion of thiamine metabolites. J. Nutr., 85:297, 1965.

Riboflavin

Journal Articles:

Horwitt, M. K.: Nutritional requirements of man, with special reference to riboflavin. Am. J. Clin. Nutr., 18:458, 1966.

Lane, M., et al.: The anemia of human riboflavin deficiency. Blood, 25:632, 1965.

Review: Genetic differences in riboflavin utilization. Nutr. Rev., 22:273, 1964.

————: Riboflavin coenzymes and congenital malformations. Nutr. Rev., 21:24, 1963.

Revlin, R. S.: Riboflavin metabolism. New Eng. J. Med., 13:626, 1970.

Windmueller, H. G., et al.: Elevated riboflavin levels in urine of fasting human subjects. Am. J. Clin. Nutr., 15:73, 1964.

Niacin

Journal Articles:

DeLange, D. J., and Joubert, C. P.: Assessment of nicotinic acid status of population groups. Am. J. Clin. Nutr., 15:169, 1964.

Goldsmith, G. A.: Niacin—antipellagra factor, hypercholesterolemic agent. JAMA, 194:167, 1965.

Horwitt, M. K.: Niacin-tryptophan requirements of man, in terms of niacin equivalents. J. Am. Dietet. A., 34:914, 1958.

Review: Bound niacin. Nutr. Rev., 19:240, 1961.

————: Fetal death from nicotinamide deficiency. Nutr. Rev., 23:58, 1964.

————: Nicotinic acid and diabetes mellitus. Nutr. Rev., 22:166, 1964.

Pyridoxine

Journal Articles:

Baker, E. M., et al.: Vitamin B_6 requirement for adult man. Am. J. Clin. Nutr., 15:59, 1964.

Bunnell, R. H.: Vitamin B_6. Science, 146:674, 1964.

Committee on Nutrition, American Academy of Pediatrics: Vitamin B_6 requirements in man. Pediatrics, 38:75, 1966.

Coursin, D. B.: Vitamin B_6 requirements. JAMA, 189:27, 1964.

Linkswiler, H.: Biochemical and physiological changes in vitamin B_6 deficiency. Am. J. Clin. Nutr., 20:547, 1967.

Mudd, S. H.: Pyridoxine-responsive genetic disease. Fed. Proc., 30:970, 1971.

Nelson, E. M.: Association of vitamin B_6 deficiency with convulsions in infants. Public Health Rep., 71:445, 1956.

Polansky, M. M., and Murphy, E. W.: Vitamin B_6 in fruits and nuts. J. Am. Dietet. A., 48:109, 1966.

Review: Pyridoxine and dental caries; human studies. Nutr. Rev., 21:143, 1963.

———: Pyridoxine dependency. Nutr. Rev., 25:72, 1967.

———: Vitamin B_6 deficiency and tryptophan metabolism. Nutr. Rev., 21:89, 1963.

———: Vitamin B_6 dependency state in infants. Nutr. Rev., 19:229, 1961.

———: Effects of insulin on carbohydrate and fat metabolism in vitamin B_6 deficiency. Nutr. Rev., 22:314, 1964.

Sauberlich, H. E.: Human requirements for vitamin B_6. Vitamins Hormones, 22:807, 1964.

Trimpter, G. W., et al.: Vitamin B_6 dependency syndromes: new horizons in nutrition. Am. J. Clin. Nutr., 22:794, 1969.

Folic Acid

Journal Articles:

Chung, A. S., et al.: Folic acid, vitamin B_6, pantothenic acid, and vitamin B_{12} in human dietaries. Am. J. Clin. Nutr., 9:573, 1961.

Herbert, V.: Studies of folate deficiency in man. Proc. Roy. Soc. Med., 57:377, 1964.

———: Folic acid. Annual Rev. Med., 16:359, 1965.

Izak, G., et al.: The effect of small doses of folic acid in nutritional megaloblastic anemia. Am. J. Clin. Nutr., 13:369, 1963.

Kane, F. J., and Lipton, M.: Folic acid and mental illness. Southern Med. J., 63:603, 1970.

Klipstein, F. A., and Lindenbaum, J.: Folate deficiency in chronic liver disease. Blood, 25:443, 1965.

Review: Folacin activity in U.S. diets. Nutr. Rev., 22:142, 1964.

———: Folic acid restriction and cancer inhibition. Nutr. Rev., 21:82, 1963.

Streiff, R. R.: Folate deficiency and oral contraceptives. JAMA, 214:105, 1970.

Velez, H., et al.: Folic acid deficiency secondary to iron deficiency in man. Am. J. Clin. Nutr., 19:27, 1966.

Vilter, R. W., et al.: Interrelationships of vitamin B_{12}, folic acid and ascorbic acid in the megaloblastic anemias. Am. J. Clin. Nutr., 12:130, 1963.

Vitale, J. J.: Present knowledge of folacin. Nutr. Rev., 24:289, 1966.

Vitamin B_{12}

Journal Articles:

Herbert, V., and Castle, W. B.: Intrinsic factor. New Eng. J. Med., 270:1181, 1964.

Herbert, V.: Nutritional requirements for vitamin B_{12} and folic acid. Am. J. Clin. Nutr., 21:743, 1968.

Mackenzie, I. L., and Donaldson, R. M.: Vitamin B_{12} absorption and the intestinal cell surface. Fed. Proc., 28:41, 1969.

Miller, D. R., et al.: Juvenile "congenital" pernicious anemia. New Eng. J. Med., 275:978, 1966.

Review: B_{12} transport in red cell membranes. Nutr. Rev., 25:248, 1967.

———: Oral B_{12} therapy of pernicious anemia. Nutr. Rev., 22:10, 1964.

———: Vitamin B_{12} deficiency in vegetarians. Nutr. Rev., 14:73, 1956.

Rivera, J. V., et al.: Anemia due to vitamin B_{12} deficiency after treatment with folic acid in tropical sprue. Am. J. Clin. Nutr., 18:110, 1966.

Spray, G. H.: Absorption of vitamin B_{12} from the intestines. Proc. Nutr. Soc., 26:55, 1967.

Stadtman, T. C.: Vitamin B_{12}. Science, 171:859, 1971.

Sullivan, L. W., and Herbert, V.: Studies on the minimum daily requirement for vitamin B_{12}. New Eng. J. Med., 272:340, 1965.

Wilson, T. H.: Intrinsic factor and B_{12} absorption—a problem in cell physiology. Nutr. Rev., 23:33, 1965.

Biotin

Journal Articles:

Bridgers, W. F.: Present knowledge of biotin. Nutr. Rev., 25:65, 1967.

Ochoa, S., and Kaziro, Y.: Biotin enzymes. Fed. Proc., 20:982, 1961.

Review: Mechanism of action of biotin-enzymes. Nutr. Rev., 21:310, 1963.

———: The role of biotin in lipid metabolism. Nutr. Rev., 20:143, 1962.

Pantothenic Acid

Pamphlet:

Zook, E. G., et al.: Pantothenic acid in foods. Agr. Handbook No. 97. U.S.D.A., Washington, D.C., 1956.

Journal Articles:

Faber, S. R., et al.: The effects of an induced pyridoxine and pantothenic acid deficiency on excretions of oxalic and xanthurenic acids in the urine. Am. J. Clin. Nutr., 12:406, 1963.

Ishiguro, K.: Studies on pantothenic acid and age. J. Am. Dietet. A., 40:450, 1962.

Review: Relation of pantothenic acid to adrenal cortical function. Nutr. Rev., 19:79, 1966.

Ascorbic Acid

Journal Articles:

Baker, E. M.: Vitamin C requirements in stress. Am. J. Clin. Nutr., 20:583, 1967.

Grewar, D.: Infantile scurvy. Clin. Pediat., 4:82, 1965.

Hodges, R. E., et al.: Clinical manifestations of ascorbic acid deficiency in man. Am. J. Clin. Nutr., 24:432, 1971.

King, C. G.: Practical and novel advances in relation to vitamin C. J. Nutr. Educa., 1:19, 1969.

———: Present knowledge of ascorbic acid. Nutr. Rev., 26:33, 1968.

Kinsman, R. A., and Hood, J.: Some behavioral effects of ascorbic acid deficiency. Am. J. Clin. Nutr., 24: 455, 1971.

Lamden, M.: Dangers of massive vitamin C intake. (Correspondence.) New Eng. J. Med., 284:336, 1971.

Lopez, A., *et al.*: Influence of time and temperature on ascorbic acid stability. J. Am. Dietet. A., 50: 308, 1967.

Merrill, A. L.: Facts behind the figures—citrus fruits values in "Handbook No. 8," revised. J. Am. Dietet. A., 44:264, 1964.

Noble, I.: Ascorbic acid and color of vegetables. Effect of length of cooking. J. Am. Dietet. A., 50:304, 1967.

Pelletier, O.: Vitamin C status of cigarette smokers and non-smokers. Am. J. Clin. Nutr., 23:520, 1970.

Review: Ascorbic acid and the common cold. Nutr. Rev., 25:228, 1967.

Rivers, J. M.: Ascorbic acid metabolism of connective tissue. N.Y. State J. Med., 65:1235, 1965.

Schwartz, F. W.: Ascorbic acid in wound healing—a review. J. Am. Dietet. A., 56:497, 1970.

Sherloch, P., and Rothschild, E. O.: Scurvy produced by a Zen macrobiotic diet. JAMA, 199:794, 1967.

DIGESTION, ABSORPTION AND METABOLISM

Books:

Davenport, H. W.: Physiology of the Digestive Tract. ed. 2. Chicago, Year Book, Medical Publishers, 1966.

Wilson, T. H.: Intestinal Absorption. Philadelphia, W. B. Saunders, 1962.

Wiseman, G.: Absorption from the Intestine. New York, Academic Press, 1964.

Journal Articles:

Bayless, T. M., and Huang, S.: Inadequate intestinal digestion of lactose. Am. J. Clin. Nutr., 22:250, 1969.

Bergstrom, B.: Absorption of fats. Proc. Nutr. Soc., 26:34, 1967.

Bowie, M. D., *et al.*: Carbohydrate absorption in malnourished children. Am. J. Clin. Nutr., 20:89, 1967.

Brown, R. R.: Biochemistry and pathology of tryptophan metabolism and its regulation by amino acids, vitamin B_6 and steroid hormones. Am. J. Clin. Nutr., 24:243, 1971.

Brown, W. D.: Present knowledge of protein nutrition. Part 3. Postgrad. Med., 41(A):119, 1967.

Christensen, H. N.: Transport of amino acids. Nutr. Rev., 21:97, 1963.

Cohen, M., *et al.*: Lipolytic activity of human gastric and duodenal juice against medium and long chain triglycerides. Gastroenterology, 60:1, 1971.

Cornblath, M., *et al.* (eds.): Carbohydrate and energy metabolism in the newborn—an international exploration. Pediatrics, 39:582, 1967.

Crane, R. K.: A perspective of digestive-absorptive function. Am. J. Clin. Nutr., 22:242, 1969.

Dahlqvist, A.: Disaccharide intolerance. JAMA, 195: 38, 1966.

———: Localization of the small-intestinal disaccharidases. Am. J. Clin. Nutr., 20:81, 1967.

Danielsson, H.: Influence of bile acids on digestion and absorption of lipids. Am. J. Clin. Nutr., 12:214, 1963.

Dragstedt, L. R.: Why does not the stomach digest itself? JAMA, 177:758, 1961.

Fisher, R. B.: Absorption of proteins. Proc. Nutr. Soc., 26:23, 1967.

Gardner, J. D., *et al.*: Columnar epithelial cell of the small intestine: digestion and transport. New Eng. J. Med., 283:1196, 1264, 1970.

Gaylor, J. L.: Inhibition of cholesterol biosynthesis. N.Y. State J. Med., 66:1097, 1966.

Go, V. L. W., and Summerskill, W. H. J.: Digestion, maldigestion and the intestinal hormones. Am. J. Clin. Nutr., 24:160, 1971.

Haenel, H.: Human normal and abnormal gastrointestinal flora. Am. J. Clin. Nutr., 23:1433, 1970.

Herman, R. H.: Mannose metabolism. I, II. Am. J. Clin. Nutr., 24:488, 566, 1971.

Herskovic, T.: Protein malnutrition and the small intestine. Am. J. Clin. Nutr., 22:300, 1969.

Holt, L. E., *et al.*: The concept of protein stores and its implication in the diet. JAMA, 181:699, 1962.

Ingelfinger, F. J.: Gastrointestinal absorption. Nutrition Today, 2:2, (March) 1967.

———: For want of an enzyme. Nutrition Today, 3:2, (Sept.) 1968.

———: Gastric function. Nutrition Today, 6:2, (Sept./Oct.) 1971.

Isselbacher, K. J.: Metabolism and transport of lipids by intestinal mucosa. Fed. Proc., 24:16, 1965.

Jacobs, F. A.: Dietary amino acid transport via lymph. Fed. Proc., 26:302, 1967.

Johnson, L. R., and Grossman, M. L.: Intestinal hormones as inhibitors of gastric secretion. Gastroenterology, 60:120, 1971.

Jukes, T. H.: Present status of the amino acid code. J. Am. Dietet. A., 45:517, 1964.

Kenworthy, R.: Influence of bacteria on absorption from the small intestine. Proc. Nutr. Soc., 26:18, 1967.

Mansford, R. L.: Recent studies on carbohydrate absorption. Proc. Nutr. Soc., 26:27, 1967.

Mao, C. C., and Jacobson, E. D.: Intestinal absorption and blood flow. Am. J. Clin. Nutr., 23:820, 1970.

Mayer, J.: Why people get hungry. Nutrition Today, 1:2, (June) 1966.

Nasset, E. S.: Role of digestive system in protein metabolism. Fed. Proc., 24:953, 1965.

Newey, H., and Smyth, D. H.: Assessment of absorptive capacity. Proc. Nutr. Soc., 26:5, 1967.

Oomen, H. A. P. C.: Interrelationship of the human intestinal flora and protein utilization. Proc. Nutr. Soc., 29:197, 1970.

Review: Amino acid transport and insulin release. Nutr. Rev., 25:41, 1967.

————: Diarrhea caused by disaccharidase deficiency. Nutr. Rev., 22:43, 1964.

————: Effect of dietary protein on proteolytic enzymes. Nutr. Rev., 22:317, 1964.

————: Factors affecting amino acid absorption. Nutr. Rev., 24:332, 1966.

————: Medium chain triglycerides in tropical sprue. Nutr. Rev., 23:71, 1965.

————: Metabolic interrelationships of dietary carbohydrate and fat. Nutr. Rev., 22:216, 1964.

————: Mobilization of liver lipids by specific plasma proteins. Nutr. Rev., 24:87, 1966.

————: Nutritional state and hormonal regulation of liver enzymes. Nutr. Rev., 24:308, 1966.

————: Regulation of gluconeogenesis. Nutr. Rev., 24:347, 1966.

————: Sucrose intolerance: An enzymatic defect. Nutr. Rev., 23:101, 1965.

————: The effect of pectin on cholesterol absorption. Nutr. Rev., 24:209, 1966.

————: Transport of amino acids. Nutr. Rev., 21:97, 1963.

Rohrer, G. V.: Human gastric mucosa: correlation of structure and function. Am. J. Clin. Nutr., 24:137, 1971.

Rosensweig, N. S., et al.: Dietary regulation of small intestine enzyme activity in man. Am. J. Clin. Nutr., 24:65, 1971.

Shiner, M.: The structure of the small intestine and some interesting relations to its function. Proc. Nutr. Soc., 26:1, 1967.

Spencer, R. P.: Intestinal absorption of amino acids. Current Concepts. Am. J. Clin. Nutr., 22:292, 1969.

Stifel, F. B., and Herman, R. H.: Histidine metabolism. Am. J. Clin. Nutr., 24:207, 1971.

Symposium on mechanisms of gastrointestinal absorption. Am. J. Clin. Nutr., 12:161, 1963.

Treadwell, C. R., et al.: Factors in sterol absorption. Fed. Proc., 21:903, 1962.

MEETING NUTRITIONAL NORMS

Books and Pamphlets:

Food For the Young Family. Home and Garden Bull. No. 85. U.S.D.A., Washington, D.C., 1971.

Your Money's Worth in Food. Home and Garden Bull. No. 183. U.S.D.A., Washington, D.C., 1970.

Journal Articles:

Brink, M. E., et al.: Nutritional values of milk compared with filled and imitation milks. Am. J. Clin. Nutr., 22:168, 1969.

Bruch, H.: The allure of food cults and nutritional quakery. J. Am. Dietet. A., 57:316, 1970.

Erhard, D.: Nutrition education for the now generation. J. Nutr. Educa., 2:135, 1971.

Kammer, J. B., and Shawhan, G. L.: Comparison of food prices in high and low-income areas. J. Home Econ., 62:56, 1970.

Lane, M. M.: Food fads. Nursing Homes, 20:22, 1971.

Leverton, R. M.: Basic nutrition concepts. J. Home Econ., 59:346, 1967.

Nagy, M.: Nutritive value of breakfast cereals. (Questions and Answers.) JAMA, 215:1994, 1971.

Ohlson, M. A., and Hart, B. P.: Influence of breakfast on total day's food intake. J. Am. Dietet. A., 47:282, 1965.

Patwardhan, V. N.: Dietary allowances—an international point of view. J. Am. Dietet. A., 56:191, 1970.

Rusoff, L. L.: The role of milk in modern nutrition. Borden's Rev. Nutr. Res., 25:17, (Apr.-Sept.) 1964.

Sabry, Z. I.: The Canadian dietary standard. J. Am. Dietet. A., 56:195, 1970.

Sebrell, W. H.: Recommended dietary allowances—1968 revision. J. Am. Dietet. A., 54:103, 1969.

————: The role of the bread-cereal group in the well-balanced diet. Borden's Rev. Nutr. Res., 27:1, (Jan.-Mar., Apr.-June) 1966.

Seidler, A. J.: Nutritional contributions of the meat group to an adequate diet. Borden's Rev. Nutr. Res., 24:29, (July-Sept.) 1963.

Stiebling, H. K.: Foods of the vegetable-fruit group—their contributions to nutritionally adequate diets. Borden's Rev. Nutr. Res., 25:51, (Oct.-Dec.) 1964.

Walker, A. R. P.: Optimal intake of nutrients. Nutr. Rev., 23:321, 1965.

REGIONAL, CULTURAL AND RELIGIOUS FOOD PATTERNS

Journal Articles:

Adolph, W. H.: Nutrition in the Near East. J. Am. Dietet. A., 30:753, 1954.

Bailey, M. A.: Nutrition education and the Spanish-speaking American. J. Nutr. Educa., 2:50, 1970.

Delgado, G., et al.: Eating patterns among migrant families. Public Health Rep., 76:349, 1961.

Hardinge, M. G., et al.: Nutritional studies of vegetarians. J. Am. Dietet. A., 48:25, 1966.

Insull, W., and Kenzaburo, T.: Diet and nutritional status of Japanese. Am. J. Clin. Nutr., 21:753, 1968.

Jerome, N. W.: Northern urbanization and food consumption patterns of southern-born Negroes. Am. J. Clin. Nutr., 22:1667, 1969.

Joseph, S., et al.: Composition of Israeli mixed dishes. J. Am. Dietet. A., 40:125, 1962.

Kight, M. A., *et al.*: Nutritional influences of Mexican-American foods in Arizona. J. Am. Dietet. A., 55: 557, 1969.

Korff, S. I.: The Jewish dietary code. Food Technology, 20:76, 1966.

Mayer, J.: The nutritional status of American Negroes. Nutr. Rev., 23:161, 1965.

Our cooking heritage: African foods. What's New in Home Economics, 35:28, 1971.

Sakr, A. H.: Dietary regulations and food habits of Muslims. J. Am. Dietet. A., 58:123, 1971.

Sanjur, D., and Scoma, A. D.: Food habits of low-income children in northern New York. J. Nutr. Educa., 2:85, 1971.

THE ECOLOGY OF FOOD

Books and Pamphlets:

Bernarde, M. A.: The Chemicals We Eat. New York, American Heritage Press, 1971.

Food Protection Committee, Food and Nutrition Board: New Developments in the Use of Pesticides. National Academy of Sciences–National Research Council Publ. No. 1082. Washington, D.C., 1963.

————: An Evaluation of Public Health Hazards from Microbiological Contamination of Foods. National Academy of Sciences–National Research Council Publ. No. 1195. Washington, D.C., 1963.

————: Chemicals Used In Food Processing. National Academy of Sciences–National Research Council Publ. No. 1274. Washington, D.C., 1965.

————: Toxicants Occurring Naturally in Foods. National Academy of Sciences–National Research Council Publ. No. 1354. Washington, D.C., 1966.

National Communicable Disease Center: Salmonella Surveillance. Report 58. U.S. Dept. H.E.W., Washington, D.C., 1967.

Protecting Our Food. Yearbook of Agriculture 1967. U.S.D.A., Washington, D.C., 1967.

Journal Articles:

Aaron, E., *et al.*: Urban salmonellosis. Am. J. Public Health, 61:337, 1971.

Adler, H. E.: Salmonella in eggs—an appraisal. Food Technology, 19:191, 1965.

Bird, K.: The food processing front of the seventies. J. Am. Dietet. A., 58:103, 1971.

Bryan, F. L.: New concepts in foodborne illness. J. Environ. Health, 31:327, 1969.

Celeste, A. C., and Shane, C. G.: Mercury in fish. FDA Papers, 4:27, 1970.

Cheng, T. C.: Parasitology and food protection. J. Environ. Health, 28:208, 1965.

Cliver, D. O.: Implications of foodborne infectious hepatitis. Public Health Rep., 81:185, 1966.

Despaul, J. E.: The gangrene organism—a food-poisoning agent. J. Am. Dietet. A., 49:185, 1966.

Eadie, G. A., *et al.*: Type E botulism. JAMA, 187: 496, 1964.

Editorial: Salmonella control. JAMA, 189:691, 1964.

————: The most deadly poison. JAMA, 187:530, 1964.

————: Carcinogen in groundnuts. Brit. Med. J., 5043:204, 1964.

Eyl, T. B.: Organic-mercury food poisoning. Current Concepts. New Eng. J. Med., 284:706, 1971.

Feuell, A. J.: Toxic factors of mould origin. Canad. Med. A. J., 94:574, 1966.

Finkel, A. J.: Mercury residue blood levels and tolerance limits in fish eaters. (Questions and Answers.) JAMA, 216:1208, 1971.

Goddard, J. L.: Incident at Selby Junior High. Nutrition Today, 2:2, (Sept.) 1967.

Koff, R. S., *et al.*: Viral hepatitis from shellfish. New Eng. J. Med., 276:703, 1967.

Lachance, P. A.: Nutrification—a new nutritional concept for new types of foods. Food Technology, 24: 100, 1970.

LaChapelle, N. C., *et al.*: A gastroenteritis outbreak of Staphylococcus aureus, type 29. Am. J. Public Health, 56:94, 1966.

Most, H.: Trichinellosis in the United States. JAMA, 162:871, 1965.

Note: Limiting temperature and humidity for production of aflatoxin by Aspergillus flavus in peanuts. Nutr. Rev., 25:286, 1967.

————: Thermostable Clostridium perfringens as the cause of a food poisoning outbreak. Nutr. Rev., 25:287, 1967.

Review: Foods and feeds as sources of carcinogenic factors. Nutr. Rev., 24:321, 1966.

Salmonella, the ubiquitous bug. FDA Papers, 1:13, (Feb.) 1967.

Snyder, R. D.: Congenital mercury poisoning. New Eng. J. Med., 284:1014, 1971.

Spensley, P. C.: Mycotoxins—a menace of moulds. Royal Soc. Health J., 90:248, 1970.

Strong, F. M.: Naturally occurring toxic factors in plants and animals used as food. Canad. Med. A. J., 94:568, 1966.

Thatcher, F. S.: Food-borne bacterial toxins. Canad. Med. A. J., 94:582, 1966.

Wogan, G. N.: Current research on toxic food contaminants. J. Am. Dietet. A., 49:95, 1966.

Zimmerman, W. J.: Current status of trichiniasis in U.S. swine. Public Health Rep., 80:1061, 1965.

Food Additives, Intentional and Accidental

Pamphlet:

Additives in Our Foods. Food & Drug Adm., U.S. Dept. H.E.W., Washington, D.C., 1966.

Journal Articles:

Council on Foods and Nutrition, A.M.A.: Radioactivity in foods. JAMA, 171:119, 1959.

Fitzhugh, O. G.: Problems related to the use of pesticides. Canad. Med. A. J., 94:598, 1966.

Food Additives: Safety of food additives continually evaluated. Public Health Rep., 81:244, 1966.

Hodges, R. E.: The toxicity of pesticides and their residues in food. Nutr. Rev., 23:230, 1965.

Johnson, P. E.: Health aspects of food additives. Am. J. Public Health, 56:948, 1966.

Jukes, T. H.: Chemical residues in foods: J. Am. Dietet. A., 59:203, 1971.

Oser, B. L.: Problems related to the use of food additives. Canad. Med. A. J., 94:604, 1966.

Philp, J. McL.: Toxicity and naturally occurring chemicals. Royal Soc. Health J., 90:237, 1970.

Smith, E. H.: Problems in the safe and effective use of pesticides in agriculture. Nutr. Rev., 22:193, 1964.

Regulations Protecting our Food Supply

Journal Articles:

Analysis of pesticide residues. FDA Papers, 1:17, (June) 1967.

Beacham, L. M.: Food standards. FDA Papers, 1:5, (July-Aug.) 1967.

Breeling, J. L.: Nutritional guidelines. The how, the why and the when. J. Am. Dietet. A., 59:102, 1971.

Cooke, J. A.: Nutritional guidelines and the labeling of foods. J. Am. Dietet. A., 59:99, 1971.

FAO/WHO Committee on Technical Basis for Legislation on Irradiated Foods: The irradiation of food. WHO Chronicle, 20:371, 1966.

FDA units and their function. FDA Papers, 4:4, (May) 1970.

Grant, J. D.: New issues in consumerism. FDA Papers, 4:15, Dec. 1970-Jan. 1971.

Howard, H. W.: Ingredient labeling. Food technology, 25:18, 1971.

Kingma, F. J.: Establishing and monitoring drug residue levels. FDA Papers, 1:9, (July-Aug.) 1967.

Milk surveillance report. J. Environ. Health, 33:350, 1971.

Roe, R. S.: FDA Food additives requirements. FDA Papers, 1:25, (May) 1967.

Somers, R. K.: New meat inspection laws for consumer protection. Public Health Rep., 84:214, 1969.

Spiher, Jr., A. T.: The GRAS list review. FDA Papers, 4:12, Dec. 1970-Jan. 1971.

What do you need on a can label? What's New in Home Economics, 34:44, 1970.

PART TWO

APPLICATION OF NUTRITION TO CRITICAL PERIODS THROUGHOUT THE LIFE CYCLE

GROWTH AND DEVELOPMENT
General
Books and Pamphlets:

Birch, H. G., and Gussow, J. D.: Disadvantaged Children: Health, Nutrition and School Failure. New York, Grune & Stratton, 1970.

Cheek, D. B.: Human Growth. Philadelphia, Lea & Febiger, 1968.

Hathaway, M. L.: Heights and weights of children and youth in the United States, Home Econ. Res. Report No. 2. Institute of Home Economics, Agricultural Research Service, U.S.D.A., Washington, D.C., 1957.

Height and weight of children in the United States, India, and the United Arab Republic. P.H.S. Publ. 1000, Series 3, No. 14. U.S. Dept. H.E.W., Washington, D.C., 1971.

McCammon, R. W.: Human Growth and Development. Springfield, Ill., Charles C Thomas, 1970.

Nutrition and Intellectual Growth in Children. Washington, D.C.: The Association for Childhood Education International, 1969.

Scrimshaw, N. S., Gordon, J. E.: Malnutrition, Learning and Behavior. Cambridge, Mass., The M.I.T. Press, 1968.

Springer, N. S.: An Annotated Bibliography—Nutrition and Mental Retardation (1964-1970). Ann Arbor, Mich., ISMR–University of Michigan, 1970.

Physical Growth and Development

Journal Articles:

Cone, T. E., Jr.: Growth problems of the adolescent. Med. Clin. N. Am., 49:357, 1965.

Corbin, C. B.: Standards of subcutaneous fat applied to percentile norms for elementary school children. Am. J. Clin. Nutr., 22:836, 1969.

Crispen, S., et al.: Nutritional status of preschool children. II. Anthropometric measurements and interrelationships. Am. J. Clin. Nutr., 21:1280, 1968.

Dayton, D. H.: Early malnutrition and human development. Children, 16:210, 1969.

Deren, J. S.: Development of structure and function in the fetal and newborn stomach. Am. J. Clin. Nutr., 24:144, 1971.

Dugdale, A. E.: An age-independent anthropometric index of nutritional status. Am. J. Clin. Nutr., 24: 174, 1971.

Dugdale, A. E., *et al.*: Patterns of growth and nutrition in childhood. Am. J. Clin. Nutr., 23:1280, 1970.

Editorial: Growth after malnutrition. Brit. Med. J., 2:495, (May 30) 1970.

Eid, E. E.: Follow-up study of physical growth of children who had excessive weight gain in first six months of life. Brit. Med. J., 2:74, (April 11) 1970.

Hathaway, M. L.: Overweight in children. J. Am. Dietet. A., 40:511, 1962.

Hurley, L. S.: Nutrients and Genes: Interactions in Development. Nutr. Rev., 27:3, 1969.

Review: Intrauterine growth. Nutr. Rev., 22:266, 1964.

———: Subsequent growth of children treated for malnutrition. Nutr. Rev., 24:267, 1966.

Nutrition and Mental Development

Journal Articles:

Abelson, P. H.: Malnutrition, learning and behavior. Science, 164:17, 1969.

Allen, D. E., *et al.*: Nutrition, family commensality and academic performance among high school youth. J. Home Econ., 62:333, 1970.

Barnes, R. H., *et al.*: Learning behavior following nutritional deprivation in early life. J. Am. Dietet. A., 51:34, 1967.

Champakam, S., *et al.*: Kwashiorkor and mental development. Am. J. Clin. Nutr., 21:844, 1968.

Cravioto, J., and Robles, B.: Evolution of adaptive and motor behavior during rehabilitation from kwashiorkor. Am. J. Orthopsychology, 35:449, 1965.

Cravioto, J., *et al.*: Nutrition, growth and neurointegrative development; an experimental ecology study. Pediatrics (Suppl.), 38:319, 1966.

Davison, A. N., and Dobbing, J.: Myelination as a vulnerable period in brain development. Brit. Med. Bull., 22:40, 1966.

Douglas, J. W. B., *et al.*: The relation between height and measured educational ability in school children of the same social class, family size and stage of sexual development. Human Biol., 37:178, 1965.

Eichenwald, H. G., and Fry, P. C.: Nutrition and learning. Science, 163:644, 1969.

Hopwood, H. H., and Van Iden, S. S.: Scholastic underachievement as related to sub-par physical growth. J. School Health, 35:377, (Oct.) 1965.

Liang, P. H., *et al.*: Evaluation of mental development in relation to early malnutrition. Am. J. Clin. Nutr., 20:1290, 1967.

Medical News: Mental retardation from malnutrition: irreversible. JAMA, 206:30, 1968.

Monckeberg, B.: Malnutrition and mental behavior. Nutr. Rev., 27:191, 1969.

Mosier, H. D., Jr.: Physical growth in mental defectives. A study in an institutionalized population. Pediatrics (Suppl.), 36:465, 1965.

Read, M. S.: Malnutrition and mental retardation. J. Nutr. Educa., 2:23, 1970.

Review: Behavioral development during recovery from nutritional marasmus. Nutr. Rev., 29:31, 1971.

———: Mental development following kwashiorkor. Nutr. Rev., 27:46, 1969.

———: The infant brain following severe malnutrition. Nutr. Rev., 27:251, 1969.

———: Undernutrition in children and subsequent brain growth and intellectual development. Nutr. Rev., 26:197, 1968.

Rosso, P., *et al.*: Changes in brain weight, cholesterol, phospholipid, and DNA content in marasmic children. Am. J. Clin. Nutr., 23:1275, 1970.

Winick, M.: Malnutrition and brain development. J. Pediat., 74:667, 1969.

Winick, M., and Rosso, P.: The effect of severe early malnutrition on cellular growth of human brain. Pediat. Res., 3:181, 1969.

NUTRITION IN PREGNANCY AND LACTATION

Books and Pamphlets:

Beaton, G. H., and McHenry, E. W.: Nutrition: A Comprehensive Treatise. Vol. III. Chap. 3. New York, Academic Press, 1966.

Committee on Maternal Nutrition, Food and Nutrition Board: Maternal Nutrition and the Course of Pregnancy. National Academy of Sciences–National Research Council, Washington, D.C., 1970.

Giroud, A.: The Nutrition of the Embryo. Springfield, Ill., Charles C Thomas, 1970.

Prenatal Care. Children's Bureau Publ. No. 4. U.S. Dept. H.E.W., Washington, D.C., 1962.

WHO: Nutrition in Pregnancy and Lactation. Tech. Report Series No. 302. Geneva, Switzerland, 1965.

Journal Articles:

Allen, C. E., *et al.*: Vigorous weight reduction during pregnancy: Nitrogen balance before and during normal gestation. JAMA, 188:392, 1964.

Applebaum, R. M.: The physician and a common sense approach to breast-feeding. Southern Med. J., 63:793, 1970.

Bartholomew, M. M., and Poston, F. E.: Effect of food taboos on prenatal nutrition. J. Nutr. Educa., 2:15, 1970.

Beal, V. A.: Breast- and formula feeding in infants. J. Am. Dietet. A, 55:31, 1969.

———: Nutritional studies during pregnancy. I. Changes in intake of calories, carbohydrate, protein and calcium. II. Dietary intake, maternal weight gain and size of infant. J. Am. Dietet. A., 58:312, 321, 1971.

Beaton, G. H.: Some physiological adjustments relating to nutrition in pregnancy. Canad. Med. A. J., 95: 622, 1966.

Beck, J.: Guarding the unborn. Today's Health, 46: 38, (Jan.) 1968.

Bruhn, C. M., and Pangborn, R. M.: Reported incidence of pica among migrant families. J. Am. Dietet. A., 58:417, 1971.

Cantlie, G. S. D., *et al.*: Iron and folate nutrition in a group of private obstetrical patients. Am. J. Clin. Nutr., 24:637, 1971.

Crosby, W. H.: Food Pica and Iron Deficiency. Arch. Intern. Med., 127:960, 1971.

Editorial: Calorie requirements of breast feeding. Brit. Med. J., 3:721, (Sept. 26) 1970.

Editorial: Pregnant weight watchers risk harm to babies. Public Health Rep., 85:964, 1970.

Edwards, C. H., *et al.*: Effect of clay and cornstarch intake on women and their infants. J. Am. Dietet. A., 44:109, 1964.

Gold, E. M.: Interconceptional care. J. Am. Dietet. A., 55:27, 1969.

Halsted, J. A.: Geophagia in man: its nature and nutritional effects. Am. J. Clin. Nutr., 21:1384, 1968.

Harfouche, J. K.: The importance of breast-feeding. J. Trop. Ped., 16:134, 1970.

Holly, R. G.: Dynamics of iron metabolism in pregnancy. Am. J. Obstet. Gynec., 93:370, 1965.

Landesman, R., and Knapp, R. C.: Diagnosis and treatment of toxemias of pregnancy. I and II. N.Y. State J. Med., 60:3830, 1960.

Larson, R. H.: Effect of prenatal nutrition on oral structures. J. Am. Dietet. A., 44:368, 1964.

Little, B.: Current concepts: Treatment of preeclampsia. New Eng. J. Med., 270:94, 1964.

Lowenstein, L., *et al.*: The incidence and prevention of folate deficiency in a pregnant clinic population. Canad. Med. A. J., 95:797, 1966.

Malnutrition during pregnancy. (Medical News.) JAMA, 212:44, 1970.

Matoth, Y., *et al.*: Studies on folic acid in infancy. 3. Folates in breast-fed infants and their mothers. Am. J. Clin. Nutr., 16:356, 1965.

Metz, J.: Folate deficiency conditioned by lactation. Am. J. Clin. Nutr., 23:843, 1970.

Meyer, H. F.: Breast-feeding in the U.S. Clin. Pediat., 7:708, 1968.

Naeye, R. L., *et al.*: Urban poverty: effects on prenatal nutrition. Science, 166:1026, 1969.

Naismith, D. J.: The foetus as a parasite. Proc. Nutr. Soc., 28:25, 1969.

Nausea of pregnancy. (Questions and Answers.) JAMA, 187:165, 1964.

Payton, E., *et al.*: Dietary habits of 571 pregnant southern Negro women. J. Am. Dietet. A., 37:129, 1960.

Pike, R. L.: Sodium intake during pregnancy. J. Am. Dietet. A., 44:176, 1964.

Pike, R. L., and Gursky, D. S.: Further evidence of deleterious effects produced by sodium restriction during pregnancy. Am. J. Clin. Nutr., 23:883, 1970.

Review: Diet, detoxification, and toxemia of pregnancy. Nutr. Rev., 21:269, 1963.

————: Intrauterine growth. Nutr. Rev., 22:266, 1964.

————: Maternity care: The world situation. WHO Chronicle, 21:140, 1967.

————: Paraphagia and anemia. Nutr. Rev., 27:52, 1969.

————: Vigorous weight reduction during pregnancy. Nutr. Rev., 22:237, 1964.

Rust, H.: Food habits of pregnant women. Am. J. Nursing, 60:1636, 1960.

Schmitt, M. H.: Superiority of breast feeding—fact or fancy? Am. J. Nursing, 70:1488, 1970.

Seifert, E.: Changes in beliefs and food practices in pregnancy. J. Am. Diet. A., 39:455, 1961.

Semmens, J. P.: Implications of teen-age pregnancy. Obstet. Gynec., 26:77, 1965.

Smith, F.: Dietary habits of girls pregnant at 16 or under. Public Health Rep., 84:213, 1969.

Sodium intake in pregnancy: two views. JAMA, 200: 42, 1967.

Stevens, H. A., and Ohlson, M. A.: Nutritive value of the diets of medically indigent pregnant women. J. Am. Dietet. A., 50:290, 1967.

Streiff, R. R., and Little, A. B.: Folic acid deficiency in pregnancy. New Eng. J. Med., 276:776, 1967.

Thomson, A. M., *et al.*: The energy cost of human lactation. Brit. J. Nutr., 24:565, 1970.

Widdowson, E. M.: How the foetus is fed. Proc. Nutr. Soc., 28:17, 1969.

Woody, D. C., and Woody, H. B.: Management of breast feeding. J. Pediat., 68:344, 1966.

NUTRITION OF INFANTS

(*See also* references under Protein, Minerals and Vitamins)

General

Books and Pamphlets:

A Practical Guide to Combating Malnutrition in the Preschool Child. Nutritional Rehabilitation through Maternal Education. New York, Appleton-Century-Crofts, 1970.

Beech-Nut, Inc.: Nutritive Values and Ingredients of Beech-Nut Baby Foods. Canajoharie, N.Y., Beech-Nut, Inc., 1969.

Fomon, S. J.: Infant Nutrition. Philadelphia, W. B. Saunders, 1967.

————: Prevention of Iron-Deficiency Anemia in Infants and Children of Preschool Age. P.H.S. Publ. No. 2085. U.S. Dept. H.E.W., Washington, D.C., 1970.

Gerber Products Co.: Nutritive Values of Gerber Baby Foods. Fremont, Mich., Gerber Products Co., 1966.

How to make a baby's formula; by terminal heat method, by aseptic method, by tap water method. Evaporated Milk Ass., Chicago, Ill.

Hunt, E. P.: Recent Demographic Trends and Their Effects on Maternal and Child Health Needs and Services. Children's Bureau, U.S. Dept. H.E.W., Washington, D.C., 1966.

Nelson, W. E.: Textbook of Pediatrics. ed. 8. Philadelphia, W. B. Saunders, 1964.

Spock, B.: Baby and Child Care. rev. ed. New York, Hawthorn Books, 1968.

Spock, B., and Lowenberg, M. E.: Feeding Your Baby and Child. New York, Pocket Books, 1955.

Willis, N. H.: Basic Infant Nutrition. Philadelphia, J. B. Lippincott, 1964.

Journal Articles:

Aykroyd, W. R.: Nutrition and mortality in infancy and early childhood: past and present relationships. Am. J. Clin. Nutr., 24:480, 1971.

Beal, V. A.: Termination of night feeding in infancy. J. Pediat., 75:690, 1969.

Filer, L. J., Jr.: Modified food starches for use in infant foods. Nutr. Rev., 29:55, 1971.

————: Salt in infant foods. Nutr. Rev., 29:27, 1971.

Fomon, S. J., et al.: Relationship between formula concentration and rate of growth of normal infants. J. Nutr., 98:241, 1969.

French, J. G.: Relationship of morbidity to the feeding patterns of Navajo children from birth through 24 months. Am. J. Clin. Nutr., 20:375, 1967.

Husband, J., et al.: Gastric emptying of starch meals in the newborn. Lancet, 2:290, 1970.

Mayer, J.: Hypertension, salt intake, and the infant. Postgrad. Med., 45:229, 1969.

O'Grady, R. S.: Feeding behavior in infants. Am. J. Nursing, 71:736, (April) 1971.

Rivera, J.: The frequency of use of various kinds of milk during infancy in middle and lower income families. Am. J. Public Health, 61:277, 1971.

Rubini, M. E.: The many-faceted mystique of monosodium glutamate. (Editorial.) Am. J. Clin. Nutr., 24:169, 1971.

Whitten, C. F., et al.: Evidence that growth failure from maternal deprivation is secondary to undereating. JAMA, 209:1675, 1969.

Ziegler, E. G., and Fomon, S. J.: Fluid intake, renal solute load, and water balance in infancy. J. Pediat., 78:561, 1971.

Minerals in Infant Nutrition

Journal Articles:

Andelman, M. B., and Sered, B. R.: Utilization of dietary iron by term infants. Am. J. Dis. Child., 111: 45, 1966; 113:403, 1967.

Beal, V. A., et al.: Iron intake, hemoglobin and physical growth during the first two years of life. Pediatrics, 30:518, 1962.

Committee on Nutrition: Iron balance and requirements in infancy. Pediatrics, 43:134, 1969.

Coussins, H.: Magnesium metabolism in infants and children. Postgrad. Med., 46:135, 1969.

Editorial: Iron deficiency in infants. JAMA, 195:175, 1966.

Filer, L. J., and Martinez, G. A.: Calorie and iron intake by infants in the United States: an evaluation of 4000 representative six-month olds. Clin. Pediat., 2:470, 1963.

Krupke, S. S., and Sanders, E.: Prevalence of iron-deficiency anemia among infants and young children seen at rural ambulatory clinics. Am. J. Clin. Nutr., 23:716, 1970.

Review: Calcium deficiency in malnourished infants. Nutr. Rev., 23:164, 1965.

Vitamins in Infant Nutrition

Journal Articles:

Bakwin, M.: The overuse of vitamins in children. J. Pediat., 59:154, 1961.

Committee on Nutrition: Infantile scurvy and nutritional rickets in the U.S. Pediatrics, 29:646, 1962.

Fomon, S. J., et al.: Influence of vitamin D on linear growth of normal full-term infants. J. Nutr., 88:345, 1966.

Herting, D. C., and Drury, E. E.: Vitamin E content of milk, milk products and simulated milks: Relevance to infant nutrition. Am. J. Clin. Nutr., 22: 147, 1969.

Ossofsky, H. J.: Infantile scurvy. Am. J. Dis. Child., 109:173, 1965.

Addition of Solid Foods

Journal Articles:

Anderson, T. A., and Fomon, S. J.: Commercially prepared infant cereals: Nutritional considerations. J. Pediat., 78:788, 1971.

————: Commercially prepared strained and junior foods for infants: nutritional considerations. J. Am. Dietet. A., 58:520, 1971.

Beal, V. A.: On the acceptance of solid foods and other food patterns of infants and children. Pediatrics, 20:448, 1957

Committee on Nutrition: On the feeding of solid foods to infants. Pediatrics, 21:685, 1958.

Fomon, S. J., et al.: Acceptance of unsalted strained foods by normal infants. J. Pediat., 76:242, 1970.

Jelliffe, D. B.: Commerciogenic malnutrition. Food Technology, 25:55, 1971.

McIntosh, E. M.: Let's talk about baby foods. What's New in Home Economics, 35:25, 1971.

Review: Solid foods in the nutrition of young infants. Nutr. Rev., 25:233, 1967.

The use and care of baby's food. What's New in Home Economics, 35:93, 1971.

Milks

Journal Articles:

Berenberg, W., *et al.*: Hazards of skimmed milk, un-boiled and boiled. Pediatrics, 44:734, 1969.

Committee on Nutrition: Appraisal of nutritional adequacy of infant formulas used as cow milk substitutes. Pediatrics, 31:329, 1963.

Fomon, S. J., *et al.*: Excretion of fat by normal full-term infants fed various milk and formulas. Am. J. Clin. Nutr., 23:1299, 1970.

Jackson, R. L., *et al.*: Growth of "well-born" American infants fed human and cow's milk. Pediatrics, 33:642, 1964.

Owen, G. M.: Modification of cow's milk for infant formulas: Current practices. Am. J. Clin. Nutr., 22:1150, 1969.

Smith, C. A.: Overuse of milk in the diets of infants. JAMA, 172:567, 1960.

Protein Requirement

Journal Articles:

Effect of nitrogen intake on nitrogen balance in infants. Nutr. Rev., 20:105, 1962.

Holt, L. E., Jr.: The protein requirement of infants. J. Pediat., 54:496, 1959.

Holt, L. E., Jr., *et al.*: The concept of protein stores and its implication in diet. JAMA, 181:699, 1962.

NUTRITION OF CHILDREN AND YOUTH

(*See also* references under Proteins, Minerals, Vitamins)

General

Books and Pamphlets:

David, L.: Slimming for Teenagers. New York, Pocket Books, 1966.

György, P., and Burgess, A.: Protecting the Pre-School Child. London, Tavistock, 1965.

Heald, F. P., ed.: Adolescent Nutrition and Growth. New York, Appleton-Century-Crofts, 1969.

Hill, M. M.: Food Choices of the Teen-age Girl. New York, Nutrition Foundation, 1966.

Martin, E. A.: Nutrition Education in Action. New York, Holt, Rinehart & Winston, 1963.

McWilliams, M.: Nutrition for the Growing Years. New York, John Wiley & Sons, 1967.

Preschool Malnutrition: Primary Deterrent to Human Progress. National Academy of Sciences–National Research Council Publ. No. 1282. Washington, D.C., 1966.

Salmon, M. B.: Food Facts for Teenagers. Springfield, Ill., Charles C Thomas, 1965.

Tanner, J. M.: Growth at Adolescence. Oxford, England, Blackwell Scientific Publications, 1962.

WHO Expert Committee: Health Problems of Adolescence. WHO Publ. No. 308. Geneva, Switzerland, 1965.

Journal Articles:

Beal, V. A.: Nutrition in a longitudinal growth study. J. Am. Dietet. A., 46:457, 1965.

Blackburn, M. L.: Who turns the child "off" to nutrition? J. Nutr. Educa., 2:45, 1970.

Getty, G., and Hollinsworth, M.: Through a child's eye seeing. Nutrition Today, 2:17, (June) 1967.

The American Dietetic Association: Position paper on food and nutrition services in day-care centers. J. Am. Dietet. A., 59:47, 1971.

Watt, B., *et al.*: Energy intake of well-nourished children and adolescents. Am. J. Clin. Nutr., 22:1383, 1969.

Preschoolers

Journal Articles:

Crumrine, J. L., and Fryer, B. A.: Protein components of blood and dietary intake of preschool children. J. Am. Dietet. A., 57:509, 1970.

Dierks, E. C., and Morse, L. M.: Food habits and nutrient intakes of pre-school children. J. Am. Dietet. A., 47:292, 1965.

Eppright, E. S., *et al.*: Eating behavior of preschool children. J. Nutr. Educa., 1:16, 1969.

————: The North Central Regional study of diets of preschool. 2. Nutrition knowledge and attitudes of mothers. 3. Frequency of eating. J. Home Econ., 62:372, 407, 1970.

Fox, H. M., *et al.*: Diets of preschool children in the North Central Region. Calcium, Phosphorus and Iron. J. Am. Dietet. A., 59:233, 1971.

————: The North Central Regional study of diets of preschool children. 1. Family environment. J. Home Econ., 62:241, 1970.

Fryer, B. A., *et al.*: Diets of preschool children in the North Central Region. Calories, protein, fat and carbohydrate. J. Am. Dietet. A., 59:228, 1971.

Futrell, M. F., *et al.*: Nutritional status of Negro preschool children in Mississippi. Evaluation of HOP Index. Impact of education and income. J. Am. Dietet. A., 59:218, 224, 1971.

Gutelius, M. F.: The problems of iron deficiency anemia in preschool Negro children. Am. J. Public Health, 59:290, 1969.

Harrison, H. E.: The disappearance of rickets. Am. J. Public Health, 56:734, 1966.

Hookworm and nutrition. Postgrad. Med., 46:191, 1969.

Juhas, L.: Nutrition education and the development of language. J. Nutr. Educa., 1:12, 1969.

Kerrey, E., *et al.*: Nutritional status of preschool children. I. Dietary and biochemical findings. Am. J. Clin. Nutr., 21:1274, 1968.

Owen, G. M., and Kram, K. M.: Nutritional status of preschool children in Mississippi: Food sources of nutrients in the diets. J. Am. Dietet. A., 54:490, 1969.

Owen, G. M., *et al.*: Nutritional status of Mississippi preschool children. A pilot study. Am. J. Clin. Nutr., 22:1444, 1969.

Tepley, L. J.: Nutritional needs of the preschool child. Nutr. Rev., 22:65, 1964.

Van Duzen, J. P., *et al.*: Protein and calorie malnutrition among preschool Navajo Indian children. Am. J. Clin. Nutr., 22:1362, 1969.

The School Age Child

Journal Articles:

Agran, P.: The National School Lunch Program. J. School Health, 39:440, 1969.

Council on Foods and Nutrition, A.M.A.: Confections and carbonated beverages in schools. JAMA, 180:92, 1962.

Daniels, A. M.: Training school nurses to work with groups of adolescents. Children, 13:210, (Nov.-Dec.) 1966.

Eppright, E. S., and LeBaron, H. R.: Our responsibilities to children and youth. J. Am. Dietet. A., 38:354, 1961.

Lantis, M.: The child consumer; cultural factors influencing his food choices. J. Home Econ., 54:370, 1962.

Myers, M. L., *et al.*: A nutrition study of school children in a depressed urban district. I. Dietary findings. J. Am. Dietet. A., 53:226, 1968.

Paige, D. M.: School feeding program: who should receive what? J. School Health, 41:261, 1971.

Review: The effects of a balanced lunch program on the growth and nutritional status of school children. Nutr. Rev., 23:35, 1965.

Saratscotis, J. B., and Gordon, J.: Nutritional status of primary school pupils in Baltimore. H.S.M.H. Health Reports, 86:302, 1971.

Todhunter, E. N.: School feeding from a nutritionist's point of view. Am. J. Public Health, 60:2302, 1970.

Adolescents

Journal Articles:

Dwyer, J. T., *et al.*: Nutritional literacy of high school students. J. Nutr. Educa., 2:59, 1970.

Edwards, C. H., *et al.*: Nutrition survey of 6200 teen-age youth. J. Am. Dietet. A., 45:543, 1964.

Hampton, M. C., *et al.*: Caloric and nutrient intakes of teen-agers. J. Am. Dietet. A., 50:385, 1967.

Huenemann, R. L.: A study of teenagers: body size and shape, dietary practices and physical activity. Food and Nutrition News, 37:7, (Apr.) 1966. (Nat. Live Stock and Meat Board.)

Huenemann, R. L., *et al.*: Food and eating practices of teenagers. J. Am. Dietet. A., 53:17, 1968.

Johnson, J. A.: Nutritional aspects of adolescence. J. Pediat., 59:741, 1961.

Mitchell, H. S.: Protein limitation and human growth. J. Am. Dietet. A., 44:165, 1964.

Nutritional implications of some problems of adolescents. Dairy Council Digest, 38:25, (Sept.-Oct.) 1967.

Stare, F. J., and Dwyer, J.: An eye to the future: healthy eating for teenagers. J. School Health, 39:595, 1969.

Yoshimura, H.: Anemia during physical training (sports anemia). Nutr. Rev., 28:251, 1970.

GERIATRIC NUTRITION

Books and Pamphlets:

Howell, S. C., and Loeb, M. B.: Nutrition and aging: A Monograph for Practitioners. Gerontological Society, Washington, D.C., 1970.

Institute of Rehabilitative Medicine, New York University Medical Center: Mealtime Manual for the Aged and Handicapped. New York, Simon & Schuster (Essandess Special Editions), 1970.

Mathiasen, G.: The Golden Years—A Tarnished Myth. The National Council on Aging, Washington, D.C., 1970.

Journal Articles:

Anderson, E. L.: Eating patterns before and after dentures. J. Am. Dietet. A., 58:421, 1971.

Balsley, M., *et al.*: Nutrition in disease and stress. Geriatrics, 26:87, 1971.

Bernstein, D. S.: Prevalence of osteoporosis in high-land low-fluoride areas in North Dakota. JAMA, 198:499, 1966.

Bullamore, J. R., *et al.*: Effect of age on calcium absorption. Lancet, No. 7672:535, (Sept. 12) 1970.

Caniggia, A.: Senile osteoporosis. J. Am. Dietet. A., 47:49, 1965.

Cashman, J. W., *et al.*: Nutritionists, dietitians and Medicare. J. Am. Dietet. A., 50:17, 1967.

da Costa, F., and Moorhouse, J. A.: Protein malnutrition in aged individuals on self-selected diets. Am. J. Clin. Nutr., 22:1618, 1969.

Dibble, M. V., *et al.*: Evaluation of the nutritional status of elderly subjects, with a comparison of Fall and Spring. J. Am. Geriat. Soc., 15:1031, 1967.

Eckerstrom, S.: Clinical aspects of metabolism in the elderly. Geriatrics, 21:161, 1966.

Gordon, B. M.: A feeding plan for geriatric patients. Hospitals, 39:92, (Apr. 16) 1965.

Guggenheim, K., and Margulee, I.: Factors in the nutrition of elderly people living alone or as couples and receiving community assistance. J. Am. Geriat. Soc., 13:561, 1965.

Hegsted, D. M.: Nutrition, bone and calcified tissue. J. Am. Dietet. A., 50:105, 1967.

Henriksen, B., and Cate, H. D.: Nutrient content of food served vs. food eaten in nursing homes. J. Am. Dietet. A., 59:126, 1971.

Jernigan, A. K.: Home delivered meals as a hospital service. Hospitals, 43:90, (Sept. 16) 1969.

Joering, E.: Nutrient contribution of a meals program for senior citizens. J. Am. Dietet. A., 59:129, 1971.

Lukaczer, M.: Lessons for the federal effort against hunger and malnutrition—from a case study. Am. J. Public Health, 61:259, 1971.

McCarthy, L. W.: Motivate . . . don't manipulate. Nursing Homes, 20:36, 1971.

Nutrition and eating problems of the elderly . . . Current comment. J. Am. Dietet. A., 58:43, 1971.

Patients drink beer in hospital pub. (Medical News.) JAMA, 212:1790, (June 15) 1970.

Pelcovits, J.: Nutrition for older Americans. J. Am. Dietet. A., 58:17, 1971.

Roman, E.: New foods to serve. Nursing Homes, 20:14, 1971.

Sebrell, W. H.: It's not age that interferes with nutrition of the elderly. Nutrition Today, 1:15, (June) 1966.

Settle, E.: Correction of malnutrition in the aged; comparative efficacy of an anabolic hormone and enzyme vitamin complex. Geriatrics, 21:173, 1966.

Stone, V.: Give the older person time. Am. J. Nursing, 69:2124, 1969.

Swanson, P.: Adequacy in old age: I. Role of nutrition. II. Nutrition education program for the aging. J. Home Econ., 56:651, 728, 1964.

Tappel, A. L.: Will antioxidant nutrients slow aging processes? Geriatrics, 23:97, 1968.

Watkin, D. M.: Nutrition of older people. Am. J. Public Health, 55:548, 1965.

Weiner, M. F.: A practical approach in encouraging geriatric patients to eat. J. Am. Dietet. A., 55:384, 1969.

PART THREE

DIET IN DISEASE

(It is suggested that the bibliography under Nutrition and the references and Supplementary Readings quoted in each chapter also be consulted.)

GENERAL REFERENCES

Books:

Beeson, P. B., and McDermott, W.: Cecil-Loeb Textbook of Medicine. ed. 13. Philadelphia, W. B. Saunders, 1971.

Bruner, J. S.: The Process of Education. Cambridge, Mass. Harvard University Press, 1965.

Goodman, L., and Gilman. A.: Pharmacological Basis of Therapeutics. ed. 4. New York, Macmillan, 1970.

Guyton, A. C.: Textbook of Medical Physiology. ed. 4. Philadelphia, W. B. Saunders, 1971.

————: Function of the Human Body. ed. 3. Philadelphia, W. B. Saunders, 1969.

Lillienfeld, A. M., and Gifford, A. J.: Chronic Diseases and Public Health. Baltimore, The Johns Hopkins Press, 1966.

Nelson, W. E.: Textbook of Pediatrics. ed. 9. Philadelphia, W. B. Saunders, 1969.

Turner, D.: Handbook of Diet Therapy. ed. 5. Chicago, University of Chicago Press, 1970.

Diet Manuals:

Mayo Clinic Diet Manual. ed. 4. Philadelphia, W. B. Saunders, 1971.

(*See also* Diet Manuals from medical centers, state and local dietetic associations, and state health departments.)

Journals:

American Journal of Clinical Nutrition
American Journal of Nursing
American Journal of Public Health
Diabetes
Gastroenterology
Hospitals
Journal of Chronic Disease
Journal of Home Economics
Journal of Pediatrics
Journal of the American Dietetic Association
Journal of the American Medical Association
Lancet
New England Journal of Medicine
Nursing Outlook
Nutrition Reviews
Pediatrics
Postgraduate Medicine
Today's Health

THE PATIENT AND HIS NUTRITIONAL PROBLEMS; ROUTINE HOSPITAL DIETS

General

Books:

Benjamin, A.: The Helping Interview. Boston, Houghton Mifflin Co., 1969.

Bermosk, L. S., and Mordan, M. J.: Interviewing in Nursing. New York, Macmillan, 1964.

Food Customs of New Canadians. Toronto, Toronto Nutrition Committee, 1967.

Garrett, A.: Interviewing—Its Principles and Practices. New York, Family Service Association of America, 1942.

Gift, H. H., Washborn, M. B., and Harrison, G. G.: Nutrition, Behavior, and Change. Englewood Cliffs, N.J., Prentice-Hall, 1972.

Kosa, J., Antonovsky, A., and Zola, I. K. (eds.): Poverty and Health: A Sociological Analysis. Cambridge, Mass., Harvard University Press, 1969.

Mead, M.: Food Habits Research: Problems of the 1960's. National Academy of Sciences–National Research Council Publ. No. 1225. Washington, D.C., 1964.

Journal Articles:

Grant, M., and Earl, L. B.: Nutrition problems and programs in the District of Columbia. J. Am. Dietet. A., 55:112, 1969.

Hegsted, D. M.: Nutritional requirements in disease. J. Am. Dietet. A., 56:303, 1970.

Knoll, A. P.: Menu planning for the geriatric patient. Hospitals, 45:64, (Jan. 1) 1971.

Moreland, P. L., and Lawson, C. H.: For contract food service management. Hospitals, 44:105, (Jan. 1) 1970.

Meyers, W. W.: For the hospital food service manager. Hospitals, 44:104, (Jan. 1) 1970.

Phillips, M. G.: Nutrition opportunities in specialized health areas. J. Am. Dietet. A., 54:348, 1969.

Tarnower, W.: Psychological needs of the hospitalized patient. Nurs. Outlook, 13:28, (July) 1965.

Vaughn, M. E.: An agency nutritionist looks at home health care under medicare. J. Am. Dietet. A., 51:146, 1967.

Youland, D. M., et al.: Nutrition services in home health agencies. J. Am. Dietet. A., 56:111, 1970.

Meaning of Food

Journal Articles:

Babcock, C. G.: Attitudes and the use of food. J. Am. Dietet. A., 38:546, 1961.

Brozek, J.: Research on diet and behavior. J. Am. Dietet. A., 56:321, 1970.

Cassel, J.: Social and cultural implications of food and food habits. Am. J. Public Health, 47:732, 1957.

Fathauer, G. H.: Food habits—an anthropologist's view. J. Am. Dietet. A., 37:335, 1960.

Jerome, N. W.: Northern urbanization and food consumption patterns of southern-born Negroes. Am. J. Clin. Nutr., 22:1667, 1969.

Manning, M. L.: The psychodynamics of dietetics. Nurs. Outlook, 13:57, 1965.

Pumpian-Mindlin, E.: The meanings of food. J. Am. Dietet. A., 30:576, 1954.

Teaching the Patient

Journal Articles:

Craig, D. G.: Guiding the change process in people. J. Am. Dietet. A., 58:22, 1971.

Johnson, D.: Effective diet counseling begins early in hospitalization. Hospitals, 41:94, 1967.

Matthews, L. I.: Principles of interviewing and patient counseling. J. Am. Dietet. A., 50:469, 1967.

Morris, E.: How does a nurse teach nutrition to patients? Am. J. Nursing, 60:67, (Jan.) 1960.

Paynich, M. L.: Cultural barriers to nurse communication. Am. J. Nursing, 64:87, (Feb.) 1964.

Storlie, F.: A philosophy of patient teaching. Nurs. Outlook, 19:378, 1971.

Vargas, J. S.: Teaching as changing behavior. J. Am. Dietet. A., 58:512, 1971.

FOOD AND FOOD COMPOSITION

Books:

Corinne Netzer: The Brand Name Calorie Counter. New York, Dell Publishing Co., 1969.

Nutritive Values of Foods. Home and Garden Bulletin No. 72. USDA, Washington, D.C., 1970.

Journal Articles:

Butz, E. L.: Our daily bread. J. Am. Dietet. A., 56:107, 1971.

Call, D. L., and Hayer, M. G.: Reaction of nutritionists to nutrient labeling of foods. Am. J. Clin. Nutr., 23:1347, 1970.

Feeley, R. M., and Watt, B. K.: Nutritive value of foods distributed under USDA food assistance programs. J. Am. Dietet. A., 57:528, 1970.

Gormican, A.: Inorganic elements in foods used in hospital menu. J. Am. Dietet. A., 56:397, 1970.

Merrill, A. L.: Citrus fruit values in "Handbook No. 8," revised. J. Am. Dietet. A., 44:264, 1964.

Rubini, M. E.: Filled milk and artificial milk substitutes. Am. J. Clin. Nutr., 22:163, 1969.

Standal, B. R., et al.: Fatty acids, cholesterol, and proximate analysis of some ready-to-eat foods. J. Am. Dietet. A., 56:392, 1970.

Watt, B. K.: Concepts in developing a food composition table. J. Am. Dietet. A., 40:297, 1962.

WEIGHT CONTROL

Books:

Leverton, R. M.: Food Becomes You. ed. 3. Ames, Iowa, Iowa State University Press, 1965.

Mayer, J.: Overweight: Causes, Cost, and Control. Englewood Cliffs, N. J., Prentice-Hall, 1968.

Obesity and Health. Public Health Service, Division of Chronic Diseases, U.S. Dept. H.E.W., 1966.

Wyden, P.: The Overweight Society. New York, William Morrow and Co., 1965.

Overweight

Journal Articles:

Bruch, H.: The emotional significance of the preferred weight. Am. J. Clin. Nutr., 5:192, 1957.

————: Psychological aspects of obesity in adolescents. Am. J. Public Health, 48:1349, 1958.

Bullen, B. A., *et al.*: Physical activity of obese and non-obese adolescent girls. Am. J. Clin. Nutr., 14: 211, 1964.

Cheek, D. B., *et al.*: Overgrowth of lean and adipose tissue in adolescent obesity. Pediat. Res., 4:268, 1970.

Dwyer, J. T., and Mayer, J.: Biases in counting calories. J. Am. Dietet. A., 54:305, 1969.

————: Potential dieters: who are they? J. Am. Dietet. A., 56:510, 1970.

Eid, E. E.: Follow-up study of physical growth of children who had excessive weight gain during first six months of life. Brit. Med. J., 2:74, 1970.

The feeding center and body weight regulation. Nutr. Rev., 28:216, 1970.

Hirsh, J., and Knittle, J. L.: Cellularity of obese and nonobese human adipose tissue. Fed. Proc., 29: 1516, 1970.

Huenemann, R. L.: Consideration of adolescent obesity as a public health problem. Public Health Rep., 83:491, 1968.

Kalkhoff, R., and Ferrow, C.: Metabolic differences between obese overweight and muscular overweight men. New Eng. J. Med., 284:1236, 1971.

Leveille, G. A.: Adipose tissue metabolism: influence of periodicity of eating and diet composition. Fed. Proc., 29:1294, 1970.

Rabinowitz, D.: Some endocrine and metabolic aspects of obesity. Ann. Rev. Med., 21:241, 1970.

Rubin, R.: Body image and self-esteem. Nurs. Outlook, 16:20, 1968.

Schachter, S.: Obesity and eating. Science, 161:751, 1968.

Seltzer, C., and Mayer, J.: A simple criterion of obesity. Postgrad. Med., 38:A101, 1965.

Speckman, E. W., *et al.*: The effect of nutrition on body composition. Nutr. Rev., 25:1, 1967.

Stunkard, A., *et al.*: The management of obesity: patient self-help and medical treatment. Arch Int. Med., 125:1067, 1970.

Stunkard, A., and Mendelson, M.: Disturbances in body image of some obese persons. J. Am. Dietet. A., 38:328, 1961.

Wolff, K.: Eating habits and emotional problems. J. Am. Dietet. A., 54:318, 1969.

Young, C. M.: Some comments on the obesities. J. Am. Dietet. A., 45:134, 1964.

————: Management of the obese patient. JAMA, 186:903, 1963.

Anorexia Nervosa

Journal Articles:

Farquharson, R. F., and Hyland, H. H.: Anorexia nervosa: the course of 15 patients treated from 20 to 30 years previously. Canad. Med. A. J., 94:411, 1966.

Sours, J. A.: Clinical studies in anorexia nervosa syndrome. N.Y. State J. Med., 68:1363, 1968.

DIABETES MELLITUS

Books:

Ellenberg, M., and Rifkin, H.: Diabetes Mellitus: Theory and Practice. New York, McGraw-Hill, 1970.

Rosenthal, H., and Rosenthal, J.: Diabetic Care in Pictures. ed. 4. Philadelphia, J. B. Lippincott, 1968.

Adult Diabetes

Journal Articles:

Albrink, M. J., and Davidson, P. C.: Dietary therapy and prophylaxis of vascular disease in diabetes. Med. Clin. N. Am., 55:877, 1971.

Cole, H. S., and Camerini-Davalos, R. A.: Diet therapy in diabetes mellitus. Med. Clin. N. Am., 54: 1577, 1970.

Danowski, T. S.: Therapies of diabetes mellitus. Postgrad. Med., 45:137, (Apr.) 1969.

Felig, P., and Bondy, P. K. (eds.): Symposium on diabetes mellitus. Med. Clin. N. Am., 55:791-1075, 1971.

Jerrigan, A. K.: Diabetic patients require education and understanding. Hospitals, 44:77, (Apr. 1) 1970.

Kalkhoff, B. K., *et al.*: Metabolic effects of weight loss in obese subjects. Changes in plasma substrate levels, insulin and growth hormone response. Diabetes, 20:83, 1971.

Knowles, H. C., Jr.: Prevalence and development of diabetes. Fed. Proc., 27:945, 1968.

Murawski, B. J., *et al.*: Personality patterns in patients with diabetes mellitus of long duration. Diabetes, 19:259, 1970.

Podolsky, S.: Special needs of diabetics undergoing surgery. Postgrad. Med., 45:128, (Feb.) 1969.

Sharky, T. P.: Diabetes mellitus. Present problems and new research. J. Am. Dietet. A., 58:201-209; 336-344; 422-444; 528-537, 1971.

Stone, D. B.: A rational approach to diet and diabetes. J. Am. Dietet. A., 46:30, 1965.

Watkins, J. D., and Moss, F. T.: Confusion in the management of diabetes. Am. J. Nursing, 69:521, 1969.

Diabetes and Pregnancy

Journal Articles:

Garnet, J. D.: Pregnancy in women with diabetes. Am. J. Nursing, 69:1900, 1969.

McLendon, H., and Bottomy, J. R.: A critical analysis of the management of pregnancy in diabetic women. Am. J. Obstet. Gynec., 80:641, 1960.

Juvenile Diabetes

Journal Articles:

Drash, A.: Diabetes mellitus in childhood: A review. J. Pediat., 78:919, 1971.

Kaufman, R. V., and Hersher, B.: Body image changes in teen-age diabetics. Pediatrics, 48:123, 1971.

Knowles, H. C., *et al.*: The course of juvenile diabetes treated with unmeasured diet. Monograph. Diabetes, 14:239, 1965.

Koski, M. L.: The coping process in childhood diabetes. Acta Pediat. Scand., Supplement, 198:1, 1969.

Moore, M. L.: Diabetes in children. Am. J. Nursing, 67:104, 1967.

Moss, J. M.: Management of juvenile diabetes. Gen. Pract., 38:78, 1968.

Schwartz, R.: The critically ill child: diabetic keto acidosis and coma. Pediatrics, 47:902, 1971.

Weil, W. B., Jr.: Juvenile diabetes mellitus. New Eng. J. Med., 278:829, 1968.

Teaching the Diabetic Patient

Journal Articles:

Anderson, R. S., *et al.*: Evaluation of clinical, cultural and psychosomatic influences in the teaching and management of diabetic patients. Am. J. Med. Sci., 245:682, 1963.

Collier, B. N., and Etzwiler, D. D.: Comparative study of diabetes knowledge among juvenile diabetics and their parents. Diabetes, 20:51, 1970.

Etzwiler, D. D.: Who's teaching the diabetic? Diabetes, 16:111, 1967.

FORECAST. Published monthly by the American Diabetes Assn., 18 East 48th Street, New York, N.Y. 10017. $2.00 per year.

Skiff, A. W.: Programmed instruction and patient teaching. Am. J. Public Health, 55:409, 1965.

Spiegel, A. D.: Programmed instructional materials for patient education. J. Med. Educa., 42:958, 1967.

Tani, G. S., and Hankin, J. H.: A self-learning unit for patients with diabetes. J. Am. Dietet. A., 58:311, 1971.

Williams, T. F., *et al.*: The clinical picture of diabetic control, studied in four settings. Am. J. Public Health, 57:441, 1967.

————: Dietary errors made at home by patients with diabetes. J. Am. Dietet. A., 51:19, 1967.

CARDIAC DISEASE
General

Books:

Somerville, W. (ed.): Paul Wood's Diseases of the Heart and Circulation, ed. 3. Philadelphia, J. B. Lippincott, 1968.

Dietary Fat and Human Health: A Report of the Food and Nutrition Board, National Academy of Sciences–National Research Council Publ. No. 1147. Washington, D.C., 1966.

Journal Articles:

Adlin, E. V., *et al.*: Dietary salt intake in hypertensive patients with normal and low plasma renin activity. Am. J. Med. Sci., 261:67, 1971.

Brown, W. J., Jr., *et al.*: Exchangeable sodium and blood volume in normotensive and hypertensive humans on high and low sodium intakes. Circulation, 43:508, 1971.

Carter, A. B.: Hypertension—its causes and treatment. Nurs. Times, 67:531, 1971.

Conn, J. W.: Hypertension, the potassium ion and impaired carbohydrate tolerance. New Eng. J. Med., 273:1135, 1965.

Cooper, G. R., and Heap, B.: Sodium ion in drinking water. II. Importance, problems, and potential applications of sodium-ion-restricted therapy. J. Am. Dietet. A., 50:37, 1967.

Elliott, G. B., and Alexander, E. A.: Sodium from drinking water as an unsuspected cause of cardiac decompensation. Circulation, 23:562, 1961.

Farag, S. A., and Mozar, H. N.: Preventing recurrences of congestive heart failure. J. Am. Dietet. A., 51:26, 1967.

Hartroft, W. S.: The nutritional aspects of hypertension and its reversibility. Am. J. Public Health, 56:462, 1966.

Heap, B., and Robinson, C.: New booklets for patients on sodium restriction. J. Am. Dietet. A., 34:277, 1958.

Kohner, E. M., *et al.*: Effect of diuretic therapy on glucose tolerance in hypertensive patients. Lancet, 1:986, 1971.

Kuchel, O., *et al.*: Hypertension and peptic ulcer. Lancet, 1:652, 1971.

Schroeder, H. A.: Municipal drinking water and cardiovascular death rates. JAMA, 195:81, 1966.

Weller, J. M., and Hoobler, S. W.: Salt metabolism in hypertension. Ann. Int. Med., 50:106, 1959.

White, J. M., *et al.*: Sodium ion in drinking water. I. Properties, analysis, and occurrence. J. Am. Dietet. A., 50:32, 1967.

Atherosclerosis

Journal Articles:

Brown, H. B., *et al.*: Design of practical fat-controlled diets. Foods, fat composition and cholesterol content. JAMA, 196:205, 1966.

Christakis, G., *et al.*: The anti-coronary club: a dietary approach to the prevention of coronary heart disease—a seven year report. Am. J. Public Health, 56:299, 1966.

Dayton, S., *et al.*: Can change in the American diet prevent coronary heart disease? Am. J. Dietet. A., 46:20, 1965.

————: A controlled clinical trial of a diet high in unsaturated fat in preventing complications of atherosclerosis. Circulation, 40: Suppl. 11, 1969.

————: Prevention of coronary heart disease and other complications of atherosclerosis by modified diet. Am. J. Med., 46:751, 1969.

Epstein, F. H.: The epidemiology of coronary heart disease. J. Chron. Dis., 18:735, 1965.

Frederickson, D. S., *et al.*: Fat transport in lipoproteins—an integrated approach to mechanisms and disorders. New Eng. J. Med., 276:34, 94, 148, 215, 273, 1967.

Grande, R.: Dietary carbohydrates and serum cholesterol. Am. J. Clin. Nutr., 20:176, 1967.

Heaton, K. W.: Sugar consumption and myocardial infarction. Lancet, 1:185, 1971.

Jepson, E. M., *et al.*: Treatment of essential hyperlipidemia. Lancet, 1:131, 1971.

Kannel, W. B., *et al.*: The coronary profile: 12-year follow-up in the Framingham study. J. Occup. Med., 9:611, 1967.

Keys, A. (ed.): Coronary heart disease in seven countries. Am. Heart Association Monograph 29. Circulation, 41: Suppl. 1, 1970.

Keys, A., *et al.*: Mortality and coronary heart disease among men studied for 23 years. Arch. Intern. Med., 128:201, 1971.

Lees, R., and Wilson, D. E.: The treatment of hyperlipidemia. New Eng. J. Med., 284:186, 1971.

Leren, P.: The Oslo diet-heart study: Eleven-year report. Circulation, 42:935, 1970.

Levy, R. I., and Fredrickson, D. S.: Diagnosis and management of hyperlipoproteinemia. Am. J. Cardiol., 22:576, 1968.

Levy, R. I., and Glucek, C. J.: Hypertriglyceridemia, diabetes mellitus, and coronary vessel disease. Arch. Intern. Med., 123:220, 1969.

Lewis, L. A., *et al.*: Ten years' dietary treatment of primary hyperlipidemia. Geriatrics, 25:64, 1970.

National Diet-Heart Study Research Group: The national diet-heart study final report. Circulation, 37: Suppl. 3, 1968.

Phillips, J. A., and Vail, G. E.: Effect of heat on fatty acids. J. Am. Dietet. A., 50:116, 1967.

Spain, D. M.: Atherosclerosis. Sci. Am., 215:48, 1966.

Zukel, M. C.: Revising booklets on fat-controlled meals. Background information on nutrient composition. J. Am. Dietet. A., 54:20, 1969.

————: Appraising and revising educational health materials. A look at the booklets for "Planning Fat-Controlled Meals." J. Am. Dietet. A., 54:25, 1969.

RENAL DISEASE

Book:

Pitts, R. F.: Physiology of the Kidney and Body Fluids. Chicago, Year Book Medical Publishers, 1968.

Journal Articles:

Berlyne, G. M.: Nutrition in renal failure. Nut. Rev., 27:219, 1969.

————: Aminoacid loss in peritoneal dialysis. Lancet, 1:1339, 1967.

Blagg, C. R.: Home hemodialysis: six years' experience. New Eng. J. Med., 283:1126, 1970.

Coburn, J. W., *et al.*: Rapid appearance of hypercalcemia with initiation of hemodialysis. JAMA, 210:2276, 1969.

Comty, C. M.: Long-term dietary management of dialysis patients. J. Am. Dietet. A., 53:439, 1968.

Downing, S. R.: Nursing support in early renal failure. Am. J. Nursing, 69:1212, 1969.

Edwards, M., *et al.*: Iron therapy in patients on maintenance hemodialysis. Lancet, 2:491, 1970.

Erslev, A. J.: Anemia of chronic renal disease. Arch. Intern. Med., 126:774, 1970.

Freeman, R. M., and Bulechek, G. M.: Programmed instruction: an approach to dietary management of dialysis patients. Am. J. Clin. Nutr., 21:613, 1968.

Giordano, C., *et al.*: Incorporation of urea 15 N in amino acids of patients with chronic renal failure on a low nitrogen diet. Am. J. Clin. Nutr., 21:394, 1968.

Giovannetti, S., and Maggiore, Q.: A low nitrogen diet with proteins of high biological value for severe uremia. Lancet, 1:1000, 1964.

Giovannetti, S., *et al.*: Implications of diet therapy. Arch. Intern. Med., 126:900, 1970.

Kahn, H. D.: Effect of cranberry juice on urine—implications for therapy of urinary tract infection and calculi. J. Am. Dietet. A., 51:251, 1967.

Kopple, J., *et al.*: Evaluating modified protein diet for uremia. J. Am. Dietet. A., 54:481, 1969.

Levin, S.: Diet and infrequent peritoneal dialysis in chronic uremia. Am. J. Clin. Nutr., 21:613, 1968.

Levinsky, N. G.: Acute renal failure. New Eng. J. Med., 274:1016, 1966.

Mayer, J.: Nutrition and renal calculi. Postgrad. Med., 46:209, 1969.

Merril, J. P., and Hampers, C. L.: Uremia. New Eng. J. Med., 282:953, 1014, 1970.

Pendas, J. P.: Dietary management in chronic hemodialysis. Am. J. Clin. Nutr., 21:638, 1968.

Shinaberger, J. H., and Ginn, H. E.: Low protein, high essential amino acid diet for nitrogen equilibrium in chronic dialysis. Am. J. Clin. Nutr., 21:618, 1968.

Sullivan, J. F., and Eisenstein, A. B.: Ascorbic acid depletion in patients undergoing chronic hemodialysis. Am. J. Clin. Nutr., 23:1339, 1970.

Tsaltas, T. T.: Dietetic management of uremic patients: I. Extraction of potassium from foods for uremic patients. Am. J. Clin. Nutr., 22:490, 1969.

Wright, P. L., *et al.*: Effectiveness of modified Giovannetti diet compared with mixed low protein diet. Metabolism, 19:201, 1970.

Wright, R. G., *et al.*: Psychological stress during hemodialysis for chronic renal failure. Ann. Intern. Med., 64:611, 1966.

GASTROINTESTINAL DISEASE

Books:

Ingelfinger, F. J.: Let the ulcer patient enjoy his food. *In* Ingelfinger, F. J. (ed.): Controversy in Internal Medicine. Philadelphia, W. B. Saunders, 1966.

Roth, J. L. A.: The ulcer patient should watch his diet. *In* Ingelfinger, F. J. (ed.): Controversy in Internal Medicine. Philadelphia, W. B. Saunders, 1966.

Spiro, H. M.: Clinical Gastroenterology. New York, Macmillan, 1970.

Peptic Ulcer

Journal Articles:

ADA position paper on bland diet in the treatment of chronic duodenal ulcer disease. J. Am. Dietet. A., 59:244, 1971.

Buchman, E., et al.: Unrestricted diet in the treatment of duodenal ulcer. Gastroenterology, 56: 1016, 1969.

Caron, H. S., et al.: Objective assessment of cooperation with an ulcer diet: relation to antacid intake and to assigned physician. Am. J. Med. Sci., 261:61, 1971.

Fordtran, J. S.: Acid rebound. New Eng. J. Med., 279:900, 1968.

Hartroft, W. S.: The incidence of coronary artery disease in patients treated with the Sippy diet. Am. J. Clin. Nutr., 15:205, 1964.

Joint Committee, American Dietetic Association and American Medical Association: Diet as related to gastrointestinal function. J. Am. Dietet. A., 38: 425, 1961.

Kirsner, J. B.: Peptic ulcer: a review of recent literature on various clinical aspects. Part II. Gastroenterology, 54:945, 1968.

Piper, D. W.: Milk in treatment of gastric disease. Am. J. Clin. Nutr., 22:191, 1969.

Malabsorption

Journal Articles:

Bayless, T. M., and Christopher, N. L.: Disaccharidase deficiency. Am. J. Clin. Nutr., 21:181, 1969.

Bolin, T. D., and Davis, A. E.: Primary lactase deficiency: genetic or acquired. Am. J. Dig. Dis., 15:679, 1970.

Christopher, N. L., and Bayless, T. M.: Role of the small bowel and colon in lactose-induced diarrhea. Gastroenterology, 60:845, 1971.

Gray, G. M.: Intestinal digestion and maldigestion of dietary carbohydrates. Ann. Rev. Med., 22: 391, 1971.

Greenberger, N. J., and Skillman, T. G.: Medium-chain triglycerides. Physiological considerations and clinican implications. New Eng. J. Med., 280:1045, 1969.

Huang, S. S., and Bayless, T. M.: Lactose intolerance in healthy children. New Eng. J. Med., 276: 1283, 1967.

Rubin, W.: Celiac disease. Am. J. Clin. Nutr., 24:91, 1971.

Schwartz, M. K., et al.: The effect of gluten-free diet on fat, nitrogen, and mineral metabolism in patients with sprue. Gastroenterology, 54:791, 1968.

Shatin, R.: Evolution and lactase deficiency. Gastroenterology, 54:992, 1968.

Symposium: Malabsorption. Fed. Proc., 26:1388-1431, 1967.

Toskes, P. P., et al.: Vitamin B_{12} malabsorption in pancreatic insufficiency. New Eng. J. Med., 284: 627, 1971.

Welsh, J. D., et al.: Studies of lactose intolerance in families. Arch. Intern. Med., 122:315, 1968.

Regional Enteritis

Journal Articles:

Crohn, B. B.: Current status on therapy in regional enteritis. JAMA, 166:1479, 1958.

Roy, A. D., et al.: Effect of diet on the trypsin and chymotrypsin output in the stools of patients with an ileostomy. Gastroenterology, 53:584, 1967.

Ulcerative Colitis

Journal Articles:

Chalfin, D., and Holt, P. R.: Lactase deficiency in ulcerative colitis, regional enteritis and viral hepatitis. Am. J. Dig. Dis., 12:81, 1967.

Lapore, M. J.: The importance of emotional disturbances in chronic ulcerative colitis. JAMA, 191:819, 1965.

Truelove, S. C.: Medical management of ulcerative colitis. Brit. Med. J., 1:605, 1968.

Watkinson, G.: The medical management of ulcerative colitis. Postgrad. Med., 44:696, 1968.

Liver Disease

Journal Articles:

Gabuzda, G. J.: Cirrhosis, ascites and edema. Gastroenterology, 58:546, 1970.

Kudzma, D. J., et al.: Alcoholic hyperlipidemia: induction by alcohol but not by carbohydrate. J. Lab. Clin. Med., 77:384, 1971.

Marin, G. A., et al.: Studies of malabsorption occurring in patients with Laennec's cirrhosis. Gastroenterology, 56:727, 1969.

Peters, R. S., et al.: Use of a diet supplement in Laennec's cirrhosis. Gastroenterology, 54:872, 1968.

Rubin, E., and Lieber, C. S.: Malnutrition and liver disease—an overemphasized relationship. Am. J. Med., 45:1, 1968.

Sarles, H., et al.: Diet, cholesterol gallstones and the composition of bile. Am. J. Dig. Dis., 15: 251, 1970.

Small, D. M.: Gallstones. New Eng. J. Med., 279: 588, 1968.

Symposium: Nutrition and liver disease. Am. J. Clin. Nutr., 23:447-499; 581-625, 1970.

SURGERY

Journal Articles:

Buchwald, H.: The dumping syndrome and its treatment. A review and presentation of cases. Am. J. Surgery, 116:81, 1968.

Dudrick, S. J., *et al.*: Long-term total parenteral nutrition with growth, development, and positive nitrogen balance. Surgery, 64:134, 1968.

Machella, T. E.: Mechanism of the post-gastrectomy dumping syndrome. Gastroenterology, 54:721, 1968.

Mulcare, D. B., *et al.*: Effect of diet on malabsorption after small-bowel by-pass. J. Am. Dietet. A., 57:331, 1970.

Nutritional disturbances after partial gastrectomy. Nutr. Rev., 26:140, 1968.

Schwartz, P. L.: Ascorbic acid in wound healing— a review. J. Am. Dietet. A., 56:497, 1970.

Shils, M. E., *et al.*: Long-term parenteral nutrition through an external arteriovenous shunt. New Eng. J. Med., 283:431, 1970.

Shultz, K. T., *et al.*: Mechanism of postgastrectomy hypoglycemia. Arch. Intern. Med., 128:240, 1971.

Thompson, W. R., *et al.*: Use of the "space diet" in the management of a patient with extreme short bowel syndrome. Am. J. Surgery, 117:449, 1969.

Total parenteral nutrition. Nutr. Rev., 28:286, 1970.

Weser, E.: Intestinal adapation to small bowel resection. Am. J. Clin. Nutr., 24:133, 1971.

SPECIAL PROBLEMS

Journal Articles:

Cole, D.: Feeding allergic patients. Hospitals, 45:95, (Feb. 16) 1971.

Davenport, H. W.: Salicylate damage to the gastric mucosal barrier. New Eng. J. Med., 276:1307, 1967.

Dobbins, W. O.: Drug-induced steatorrhea. Gastroenterology, 54:1193, 1968.

Mayer, J.: Nutrition and gout. Postgrad. Med., 45: 277, 1969.

FEEDING THE HANDICAPPED

Books:

Committee On Children With Handicaps: The Pediatrician and the Child With Mental Retardation. Evanston, Ill., American Academy of Pediatrics, 1971.

Klinger, J. L., *et al.*: Mealtime Manual for the Aged and Handicapped. New York, Simon & Shuster, 1970.

DISEASE OF INFANTS AND CHILDREN

Books:

Fomon, S. J.: Infant Nutrition. Philadelphia, W. B. Saunders, 1967.

Gardiner, L. I. (ed.): Endocrine and Genetic Diseases of Childhood. Philadelphia, W. B. Saunders, 1969.

Hsia, D. Y.: Inborn Errors of Metabolism, Part I, Clinical Aspects. Chicago, Year Book Medical Publishers, 1966.

Inborn Errors of Metabolism—General

Journal Articles:

Craig, J. W.: Present knowledge of nutrition in inborn errors of metabolism. Nutr. Rev., 26:161, 1968.

Efron, M. L.: Aminoaciduria. New Eng. J. Med., 272:1059, 1965.

Holtzman, N. A.: Dietary treatment of inborn errors of metabolism. Ann. Rev. Med., 21:335, 1970.

Howell, R. R.: Inborn errors of metabolism: some thoughts about their basic mechanisms. Pediatrics, 45:901, 1970.

Scriver, C. R.: Mutants: consumers with special needs. Nutr. Rev., 29:155, 1971.

Amino Acid Metabolism—Phenylketonuria

Journal Articles:

Acosta, P. B., *et al.*: Mothers' dietary management of PKU children. A survey. J. Am. Dietet. A., 53: 460, 1968.

Berman, J. L., and Ford, R.: IQ's and intelligence loss in patients with PKU and some variant states. J. Pediat., 77:765, 1970.

Berry, H. K., *et al.*: Amino acid balance in the treatment of phenylketonuria. J. Am. Dietet. A., 58: 210, 1971.

Fisch, R. O., *et al.*: Responses of children with phenylketonuria to dietary treatment. J. Am. Dietet. A., 58:32, 1971.

Hunt, M. H., *et al.*: Nutritional management in phenylketonuria. Am. J. Dis. Child., 122:1, 1971.

Koch, R., *et al.*: An approach to management of phenylketonuria. J. Pediat., 76:815, 1970.

Perry, T. L., *et al.*: Glutamine depletion in phenylketonuria: A possible cause of mental defect. New Eng. J. Med., 282:761, 1970.

Saunders, C.: Phenylketonuria 1969. Postgrad. Med., 46:159, 1969.

Smith, B. A., and Waisman, H. A.: Adequate phenylalanine intake for optimum growth and development in the treatment of phenylketonuria. Am. J. Clin. Nutr., 24:423, 1971.

Sutherland, B. S., *et al.*: Growth and nutrition in treated phenylketonuric patients. JAMA, 211:270, 1970.

Wong, R. G., *et al.*: Mineral balance in treated phenylketonuric children. J. Am. Dietet. A., 57: 229, 1970.

Other Amino Acids

Journal Articles:

Goodman, S. I., *et al.*: The treatment of maple syrup urine disease. J. Pediat., 75:485, 1969.

Harries, J. T., *et al.*: Low proline diet in type I hyperprolinemia. Arch. Dis. Child., 46:72, 1971.

Hill, A., *et al.*: Dietary treatment of tyrosinosis. J. Am. Dietet. A., 56:308, 1970.

La Du, B. N.: The enzymatic deficiency in tyrosinemia. Am. J. Dis. Child., 113:54, 1967.

Perry, T. L., *et al.*: Treatment of homocystinuria with a low-methionine diet, supplemental cystine, and a methyl donor. Lancet, 2:474, 1968.

Rosenberg, L. E., *et al.*: Methymalonic aciduria. New Eng. J. Med., 278:1319, 1968.

Roth, H., and Segal, H.: The dietary management of leucine-induced hypoglycemia with a report of a case. Pediatrics, 34:831, 1964.

Sass-Kortsak, A., *et al.*: Conference on hereditary tyrosinemia. Observations on treatment in patients with tyrosiluria. Canad. Med. A. J., 97:1089, 1967.

Schimke, R. N.: Low methionine diet treatment of homocystinuria. Ann. Intern. Med., 70:642, 1969.

Snyder, R. D., and Robinson, A.: Leucine-induced hypoglycemia. Am. J. Dis. Child., 113:566, 1967.

Snyderman, S. W., *et al.*: Maple syrup urine disease with particular reference to dietotherapy. Pediatrics, 34:454, 1964.

Westall, R. G.: Dietary treatment of a child with maple syrup urine disease. Arch. Dis. Child., 38:485, 1964.

Carbohydrates

Journal Articles:

Hansen, R. G.: Hereditary galactosemia. JAMA, 208:2077, 1969.

Koch, R., *et al.*: Nutritional therapy of galactosemia. Clin. Pediat., 4:571, 1965.

Fatty Acids

Journal Articles:

Sidbury, J. B., *et al.*: An inborn error of short-chain fatty acid metabolism. J. Pediat., 70:8, 1967.

Gastrointestinal Disease

Journal Articles:

Cystic Fibrosis

di Sant' Agnese, P., *et al.*: Cystic fibrosis of the pancreas. New Eng. J. Med., 277:1287, 1344, 1399, 1967.

Handwerger, J., *et al.*: Glucose tolerance in cystic fibrosis. New Eng. J. Med., 281:451, 1969.

McCollum, A. T.: Cystic fibrosis: economic impact upon the family. Am. J. Public Health, 61:1335, 1971.

Shwachman, H., *et al.*: Studies in cystic fibrosis: report of 130 patients diagnosed under 3 months of age over a 20-year period. Pediatrics, 46:335, 1970.

Wiehoffen, D. M., and Pringle, D. J.: Dietary intake and food tolerances of children with cystic fibrosis. J. Am. Dietet. A., 54:206, 1969.

Other G. I. Problems

Lebenthal, E., *et al.*: Glucose-galactose malabsorption in an Oriental-Iraqi Jewish family. J. Pediat., 78:844, 1971.

Sultz, H. A., *et al.*: The epidemiology of peptic ulcer in childhood. Am. J. Public Health, 60:492, 1970.

Failure to Thrive

Journal Articles:

Ablett, J. G., and McCance, R. A.: Energy expenditure of children with Kwashiorkor. Lancet, 2:517, 1971.

Krieger, I., and Chen, Y. C.: Calorie requirements for weight gain in infants with failure due to maternal deprivation, undernutrition, and congenital disease. Pediatrics, 44:647, 1969.

Formulas

Journal Articles:

Berenberg, W., *et al.*: Hazards of skimmed milk, unboiled and boiled. Pediatrics, 44:734, 1969.

Coodin, F. J., *et al.*: Formula fatality. Pediatrics, 47:438, 1971.

Jung, A. L., *et al.*: Extreme hyperosmolality and "transient diabetes" due to inappropriately diluted infant formula. Am. J. Dis. Child., 118:859, 1969.

Prematurity

Journal Articles:

Babson, S. G., and Bramhill, J. L.: Diet and growth in the premature infant. J. Pediat., 74:890, 1969.

Snyderman, S. E., *et al.*: The protein requirement of the premature infant. I. The effect of protein intake on the retention of nitrogen. J. Pediat., 74:872, 1969.

Goldman, H. I., *et al.*: Clinical effects of two different levels of protein intake on low-birth-weight infants. J. Pediat., 74:881, 1969.

Renal Failure

Journal Articles:

Dobrin, R. S., *et al.*: The critically ill child: acute renal failure. Pediatrics, 48:286, 1971.

Simmons, J. M., *et al.*: Relation of calorie deficiency to growth failure in children on hemodialysis and the growth response to calorie supplementation. New Eng. J. Med., 285:653, 1971.

Glossary

acetone bodies (as′e-tōn). Acetone, acetoacetic acid and beta-hydroxybutyric acid. Called also ketone bodies. (See *ketosis,* defined below.)

acidosis (as′ĭ-do′sis). A pathological condition resulting from an accumulation of acid or loss of base in the body, and characterized by increase in hydrogen ion concentration.

aflatoxins (a′flah-tok′sin). Group of toxic substances produced by certain molds which grow on peanuts and cereals and which have toxic and carcinogenic effects in many animal species.

albuminuria (al′bu-mĭ-nu′ri-ah). The presence of the protein albumin in the urine.

alginate (ăl′jĭ-nāt). A compound made from marine kelp which forms a viscous solution or a gel.

alkaline reserve (al′kah-lĭn). Alkaline or basic material available in the body to neutralize acids.

alkalosis (al′kah-lo′sis). A pathological condition resulting from accumulation of base or loss of acid in the body and characterized by a decrease in hydrogen ion in the body.

allergen (al′er-jen). Any substance capable of inducing allergy.

alpha-ketoglutaric acid (ke′to-gloo-tar′ik). Intermediary product in the Krebs cycle.

amino acid (a-me′no as′id). An organic compound containing nitrogen known as the building blocks of the protein molecule.

amylase (am′ĭ-lās). A pancreatic enzyme that digests starch, as ptyalin in the saliva.

amylopectin (am′i-lo-pek′tin). The branched chain insoluble form of starch which stains violet red with iodine and forms a paste with hot water.

amylose (am′ĭ-lōs). The straight chain soluble form of starch which stains blue with iodine and does not form a paste with hot water.

anabolism (ah-nab′o-lizm). Term applied to that phase of metabolism which synthesizes new molecules, especially protoplasm.

anions (an′i-on). An ion carrying a negative charge. Since unlike forms of electricity attract each other, it is attracted by, and travels to, the anode or positive pole. The anions include all the non-metals, the acid radicals, and the hydroxyl ion.

antihemorrhagic (an′ti-hem′o-raj′ik). Preventing hemorrhage. Often applied to vitamin K.

antineuritic (an′ti-nu-rit′ik). Counteracting neuritis. Often applied to thiamine.

antioxidant (an′ti-ok′se-dant). A substance that prevents or delays oxidation. Often applied to vitamin E.

antirachitic (an′ti-rah-kit′ik). Preventive, curative or corrective of rickets. Often applied to vitamin D.

antiscorbutic (an′ti-skor-bu′tik). Preventing or curing scurvy. Often applied to ascorbic acid.

antivitamin (an′ti-vi′ta-min). Any substance that prevents normal metabolic functioning of vitamins by making them unabsorbable or ineffective.

apoenzyme (ap′o-en′zīm). The protein portion of an enzyme to which the prosthetic group or coenzyme is attached. The coenzyme may be a vitamin.

ascorbic acid (a-skor′bik). Vitamin C, deficiency of which is a causative factor in scurvy.

aspergillus flavus (as′per-jil′us fla-vus). A group of molds found on corn, peanuts and certain grains when improperly dried and stored; source of aflatoxin.

autosomal (au′to-so′mal). Pertaining to an autosome, a paired chromosome, not a sex chromosome.

avidin (av′i-din). A proteinlike antivitamin isolated from egg white; antagonist of biotin.

avitaminosis (a-vi′ta-min-o′sis). A condition due to the lack or the deficiency of a vitamin in the diet, or to lack of absorption or utilization of it.

base (bās). A substance which combines with acids to form neutral compounds.

biotin (bi′o-tin). A member of the vitamin B complex.

botulism (bot′u-lizm). Poisoning from the toxin produced by the organism *Clostridium botulinum.* The toxin has a selective action on the nervous system.

calciferol (kal-sif′er-ol). Vitamin D₂, produced by irradiating ergosterol.

calcification (kal′si-fi-ka′shun). Process by which organic tissue becomes hardened by a deposit of calcium salts.

calorimeter (kal'o-rim'e-ter). An instrument for measuring the heat change in any system (such as the types pictured in Chapter 5, one of which is used to measure the amount of heat produced by the body), and the bomb calorimeter used to measure the calorie (energy) value of foods.

carotene (kar'o-tēn). A yellow pigment which exists in several forms; alpha, beta and gamma carotene are provitamins which may be converted into vitamin A in the body.

carotenoid (kah-rot'e-noid). Pertaining to a number of compounds related to carotene. They are primarily yellow pigments.

carrageenin (kar'ah-gēn'in). From carrageen (Irish moss); the commercial colloid extract from the moss which forms a gel.

casein (ka'se-in). The principal protein of milk, the basis of cheese.

catabolism (kah-tab'o-lizm). That aspect of metabolism which converts nutrients or complex substances in living cells into simpler compounds, with the release of energy.

cation (kat'i-on). An ion carrying a positive charge which is attracted to the negative pole or cathode. (See anion above.) Cations include all metals and hydrogen.

cheilosis (ki-lo'sis). A condition marked by lesions on the lips and cracks at the angles of the mouth.

cholecalciferol (ko'le-kal-sif'er-ol). Vitamin D_3 derived from dehydrocholesterol.

cholesterol (ko-les'ter-ol). The most common member of the sterol group, defined below. It is a precursor of vitamin D and closely related to several hormones in the body. It constitutes a large part of the most frequently occurring type of gallstones, and occurs in atheroma of the arteries.

choline (ko'lēn). A component of lecithin. Necessary for fat transport in the body. Prevents the accumulation of fat in the liver.

chromatin (kro'mah-tin). The more stainable portion of the cell nucleus: contains the chromosomes.

chylomicrons (ki'lo-mi'kron). Particles of emulsified lipoproteins containing primarily triglycerides from dietary fat and very little protein.

chymotrypsin (ki'mo-trip'sin). One of the proteolytic enzymes of the pancreatic juice.

citrovorum factor (sit'ro-vo'rum fak'ter). A biologically active form of folic acid (folinic acid).

clostridium (klos-trid'e-um). A genus of schizomycetes, an anaerobic spore-forming rod-shaped bacterium, *C. perfringens* (and other species) a cause of gangrene.

cobalamin (co-bal'a-min). The basic molecule of vitamin B_{12} several compounds of which have vitamin activity.

collagen (kol'a-jen). The main protein constituent of connective tissue and of the organic substance of bones; changed into gelatin by boiling.

colloidal (ko-loi'dal). Pertaining to a colloid, which is a substance containing tiny, solid, evenly dispersed particles not dissolved in the medium, but which will not settle out.

congenital (kon-jen'i-tal). Existing at or before birth.

creatine (kre'a-tin). A nitrogenous end product of muscle metabolism.

creatinine (kre-at'i-nin). A basic substance, creatine anhydride, derived from creatine.

cyanocobalamin (si'ah-no-ko-bal'ah-men). Vitamin B_{12}, a dark red compound containing cobalt and a cyanide group.

cyclamate (si'kla-māt). Sodium or calcium cyclamate, known as Sucaryl, used as an artificial sweetener. Use prohibited by FDA.

cystine (sis'tin). A nonessential amino acid containing sulfur.

cystinuria (sis'ti-nu're-ah). The occurrence of excessive cystine in the urine.

deaminization (de-am'in-i-za'shun). The process of metabolism by which the nitrogen portion (amine group) is removed from amino acids.

dehydration (de'hi-dra'shun). Removal of water from food or tissue; or the condition that results from undue loss of water.

DHEW. United States Department of Health, Education, and Welfare.

disaccharidase (di-sak'ah-ri-das). An enzyme which hydrolyzes disaccharides.

disaccharide (di-sak'a-rid). Any one of the sugars which yields two single sugars on hydrolysis.

DNA, deoxyribonucleic acid (de-ok'se-ri'bo-nu-kle'ik). Found in the nucleus of living cells; functions in the transfer of genetic characteristics.

dyssebacea (dis'se-ba'shea). Disorder of the sebaceous follicles often seen in riboflavin deficiency.

electrolyte (e-lek'tro-līt). The ionized form of an element. Common electrolytes in the body are sodium, potassium and chloride.

endogenous (en-doj'e-nus). Originating within the organism, e.g. nutrients synthesized in intermediary metabolism.

endosperm (en'do-sperm). The nutritive substance within the embryo sac of plants.

enteropathy (en'ter-op'ah-the). Any disease of the intestine.

enzyme (en'zīm). A substance, usually protein in nature and formed in living cells, which brings about chemical changes.

ergocalciferol (er'go-kal-cif'er-ol). Vitamin D_2 derived from ergosterol. (See *calciferol*.)

ergosterol (er-gos'ter-ol). A sterol found in plant and in animal tissues which, on exposure to ultraviolet light, is converted into vitamin D_2. (See *sterol*.)

exogenous (eks-oj'e-nus). Originating outside the organism, e.g. nutrients in food.

FAO. Food and Agriculture Organization of the United Nations, Headquarters in Rome, Italy.

fatty acids (fat′e as′ids). The organic acids which combine with glycerol to form fat.

favism (fa′vism). An acute hemolytic anemia due to contact with the fava or broad bean.

FDA. Food and Drug Administration of the Public Health Service, U.S. Department of Health, Education and Welfare, Washington, D.C.

ferritin (fer′i-tin). An iron-containing protein: the form in which iron is stored in the liver, spleen, intestinal mucosa and reticuloendothelial cells.

flavoproteins (fla′vo-pro′te-in). Compounds containing riboflavin, certain nucleotides and proteins. They are important as enzymes in the Krebs cycle.

folacin (fo′la-sin). Another term for folic acid.

folic acid (fo′lic as′id). A vitamin of the B complex group, known also as pteroylglutamic acid or folacin.

folinic acid (fo-lin′ik). A folic acid derivative closely related to the true enzyme, also called "citrovorum factor."

formiminoglutamic acid (FIGLU) (form-im′i-no′gluta′mik). Intermediary product of histidine metabolism. Since folic acid is necessary for its breakdown, the urinary excretion of FIGLU may be measured to determine folic acid status.

galactose (gah-lak′tos). A monosaccharide derived from lactose by hydrolysis.

galactose-1-phosphate (gas-lak′tos). An intermediate product of galactose metabolism.

galactosemia (gah-lak′to-se′me-ah). A hereditary condition characterized by excess galactose in the blood.

genes (jēns). Units of hereditary DNA, carried by chromosomes.

gliadin (gli′a-din). One of the proteins found in the gluten of cereal grains.

gluten (gloo′ten; -t′n). A protein found in many cereal grains.

glyceride (glis′er-īd). A compound formed when glycerol and an acid are combined.

glycogen (gli′ko-jen). A carbohydrate, similar in composition to the amylopectin form of starch. In this form, carbohydrate is stored in the liver and the muscles.

hemicellulose (hem′e-sel′u-los). A complex carbohydrate similar to cellulose found in the cell wall of plants; indigestible but absorbs water, thereby stimulating laxation.

hexose (hek′sos). A single sugar containing six carbon atoms.

histidine (his′ti-din). An amino acid required by growing animals.

homogenized (ho-moj′e-nizd). Made homogeneous. Usually applied to dispersing milk fat in such fine globules that cream will not rise to the top.

hydrogenation (hi′dro-jen-a′shun). The process of introducing hydrogen into a compound, as when oils are hydrogenated to produce solid fats.

hydrolysate (hi-drol′i-sat). A product of hydrolysis. Often applied to protein hydrolysate.

hydrolysis (hi-drol′i-sis). A chemical reaction in which decomposition is due to the incorporation and splitting of water, resulting in the formation of two new compounds.

hydroxyproline (hi-drok′se-pro′lin). An amino acid which occurs in structural proteins, primarily collagen.

hypercalcemia (hi′per-kal-se′me-ah). An excess of calcium in the blood.

hypercholesteremia (hi′per-ko-les′ter-e′me-a). Excess of cholesterol in the blood.

hyperglycemia (hi′per-gli-se′me-a). An increase in the blood sugar level above normal.

hyperlipemia (hi′per-li-pe′me-a). Excess of fat or lipids in the blood.

hyperlipidemia (hi′per-lip-i-de′me-ah). An excess of lipids in the blood.

hyperlipoproteinemia (hi′per-lip′o-pro′te-in-e′me-ah). An excess of lipoprotein in the blood.

hyperplasia (hi′per-pla′zhe-a). Increase in number of normal cells in normal arrangement in a tissue.

hypertrophy (hi-per′tro-fe). Increase in cell size.

hyperuricemia (hi′per-u′ri-se′me-ah). Excess of uric acid in the blood.

hypervitaminosis (hi′per-vi′ta-min-o′sis). A condition due to an excess of one or more vitamins.

hypoalbuminemia (hi′po-al-bu′min-e′me-a). Abnormally low albumin content of the blood.

hypocalcemia (hi′po-kal-se′me-a). Abnormally low blood calcium.

hypoglycemia (hi′po-gli-se′me-a). A decrease in the blood sugar level below normal.

hypoproteinemia (hi′po-pro′te-in-e′me-a). A decrease in the normal quantity of serum protein in the blood.

idiopathic (id′i-o-path′ik). Self-originated; occurring without known cause.

inositol (in-o′si-tol). A member of the vitamin B complex.

isoleucine (i′so-lu′sin). An essential amino acid.

isotopes (i′so-tope). Two or more chemical elements which have the same atomic number and identical chemical properties, but which differ in atomic weight or in the structure of the nucleus.

ketogenic (ke′to-jen′ik). Capable of being converted into ketone bodies. Ketogenic substances in metabolism are the fatty acids and certain amino acids.

ketone bodies (ke′tōn). Acetoacetic acid, β-hydroxybutyric acid and acetone.

ketosis (ke-to′sis). A condition in which there is an accumulation in the body of the ketone bodies as a result of incomplete oxidation of the fatty acids.

kwashiorkor (kwa-shi-or′ker). A severe protein-calorie deficiency disease occurring in small children. Endemic in many parts of the world.

lecithin (les′i-thin) . A phospholipid containing glycerol, fatty acids, phosphoric acid and choline.

leucine (lu′sin). An essential amino acid.

linoleic acid (lin′o-le′ik as′id). A polyunsaturated fatty acid essential for nutrition.

linolenic acid (lin′o-le′nik as′id). A polyunsaturated fatty acid.

lipase (li′pās; lip′ās). An enzyme that digests fat.

lipid (lip′id), **lipoid** (lip′oid). Fat or fatlike substances.

lipoprotein (lip′o-pro′te-in). Combination of a protein with a fat, found in both animal and plant tissues.

lipotrophic (lip′o-trop′ik) . Applied to substances essential for fat metabolism.

lysosomes (li′so-sōms). Membranous structures in cytoplasm which contain hydrolytic enzymes.

malabsorption syndrome (mal′ab-sorp′shun). A group of symptoms which result from the inability to digest or absorb food in the intestinal tract.

marasmus (ma-raz′mus). Wasting and emaciation, especially in infants due to underfeeding or disease.

melanin (mel′ah-nin). The dark amorphous pigment of the skin, hair and certain other tissues which derives from tyrosine metabolism.

menadione (me-an-di′on). Synthetic vitamin K.

metabolism (me-tab′o-lizm). General term to designate all chemical changes which occur in food nutrients after they have been absorbed from the gastrointestinal tract and to the cellular activity involved in utilizing these nutrients.

methionine (meth-i′o-nin). An essential amino acid containing sulfur.

mitochondria (mit′o-kron′dre-ah). Small granules or rod-shaped structures in the cell.

monosaccharide (mon′o-sak′a-rid). A simple sugar which cannot be decomposed by hydrolysis.

mono-unsaturated (mon′o-un-sat′u-rat-ed). An organic compound such as a fatty acid in which two carbon atoms are united by a double bond.

mucopolysaccharide (mu′ko-pol′e-sak′ah-rid). A group of polysaccharides which contains hexosamine, which may or may not be combined with protein and which, dispersed in water, form many of the mucins.

mucoprotein (mu′ko-pro′te-in). Substance containing a polypeptide chain and disaccharides, found in mucous secretions of the digestive glands.

mucoviscidosis (mu′ko-vi-si-do′sis). The hereditary condition more often called cystic fibrosis or pancreatic fibrosis.

naphthoquinone (naf′tho-kwin′on). A derivative of quinone; some of these derivatives have vitamin K activity.

NAS–NRC. National Academy of Science–National Research Council, Washington, D.C.

niacin (ni′a-sin). A member of the vitamin B complex, formerly known as nicotinic acid. An antipellagra factor.

niacinamide (ni′ah-sin-am′id). Nicotinamide, the amide derivative of nicotinic acid (niacin).

NRC–RDA. National Research Council–Recommended Dietary Allowances.

nucleoprotein (nu′kle-o-pro′tein). The conjugated protein found in the nuclei of cells.

nucleotide (nu′kle-o-tid). Compound containing a sugar-phosphate component and a purine or pyrimidine base.

nutrient (nu′tre-ent). An organic or inorganic substance in food which is digested and absorbed in the gastrointestinal tract and utilized in intermediary metabolism.

oleic acid (o-le′ik). A monounsaturated fatty acid.

opsin (op′sin). Protein compound which combines with retinal, vitamin A aldehyde, to form rhodopsin, visual purple.

osteomalacia (os′te-o-ma-la′she-a). Softening of the bone due to loss of calcium. Occurs chiefly in adults.

osteoporosis (os′te-o-po-ro′sis). Abnormal porousness or rarefaction of bone due to failure of the osteoblasts to lay down bone matrix, and occurring when resorption dominates over mineral deposition.

oxaluria (ok′sah-lu′re-ah). The presence of an excess of oxalic acid or of oxalates in the urine.

oxidation (ok′si-da′shun). A chemical process by which a substance combines with oxygen. Chemically it is an increase of positive charges on an atom through the loss of electrons.

pantothenic acid (pan′to-then′ik). A member of the vitamin B complex.

para-aminobenzoic acid (PABA) (par′a-a-men′no-ben-zo′ik as′id). A part of pteroylglutamic acid, one of the forms of folic acid.

pentose (pen′tos). A single sugar containing five carbon atoms. Ribose is a pentose.

peptide (pep′tid). A compound of two or more amino acids containing one or more peptide groups. Peptides are formed as intermediary products of protein digestion.

pesticide (pes′ti-sid). A poison used to destroy pests of any sort. The term includes fungicides, insecticides and rodenticides.

phenylalanine (fen′il-al′a-nen; nin). An essential amino acid.

phenylketonuria (PKU) (fen′il-ke′ton-nu′re-ah). An inborn error of the metabolism of phenylalanine; phenylpyruvic acid appears in the urine.

phenylpyruvic acid (fen′il-pi-ru′vik). An intermediate product in phenylalanine metabolism.

phospholipid (fos'fo-lip'id). A fat in which one fatty acid is replaced by phosphorus and a nitrogenous compound.

phosphorylation (fos'for-i-la'shun). The process of introducing the trivalent phosphate group into an organic molecule. The phosphate donor is usually ATP.

polysaccharide (pol'e-sak'ah-rid). A complex carbohydrate which contains more than four molecules of monosaccharides combined with each other.

polyunsaturated (pol'e-un-sat'u-rat'ed). An organic compound such as a fatty acid in which there is more than one double bond.

precursor (pre-kur'ser). A substance which is converted into another; e.g. β carotene to vitamin A.

protease (pro'te-as). An enzyme that digests protein.

protein hydrolysate (pro'te-in hi-drol'i-zat). A solution containing the constituent amino acids of an artificially digested protein, usually milk or beef protein.

proteinuria (pro'te-i-nu're-a). Presence of protein in the urine.

proteolytic (pro'te-o-lit'ik). Effecting the digestion of proteins.

provitamin (pro-vi'ta-min). The forerunner of a vitamin. Provitamin A is carotene.

pteroylglutamic acid (ter-ol-glu-tam'ic as'id). (See *folic acid.*)

ptyalin (ti'a-lin). The starch splitting enzyme amylase of saliva.

purine(s) (pu'rēn). End products of nucleoprotein metabolism.

pyridoxine (pi'ri-dok'sin). Vitamin B_6, a member of the vitamin B complex.

pyrophosphate (pi'ro-fos'fāt). Any salt of phosphoric acid containing two phosphate groups.

rachitogenic (rah-kit'o-jen'ik). Capable of causing rickets.

RAD. A unit of measurement of absorbed doses of ionizing radiation.

rennin (ren'in). The milk-curdling enzyme of the gastric juice.

retinal (ret'i-nal). The aldehyde form of vitamin A which is necessary for the synthesis of rhodopsin, visual purple.

retinoic acid (ret'i-no-ic). The acid form of vitamin A.

retinol (ret'i-nol). The chemical term for vitamin A alcohol.

retinyl (ret'i-nel). Refers to the vitamin A portion of the ester form of the vitamin. Retinyl palmitate is hydrolyzed to vitamin A alcohol (retinol) and palmitic acid in the gastrointestinal tract.

rhodopsin (ro-dop'sin). Visual purple, formed in the rods of the retina by combining the protein opsin and vitamin A aldehyde. It is necessary for scotopic vision.

riboflavin (ri'bo-fla'vin). Heat-stable factor of B complex, sometimes called vitamin B_2.

ribonucleic acid (RNA) (ri-bo-nu'kle-ik). A nucleic acid replicated from DNA and found in cytoplasm.

saccharine (sak'ah-rin). An intensely sweet, white crystalline compound used as a substitute for ordinary sugar. It has no food value.

safflower oil (saf'flou'er). An edible oil from the seeds of the safflower plant, *Carthamus tinctorius;* high in linoleic acid.

saponification (sa-pon'i-fi-ka'shun). The splitting of fat by an alkali, yielding glycerol and soap. This may occur during the digestion of fat.

sodium benzoate (so'de-um ben'zo-āt). A salt of benzoic acid used as a preservative in foods.

sphingomyelin (sfing'go-mi'e-lin). A phospholipid found primarily in brain and lung tissue as a constituent of the myelin sheaths.

stachyose (stak'e-os). An indigestible tetrasaccharide containing galactose.

stearic acid (ste'a-rik). A saturated fatty acid.

steatorrhea (ste'a-to-re'a). Presence of an excess of fat in the stools.

sterol (ster'ol). Fat-soluble substance with a complex molecular structure.

substrate (sub'strāt). A substance upon which an enzyme acts.

succinic acid (suk-sin'ik). Intermediary product in metabolism.

suet (su'et). Hard fat of beef or mutton.

synthesis (sin'the-sis). The process of building up a chemical compound.

thiamine (thi'am-in). Vitamin B_1. Antineuritic factor, member of the B complex.

thyrocalcitonin (thi'ro-cal'ci-to'nin). A thyroid hormone which prohibits release of calcium from bone.

tocopherol (to-kof'er-ol). An alcohol-like substance, several forms of which have vitamin E activity.

transamination (trans'am-i-na'shun). The transferring of an amino group from an amino acid to another compound. By this process the body is able to synthesize the nonessential amino acids as well as form urea. A vitamin B_6-containing enzyme is necessary for this reaction.

transferrin (trans-fer'in). A protein compound found in the blood stream which transports iron to the bone marrow for hemoglobin synthesis, to the liver or spleen for storage or to the other tissues for their use.

trichinosis (trik'i-no'sis). A disease due to infection with trichinae—parasites found in raw pork.

tularemia (too'la-re'me-ah). A disease of rodents, resembling plague, which is transmitted by the bites of flies, fleas, ticks and lice and may be acquired by man through handling of infected animals.

tyrosine (ti-ro′sin). A nonessential amino acid.

UNESCO. United Nations Educational, Scientific and Cultural Organization. Headquarters, Paris, France.

urea (u-re′a). The chief nitrogenous end product of protein metabolism in the body.

USDA. United States Department of Agriculture.

valine (val′in). An essential amino acid.

viosterol (vi-o′ster-ol). A solution of irradiated ergosterol in oil; vitamin D_2.

Wernicke-Korsakoff syndrome (ver′ni-ke–kor-sak′of). A psychosis which is usually based on chronic alcoholism, probably due to prolonged thiamine deficiency.

WHO. World Health Organization of the United Nations, Headquarters, Geneva, Switzerland.

xerophthalmia (ze′rof-thal′mi-a). A dry and lusterless condition of the conjunctiva of the eyes resulting from a vitamin A deficiency.

zein (ze′in). A protein obtained from corn.

Index

Page numbers in *italics* refer to illustrations and tabular material.